Gastrointestinal and Colorectal Anesthesia

Gastrointestinal and Colorectal Anesthesia

Edited by

Chandra M. Kumar
The James Cook University Hospital
Middlesbrough, U.K.

Mark Bellamy
St. James's University Hospital
Leeds, U.K.

informa
healthcare

New York London

Informa Healthcare USA, Inc.
52 Vanderbilt Avenue
New York, NY 10017

International Standard Book Number-10: 0-8493-4073-X (Hardcover)
International Standard Book Number-13: 978-0-8493-4073-4 (Hardcover)

Library of Congress Cataloging-in-Publication Data

Gastrointestinal and colorectal anesthesia/ edited by Chandra Kumar, Mark Bellamy.
    p. ; cm.
Includes bibliographical references and index.
ISBN-13: 978-0-8493-4073-4 (hardcover : alk. paper)
ISBN-10: 0-8493-4073-X (hardcover : alk. paper)
1. Anesthesia in gastroenterology I. Kumar, Chandra M. II. Bellamy, Mark C.
[DNLM: 1. Anesthesia--methods 2. Digestive System Surgical Procedures. WI 900 G2572 2006]

RD87.3.G37G37 2006
617.9'6743--dc22   2006046569

Visit the Informa Web site at
www.informa.com

and the Informa Healthcare Web site at
www.informahealthcare.com

Foreword

Medicine in all of its component specialties continues to advance. The continuing development of new and improved techniques of anesthesia and perioperative care has to match changes in other fields. The present impressive record for low morbidity, mortality, and complication rates due to anesthesia can only be achieved by regular updates and authoritative texts. State-of-the-art textbooks are one key element in this process, and a new book should be viewed with delight; particularly one that is as scholarly as this one. A major part of surgical practice is encompassed by the surgical specialties of gastrointestinal and colorectal practice in its broadest sense.

Of course, all existing general anesthesia texts contain sections concerning gastrointestinal and colorectal topics. What we have long needed, though, is an authoritative text devoted to these areas of practice. Now we have it.

The importance of the anesthetist in perioperative care cannot be too greatly emphasized. Correct patient selection and procedure planning can only be optimized by a team approach and together with the surgeon; the anesthetist forms the core of the team. A thorough understanding of the underlying physiology of the gastrointestinal tract is important and a logical starting place for this book. Surgical considerations, outcomes, and morbidity prediction are key and are covered in the following chapters. I am particularly pleased to see whole chapters devoted to preassessment, preoptimization, and perioperative fluid management—all crucial areas and ones that are sadly often inadequately considered.

Much of modern surgical practice is undertaken using cameras, fiber optics, and display screens. Three-dimensional goggles, head-up displays, and robotics are just around the corner. These varied endoscopic techniques are continually widening the limits of surgical practice and bringing with them new frontiers for the anesthetist, each with their own individual considerations. Not only that, but the drive for expanding the "basket" of procedures that can be undertaken on an ambulatory basis seems almost unstoppable (not that it should be curtailed). Sedation, regional block, or general anesthesia? These are all covered in this book. With this drive to everything ambulatory comes the need to push back the boundaries on recovery, postoperative analgesia, and postoperative nausea and vomiting—all vitally important topics given their own space in this book.

Of course, one would expect all of the "usual" chapters to be present, and the reader will not be disappointed. They are all there—hepatobiliary, pancreatic, gastric, bariatric, intestinal, colorectal, etc. Relevant endocrine conditions are also included. It is difficult to see what might be missing. I certainly could not find anything important which had been omitted.

I can see this book being a valuable addition to the library of any anesthetist who regularly works with gastrointestinal and colorectal surgeons. Not only that, but it will also be of value to nonmedical anesthetists, theatre practitioners, nurses, and even surgeons. I am honored to have been asked to be a (very small) part of it.

Brian J. Pollard

Preface

Anesthetists usually acquire skills of anesthesia for gastrointestinal and colorectal surgery from their peers during training. The techniques are later modified and adopted depending on the circumstances and opportunities available. The purpose of this book is to improve the perioperative management of patients undergoing gastrointestinal and colorectal surgery. Anesthesia for gastrointestinal and colorectal surgery is not comprehensively covered in any textbook: While much topical material has recently appeared in journals, it has been scattered. In this book, we have brought this material together in a cohesive and organized fashion.

The material in this book has been collated and written by acknowledged international experts skilled in specific areas relating to gastrointestinal and colorectal surgery.

This book will be the most comprehensive and up-to-date collection of material in the field. The multiple authors provide authoritative information on a broad and comprehensive scale that is not possible in a single medical institution. Each chapter aims to provide the scientific and clinical basis for anesthetic practice.

This book will appeal to all practicing anesthetists, as well as to trainees in anesthesia and surgery, clinical specialist nurses, and other health-care professionals involved in the care of patients undergoing gastrointestinal and colorectal surgery.

Chandra M. Kumar
Mark Bellamy

Contents

Contributors

Gareth L. Ackland   Portex Institute for Anesthesia and Critical Care Medicine, Institute of Child Health, University College London, London, U.K.

Mark Bellamy   Intensive Care Unit, St. James's University Hospital, Leeds, U.K.

John C. Berridge   Department of Anesthetics, The General Infirmary at Leeds, Leeds, U.K.

Andrew Berrill   Department of Anesthesia, St. James's University Hospital, Leeds, U.K.

Tim Brown   Department of Surgery, St. Mark's Hospital, London, U.K.

Lennart Christiansson   Department of Anesthesiology, University Hospital, Uppsala, Sweden

Graham P. Copeland   North Cheshire Hospitals, National Health Service Trust, Warrington, Cheshire, U.K.

David M. Cressey   Department of Perioperative and Critical Care, Freeman Hospital, Newcastle upon Tyne, U.K.

Mervyn H. Davies   Liver Unit, St. James's University Hospital, Leeds, U.K.

Peter A. Davis   Department of Upper Gastrointestinal Surgery, The James Cook University Hospital, Middlesbrough, U.K.

Terry T. Durbin   Department of Anesthesiology, The Pennsylvania College of Medicine, and The Milton S. Hershey Medical Center, Hershey, Pennsylvania, U.S.A.

Korat Farooq   Department of Anesthesia, York Hospital, York, U.K.

Irwin Foo   Department of Anesthesia, Critical Care and Pain Medicine, Western General Hospital, Edinburgh, U.K.

Vikram Garoud   Department of Surgery, The James Cook University Hospital, Middlesbrough, U.K.

Steven Gayer   Department of Anesthesiology, University of Miami Miller School of Medicine, Miami, Florida, U.S.A.

Bussa R. Gopinath   Department of Upper Gastrointestinal Surgery, The James Cook University Hospital, Middlesbrough, U.K.

George M. Hall   Department of Anesthesia and Intensive Care Medicine, St. George's University of London, London, U.K.

Timothy Jackson   Department of Anesthesia, St. James's University Hospital, Leeds, U.K.

Iain Jones   Department of Anesthesia, St. James's University Hospital, Leeds, U.K.

Chandra M. Kumar   Department of Anesthesia, The James Cook University Hospital, Middlesbrough, U.K.

Frank Loughnane   Department of Anesthesia, St. James's University Hospital, Leeds, U.K.

Andrew B. Lumb   Department of Anesthetics, St. James's University Hospital, Leeds, U.K.

Damien Mantle   Department of Anesthesia, Critical Care and Pain Medicine, Western General Hospital, Edinburgh, U.K.

Hamish A. McLure   Department of Anesthesia, St. James's University Hospital, Leeds, U.K.

Stuart D. Murdoch   Department of Anesthesia, St. James's University Hospital, Leeds, U.K.

Dave Murray   Cleveland School of Anesthesia, The James Cook University Hospital, Middlesbrough, U.K.

Monty G. Mythen   Portex Institute for Anesthesia and Critical Care Medicine, Institute of Child Health, University College London, London, U.K.

Udvitha C. Nandasoma   Liver Unit, St. James's University Hospital, Leeds, U.K.

Ian Nesbitt   Department of Perioperative and Critical Care, Freeman Hospital, Newcastle upon Tyne, U.K.

Grainne Nicholson   Department of Anesthesia and Intensive Care Medicine, St. George's University of London, London, U.K.

Susan M. Nimmo Department of Anesthesia, Critical Care and Pain Medicine, Western General Hospital, Edinburgh, U.K.

Howard Palte Department of Anesthesiology, University of Miami Miller School of Medicine, Miami, Florida, U.S.A.

Johan Raeder Department of Anesthesia, Ullevaal University Hospital, Oslo, Norway

Anil Reddy Department of Surgery, The James Cook University Hospital, Middlesbrough, U.K.

Heinz E. Schulenburg Department of Anesthesia, St. James's University Hospital, Leeds, U.K.

Ian H. Shaw Department of Anesthesia and Intensive Care, Newcastle General Hospital, Newcastle upon Tyne, U.K.

Chris P. Snowden Department of Perioperative and Critical Care, Freeman Hospital, Newcastle upon Tyne, U.K.

Elizabeth C. Storey Department of Anesthetics, St. James's University Hospital, Leeds, U.K.

Robert Thomas Intensive Care Unit, St. James's University Hospital, Leeds, U.K.

Ian H. Warnell Department of Anesthesia and Intensive Care, Newcastle General Hospital, Newcastle upon Tyne, U.K.

R. Jonathan T. Wilson Department of Anesthesia, York Hospital, York, U.K.

Robert Wilson Department of Surgery, The James Cook University Hospital, Middlesbrough, U.K.

Al Windsor Department of Surgery, University College Hospital, London, U.K.

1

Physiology of the Gastrointestinal Tract Including Splanchnic Blood Flow and Tonometry

Gareth L. Ackland and Monty G. Mythen
Portex Institute for Anesthesia and Critical Care Medicine, Institute of Child Health, University College London, London, U.K.

INTRODUCTION

The primary functions of the gastrointestinal (GI) system are the digestion/absorption of nutrients and the elimination of waste material (Table 1). A 70-kg adult consumes approximately 800 to 1000 g of food and 1200 to 1500 mL of water per day, while excreting approximately 50 g of undigested material and 100 mL of water per day.

The GI tract carries out many other functions, some of which become critical to shaping perioperative outcome and so these receive more attention (1). Whereas the critical role that the GI tract plays during the perioperative period is not necessarily specific to GI surgery, several features of intra-abdominal surgical intervention have important effects on GI physiology, which may impair the physiological responses to concomitant pathological challenges. To help understand the challenges presented during GI surgery, the normal GI physiology and responses to pathophysiological changes are considered. Potential mechanisms are also highlighted that contribute to postoperative GI tract dysfunction, which is the most common source of morbidity and is associated with decreased survival and increased length of hospital stay (Fig. 1) (2).

HEPATOSPLANCHNIC CIRCULATION (3,4)

The hepatosplanchnic circulation receives 30% of total cardiac output, consuming 20% to 35% of total body oxygen consumption, even though it supplies organs that account for only 5% of body weight. Importantly, in contrast to all other splanchnic organs, the liver receives blood from an artery and a vein, which has unique consequences for the relationship between hepatic blood and oxygen supply during low flow conditions. With increasing age, splanchnic blood flow declines both absolutely and as a fraction of total cardiac output. Increasing oxygen extraction can help to maintain oxygen consumption when oxygen supply decreases. However, because

Table 1 Functions of the Gastrointestinal Tract

Mouth	Chewing, lubrication, addition of salivary amylase to food
Pharynx and esophagus	Swallowing
Stomach	Storage, initiation of digestion
Small intestine	Digestion and absorption
Pancreas	Digestive enzymes, pH optimization
Liver and gall bladder	Bile salts for emulsification of fat
Large intestine	Storage and concentration of undigested food
Rectum	Defecation

hepatosplanchnic metabolic needs are already high under normal conditions, oxygen extraction is increased compared with other tissues. This high demand may result in impaired liver function when hepatosplanchnic oxygen extraction exceeds 70% to 80%.

During low blood-flow states, major reductions in splanchnic blood flow and volume occur (5). However, different etiologies of low blood flow are associated with differential effects on cardiac output and hepatosplanchnic perfusion. In hemorrhage, hepatosplanchnic blood flow decreases more than the cardiac output, whereas in cardiogenic shock, hepatosplanchnic blood flow and cardiac output decrease

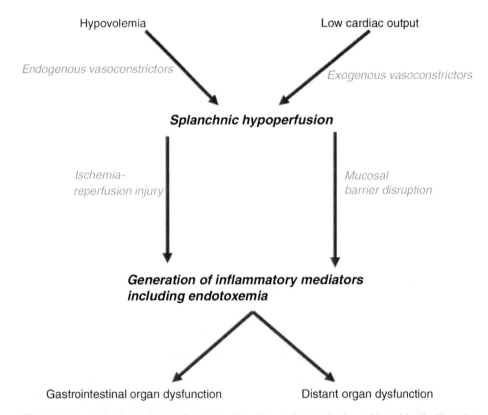

Figure 1 Impaired gastrointestinal tract function perioperatively and in critically ill patients is strongly associated with morbidity and mortality. Because the gut is a reservoir of inflammatory mediators and bacteria, mucosal barrier breakdown is a potent cause of local and distant organ dysfunction. *Source*: From Ref. 6.

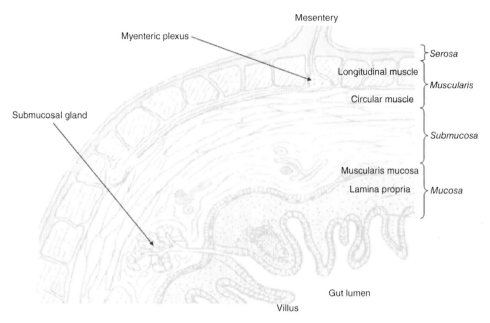

Figure 2   Cross-sectional anatomy of gastrointestinal tract.

in parallel. Mucosal barrier breakdown is an ever-present threat during these types of insults, owing to an oxygen countercurrent exchange mechanism in absorptive villi of the small intestine. These villi are particularly susceptible to deleterious circulatory or hypoxic changes. The countercurrent exchange mechanism renders cells relative hypoxic at the luminal tip compared with those at its base, even under normal conditions. Thus, at times of hypoperfusion or cellular stress (inflammation and trauma), this tissue has relatively little reserve and is vulnerable to local and/or systemic insults such as hemorrhage or tissue hypoxia.

There are two critical components in understanding the physiology of the hepatosplanchnic circulation: the unique architecture of the hepatic vasculature and the microvasculature of the mesenteric circulation (Fig. 2).

GASTROINTESTINAL MICROVASCULATURE

The intestinal microvasculature is arranged in the form of three parallel circuits supplying blood to the mucosa, submucosa, and muscularis propria. Each of these parallel circuits comprises five components arranged in series (Fig. 3). Resistance arterioles regulate blood flow to the splanchnic bed, so that at constant hydrostatic pressure flow is inversely proportional to resistance. In conjunction with precapillary arteriolar sphincters, these resistance arterioles are able to autoregulate and partially compensate for reductions in blood flow, although such a mechanism has received rather less investigation than similar mechanisms in the kidney or brain. As well as maintaining liver and gut perfusion, the splanchnic bed also acts as a "circulatory sink." Forty percent of the mesenteric circulation is contained in venules, which act as high-capacitance vessels. In combination with the mesenteric collecting veins, the venules contain up to 30% of the body's total blood volume. These two mechanisms

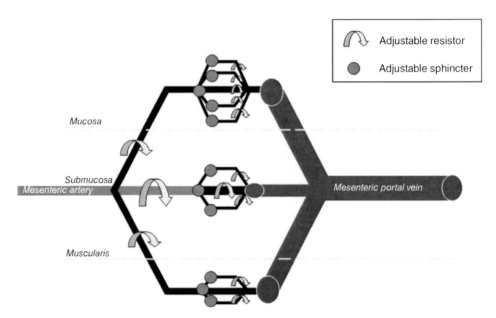

Figure 3 Control of gastrointestinal microvasculature is dependent on parallel series of arteriolar resistors, precapillary sphincters, and high-capacitance capillaries and venules.

are of paramount importance in allowing routine hemodynamic challenges to be met, such as exercise, feeding, and large fluid shifts. The mucosa and submucosa receive approximately 70% of total gut blood flow, of which the main site (superficial villus) receives half.

Microvascular adaptation permits oxygen uptake only to be dependent on blood flow at very low blood flow. Oxygen consumption is maintained during periods of impaired oxygen delivery by increasing oxygen extraction through the recruitment of a relatively underperfused, extensive network of collatoral capillary beds. Mucosal permeability seems, therefore, to be protected to a large degree, only becoming compromised when oxygen uptake falls below 50%. Human studies suggest that oxygen supply dependency may occur with as little as 30% reduction in GI blood flow, with mucosal supply dependency (identified using continuous flow gastric tonometry) occurring before global splanchnic supply dependency can be identified [using portal venous carbon dioxide (CO_2) measurement]. Tonometry data from human studies suggest that the mucosa may respond differently to reduced oxygen delivery depending on the cause. Although stagnant hypoxia is readily detected, sensitivity to anemic hypoxia appears to be much lower.

A further protective mechanism is afforded by the hepatic arterial buffer response, which serves to maintain liver blood flow under conditions of low mesenteric blood flow through the hydrodynamic interaction between the portal venous and hepatic arterial blood flow. Branches of the hepatic arterial system and portal vein are anatomically apposed, situated in the space of Mall. The proposed mechanism of the hepatic arterial buffer response centers on this close anatomical apposition, whereby accumulation of adenosine at times of decreased portal venous blood flow produces a compensatory dilatation of the hepatic arteries. Both experimentally and clinically (in liver transplant patients), increases in hepatic arterial blood flow compensate for 10% to 25% of portal venous blood flow reduction. Different etiologies of low-flow states reveal varying adaptations of the hepatic vasculature, as explored in an experimental porcine model. During isolated abdominal blood-flow reduction, hepatic oxygen consumption and portal venous and hepatic arterial blood flow decreases; whereas in cardiac tamponade and mesenteric ischemia, portal venous flow reduction occurs with a concomitant increase in hepatic arterial blood flow, thereby maintaining hepatic oxygen consumption. However, prolonged and severe systemic hypoperfusion (through cardiac tamponade) abolishes the ability of the hepatic arterial blood flow to compensate for decreased portal venous flow.

NEURAL CONTROL OF THE GASTROINTESTINAL TRACT (7,8)

The tone of the mesenteric vasculature depends on the complex balance between neurally mediated sympathetic vasoconstriction, the local action of vasoregulatory substances that are under the influence of the apparently paradoxically named "sensory-motor" nerves, the parasympathetic cholinergic nerve supply, the enteric nervous system, and endothelium-derived agents (Fig. 4). Neural control of the GI tract involves multiple components, including central nervous system, spinal cord, prevertebral sympathetic ganglia, and the enteric nervous system. Nutrients in the gut lumen act through a number of different feedback mechanisms, dependent on extrinsic intestinal afferent innervation, to alter gut motility, inhibit gastric emptying, and modulate pancreatic and gallbladder enzyme production. Both intraluminal mechanical and chemical stimuli activate vagal and spinal afferents. Furthermore, different macronutrients (protein, lipids, and carbohydrate) may activate specific afferent pathways, although this seems to be an indirect pathway via the release of peptides and other hormones located in intestinal mucosal entero-endocrine

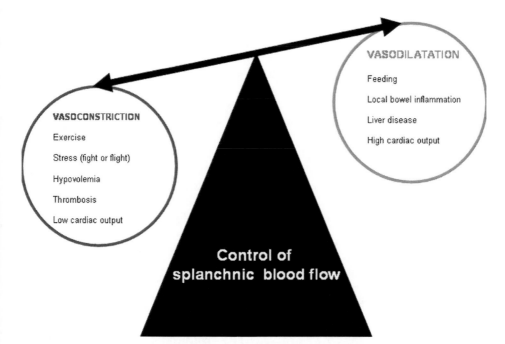

Figure 4 Gastrointestinal blood supply depends on a dynamic balance between vasodilatation and vasoconstriction during both health and disease.

cells. An important example of such a mediator is the hormone cholecystokinin (CCK), which mediates intestinal lipid inhibition of gastric emptying through a vagal capsaicin-sensitive afferent pathway. CCK also inhibits pancreatic and acid secretion. Other principal hormones include gastrin, which stimulates gastric acid secretion and intestinal motility, and secretin, which potentiates the actions of CCK. Over 100 hormonally active peptides have been identified, with a variety of intra- and extra-GI sites of either location and/or action. Knowledge of the actions of these mediators is rapidly changing, but several exhibit multiple actions including roles as metabolic hormones, neurotransmitters, and long-acting growth factors.

Enteric Nervous System (9)

The enteric nervous system is a part of the autonomic nervous system, containing an estimated 100 million neurones that occur most densely in the myenteric plexus, one of the three major ganglionated plexuses [myenteric (Auerbach's), submucosal (Meissner's), and the mucosal plexus] and several aganglionated plexuses. The myenteric plexus is positioned between the outer longitudinal and circular muscle layers throughout the digestive tract, from the esophagus to the rectum. The submucous plexus is positioned in the submucosa, being prominent in the intestines only. Nonganglionated plexuses also supply all the layers of the gut. At least 16 phenotypically distinct neuronal populations have been identified and classified according to morphology, electrical properties, neurotransmitter/neuromodulator content, and functional properties (Table 2).

The average ratio of sensory neurones, interneurones, and motor neurones is 2:1:1. Varying proportions of these neurones are activated during different reflexes. In addition to neurones, enteric ganglia contain glial cells that resemble astrocytes of the central nervous system. Despite considerable cross talk with the central nervous system, the enteric nervous system is capable of integrating and coordinating motility, secretions, blood flow, and immune responses into organized patterns of behavior through local neural reflexes. The essentially independent function of the enteric nervous system, first recognized by Bayliss and Starling who reported peristalsis in isolated gut segments, has led to the title "Little Brain of the Gut." For example, gastric motility initiates the gastroileac reflex that increases the motility of the terminal ileum and increases the rate of emptying of chyme through the ileocaecal sphincter into the large intestine. Distention of the terminal ileum initiates the ileogastric reflex, which decreases gastric motility. Overextension of any part of the intestine stimulates the intestinal reflex, which inhibits motility in the remaining intestine. Distention or contraction of the terminal ileum reflexively relaxes the ileocaecal sphincter to facilitate emptying of the ileum. In contrast, distention of the cecum causes the sphincter to contract; this prevents further emptying and reflux of chyme and colonic bacteria back into the ileum.

Table 2 Classification of Enteric Neurones

Morphology	Dogiel types I–VII
Electrical	Synaptic and after-hyperpolarization
Chemical	Transmitters and other markers
Functional	Sensory, interneuron, motor (muscle), secretomotor

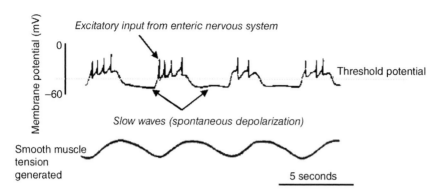

Figure 5   Neurophysiological and contractile characteristics of gastrointestinal smooth muscle.

    The GI tract displays distinct contractile patterns. Gut motility is partly deter-
mined by several types of "pacemaker cells" (the interstitial cells of Cajal), which
underlie rhythmic changes in membrane potential observed in smooth muscle
throughout the GI tract. The frequency of these rhythmic slow waves varies throughout the GI tract, from approximately 3/min in the stomach, 12/min in the duodenum,
and approximately 8/min in the terminal ileum. If suitable excitatory input from
closely apposed enteric neurones occurs, pacemaker cells entrain the surrounding,
electrically coupled cells of the circular and longitudinal muscle layers, and action
potentials are generated on top of the pacemaker driven, slow wave form (Fig. 5).
Because the resistance to current spread through cytoplasm is much less than the
resistance to current flow between adjacent cells, the wave of depolarization spreads
most rapidly in the direction of the long axis of the smooth muscle cells. Thus,
depolarization is propagated primarily in a longitudinal direction in the longitudinal
muscle layer, and in a circular fashion in the circular layer.
    During fasting, peristalsis is minimal. Every 75 to 90 minutes a strong peristaltic
wave of contraction is initiated in the stomach or duodenum and then propagated to
the terminal ileum. This pattern of activity is referred to as the migrating myoelectric
complex (MMC), which may help clear accumulated fluid from the stomach and intestine and prevent migration of colonic bacteria into the small intestine. Pacemaker cells
also demonstrate plasticity: experimentally, their function can be partially restored
over time after certain environmental insults, such as bowel obstruction. With age,
enteric nervous system neurons decline throughout the GI tract. Most studies have
identified cholinergic neurones as being the most vulnerable whereas the numbers
of nitrergic neurones decline less. These findings are consistent with the clinical observation that GI transit time is markedly reduced with age, occurring in over 25% of
individuals older than 65 years. Increased free radical generation and loss of protective
neurotrophic factors have been implicated. Whether the level or pattern of expression
of neuronal proteins changes during ageing is unknown.

NEUROTRANSMITTERS

The strength of smooth muscle contraction is modulated by both extrinsic mechanism
and intrinsic mechanism, involving a variety of hormones (e.g., gastrin depolarizes),
neurotransmitters (acetylcholine depolarizes; norepinephrine hyperpolarizes), and stretching of smooth muscle cells (depolarization). Neuromodulators including calcitonin
gene–related peptide, nitric oxide (NO), vasoactive intestinal peptide, substance P,

and cyclooxygenase-2 pathway–derived prostaglandins also inhibit GI motility. Norepinephrine is the key sympathetic-mediated vasoconstrictor acting with the cotransmitters adenosine triphosphate (ATP) and neuropeptide Y. The vasodilatory calcitonin gene–related peptide is the main neurotransmitter released at sensory-motor nerves, among many other putative agents. The enteric nervous system includes the nonadrenergic, noncholinergic system that supplies perivascular myenteric nerves. NO is a putative neurotransmitter in this system, in addition to the well-established endothelium-derived role in maintaining basal vascular tone. NO inhibits the synthesis and potent vasoconstrictor action of another endothelial derived factor, endothelin-1, a mediator of tonic vasoconstriction. Flow characteristics within the splanchnic circulation may also play a role under some circumstances, such as pulsatile versus nonpulsatile cardiopulmonary bypass.

CENTRAL NERVOUS SYSTEM CONTROL OF THE GASTROINTESTINAL SYSTEM

The sympathetic nervous system (derived from T5 and below) is an important source of inhibition of GI motility. Adrenergic stimulation is triggered by a number of stimuli including GI afferent sensory neurones forming an inhibitory sympathetic reflex. Both alpha-1 and alpha-2 receptor subtypes impair gut motility, but alpha-2 agonists are particularly potent at inhibiting MMCs. Since 1899, GI physiologists have appreciated that sympatholysis improves intestinal motility, through early experiments involving sectioning of the splanchnic nerves. The key brainstem coordinator of the parasympathetic nervous system that controls gut motility is the dorsal vagal complex, comprising the dorsal motor nucleus of the vagus, nucleus tractus solitarius, area postrema, and nucleus ambiguus. The dorsal vagal complex integrates pathways of the brain and the enteric circuits, and is responsible for the control and coordination of the behavior of the muscular, secretory, and circulatory systems. Sensory vagal afferent fibers from the upper GI tract synapse in the dorsal motor nucleus of the vagus and the nucleus tractus solitarius, mediating nonpainful physiological sensations. The pattern of brain activation to gut stimulation suggests that projections from both vagal and spinal afferents are involved in mediating sensation and pain, although such gut sensation is only represented vaguely in the somatosensory cortices. The dorsal vagal outflow center also receives several descending projections from higher centers, including pathways from the frontal cerebral cortex, stria terminalis, paraventricular nucleus of the hypothalamus, and the central nucleus of the amygdala.

The dorsal vagal complex is topographically organized, being divided along the longitudinal axis into three columns innervating different regions of the GI tract. The middle column projects to the stomach, the lateral column to the intestine and cecum, and the medial column to the pancreas, although other regions of the gut, including the duodenum, receive innervation from multiple columns. Vagal efferent neurones of the motor pathways are parasympathetic preganglionic neurones. A variety of central effects, primarily on the upper GI tract, are mediated through these neurones, including relaxation of the proximal stomach, enhancement of gastric peristalsis, and promotion of gastrin secretion. The dorsal vagal complex also controls the vagovagal reflex, which subserves a wide range of GI functions (Table 3).

Hence, disruption of the vago-vagal pathways may result in marked disturbances of GI functions. After chronic vagotomy, however, the digestive functions of the GI tract are well preserved, confirming autonomy of the enteric nervous

Table 3 Functions of the Vago-Vagal Reflex

Gastric relaxation in response to esophageal, gastric, or duodenal distension
Chemical stimulation of the duodenum with acid or hyperosmolar solution
   inhibits gastric motility (causing postprandial delay in gastric emptying)
Control of food intake
Control of gastric and pancreatic secretion

---

system. Whereas the enteric nervous system in the upper regions of the GI tract receives parasympathetic and sensory innervation via the vagus nerve, most enteric neurones do not receive direct vagal connections. Vagal efferent fibers divide into esophageal and anterior and posterior vagal trunks, which indirectly innervate the small bowel by communication with the enteric nervous system. Transmission from vagal input neurones to enteric neurones is mediated principally by acetylcholine acting on nicotinic cholinergic receptors, but several other transmitters are involved in these processes. For example, exposure of the dorsal vagal nucleus to serotonin, thyrotropin-releasing hormone, and vasopressin results in increased gastric acid secretion and motility. Motility, secretion, and blood flow are controlled in the distal colon and rectum by the pelvic nerves.

NEUROIMMUNE INTERACTIONS

Both central and enteric nervous systems demonstrate neuroimmune interactions, which have important clinical implications. The complexity of neuroimmune interactions and their effect on gut physiology is exemplified by numerous experimental observations that bowel manipulation compounds gut dysmotility and inflammation but is not the sole cause of them. There are important central and local neural interactions that may act in concert or serve to counteract each other. In the central nervous system, circumventricular organs (including the area postrema) permit systemically circulating inflammatory cytokines, such as tumor necrosis factor alpha, to act upon the neural circuitry of the medullary dorsal vagal complex. Gut stasis, nausea, and vomiting may result from this interaction. Vagal afferents also detect inflammatory mediators directly. The enteric nervous system is also profoundly affected by immune mediators. Smooth muscle contractility and neurotransmitter release are both affected during inflammation, with persistent changes after the resolution of inflammation and/or healing. Sustained gut afferent nerve stimulation through a variety of mediators provokes local release of substance P and calcitonin group–related peptide, with consequent amplification of inflammation by activation of local mast cells. In addition, the same afferent pathways form a sympathoinhibitory reflex.

   Local actions of either circulating inflammatory mediators or direct bowel manipulation induce a local inflammatory reaction, all of which are implicated in the mechanism underlying postoperative ileus. Immune mediators may either excite neurons within the gut wall directly or sensitize them to physiological or pathological stimuli. This is a two-way process because enteric neurons also innervate Peyers patches and receptors for enteric neurotransmitters are located on lymphocytes in the lamina propria of the mucosa. Direct bowel manipulation may result in a loss of mucosal integrity, allowing the translocation of gut luminal contents that can act synergistically, either locally or systemically, to compound any inflammatory reaction. Endotoxemia is common during many clinical scenarios, ranging from major surgery to cardiac failure. In both animal models and human studies, endotoxin has repeatedly been demonstrated to cause both gut motor dysfunction and loss of mucosal integrity. Bowel manipulation also directly and/or indirectly alters neuronal and neurohumoral signaling via local and central pathways, with consequent abnormal gut motility.

METABOLIC INTERACTIONS

Surprisingly, experimental data show that systemic hypoxemia does not alter mucosal blood flow, blood volume, and splanchnic blood flow, but the effect on mucosal acidosis is rather more unclear. Whether the duration, severity, or type of hypoxia affects GI blood flow and mucosal integrity remains unclear. However, both metabolic and respiratory acidosis impair gastric emptying. Although electrolyte disturbances are implicated in impaired GI homeostasis, systematic exploration of this assertion is lacking. More robust data from the literature on diabetes indicate that relatively mild hyperglycemia delays gastric emptying, whereas the reverse is true of hypoglycemia. Both hypothermia and hyperthermia are associated with reduced perfusion of the GI tract; but due to several confounding factors, it is difficult to ascribe specific effects of changes in temperature to alterations in GI physiology.

CLINICAL MEASUREMENT OF SPLANCHNIC BLOOD FLOW (10)

Gastric Tonometry

A variety of techniques to assess GI perfusion have been developed. Several methods measure portal blood flow or total liver blood flow either directly or indirectly. These include plasma indocyanine green clearance and portal vein catheterization with measurement of blood flow, oxygen saturation, and lactate. However, the most widely used method for assessing GI perfusion in routine clinical practice is GI tonometry (Fig. 6). Gastric tonometry is the most widely used variant of this technique, although in studies, tonometry has been used to assess regional perfusion in the colon (humans) and esophagus (animals).

Gastric tonometry assumes that as local gut perfusion is compromised, anaerobic metabolism ensues with the generation of lactic acid and CO_2. When GI blood flow is reduced by restriction of superior mesenteric artery blood flow in the absence of the hormonal milieu that occurs with systemic hypovolemia, mucosal pH decreases (CO_2 increases) only when flow is less than 50% of baseline. However, this relationship may not hold in hypovolemia and shock, where vasoactive mediators released in response to decreased intravascular volume are likely to have significant effects on the microcirculation. Although the assumption is made that the CO_2 is of (vulnerable) mucosal origin, and this is supported by histological damage to the mucosa in shocked patients, it is possible that the CO_2 could be derived from the serosal or muscular levels of the GI tract. Early gastric tonometry studies were based on saline tonometry in order to measure (mathematically derived) gastric mucosal pH. This technique was prone to errors and intra- and interobserver inconsistencies. Mathematical derivation of gastric pH assumed that mucosal bicarbonate was the same as arterial bicarbonate, which may reflect its initial impressive predictive value because it was partly reflecting systemic acid–base balance [i.e., because pH, arterial

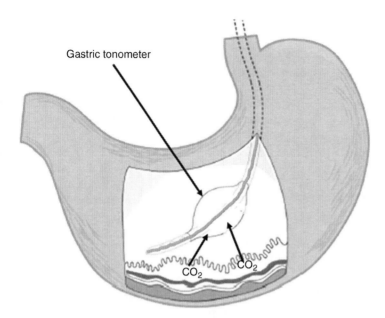

Gastric tonometer

CO_2 CO_2

Figure 6 Gastrointestinal tonometry in the stomach allows a surrogate marker of hepatos-planchnic blood flow to be measured clinically.

PCO_2 ($PaCO_2$), and peak end-tidal (Pet) CO_2 have been referenced to gastric muco-sal PCO_2 ($PgCO_2$), the latter obviating the need for arterial sampling (Fig. 7)]. The measurement of Pg-etCO$_2$ difference is not affected by systemic acid–base status, although changes in alveolar dead space complicate interpretation of the $PgCO_2$ gap (Fig. 7). In the absence of population- and pathology-specific data, consensus opinion suggests that a $PgCO_2$ gap of greater than 2 kPa is abnormal.

There are several other potential confounding factors, including temperature (when differences in temperature occur between CO_2 measured in the gaseous phase in the stomach but indexed against arterial CO_2 measured in the liquid phase). The Haldane effect may also explain elevated gastric CO_2 levels in certain situations where increased oxygen extraction occurs in the absence of decreased perfusion. Local metabolic factors that alter the position of the hemoglobin–CO_2 dissociation curve could result in changes in measured gastric CO_2 in the absence of any altera-tion in local CO_2 production. The presence of drugs such as ranitidine also influences gastric CO_2, because gastric luminal CO_2 production partly reflects the reflux buffer-ing of gastric acid. Finally, alterations in substrate metabolism in the GI mucosa may also influence CO_2 production. For example, a lower gastric pHi was observed in swine that were hemorrhaged and resuscitated with a hemoglobin substitute pre-sented in a maltose-containing preparation than those that were resuscitated with a nonsugar-containing preparation.

$$pHi = pHa - 0.015 \times (T - 37) \times$$
$$\log_{10} \frac{PaCO_2 \times 10^{0.019(T - 37)}}{PrCO_2}$$

Figure 7 Formula used for calculation of gastric-to-arterial PCO_2 difference (Pg-aCO$_2$), with correction for body temperature.

CLINICAL STUDIES

In healthy volunteers, the only detector of controlled hemorrhagic hypovolemia (after 10–15% of circulating volume was withdrawn) was an increase in the $PgCO_2$ gap, with no changes in commonly measured hemodynamic variables, such as heart rate and arterial blood pressure. Several perioperative studies, in general and cardiac surgical patients, have consistently shown that an increased tonometric CO_2 gap is associated with longer hospital stay. Similarly, several authors have demonstrated in critically ill patients that a persistently abnormal pHi or Pr-aCO$_2$ value during the first 24 hours after intensive care unit admission is associated with increased mortality. As yet, no randomized clinical trials have been undertaken to challenge the gut hypoperfusion hypothesis by using goal-directed therapy or other therapeutic strategies to manipulate the Pg-aCO$_2$ gap below levels associated with poor outcome in observational studies. In studies of trauma and intensive care patients where pHi has been targeted, mixed results have been observed, although these studies have been beset by methodological problems. However, patients in whom the pHi gap was elevated at the time of admission were often resistant to therapeutic intervention. Despite this, in surgical patients, preemptive administration of fluid targeted to optimize stroke volume improves gut perfusion (as measured by tonometry) and postoperative outcome (morbidity and length of hospital stay).

SUMMARY

Understanding the physiology of the GI tract remains a challenge, given the neurophysiological complexity and local and systemic interactions of many critical mediators. Ongoing research continues to yield novel and potentially clinically important findings. The high cost of GI-related pathophysiology continues to drive translation of new research findings from the laboratory to the bedside. This requires an integrative approach from both basic and clinical scientists.

REFERENCES

1. Ackland G, Grocott MP, Mythen MG. Understanding gastrointestinal perfusion in critical care. Crit Care 2000; 4:269–281.
2. Mythen MG. Postoperative gastrointestinal tract dysfunction. Anesth Analg 2005; 100(1):196–204.
3. Richardson PD, Withrington PG. Physiological regulation of the hepatic circulation. Annu Rev Physiol 1982; 44:57–69.
4. Takala J. Determinants of splanchnic blood flow. Br J Anaesth 1996; 77:50–58.
5. Ceppa EP, Fuh KC, Bulkley GB. Mesenteric hemodynamic response to circulatory shock. Curr Opin Crit Care 2004; 9:127–132.
6. Dantzker D. The gastrointestinal tract. The canary of the body? JAMA 1993; 270: 1247–1248.
7. Ralevic V. Splanchnic circulatory physiology. Hepatogastroenterology 1999; 46(suppl 2): 1409–1413.
8. Rehfeld JH. A centenary of gastrointestinal endocrinology. Horm Metab Res 2004; 36(11–12):735–741.
9. Hansen MB. The enteric nervous system I: organisation and classification. Pharmacol Toxicol 2003; 92(3):105–113.
10. Hamilton MA, Mythen MG. Gastric tonometry: where do we stand? Curr Opin Crit Care 2001; 7(2):122–127.

2

Surgical Considerations in Upper Gastrointestinal Surgery

Bussa R. Gopinath and Peter A. Davis
Department of Upper Gastrointestinal Surgery, The James Cook University Hospital, Middlesbrough, U.K.

Chandra M. Kumar
Department of Anesthesia, The James Cook University Hospital, Middlesbrough, U.K.

INTRODUCTION

This chapter includes a few major surgical procedures at a basic level. It is beyond the scope of this book to cover all surgical procedures on the upper gastrointestinal tract. Readers are encouraged to read excellent published textbooks of surgery for further details (1–5). It is intended for anesthesia personnel to understand the steps required in a specific surgical procedure so that appropriate anesthetic technique can be utilized at the appropriate stage of surgery.

ESOPHAGECTOMY

Carcinoma of the esophagus is more common in men and usually presents later in life. Certain disorders such as achalasia, the Plummer–Vinson syndrome, and caustic burns of the esophagus are associated with higher incidence of carcinoma. Tumors can occur in any part of the esophagus but are most common in the lower third. They typically present with a short history of progressive dysphagia. There may be regurgitation of food or liquid, or blood-stained vomiting.

Assessment

Diagnosis is confirmed by endoscopy and biopsy. The extent of the disease is staged with chest and abdominal computed tomography (CT), endoluminal ultrasound, and positron emission tomogram scan. Pulmonary function tests, electrocardiogram, and nutritional assessment to assess fitness for major surgery should be performed. The patient may require a supplemental diet or intravenous nutrition to correct malnutrition. The patient is fully assessed for fitness for surgery and anesthesia (Chapters 7 and 11).

Surgery

Surgical resection for carcinoma of the esophagus is contemplated in patients with potentially operable tumor without metastases. It necessitates a two-stage (Ivor-Lewis) esophagectomy with gastric replacement of the esophagus. The colon or jejunum may be used as the conduit in the absence of the stomach, which is the most commonly used as conduit.

Relevant Anatomy

The esophagus is 25 to 26 cm long and extends from the cricopharyngeus muscle in the neck to the stomach just below the diaphragm. As it passes through the superior mediastinum, it lies behind the left main bronchus and in front of the thoracic aorta. It continues through the posterior mediastinum on the vertebral bodies to the left of the midline to pierce the diaphragm surrounded by the crura. A short segment of intra-abdominal esophagus joins the proximal stomach at the gastroesophageal junction.

The skills of an experienced and dedicated anesthetist are essential. The patient is anesthetized and intubated with a double-lumen endotracheal tube (Chapter 11). A nasogastric tube is inserted with the tip in the upper esophagus. The patient is placed supine during the first abdominal stage, and then turned to full left lateral position during the second thoracic stage.

Technique

Upper midline incision from xiphisternum to umbilicus is required during the abdominal stage. A midline laparotomy is carried out and a thorough inspection performed to exclude metastatic disease, which would preclude resection. The stomach is mobilized to allow it to be transposed into the chest. The gastrocolic omentum is divided, preserving the right gastroepiploic arcade with the greater curve. The stomach is separated from the spleen by division of the short gastric vessels. The lesser omentum is divided and the gastroesophageal junction mobilized completely at the hiatus. The stomach is retracted in a cephalad direction to allow division of adhesions in the lesser sac and ligation and division of the left gastric vessels.

The duodenum is mobilized by Kocher's maneuver to allow the pylorus to be brought up to the hiatus without tension. To facilitate gastric emptying in a vagotomized stomach, a pyloroplasty is performed. A feeding jejunostomy is inserted to allow enteral feeding in the recovery period. The abdomen is closed and the patient turned from supine to left lateral position for the thoracic stage.

A right-sided thoracotomy is performed through the fifth intercostal space. The lung is deflated to allow exposure to the thoracic cavity. The inferior pulmonary ligament is divided to mobilize the lung from esophagus. The azygos vein is ligated and divided as it arches over the esophagus. The mediastinal pleura is incised over the esophagus, and the segmental vessels from the aorta are ligated and divided. The esophagus is mobilized from above the site of the tumor down to the hiatus with the excision of fascia, lymph nodes, and connective tissue. The mobilized stomach is drawn into the chest. A linear stapler is used to divide the stomach from the angle of His to the lesser curvature. Anastomosis between the proximal esophagus and mobilized stomach is made using either a circular stapler or a hand-sewn technique. Two chest drains, one basal and one apical, are placed, and the lung is reinflated. The chest is closed using appropriate suture materials.

Intraoperative Care

A meticulous anesthetic technique (Chapter 11) by an experienced, dedicated anesthetist is of paramount importance.

Postoperative Care

Usually, the patient is extubated at the end of the procedure and managed in the intensive care unit or high dependency unit. Sometimes, extubation is not feasible depending on the clinical condition of the patient, and a prior arrangements must be made for an intensive care unit bed with elective ventilation (Chapter 27). Good analgesia technique without excessive sedation is essential, and thoracic epidural analgesia is the norm. Regular chest physiotherapy is advocated. An intercostal drain is present, and this is connected to an underwater sealed drainage bottle. The nasogastric tube is aspirated hourly, and the jejunal feeding may be started after 24 hours. Electrolyte balance must be maintained and corrected. A water-soluble contrast swallow is performed to check the anastomosis for leaks and gastric emptying on the fifth or sixth postoperative day. If this is satisfactory, drains are removed and oral nutrition is started.

Complications

Chest infection can occur but this can be minimized by aggressive physiotherapy and selective brochoscopy and lavage. Anastomotic leakage, mediastinitis, empyema, and chylothorax are known to occur. There is often a delayed gastric emptying. Management of postoperative complications is included in Chapter 11.

SURGERY FOR GASTRIC NEOPLASM

Gastric neoplasm may be epithelial or mesenchymal in origin. Adenocarcinoma, leiomyoma, and primary gastric lymphoma are encountered in clinical practice. The surgical approach to gastric cancer is dictated by the site and extent of the tumor, patient's age, and physical status. The extent of resection depends on the location of the tumor and the attainment of clear margins. Surgery usually involves total or partial gastric resection of the primary lesion and associated lymphadenectomy. Distal gastrectomy is performed for tumors in the antrum or gastric body and total gastrectomy for those in the proximal stomach. If the tumor has breached the submucosa, there may be an extensive lateral spread requiring more radical surgery, such as splenectomy, distal pancreatectomy, and extended wide resection. Patients with locally advanced disease with antral tumors causing gastric outlet obstruction or bleeding may undergo palliative gastrectomy or an appropriate bypass surgery.

Assessment

Diagnosis is confirmed by endoscopy and biopsy, the extent of disease staged by chest and abdominal CT, endoluminal ultrasound, and laparoscopy. Hematological investigations may reveal underlying iron deficiency anemia or deranged liver functions. Anemia is corrected, and blood must be crossmatched and grouped should the need arise during surgery. Patients may have features of gastric outlet obstruction, showing features of electrolyte abnormalities and malnourishment. Patient is assessed by anesthesia personnel before surgery (Chapter 7).

Surgery

Relevant Anatomy

The stomach lies in the epigastrium and left hypochondrium. It comprises the cardia, body, and antrum. It receives blood supply from the celiac axis from the left gastric, right gastric, right and gastroepiploic, and short gastric vessels.

Technique

Routine monitors are attached, and an invasive blood pressure monitoring may be essential depending on the patient's clinical condition (Chapter 12). Staging laparoscopy is usually performed just before major surgery for staging of the disease process. Sometimes, staging laparoscopy is also performed before proceeding to major surgery. Anesthetic technique is tailored accordingly. Full details of anesthetic technique are included in Chapter 12. Ventilation is controlled, and neuromuscular blocking drugs are used to relax abdominal muscles and to gain easy access to the abdominal cavity. A nasogastric tube is inserted, and the tip position in stomach is checked and then secured. The patient is placed supine on the operating table, and both arms and legs are secured using pads. A definite surgery may be abandoned any time if circumstances dictate so.

Upper midline incision from xiphisternum to umbilicus is the most commonly used incision but a rooftop incision is also favored by some. Laparotomy is carried out and a thorough inspection performed to exclude metastatic disease, which would preclude resection. The gastrocolic omentum is mobilized from the transverse colon, and adhesions in the lesser sac divided between the pancreas and stomach. The right gastroepiploic pedicle is divided below the duodenum. The right gastric pedicle is divided on the lesser curvature.

The duodenum is divided just distal to the pylorus with linear stapler, and the stomach retracted in cephalad direction. The left gastric pedicle is ligated and divided. Regional nodes and connective tissue are removed en bloc. The lesser omentum is divided up to the gastroesophageal junction.

Distal Gastrectomy.   The stomach is divided using a linear stapler from the left gastroepiploic territory on the greater curvature toward the gastroesophageal junction on the lesser curvature, ensuring clear margins from the tumor. A gastrojejunal anastomosis is fashioned between the proximal stomach remnant and a Roux-en-Y jejunal loop to reestablish continuity. The abdomen is closed in multiple layers using appropriate materials. It is not unusual to insert a drain.

Total Gastrectomy.   Mobilization of the greater curvature is completed by ligation and division of the short gastric vessels. The gastroesophageal junction is mobilized completely at the hiatus. The esophagus is divided above the tumor, and an esophagojejunal anastomosis is fashioned between the esophagus and a Roux-en-Y jejunal loop using either a circular stapler or a hand-sewn technique. A feeding jejunostomy is inserted to allow enteral feeding in the recovery period. The abdomen is closed in multiple layers using appropriate materials. It is not unusual to insert a drain.

Intraoperative Care

Patients are usually fragile, and surgery may be prolonged. Intraoperative and anesthetic management is discussed in detail elsewhere (Chapter 12). Complications related to surgery may occur, including blood loss, particularly if surgery involves splenectomy or other major surgical dissection.

Postoperative Care

The patient is usually extubated at the end of the procedure and nursed in a critical area of the ward. Good analgesia without excessive sedation is essential, and epidural analgesia is the norm (Chapter 12). Regular chest physiotherapy is employed. The nasogastric tube is aspirated hourly. Jejunal feeding may be started after 24 hours. The nasogastric tube is removed, and the patient is slowly given oral nutrition after five days. In the case of total gastrectomy, a water-soluble contrast swallow is performed to check the anastomosis for leaks on the fifth or sixth postoperative day. Vitamin B12 injection is given before discharge.

Complications

Chest infection may occur which can be minimized by aggressive physiotherapy, anastomotic leakage, or duodenal stump leakage may occur. Postgastrectomy syndrome may occur (Chapter 12).

GASTROESOPHAGEAL REFLUX SURGERY

The reflux of gastric contents into the esophagus probably occurs intermittently in everyone, particularly after eating. However, the esophagus usually reacts to this by initiating a peristaltic wave that clears its contents back into the stomach. When symptoms such as burning retrosternal pain appear, this condition is called gastroesophageal reflux. The condition is usually associated with overeating, smoking, and excessive alcohol intake. There is a strong association between gastroesophageal reflux and hiatus hernia, but each condition can occur on its own.

Factors tending to cause gastroesophageal reflux include negative intrathoracic pressure, positive intra-abdominal pressure, and a failure of the normal esophagogastric closing mechanism, such as in hiatus hernia. In sliding hiatus hernia, a diffuse weakness of the phrenoesophageal ligament during contraction of the longitudinal muscles of the esophagus is present, and the esophagogastric junction slides upwards through the widened hiatus. Herniation tends to be progressive. In para-esophageal hernia, the phrenoesophageal ligament gives way at one point, usually posteriorly at its weakest point. Rarely, the stomach becomes irreducibly fixed above the iaphragm. Occasionally, the colon or small bowel may enter the sac.

Adults usually present with symptoms resulting from reflux esophagitis, due to the presence of hiatus hernia and contents in the posterior mediastinum.

Surgical management of gastroesophageal reflux disease is indicated in patients who do not want lifelong medication (symptoms are only partially controlled in spite of full medication), who cannot tolerate medications, and who develop complications of reflux disease (stricture, Barrett's oesophagus, and aspiration secondary to regurgitation).

Assessment

Endoscopy is performed to exclude other pathologies and assess the degree of esophagitis. Esophageal manometry is carried out to exclude motility disorder and 24-hour pH monitoring is used to assess the degree of reflux and relationship to symptoms. Full anesthetic assessment is done before surgery (Chapter 7).

Surgery

Principles underlying surgical treatment of hiatus hernia are reduction of the esophagogastric junction to its normal intra-abdominal position, narrowing of the widened esophageal hiatus, and anchoring of the reduced esophagogastric junction.

Relevant Anatomy

The esophagus passes through the diaphragm at the level of T10, and the fibres of the right crus loop around it. The esophagus enters the stomach at the cardia. The normal intra-abdominal esophagus is approximately 2 cm long and on its surface lie the anterior and posterior vagi. It is enveloped between two leaves of peritoneum, continuous with the lesser omentum and gastrosplenic ligament. Lying in front of the gastroesophageal junction is the left lobe of the liver.

Technique

The surgery can be performed either via an open route or through a laparoscope. Open operation can be undertaken via either the abdominal or the thoracic route (Chapter 14). Most operations today are undertaken abdominally because the morbidity is substantially less through this route. Since the advent of laparoscopic surgery, more patients with less severe symptoms are subjected to surgery. Anesthetic management in these procedures is included elsewhere (Chapters 14 and 17).

The patient is placed in the lithotomy position. The surgeon stands between the patient's legs. An endoscope or a wide-bore bougie is inserted into the esophagus in order to prevent too tight a wrap. Usual laparoscopy is performed, and the required number of operating ports is introduced. A retractor is inserted to elevate the liver away from the hiatus. A laparoscopic inspection of the peritoneal cavity is carried out. The esophagus is dissected from the hiatus, and gastrohepatic and gastrosplenic ligaments are divided. This may involve division of short gastric vessels. A loose posterior 360° fundal wrap is performed, and the stomach wall sutured to the esophagus. The diaphragmatic crura are closed posteriorly, and the diaphragm sutured to the gastric wrap.

Intraoperative Care

Patients must be deeply anesthetized, and judicious use of muscle relaxant is advocated. Injury to any intra-abdominal organ is possible. A gastroscope is left in situ, and repeated gastroscopy may be required. Full details of intraoperative care in these patients are dealt elsewhere (Chapters 14 and 17). A wide-bore nasogastric tube is inserted and properly secured at the end of the surgery after removing the gastroscope.

Postoperative Care

Regular antiemetic for 24 hours is administered to minimize the chance of vomiting and disruption to the wrap. Management of analgesia is dealt with elsewhere (Chapter 25). Patients are allowed clear fluids after 12 hours and a soft diet for three to four weeks is recommended.

LAPAROTOMY FOR PERFORATED PEPTIC ULCER

Improved medical management has reduced the incidence of perforated peptic ulcer, although it remains a common cause of peritonitis. In the majority of cases, surgery is advisable unless the patient is unfit. The conservative measures include intravenous fluids, antibiotics, proton pump inhibitors (lansoprazole), and nasogastric suction.

Assessment

Patients present with abdominal pain and generalized peritonitis. Presence of free gas under the diaphragm on erect X ray is helpful in making the diagnosis of a perforation. Patients should receive intravenous resuscitation fluid and a urethral catheter should be inserted; antibiotics and nasogastric aspiration are started prior to surgery. The patient is assessed and resuscitated with appropriate intravenous fluid (Chapter 7).

Surgery

The principle is to close the perforation with interrupted full-thickness sutures and cover the area with the greater omentum.

Relevant Anatomy

The majority of perforations occur through the anterior wall of the first part of the duodenum. The first part of the duodenum is suspended in continuity with the stomach from the liver by lesser omentum becoming retroperitoneal in its second part. Prepyloric vein of Mayo demarcates plyorus and duodenum.

Technique

The patient is placed supine on the table with a nasogastric tube sited in the stomach. Upper midline incision from xiphisternum to umbilicus is used. The peritoneal cavity is cleared of food residue and bile with suction and lavage. A laparotomy is performed to identify the site of the perforation, which is packed off with large swabs. The perforation is closed with interrupted full-thickness sutures. A pedicle of greater omentum is placed over the area and secured. The abdomen is closed using appropriate techniques with suture materials of choice, preceded by lavage and placement of a silicone drain.

Intraoperative Care

Usual intraoperative anesthetic care like in other abdominal surgeries applies (Chapter 24).

Postoperative Care

Depending upon patient's progress, amount and quantity of gastric aspirate, the nasogastric tube is removed and oral nutrition started. Routine postoperative care is required. Adequate hydration is maintained until nutrition starts. Antibiotics are usually administered, and a proton pump inhibitor is prescribed for at least eight weeks. Patients usually receive anti-*Helicobacter* therapy as well.

Complications

Intra-abdominal abscess, leakage from the perforation site, or reperforation can occur in the immediate postoperative period, requiring anesthesia. Gastric outlet obstruction from scarring and oedema may occur in long term.

LAPAROTOMY FOR GASTRODUODENAL BLEEDING

Gastrointestinal hemorrhage is a potentially life-threatening condition. Failure to respond to medical management with recurrent or continual bleeding is an indication for endoscopy and urgent surgery. If patients are elderly, any excessive blood loss is not tolerated. Bleeding can occur from gastric ulcer, gastric tumors, Mallory–Weiss tear, etc. The ulcer may be adherent posteriorly to the pancreas and may have eroded the splenic artery.

Assessment

Adequate resuscitation is essential before surgery. Adequate blood transfusion may be required. Appropriate investigations are carried out, and clotting abnormalities (if any) are corrected.

Surgery

The main aim is to find the bleeding point and stop bleeding by ligation, or resection.

Relevant Anatomy
Anatomy is as described above.

Technique
The patient is placed supine with a nasogastric tube sited with its tip in the stomach. An incision is made in the upper midline from xiphisternum to umbilicus. A pyloroduodenotomy is made and the source of bleeding is confirmed. The duodenum is mobilized by Kocher's maneuver if needed. In the case of bleeding duodenal ulcer, a longitudinal duodenotomy is performed. A spurting vessel such as gastroduodenal artery is usually visible at the base of an ulcer. This is underrun using interrupted sutures to achieve hemostasis. The pyloroduodenotomy can then be closed. If a gastric ulcer is bleeding, a subtotal gastrectomy that includes the ulcer may be necessary (as distal gastrectomy). The abdomen is closed, and a silicone drain is placed.

Intraoperative Care

Anesthetic management is like in any other major abdominal surgery (Chapter 24).

Postoperative Care

The patient is monitored for signs of recurrent gastrointestinal hemorrhage. The nasogastric tube remains in situ for five days, and oral nutrition is started slowly. Adequate analgesia is provided (Chapter 25). Patients should receive proton pump inhibitor in the postoperative period for at least eight weeks.

Complications

Recurrent gastrointestinal bleeding and leakage from duodenotomy or gastric suture lines may occur.

CHOLECYSTECTOMY

The most common disease of the gall bladder is caused by gall stones. A gall stone gives rise to symptoms when it moves. Movement may result in obstruction of the cystic duct with resultant acute cholecystitis. Stones may also migrate to the common bile duct causing obstruction to the main outflow of bile from the liver.

    The surgical management of gall bladder pathology has changed. Ultrasound allows accurate diagnosis of gall stones as well as the presence of complications, such as acute cholecystitis, obstructive jaundice/cholangitis, and pancreatitis. Such accurate diagnosis allows earlier surgical intervention. Bile duct imaging technique allows both diagnosis and treatment of one of the major complications of gall stones, obstructive jaundice. The timing of surgical interventions keeps changing, and urgent cholecystectomy is now a common practice after acute cholecystitis.

Assessment

The diagnosis of gall bladder pathology is confirmed by ultrasound. The presence of choledocholithiasis should be sought on the basis of history of jaundice, abnormal liver function tests, or ductal dilatation on ultrasound. In these cases, preoperative magnetic resonance cholangiopancreatography (MRCP) is performed, and if necessary, the common bile duct cleared by endoscopic retrograde cholangiopancreatography (ERCP). Anesthetic assessment details can be found in Chapter 7.

Surgery

The aim of surgery is to remove gall bladder and gall stones that may be present in the cystic duct or common bile duct.

Relevant Anatomy

The anatomy of the biliary tree and porta hepatis is variable. The gall bladder comprises a fundus, body, and neck. The neck may be dilated if a stone is impacted. The cystic duct arises from the neck of the gall bladder and passes medially, joining the common hepatic duct to form the common bile duct. The cystic artery arises from the right hepatic artery and runs in Calot's triangle to supply the gall bladder. A fold of peritoneum envelops the gall bladder and attaches it to the liver.

Technique

Gall bladder can be removed via an open route or through a laparoscope. Open route may be required if the surgery is not feasible through laparoscopic route.

    Open Cholecystectomy. The abdomen is opened usually by a right subcostal incision. The cystic duct and artery are carefully dissected and confirmed to arise and terminate, respectively, in the gall bladder. The cystic duct and artery are ligated, and the gall bladder is removed from the bed of the liver. Many surgeons still place a drain to the gall bladder bed for 24 hours. Common bile duct exploration may be required if previous attempts to remove common bile duct gall stones by noninvasive procedures have failed.

Laparoscopic Cholecystectomy. Laparoscopic cholecystectomy is one of the most common surgical operations. In most series, the conversion rate is between 2% and 5%.

The patient is placed supine, anesthetized, and intubated, with a nasogastric tube sited with its tip in the stomach. The patient is then placed in reverse Trendelenburg position. The surgeon's position during the operation varies; usually, the surgeon stands on the patient's left. A 1-cm incision is made below the umbilicus through the linea alba and under direct vision, and a wide-bore cannula is inserted. A pneumoperitoneum is introduced to a pressure between 12 and 15 mmHg, and a laparoscope introduced. A further 10-mm and two 5-mm ports are inserted under vision for grasping and exposing the gall bladder. A grasping forceps is used to elevate the gall bladder fundus, while dissection of Calot's triangle is performed using a diathermy hook starting laterally. The principles and techniques are the same as that of open procedure. No structures are ligated until the anatomy is clear. It may be necessary to perform a cholangiogram. The gall bladder is dissected from the liver using diathermy. The gall bladder is removed from the abdomen in a bag.

Intraoperative Care

Anesthetic management of open cholecystectomy is similar to that of any other major abdominal surgery. Anesthetic management of laparoscopic cholecystectomy is discussed in Chapter 17. The nasogastric tube is usually removed after surgery. Some surgeons prefer to use intra-abdominal drain, in which case the end tip is positioned near the gall bladder bed.

Bile leakage, hemorrhage from gall bladder bed, slipped ligaclip, and iatrogenic bile duct injury are known to occur. Open surgery may be required at any time and the situation may be very demanding. Blood loss may be excessive and organ damage may occur. Both anesthesia and operating room teams should always be ready to deal with the situation.

Postoperative Care

The patient is usually mobile and allowed to drink and eat as soon as possible after laparoscopic cholecystectomy. Analgesic management is dealt with in Chapter 25. Postoperative nausea and vomiting may occur (Chapter 26). The patients are usually discharged home after 24 hours but longer after open operation.

Complications

Chest infection, hemorrhage, bile leakage, deep vein thrombosis, etc. may occur, particularly after open cholecystectomy. Patients who have jaundice may develop postoperative renal failure.

REFERENCES

1. Dunn DC, Rawlinson N. Surgical Diagnosis, a Guide to General Surgical Care. Oxford: Blackwell Scientific Publications, 1991.

2. Clunie GJA, Tjandra JJ, Francis DMA. Textbook of Surgery. Victoria: Blackwell Sciences Pvt Ltd, 1997.
3. Colmer MR. Moroney's Surgery for Nurses. Edinburgh: Churchill Livingstone, 1986.
4. Griffin MS, Raimes SA. Upper Gastrointestinal Surgery: A Companion to Specialist Surgical Practice. 2nd ed. London: Saunders (W.B.) Co. Ltd, 2001.
5. Jaffe RA, Samuels SI. Anesthesiologist's Manual of Surgical Procedures. Philadelphia: Lippincott Williams & Watkins, 2004.

3
Surgical Considerations in Lower Gastrointestinal Surgery

Tim Brown
Department of Surgery, St. Mark's Hospital, London, U.K.

Al Windsor
Department of Surgery, University College Hospital, London, U.K.

INTRODUCTION

Surgery on the lower gastrointestinal (GI) tract, colon, rectum, and anus ranges from minor to major surgery. Whether the surgical procedure is minor or major, it still requires careful anesthetic and surgical management. There are specific challenges related to each surgical procedure. In this chapter, no attempt has been made to discuss the requirements of minor and commonly used major surgical procedures because they have been considered in greater detail in the respective chapters. Over, the last decade, hospitals worldwide have been under increasing pressure to reduce in-patient length of stay. Surgical and anesthetic teams have responded by questioning long-held views on how to go about conducting operative and perioperative care. With this, they have developed new techniques and technologies with the aim of improving operative success and overall patient outcome (Chapters 5 and 6). To achieve this goal, the concept of the "fast-track" surgical program has been developed (Chapter 22). This has required an integrated "team-based" approach and involves anesthetic, paramedical, and surgical specialties working closely together. By identifying and treating factors that can lead to or exacerbate a physiological stress response, these teams have been shown to improve outcome and benefit patients, as well as reduce hospital in-patient stay (1). In this chapter, an attempt has been made to introduce these concepts (below) from a surgical perspective, considering newer modes of surgery and surgical thinking relating to the lower GI tract. Each concept has been dealt with in more detail in other chapters in this book.

PREOPERATIVE FASTING

General anesthesia compromises the protective laryngeal reflexes and the coughing reflex. With loss of these mechanisms, patients are at risk of aspiration of gastric contents. For this reason, elective patients have traditionally been fasted from

midnight prior to their procedure. For passive gastric reflux to occur, it is estimated that 200 mL of gastric content (2) need to be present. Patients undergoing
anesthesia, who encounter airway difficulties (e.g., intubation of the esophagus),
can, however, aspirate with much lower residual gastric volumes.

Since challenging long-held views on preoperative starvation, studies have concentrated on rates of gastric emptying and safe timing of oral intake prior to general
anesthesia. Rates of emptying of clear liquids are rapid and complete in healthy individuals, leaving a residual volume of 30 to 40 mL of fluid. The ability to drink means
that patients are able to alleviate thirst and increase their general "well-being."
Solids (including dairy liquids such as milk) take longer to empty and residue can
still be seen in the stomach four hours after a light meal. These measurements are
prolonged in patients with motility disorders (e.g., diabetes and peritonitis) and do
not apply to those patients with mechanical obstruction of the bowel. These studies
have led to guidelines recommending that clear fluids no sooner than two hours and
solids six hours prior to general anesthesia are safe (2).

Metabolic Response to Starvation and Stress

Overnight fasting stimulates the body to change its metabolic profile to facilitate a
response to starvation (Chapter 4). During this time, the exogenous supply of carbohydrate has ceased and the body relies on its endogenous reserves that have been
built up while in the "fed" state. In this early period of starvation, the body is reliant
on liver glycogen stores. As glucose levels fall, glucagon secretion from the pancreas
increases and insulin secretion and sensitivity fall, probably in an attempt to minimize peripheral uptake and therefore make it available to the brain. It has been
shown that insulin resistance has diminished by 20% after one day (3) and by
50% (4) after three days of fasting in healthy individuals. Stressful events, such as
surgical trauma and generalized sepsis, are well known to increase insulin resistance
(5). The combined effect of this with preoperative starvation puts both the critically
ill and elective surgical patient at risk of developing complications related to insulin
resistance and a catabolic state. Insulin has effects on glucose, fat, and protein
metabolism. Resistance to its actions leads to alterations in substrate metabolism
and a rise in serum glucose concentration, which is immunosuppressive.

Insulin resistance is strongly linked to adverse patient outcome in terms of both
morbidity and mortality (6). Effects of insulin resistance in a high dependency setting
can be reversed by insulin replacement therapy, and patient outcome can be improved
by attention to this detail. Aggressive insulin and glucose therapy is not feasible
for all patients, however, because this requires regular glucose monitoring as well
as tight control of infusion rates. Work by Ljungqvist et al., however, has shown that
ingestion of a carbohydrate-rich drink two hours prior to surgery is just as effective at
reducing postoperative insulin resistance (7). Because it is a clear fluid it clears rapidly
from the stomach and does not lead to problems of aspiration of gastric contents
on induction. For those patients unable to take fluids (e.g., those with bowel
obstruction), preoperative intravenous glucose infusion can similarly reverse insulin
resistance (8). There is now strong evidence that reversing insulin resistance
can improve patient outcome (6).

LAPAROSCOPIC LOWER GASTROINTESTINAL SURGERY

Laparoscopic surgery has become increasingly popular since its inception in the
early 1980s. Since the first appendicectomy was performed in 1982, technological

advances have permitted more and more procedures to be performed "through the keyhole." Lower GI surgeons are now performing colonic and rectal resections with increasing frequency, as well as rectopexy surgery for rectal prolapse. It is likely that the numbers of resections performed laparoscopically will increase as more and more surgeons are trained in this technique.

At the outset of training, as with any new procedure, there is a well-recognized learning curve (9) as the surgeon "gets to grips" with laparoscopic technique. Initially, movements may appear clumsy and without ergonomic purpose and a closed operation may take a great deal longer than its open counterpart. Anesthetists may well question the merits of persisting with such a laborious discipline; however, given time, the surgeon is seen to improve to such an extent that operative time between analogous open and closed procedures becomes similar. Once the learning curve has been overcome, laparoscopic surgery has features that make it attractive to the patient, surgeon, and anesthetist. These include less pain, prevention of postoperative ileus, smaller scars, and a shorter hospital stay (10). These advantages have infiltrated public knowledge to the extent that patients now ask specifically for their procedure to be performed by the "keyhole" method. There are, however, surgical and anesthetic considerations that are peculiar to this discipline.

Inducing Pneumoperitoneum

Access to the peritoneum is gained, usually at the umbilicus, using either a blunt port and open dissection or a sprung Verres needle ("closed technique"). Although previously widely performed, this latter technique has fallen out of favor because it may contribute to higher rates of underlying visceral or vascular injury. Many surgeons now perform the open "Hasson" technique, believing it to be safer. Using a Verres needle is, however, still considered by the Royal College of Surgeons of England to be an acceptable technique because there have been no randomized controlled trials that clearly show this to be true (11).

Once access is achieved, carbon dioxide (CO_2) is insufflated to distend the peritoneal cavity and provide a working space in which to view and carry out the proposed procedure. The insufflator has an automatic pressure sensor that maintains an intraperitoneal pressure between 12 and 14 mmHg. It automatically introduces more gas should pressure fall and stops introducing gas when the desired pressure is obtained. This pressure may be reduced if necessary. Pneumoperitoneum has a number of physiological effects on the patient.

Cardiovascular

Intra-abdominal pressure caused by the pneumoperitoneum usually exceeds vena cava pressure and can therefore obstruct venous return, with subsequent reduction in cardiac output. In healthy patients, this effect is usually well tolerated; however, patients with underlying cardiac disease may not be able to compensate. These patients must receive adequate preoperative volume loading and may benefit from lower limb pneumatic compression stockings. Gasless laparoscopy may be considered in patients with severe impairment. Air embolism is a rare but recognized phenomenon that can occur, usually on establishment of the pneumoperitoneum. A sudden reduction in blood pressure and end-tidal CO_2 concentration should lead to a high index of suspicion that this has occurred. The cause is usually inadvertent vascular puncture by a Verres needle (11).

Respiratory

The pneumoperitoneum has chemical and mechanical effects on a patient's respiratory physiology. The insufflation gas commonly used for the establishment of the pneumoperitoneum is CO_2. This is absorbed into the blood stream, leading to hypercapnia and a respiratory acidosis. For this reason, end-tidal CO_2 monitoring during laparoscopic procedures is mandatory and a high minute volume is required to maintain normocapnia (11).

Mechanically, higher intra-abdominal compartment pressures caused by the pneumoperitoneum cause mechanical splinting of the diaphragm. Also, patients undergoing lower GI procedures are often head down, causing venous congestion within the lungs and reduction in total lung volume and functional residual capacity. The lungs become stiffer and ventilation-perfusion mismatch can ensue. As with cardiovascular effects, these changes are normally well tolerated; however, those patients with poor respiratory reserve may benefit from gasless laparoscopy or the use of inert insufflation gases such as helium.

There are, however, advantages to respiratory physiology brought about by laparoscopic procedures. Postoperative pain is lower after laparoscopic procedures when compared to open procedures; as a result, patients find deep breathing and mobilization easier. This reduces atelectasis and infective complications and helps prevent possible thromboembolic disease (11).

Mode of Anesthesia and Patient Position

Lower GI surgery utilizes approaches to the peritoneal cavity, the retroperitoneal space, and the perianal region. Careful positioning of a patient can make a great deal of difference to the ease of a particular procedure. Adequate analgesia, commencing prior to the painful stimulus, reduces the neuroendocrine stress response by blocking central nociceptive pathways (12).

Lower GI procedures are carried out in the supine, lithotomy ("legs up"), Lloyd–Davis (legs up, head down), left lateral (decubitus), or prone position. Each of these positions has advantages and disadvantages; therefore communication between surgeon and anesthetist is essential in order that the patient receives the safest operation with optimal access. Local, regional, and general anesthesia render these regions amenable to surgery.

Local Anesthesia

It has been estimated that up to 90% of perianal procedures can occur on an ambulatory, day-patient basis (13). For this to occur, it is necessary that the anesthetic be short acting, leave minimal side effects, allow the patient to mobilize early without difficulty, and have a low complication rate. General anesthetic is associated with nausea, hypotension, vomiting, and urinary retention, as well as complications associated with intubation of the upper airway. Regional anesthesia, although providing excellent postprocedure analgesia, affects motor function of the lower limbs and, if continuous, causes problems with patient mobility. Local anesthesia has been shown to be effective and safe, especially in the setting of "so-called" ambulatory surgical units. It allows adequate analgesia, minimal complications, and accelerated patient discharge (14).

The perineum is supplied by the bilateral, pudendal nerves (S2, 3, and 4). These branch to form the inferior rectal nerves (external anal sphincter and perianal skin); perineal nerves (sphincter urethrae, bulbospongiosus, ischiocavernosus, and peroneus muscles, and skin over posterior two-third of scrotum or labium majus), and the dorsal nerves of the clitoris or penis (skin over clitoris or most of penis).

Course of Pudendal Nerve. The nerve exits the foramina of S2, 3, and 4. It leaves the pelvis through the greater sciatic foramen, inferior to piriformis. It winds around the ischial spine to enter the ischiorectal fossa through the lesser sciatic foramen. As it runs along the lateral side wall within a fascial sheath formed by the obturator internus fascia (Alcock's canal), it divides into its terminal branches, which run through the ischioanal space to reach the structures that they supply.

Because the nerves run a relatively superficial course, they can be blocked by local anesthesia. This can be via a perineal field block, ischiorectal fossa block, or a formal pudendal nerve block. Whichever technique is used, the surgical requirement is that the perianal skin and anal mucosa be insensate and the sphincter complex relaxed.

To access the nerve fibres, it is necessary to introduce a needle into the perineal skin. This has a high sensory nerve fibre density and so is exquisitely tender. Strategies have evolved to facilitate this problem using short-acting benzodiazepines, topical anesthetic creams, and short-acting intravenous anesthetic agents with inhalational anesthesia. These techniques have been shown to be safe as well as effective and a number of units worldwide are now using them as routine (14).

Regional Anesthesia

This offers an improvement over local anesthesia in the quality of perineal block that can be achieved as well as in providing an alternative to those patients who prefer not to have procedures performed under local anesthesia. It provides excellent postoperative analgesia for in-patients and so is commonly combined with general anesthesia for this purpose. The technique can be used for day-case procedures provided short-acting agents are used and the surgeon can be relied upon to finish when he says he will. It should be noted that postoperative urinary retention is a particular side effect, as are hypotension, headache, and backache. The use of epidural anesthesia has been shown to reduce the amount of opioid analgesia that the patient requires. Opioids are associated with postoperative nausea and vomiting as well as postoperative ileus. Reduction in the amount of opioid use results in an earlier return to normal gut function and earlier enteral feeding. This has been shown to reduce infective complications and systemic inflammatory response (12).

General Anesthesia

From the surgeon's perspective, general anesthesia is safe and reliable. It provides rapid access to the operative field, and swift recovery. Patients usually suffer minimal side effects. It is suitable for major lower GI cases as well as minor "ambulatory" cases. It is rapid in onset and recovery but needs to be combined with other techniques for management of postoperative analgesia. Patients undergoing anorectal procedures performed under general anesthesia and carried out in the prone position are at greater risk of suffering airway difficulties. Should these occur, airway management can be more hazardous given the difficulty of access to the oropharynx.

BOWEL PREPARATION

This is currently an area of controversy in colorectal surgery. Traditionally, patients undergoing procedures on the distal colon, rectum, and perineum would receive a vigorous mechanical catharsis—the idea being that a clean bowel will lower rates of wound infection, peritoneal contamination, and anastomotic breakdown. The process involves ingestion of a large volume of osmotically active fluid with or without prokinetic agents such as senna. The process is continued, traditionally, until the patient is passing clear fluid per rectum.

Ingestion of such osmotically active fluid is unpleasant physically, with thirst, recurrent episodes to the lavatory, and physiological side effects. In healthy individuals, these are well tolerated and thought to be acceptable in this cohort (15); however, effects on medically or nutritionally compromised patients are more difficult to assess and may be responsible for morbidity and mortality. As yet, there are no powerful randomized controlled trials that clearly define the situation.

What has been established (but is still subject to surgeon preference) is that open operations on the right colon and perineum do not require preparation—formerly because there is no added risk of leak or infection; latterly because inadequate bowel preparation causes liquid stool, which obscures the operative site and potentially hinders the procedure. In cases involving the perineum, adequate preparation is achieved with a single phosphate enema prior to arriving in the operating room. As an exception to this, laparoscopic surgeons operating on any part of the colon may prefer that the whole bowel is purged because the bowel is lighter and can be manipulated more easily with laparoscopic instruments when empty.

CONCLUSION

It can be seen that in recent years, exciting progress has been made in the field of perioperative care and surgical technology. Advances in the biology surrounding the metabolic stress response and inflammatory processes at play in surgical and critically ill patients are being successfully translated into clinical practice. Researchers' efforts are being rewarded with improved clinical outcome in a wide range of surgical disciplines and lower GI surgery is no exception. The future should see these techniques being adopted widely, facilitated by dedicated, multidisciplinary perioperative care teams.

REFERENCES

1. Basse L, Thorbol JE, Lossl K, et al. Colonic surgery with accelerated rehabilitation or conventional care. Dis Colon Rectum 2004; 47(3):271–272.
2. Ljungqvist O, Soreide E. Preoperative fasting. Br J Surg 2003; 90(4):400–406.
3. Nygren J, Thorell A, Brismar K, et al. Short-term hypocaloric nutrition but not bed rest decrease insulin sensitivity and IGF-I bioavailability in healthy subjects: the importance of glucagon. Nutrition 1997; 13(11–12):945–951.
4. Svanfeldt M, Thorell A, Brismar K, et al. Effects of 3 days of "postoperative" low caloric feeding with or without bed rest on insulin sensitivity in healthy subjects. Clin Nutr 2003; 22(1):31–38.
5. Thorell A, Nygren J, Ljungqvist O. Insulin resistance: a marker of surgical stress. Curr Opin Clin Nutr Metab Care 1999; 2(1):69–78.
6. Ljungqvist O, Nygren J, Soop M, et al. Metabolic perioperative management: novel concepts. Curr Opin Crit Care 2005; 11(4):295–299.
7. Nygren J, Soop M, Thorell A, et al. Preoperative oral carbohydrates and postoperative insulin resistance. Clin Nutr 1999; 18(2):117–120.
8. Ljungqvist O, Thorell A, Gutniak M, et al. Glucose infusion instead of preoperative fasting reduces postoperative insulin resistance. J Am Coll Surg 1994; 178(4):329–336.

9. Shah PR, Joseph A, Haray PN. Laparoscopic colorectal surgery: learning curve and training implications. Postgrad Med J 2005; 81(958):537–540.

10. Veldkamp R, Kuhry E, Hop WC, et al. Colon cancer Laparoscopic or Open Resection Study Group (COLOR). Laparoscopic surgery versus open surgery for colon cancer: short-term outcomes of a randomised trial. Lancet Oncol 2005; 6(7):477–484.

11. Neudecker J, Sauerland S, Neugebauer E, et al. The European Association for endoscopic surgery clinical practice guideline on the pneumoperitoneum for laparoscopic surgery. Surg Endosc 2002; 16(7):1121–1143.

12. Kehlet H, Dahl JB. Anaesthesia, surgery, and challenges in postoperative recovery. Lancet 2003; 362(9399):1921–1928.

13. Smith LE. Ambulatory surgery for anorectal diseases: an update. South Med J 1986; 79(2):163–166.

14. Read TE, Henry SE, Hovis RM, et al. Prospective evaluation of anesthetic technique for anorectal surgery. Dis Colon Rectum 2002; 45(11):1553–1558.

15. Holte K, Nielsen KG, Madsen JL, et al. Physiologic effects of bowel preparation. Dis Colon Rectum 2004; 47(8):1397–1402.

4

Stress Response During Surgery

Grainne Nicholson and George M. Hall
Department of Anesthesia and Intensive Care Medicine,
St. George's University of London, London, U.K.

INTRODUCTION

The stress response refers to the series of hormonal, inflammatory, and metabolic and psychological changes that occur in response to trauma or surgery. Surgery serves as a useful model of the stress response because the changes that occur can be observed from a well-defined starting point, but similar features occur in trauma burns, severe infection, and strenuous exercise (1). Catabolic changes predominate with suppression of anabolic hormones and resultant substrate mobilization. Muscle protein loss occurs, leading to a negative nitrogen balance; salt and water retention is also an important feature. Generally, the response of the body is in proportion to the severity of the insult or trauma. For example, intra-abdominal surgery has a greater impact than superficial skin surgery.

The changes that occur with the stress response have probably evolved as a means to aid survival by mobilizing metabolic substrates, preventing ongoing tissue damage, destroying infective organisms, and activating repair processes. The benefits may not be obvious to modern medicine when physiological changes can be more easily corrected; they might even have a detrimental effect. Research has focused in recent years on modifying the surgical stress response with the aim of improving patient outcome.

HORMONAL ASPECTS OF THE STRESS RESPONSE

The hypothalamic-pituitary-adrenal (HPA) axis and the sympathetic nervous system are activated by afferent neuronal input from the operative site, both somatic and autonomic, and by the release of cytokines from the damaged area. The increased pituitary hormone secretion has secondary effects on target organs, and the magnitude of the response is proportional to the severity of the trauma. There is a failure of the normal feedback mechanisms that control hormone secretion. Enhanced secretion of catabolic hormones predominates, whereas, anabolic hormone secretion, such as insulin and testosterone, is suppressed.

Sympathoadrenal Response

Hypothalamic activation of the sympathetic autonomic nervous system results in increased secretion of catecholamines from the adrenal medulla and release of norepinephrine from presynaptic nerve terminals. Norepinephrine serves predominantly as a neurotransmitter, but some of that released from nerve terminals spills over into the circulation. This increased sympathetic activity results in the well-recognized cardiovascular effects of tachycardia and hypertension. In addition, the function of certain visceral organs, including the liver, pancreas, and kidneys is modified directly by efferent sympathetic stimulation and by circulating catecholamines (2). Renin is released from the kidneys, leading to the conversion of angiotensin I to angiotensin II. The latter stimulates the secretion of aldosterone from the adrenal cortex, which, in turn, increases sodium absorption from the distal convoluted tubule of the kidney.

Cortisol

The onset of surgery is associated with the rapid secretion of adrenocorticotrophin (ACTH) from the anterior pituitary in response to corticotrophin-releasing hormone (CRH) from the hypothalamus. Arginine vasopressin (AVP) also plays an important role in the control of ACTH secretion during stress.

ACTH acts on the adrenal gland to stimulate cortisol secretion. Feedback inhibition by cortisol normally prevents any further increases in CRH or ACTH production. However, during surgery, the normal pituitary adrenocortical feedback mechanism is no longer effective, as both hormones remain increased simultaneously. Cortisol is a C^{21} corticosteroid with both glucocorticoid and mineralocorticoid activity (3).

Plasma cortisol concentrations increase rapidly in response to surgical stimulation and remain elevated for a variable time following surgery. The normal endogenous cortisol production is between 25 and 30 mg/day, but the amount secreted following major surgery, such as abdominal or thoracic surgery, is between 75 and 100 mg on the first day (4–6). Minor surgery such as herniorrhaphy induces less than 50 mg cortisol secretion during the first 24 hours (7). The magnitude and duration of the cortisol response reflect the severity of surgical trauma as well as the occurrence of postoperative complications. Values greater than 1500 nmol/L are not uncommon (8,9).

Cortisol has complex effects on the metabolism of carbohydrate, fat, and protein (10). It causes an increase in blood glucose concentration by stimulating protein catabolism and promoting glucose production in the liver and kidney by gluconeogenesis from the mobilized amino acids. Cortisol reduces peripheral glucose utilization by an anti-insulin effect. Glucocorticoids inhibit the recruitment of neutrophils and monocyte-macrophages into the area of inflammation (11,12) and also have well-described anti-inflammatory actions, mediated by a decrease in the production of inflammatory mediators, such as leukotrienes and prostaglandins (13). In addition, the production and action of interleukin-6 (IL-6) are inhibited by ACTH and cortisol (14).

Growth Hormone

Growth hormone–releasing hormone and somatostatin released by the hypothalamus control the secretion of growth hormone, a 191-amino acid protein. Somatostatin is also found in the endocrine pancreas, where it inhibits the secretion of insulin and other pancreatic hormones, and in the gastrointestinal tract where it is an important inhibitory gastrointestinal hormone. Growth hormone (GH), also known as somatotropin, has a major role in growth regulation. The anabolic effects of growth hormone are mediated through polypeptides synthesized in the liver, muscle, and other tissues called somatomedins or insulin-like growth factors (because of their structural similarity to insulin). In addition to its effects on growth, GH has many effects on metabolism, particularly, stimulating protein synthesis and inhibiting protein breakdown. Other metabolic effects of GH include stimulation of lipolysis and an anti-insulin effect. GH also stimulates glycogenolysis in the liver; however, hormones such as cortisol and catecholamines play a more significant role in perioperative hyperglycemia. Growth hormone has enjoyed a resurgence of interest as its potential for promoting anabolism after injury has been explored. Attempts have been made to use recombinant growth hormone, insulin-like growth factor (IGF-1), or both, to reduce muscle catabolism and improve wound healing in severely catabolic states and in critically ill patients. As yet the evidence is inconclusive (15–17). In some patients, the use of GH was associated with increased mortality (17).

β-Endorphin and Prolactin

Increased concentrations of β-endorphin during surgery reflect anterior pituitary stimulation. The secretion of prolactin is under tonic inhibitory control via prolactin-release-inhibitory-factor (dopamine), and increased prolactin secretion occurs by the release of inhibitory control. The physiological effects of increased secretion of both hormones during surgery are unknown, but they may alter immune function.

Insulin and Glucagon

Insulin is a polypeptide hormone secreted by β-cells of the pancreas. Its structure consists of a 21-amino acid and 30-amino acid peptide chain linked by disulphide cross-bridges. It is the key anabolic hormone and is normally released after food intake, when blood glucose and amino acid concentrations increase. Insulin promotes the uptake of glucose into muscle, liver, and adipose tissue and its conversion into glycogen and triglycerides. Hepatic glycogenolysis and hepatic and renal gluconeogenesis are inhibited, but at higher concentrations of insulin than those that mediate the peripheral effects.

The hyperglycemic response to surgical stress is characterized by the failure of insulin secretion to respond to the glucose stimulus (18). This is caused partly by $\alpha 2$ adrenergic inhibition of β-cell secretion and also by insulin resistance, where a normal or even elevated concentration of insulin produces a subnormal biological response. The precise mechanisms underlying the development of insulin resistance following surgery or trauma remain unclear, but do not involve simply elevated concentrations of counter-regulatory hormones, such as cortisol and excessive cytokine secretion (19). Because the clinical benefits of maintaining normal blood glucose concentrations in surgical intensive care patients have been shown by Van den Berghe et al. (20), enthusiastic attempts have been made to control perioperative hyperglycemia. It has been suggested that postoperative or posttraumatic insulin resistance can be prevented or attenuated by previous glucose loading via the oral or intravenous route (21–23).

Glucagon is produced by the α cells of the pancreas. In contrast to insulin, glucagon release promotes hepatic glycogenolysis and gluconeogenesis; it also has lipolytic activity. Concentrations increase briefly in response to surgical procedures, but it is not thought to contribute significantly to perioperative hyperglycemia.

Thyroid-Stimulating Hormone and Thyroid Hormones

Thyrotropin or thyroid-stimulating hormone (TSH) secreted by the anterior pituitary promotes the production and secretion of thyroxine (T3) and triiodothyronine (T4) from the thyroid gland. The secretion of TSH is controlled by thyrotropin-releasing hormone from the hypothalamus and by negative feedback of free T3 and T4. T3 is formed in the tissues by deiodination of T4, and it is three to five times more active than T4. Thyroid hormones stimulate oxygen consumption in most of the metabolically active tissues of the body, with the exception of brain, spleen, and anterior pituitary gland. There is rapid cellular uptake of glucose, increased glycolysis and gluconeogenesis, and enhanced carbohydrate absorption from the gut in order to fuel increased metabolic activity. Thyroxine increases lipid mobilization from adipose tissue, causing an increase in free fatty acids but a decrease in plasma cholesterol, phospholipids, and triglycerides. In physiological concentrations T3 and T4 have a protein anabolic effect, but in larger doses their effects are catabolic.

TSH concentrations increase during surgery or immediately afterwards, but this effect is not prolonged. However, there is usually a pronounced and prolonged decrease in T3 concentrations (both free and protein bound), which is due partly to the effect of cortisol, which suppresses TSH secretion. Changes in thyroid hormone metabolism may represent adaptive responses to limit increases in metabolic rate in the presence of increased sympathetic activity (24).

Gonadotrophins

The gonadotrophins luteinizing hormone (LH) and follicle-stimulating hormone (FSH) are secreted from the anterior pituitary. FSH is responsible for the development of ovarian follicles in women and maintenance of the spermatic epithelium in men. LH stimulates growth and development of the Leydig cells of the testis, which produce testosterone. Small amounts of testosterone are also produced from the adrenal cortex. In addition to its reproductive effects, testosterone has important effects on protein anabolism and growth. Following surgery, testosterone concentrations are decreased for several days, although LH concentrations show variable changes (25). Estrogen concentrations have also been shown to decrease for up to five days following surgery (26). The significance of these changes is uncertain; but the decline in testosterone secretion is another example of the failure of anabolic hormone secretion.

Arginine and Vasopressin

The posterior pituitary is an extension of the hypothalamus and secretes two hormones, AVP and oxytocin. Both hormones are synthesized in the cell bodies of the supraoptic nucleus and the paraventricular nucleus of the hypothalamus, and are transported in vesicles along the axons to coalesce into storage vesicles in the nerve terminals of the posterior pituitary. AVP is a nonapeptide with a biological half-life of 16 to 20 minutes. Vasopressin is a potent stimulator of vascular smooth muscle in vitro; but in vivo, high concentrations are required to raise the blood pressure, because vasopressin also acts at the area postrema to cause a decrease in cardiac output. Hemorrhage is a potent stimulus to vasopressin secretion. Vasopressin also causes glycogenolysis in the liver and serves as a neurotransmitter in the brain and spinal cord. Vasopressin receptors in the anterior pituitary increase ACTH release. Vasopressin exerts its antidiuretic effect by activating protein water channels in the luminal membranes of the principal cells of the collecting ducts. In addition, AVP enhances hemostasis by increasing factor VIII activity.

CYTOKINES

Cytokines are low-molecular-weight ($<80\,kDa$) heterogeneous glycoproteins, which include interleukins, interferons, and tumor necrosis factor (TNF). They are synthesized by activated macrophages, fibroblasts, and endothelial and glial cells in response to tissue injury from surgery or trauma (27). Although they exert most of their effects locally (paracrine), they can also act systemically (endocrine). Cytokines play an important role in mediating immunity and inflammation by acting on surface receptors of target cells. The most important cytokine associated with surgery is IL-6; increases occur two to four hours after the start of surgery with peak values occurring after 12 to 24 hours; the size and duration of IL-6 response reflect the severity of tissue damage (28). Cytokine secretion cannot be modified by the use of neuronal blockade (29). However laparoscopic surgical techniques result in smaller increases in IL-6 than those following conventional, open surgery (30). Circulating TNF-α and IL-1β concentrations do not change significantly unless there is malignancy or underlying chronic infection, but increases may be found locally at the site of tissue damage.

The immune and the neuroendocrine systems are closely interconnected. In surgical patients, circulating cytokines may augment pituitary ACTH secretion and consequently increase the release of cortisol, sustaining the glucocorticoid response to injury for several days. A negative feedback system exists whereby glucocorticoids decrease cytokine production by inhibiting gene expression. Thus, the cortisol response to surgery limits the severity of the inflammatory response.

IL-6 and other cytokines cause the acute phase response, which includes the production of acute phase proteins such as fibrinogen, C reactive protein (CRP), complement proteins, amyloid P component, amyloid A, and ceruloplasmin in the liver (31,32). Their function is to promote hemostasis, limit tissue damage, and enhance repair and regeneration. Synthesis of acute phase proteins occurs at the expense of decreased production of other key proteins such as albumin and transferrin. Concentrations of circulating cations such as zinc and iron decrease, partly as a result of changes in the production of transport proteins. Other important aspects of the acute phase response include fever, granulocytosis, and lymphocyte differentiation.

The acute phase response prevents further tissue damage, isolates and destroys infective organisms, activates the repair processes, and is considered an integral part of wound healing and repair.

METABOLIC CONSEQUENCES

Substrate mobilization, to provide fuel for oxidation, is an intrinsic aspect of the stress response to surgery or trauma.

Carbohydrate Metabolism

Hyperglycemia is a major feature of the metabolic response to surgery and results from an increase in glucose production and a reduction in peripheral glucose utilization. This is facilitated by catecholamines and cortisol, which promote glycogenolysis and gluconeogenesis. The increase in blood glucose is proportional to the severity of surgery or injury, for example, cataract surgery under general anesthesia causes a small increase of approximately 0.5 to 1 mmol/L (33), whereas cardiac surgery results in more marked hyperglycemia. The hyperglycemic response is enhanced by the iatrogenic effects of administration of glucose infusions and blood products. The usual mechanisms that regulate glucose production and uptake are ineffective. Catabolic hormones promote glucose production, and glucose utilization is impaired due to an initial failure of insulin secretion followed by insulin resistance. Glucose concentrations greater than 12 mmol/L increase water and electrolyte loss, impair wound and anastomotic healing, and increase infection rates (34,35).

Protein Metabolism

Initially there is an inhibition of protein anabolism, followed later, if the stress response is severe, by enhanced catabolism. Protein catabolism is stimulated by increased circulating cortisol and cytokine concentrations. The amount of protein degradation is influenced by the type of surgery and also by the nutritional status of the patient; following major abdominal surgery, up to 0.5 kg/day of lean body mass can be lost, resulting in significant muscle wasting and weight loss. Skeletal muscle protein is mainly affected but some visceral muscle protein may also be catabolized to release essential amino acids. Amino acids, particularly glutamine and alanine, are used for gluconeogenesis in the liver and renal cortex to maintain circulating blood glucose greater than 3 mmol/L, and also for the synthesis of acute phase proteins in the liver. However, albumin production is reduced, impairing the maintenance of the extracellular volume. Attempts to prevent protein loss after surgery, by providing nutritional support, enteral and parenteral, have proved disappointing (36–38). The availability of additional substrates has little effect in overcoming the inhibition of protein anabolism and preventing catabolism.

Fat Metabolism

Interestingly, few changes occur in lipid mobilization following surgery unless starvation becomes a major factor postoperatively. Plasma nonesterified fatty acids (NEFAs) and ketone body concentrations do not change significantly. Increased catecholamine, cortisol, and glucagon secretion, in combination with insulin deficiency, promote some lipolysis and ketone body production. Triglycerides are metabolized to fatty acids and glycerol; the latter is a gluconeogenic substrate. High glucagon and low insulin concentrations also promote the oxidation of NEFAs to acyl CoA, which is converted in the liver to ketone bodies (β hydroxybutyrate, acetoacetate, and acetone). These serve as a useful, water-soluble fuel source for many organs.

   The most dramatic changes in lipid metabolism are seen during cardiac surgery. Heparinization activates lipoprotein lipase, which acts on triacylglycerol to cause a dramatic increase in circulating NEFA concentrations. Circulating concentrations may exceed 2 mmol/L during cardiopulmonary bypass, which may have toxic effects on cell membranes, in particular, promoting arrhythmias. The problem is less severe with the new "cleaner" heparins.

Salt and Water

AVP secretion results in water retention and concentrated urine and potassium loss and may continue for three to five days following surgery. Renin is secreted from the juxtaglomerular cells of the kidney and converts angiotensin to angiotensin II, which in turn releases aldosterone from the adrenal cortex. Under the influence of aldosterone, sodium and water are retained from the collecting ducts and increased amounts of Na^+ are exchanged for K^+ and H^+, producing a K^+ diuresis and an increase in urine acidity.

MODIFYING THE STRESS RESPONSE

Effects of Anesthesia

Although it is a common practice to view the stress response as an inevitable consequence of surgical trauma, Kehlet has suggested that the surgical stress response is an "epiphenomenon," and decreasing the endocrine and metabolic changes that occur may reduce major perioperative morbidity (39).

Intravenous Induction Agents

Etomidate, an imidazole derivative, is a potent inhibitor of adrenal steroidogenesis. A single induction dose of etomidate will inhibit cortisol and aldosterone production for up to eight hours after pelvic surgery (40). Etomidate is often used in sick patients with limited cardiovascular reserve without adverse effects, thereby raising the question of how much circulating cortisol is required in routine surgery for cardiovascular stability. Both diazepam and midazolam have also been shown to inhibit cortisol production from isolated bovine adrenocortical cells in vitro (41). Midazolam, which has an imidazole ring in addition to its benzodiazepine structure, was found to decrease the cortisol response to peripheral surgery (42) and major upper abdominal surgery (43), and may also have a direct effect on ACTH secretion (42).

Volatile Anesthetic Agents

Volatile anesthetic agents probably have little effect on the HPA axis when used at low concentrations. No difference was found between 2.1 and 1.2 minimal alveolar concentration (MAC) halothane in obtunding the pituitary hormone and sympathoadrenal responses to pelvic surgery (44). It is likely that other volatile anesthetic agents behave similarly at clinical concentrations.

High-Dose Opioid Anesthesia

The ability of morphine to inhibit the HPA axis has been known for many years (45), but it was only in the 1970s that the use of morphine to modify the metabolic and endocrine responses to surgery was first investigated (46). Large doses of morphine, however, resulted in unacceptably prolonged recovery times. Fentanyl 50 µg/kg intravenously abolished the cortisol response to pelvic surgery (47), but 100 µg/kg was required in upper abdominal surgery (48). The inevitable penalty of this technique is profound respiratory depression for several hours postoperatively.

Regional Anesthesia

It is well recognized that complete afferent blockade, both somatic and autonomic, is necessary to prevent stimulation of the HPA axis. Thus an extensive T4-S5 dermatomal block is necessary for pelvic surgery (49), and it has been known for more than 30 years that it is very difficult in upper abdominal surgery to prevent cortisol secretion with regional anesthesia (50). However, it is worth noting that cytokine-mediated responses, which occur as a consequence of tissue trauma, are not altered by afferent neuronal blockade (29).

Whether epidural anesthesia and analgesia improve the outcome of major surgery is a long-running controversy. Proponents of the technique cite beneficial effects resulting from attenuation of the stress response, which in turn has advantages for postoperative hypercoagulability and cardiovascular, respiratory, gastrointestinal, metabolic, and immune function (51,52). Rodgers et al. concluded that epidural or spinal anesthesia results in a significant reduction in postoperative morbidity and mortality (53). However, this systematic review, which claimed a reduction in mortality of one-third that does not differ by surgical group, type of regional nerve blockade, or the use of general together with regional anesthesia, has been the subject of intense controversy with many of its conclusions being challenged. There is evidence that epidural analgesia provides better postoperative pain relief and shortens the intubation time and intensive care stay of patients undergoing specific procedures, such as abdominal aortic surgery (54). A recent randomized controlled trial found that in high-risk patients undergoing major abdominal surgery, adverse morbid outcomes were not decreased by the use of combined epidural and general anesthesia and postoperative epidural analgesia (55,56). The only significant benefit with the epidural regimen was a decreased occurrence of postoperative respiratory failure. Epidural analgesia following gastrointestinal surgery has been shown to be associated with improved pain control, a shorter duration of postoperative ileus and fewer pulmonary complications, but did not affect the incidence of anastomotic leakage, intraoperative blood loss, transfusion requirements, and risk of thromboembolism or cardiac morbidity (57). Epidural analgesia is an integral part of multimodal rehabilitation programs that also include early nutrition, mobilization, and avoidance of opiates. It is not possible to determine the precise role played by regional anesthesia in these programs (58–60).

Minimal Access Surgery

The introduction of endoscopic surgical techniques has drawn attention to the importance of the inflammatory aspects of surgery (61). Laparoscopic surgery causes less tissue damage than conventional procedures, so the increases in biochemical markers of inflammation, such as IL-6 and CRP, are not as great. For individual surgeons, increasing the annual caseload of laparoscopic surgery results in shorter hospital stays for patients, although for laparoscopic cholecystectomy this has not affected postoperative mortality (62).

The classical neuroendocrine response (increases in cortisol, glucose, and catecholamines) to abdominal surgery, such as open cholecystectomy, is not significantly altered by undertaking the operation using a laparoscopic technique. The anesthetic technique has little effect on the cytokine response, because it cannot influence tissue trauma (63,64). Combined analgesic regimens, which include high-dose steroids (prednisolone 30 mg/kg), cause a small decrease in IL-6 concentrations and the acute phase response. However, their use is precluded because of the risk of unwanted side effects, including wound dehiscence (65).

Endoscopic surgery results in a decreased acute phase response and preserves immune function compared with conventional open techniques (66). It has been recommended as the treatment of choice, instead of laparotomy, for benign pelvic disease whenever feasible (67). However, concerns have been expressed about its suitability for the treatment of malignant disease, particularly because of portsite recurrences when used in the treatment of colorectal cancer (68). Recent studies have shown that laparoscopic resection of rectosigmoid carcinoma does not jeopardize survival and disease control of patients (69) and laparoscopically assisted colectomy is more effective than open colectomy in terms of morbidity, hospital stay, tumor recurrence, and cancer-related survival (70). The mechanism for this is unknown, but it has been suggested that better immune function and reduced tumor manipulation may both contribute (70).

The effects of nonsteroidal anti-inflammatory drugs (NSAIDs) on the inflammatory response to surgery depend on the timing of their administration. When given during and after surgery, they are ineffective and must be used for 24 hours preoperatively before any beneficial effects are found (71). It has been suggested that cyclooxygenase-2 inhibitors would have a similar analgesic potency, but a better safety profile compared with older NSAIDs in terms of gastrointestinal tract and platelet function. This view has recently been challenged, particularly for patients with cardiovascular disease (72).

REFERENCES

1. Nicholson G, Hall GM. The hormonal and metabolic response to anaesthesia, surgery and trauma. In: Webster N, Galley H, eds. Anaesthesia Science. 1st ed. Oxford, United Kingdom: BMJ Books, 2006 (In press).
2. Desborough JP. The stress response to trauma and surgery. Br J Anaesth 2000; 85:109–117.
3. Orth DN, Kovacs WJ, de Bold CR. The adrenal cortex. In: Wilson JD, Foster DW, eds. Williams Textbook of Endocrinology. 8th ed. Philadelphia, Pennsylvania: WB Saunders, 1992:489–621.
4. Hardy JD, Turner MD. Hydrocortisone secretion in man: studies of adrenal vein blood. Surgery 1957; 42:194–201.
5. Hume DM, Bell CC, Bartter FC. Direct measurement of adrenal secretion during operative trauma and convalescence. Surgery 1962; 52:174–187.
6. Hume DM, Nelson DH, Miller DW. Blood and urinary 17-hydrocorticosteroids in patients with severe burns. Ann Surg 1956; 143:316–329.
7. Kehlet H. A rational approach to dosage and preparation of parenteral glucocorticoid substitution therapy during surgical procedures. Acta Anaesth Scand 1975; 19:260–264.
8. Chernow B, Alexander R, Smallridge RC, et al. Hormonal responses to graded surgical stress. Arch Int Med 1987; 147:1273–1278.
9. Traynor C, Hall GM. Endocrine and metabolic changes during surgery: anaesthetic implications. Br J Anaesth 1981; 53:153–161.
10. Desborough JP, Hall GM. Endocrine response to surgery. In: Kaufmann L, ed. Anaesthesia Review. Vol. 10. Edinburgh, United Kingdom: Churchill Livingstone, 1993:131–148.
11. Parrillo JE, Fauci AS. Mechanisms of glucocorticoid action on immune processes. Annu Rev Pharmacol Toxicol 1979; 19:179–201.

12. Balow JE, Rosenthal AS. Glucocorticoid suppression of macrophage migration inhibitory factor. J Exp Med 1973; 137:1031–1039.
13. Blackwell GJ, Carnuccio R, DiRosa M, et al. Macrocortin: a polypeptide causing the anti-phospholipase effects of glucocorticoids. Nature 1980; 287:147–149.
14. Jameson P, Desborough JP, Bryant AE, et al. The effect of cortisol suppression on inter-leukin-6 and white blood cell response to surgery. Acta Anaesth Scand 1997; 41:304–308.
15. Chwals WJ, Bistrian BR. Role of exogenous growth hormone and insulin-like growth fac-tor 1 in malnutrition and acute metabolic stress: a hypothesis. Crit Care Med 1991; 19:1317–1322.
16. Ross RJM, Miell JP, Buchanan CR. Avoiding autocannibalism. Br Med J 1991; 303:1147–1148.
17. Takala J, Ruokonen E, Webster NR, et al. Increased mortality associated with growth hormone treatment in critically ill adults. N Engl J Med 1999; 341:785–792.
18. Ljungqvist O, Nygren J, Thorell A. Insulin resistance and elective surgery. Surgery 2000; 128:757–760.
19. Strommer L, Wickbom M, Wang F, et al. Early impairment of insulin secretion in rats after surgical trauma. Eur J Endocrinol 2002; 147:825–833.
20. Van den Berghe G, Wouters P, Weekers F, et al. Intensive insulin therapy in critically ill patients. N Engl J Med 2001; 19:1359–1367.
21. Byrne CR, Carlson GL. Can posttraumatic insulin resistance be attenuated by prior glu-cose loading? Nutrition 2001; 17:332–336.
22. Thorell A, Nygren J, Ljungqvist O. Insulin resistance: a marker of surgical stress. Curr Opin Nutr Metab Care 1999; 2:69–78.
23. Ljungqvist O, Thorell A, Dutniak M, et al. Glucose infusion instead of perioperative fast-ing reduces postoperative insulin resistance. J Am Coll Surg 1994; 178:329–333.
24. Singer M, De Santis V, Viale D, et al. Multiorgan failure is an adaptive, endocrine-mediated, metabolic response to overwhelming systemic inflammation. Lancet 2004; 364:545–548.
25. Woolf PD, Hamill RW, McDonald JV, et al. Transient hypogonadotrophic hypogonad-ism caused by critical illness. J Clin Endocrinol Metab 1985; 60:444–450.
26. Wang C, Chan V, Yeung RT. Effects of surgical stress on pituitary testicular function. Clin Endocrinol 1978; 9:255–266.
27. Sheeran P, Hall GM. Cytokines in anaesthesia. Br J Anaesth 1997; 78:201–219.
28. Cruickshank AM, Fraser WD, Burns HJG, et al. Response of serum interleukin-6 in patients undergoing elective surgery of varying severity. Clin Sci 1990; 79:161–165.
29. Moore CM, Desborough JP, Powell H, et al. The effects of extradural anaesthesia on the interleukin-6 and acute phase response to surgery. Br J Anaesth 1994; 72:272–279.
30. Joris J, Cigarini I, Legrand M, et al. Metabolic and respiratory changes after cholecystect-omy performed via laparotomy or laparoscopy. Br J Anaesth 1992; 69:341–345.
31. Baumann H, Gauldie J. The acute phase response. Immunol Today 1994; 15:74–79.
32. Steel DM, Whitehead AS. The major acute phase reactants: C-reactive protein, serum amyloid P component and serum amyloid A protein. Immunol Today 1994; 15:81–88.
33. Barker JP, Vafidis GC, Robinson PN, et al. Plasma catecholamine response to cataract surgery: a comparison between general and local anaesthesia. Anaesthesia 1991; 46: 642–645.
34. Bessey PQ, Walters JM, Bier DM, et al. Combined hormonal infusion stimulates the metabolic response to injury. Ann Surg 1984; 200:264–281.
35. Mossad SB, Serkey JM, Longworth DL, et al. Coagulase-negative staphylococcal sternal wound infections after open-heart operations. Ann Thorac Surg 1997; 63:395–401.
36. The Veterans Affairs Total Parenteral Nutrition Cooperative Study Group. Perioperative total parenteral nutrition in surgical patients. N Engl J Med 1991; 325:525–532.
37. Saunders C, Nishikawa R, Wolfe B. Surgical nutrition: a review. J R Coll Surg Edinb 1993; 38:195–204.

38. Kennedy BC, Hall GM. Metabolic support of critically ill patients: parenteral nutrition to immunonutrition. Br J Anaesth 2000; 85:185–188.

39. Kehlet H. The surgical stress response: should it be prevented? Can J Surg 1991; 34: 565–567.

40. Fragen RJ, Shanks CA, Molteni A, et al. Effects of etomidate on hormonal responses to surgical stress. Anesthesiology 1984; 61:652–656.

41. Holloway CD, Kenyon CJ, Dowie LJ, et al. Effect of the benzodiazepines diazepam, des-N-methyldiazepam and midazolam on corticosteroid biosynthesis in bovine adreno-cortical cells in vitro; location of site of action. J Steroid Biochem 1989; 33:219–225.

42. Crozier TA, Beck D, Schlaeger M, et al. Endocrinological changes following etomidate or methohexital for minor surgery. Anesthesiology 1987; 66:628–635.

43. Desborough JP, Hall GM, Hart GR, et al. Midazolam modifies pancreatic and anterior pituitary hormone secretion during upper abdominal surgery. Br J Anaesth 1991; 67: 390–396.

44. Lacoumenta S, Paterson JL, Burrin J, et al. Effects of two differing halothane concentrations on the metabolic and endocrine responses to surgery. Br J Anaesth 1986; 58: 844–850.

45. McDonald RK, Evans FT, Weise VK, et al. Effects of morphine and nalorphine on plasma hydrocortisone levels in man. J Pharmacol Exp Ther 1959; 125:241–252.

46. George JM, Reier CE, Lanese RR, et al. Morphine anaesthesia blocks cortisol and growth hormone response to stress in humans. J Clin Endocrinol Metab 1974; 38: 736–741.

47. Hall GM, Young C, Holdcroft A, et al. Substrate mobilisation during surgery: a comparison between halothane and fentanyl anaesthesia. Anaesthesia 1978; 33:924–930.

48. Klingstedt C, Giesecke K, Hamberger B, et al. High and low dose fentanyl anaesthesia, circulatory and plasma catecholamine responses during cholecystectomy. Br J Anaesth 1987; 59:184–188.

49. Engquist A, Brandt MR, Fernandes A, et al. The blocking effect of epidural analgesia on the adrenocortical and hyperglycaemic responses to surgery. Acta Anaesth Scand 1977; 21:330–335.

50. Bromage PR, Shibata HR, Willoughby HW. Influence of prolonged epidural blockade on blood sugar and cortisol responses to operations on the upper part of the abdomen and thorax. Surg Gynecol Obstet 1971; 132:1051–1056.

51. Rigg JRA. Does regional blockade improve outcome after surgery? Anaesth Int Care 1991; 19:404–411.

52. Liu S, Carpenter RL, Neal JM. Epidural anaesthesia and analgesia: their role in post-operative outcome. Anesthesiology 1995; 82:1474–1506.

53. Rodgers A, Walker S, Schug S, et al. Reduction of postoperative mortality and morbidity with epidural and spinal anaesthesia: results from overview of randomised trials. Br Med J 2000; 321:1493–1497.

54. Park WY, Thompson JS, Lee KK. Effect of epidural anesthesia and analgesia on peri-operative outcome: a randomized, controlled veterans affairs cooperative study. Ann Surg 2001; 234:560–571.

55. Rigg JRA, Jamrozik K, Myles PS, et al. Epidural anaesthesia and analgesia and outcome of major surgery: a randomised trial. Lancet 2002; 359:1276–1282.

56. Peyton PJ, Myles PS, Silbert BS, et al. Perioperative epidural analgesia and outcome after major abdominal surgery in high-risk patients. Anesth Analg 2003; 96:548–554.

57. Fotiadis RJ, Badvie S, Weston MD, et al. Epidural analgesia in gastrointestinal surgery. Br J Surg 2004; 91:828–841.

58. Kehlet H, Wilmore DW. Mutimodal strategies to improve surgical outcome. Am J Surg 2002; 183:630–641.

59. Holte K, Kehlet H. Epidural anaesthesia and analgesia-effects on surgical stress responses and implications for postoperative nutrition. Clin Nutr 2002; 21:199–206.

60. Kehlet H, Dahl JB. Anaesthesia, surgery and challenges in postoperative recovery. Lancet 2003; 362:1921–1928.
61. Kehlet H. Surgical stress response: does endoscopic surgery confer an advantage? World J Surg 1999; 23:801–807.
62. McMahon AJ, Fischbacher CM, Frame SH, et al. Impact of laparoscopic cholecystectomy: a population-based study. Lancet 2000; 356:1632–1637.
63. Brix-Christensen V, Tonnesen E, Sorensen IJ, et al. Effects of anaesthesia based on high versus low doses of opioids on the cytokine and acute-phase protein responses in patients undergoing cardiac surgery. Acta Anaesth Scand 1998; 42:63–70.
64. Schneemilch CE, Schilling T. Effects of general anaesthesia on inflammation. Best Pract Res Clin Anaesth 2004; 18:493–507.
65. Schulze S, Sommer P, Biggler D. Effect of combined prednisolone, epidural analgesia and indomethacin on the systemic response after colonic surgery. Arch Surg 1992; 127:325–331.
66. Buunen M, Gholghesaei M, Veldkamp R, et al. Stress response to laparoscopic surgery. Surg Endosc 2004; 18:1022–1028.
67. Marano R, Margutti F, Catalanao GF, et al. Stress responses to endoscopic surgery. Curr Opin Obstet Gynaec 2000; 12:303–307.
68. Weiss EG, Wexner SD. Laparoscopic port site recurrences in oncological cancer—a review. Ann Acad Med Singapore 1996; 25:694–698.
69. Leung KL, Kwok SPY, Lam SCW, et al. Laparoscopic resection of rectosigmoid carcinoma: prospective randomised trial. Lancet 2004; 363:1187–1192.
70. Lacy AM, Garcia-Valdecassas JC, Delgado S, et al. Laparoscopic-assisted colectomy versus open colectomy for treatment of non-metastatic colon cancer: a randomised trial. Lancet 2002; 359:2224–2229.
71. Chambrier C, Chassard D, Bienvenu J, et al. Cytokine and hormonal changes after cholecystectomy. Effect of ibuprofen pre-treatment. Ann Surg 1996; 224:178–182.
72. Topol EJ, Falk GW. A coxib a day won't keep the doctor away. Lancet 2004; 364:639–640.

5

Measurement and Prediction
of Surgical Outcomes

Graham P. Copeland
North Cheshire Hospitals, National Health Service Trust, Warrington, Cheshire, U.K.

INTRODUCTION

Clinicians have probably struggled with the capricious nature of predicting surgical outcome for hundreds of years. If one wanders off the beaten track to the basement of the Louvre in Paris, one will come across a black diorite plinth inscribed with hieroglyphics from the time of King Hammurabi of Babylon (Fig. 1). As early as 1750 B.C., he issued edicts aimed at practicing clinicians, the best known of which is:

> If a surgeon operates on a free man and the man dies or goes blind then the surgeon should have his hand cut off.
> If a surgeon operates on a slave and the slave dies then it is the responsibility of the surgeon to replace the slave.

It would appear at first sight that little has changed over the intervening 4000 years, but the introduction of general and regional anesthesia has introduced other clinicians to the "surgeon's risk." In the present litigious climate, there is no doubt that the surgeon and the anesthetist are equally responsible for delivering the best possible operative and perioperative care for patients. Good clinicians were aware of this long before lawyers and legislators came on the scene.

Clearly, a number of factors can influence the outcome of the surgical endeavor. The quality and experience of the surgeon and their anesthetist preparing the patient for surgery, and subsequent performance can have a significant effect on the outcome from surgical intervention. However, patients themselves often bring with them the major prognostic factor with regard to subsequent outcome—that of their physiological fitness. This may be reflected in their chronic disease status or the acute physiological disturbance caused by their acute illness. Finally, the procedure itself will have a major effect on surgical outcome.

All these variables are amenable to change. We can expand our clinical knowledge to encompass new procedures. We can contract our practice to those areas in which we can excel. We may be able to improve a patient's chronic disease status or devise new methods of anesthesia to minimize risk in particular patients, or we may be able to amend a patient's acute physiological disturbance. We can even alter the

45

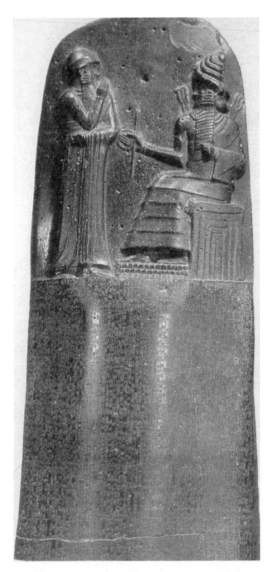

Figure 1 Black diorite stone depicting King Hammurabi of Babylon receiving his laws from the Sun-god. Inscribed in about 1750 B.C., the stone was found in Susa and now stands in the Louvre, Paris.

magnitude of our surgical intervention to a certain degree. It was with these thoughts in mind, rather than fear of lawyers and legislators, that clinicians were led to look at methods for measuring and predicting the outcome from surgical intervention.

TECHNIQUES FOR ASSESSING OUTCOME

Most experienced surgeons and anesthetists are able, accepting wide confidence limits, to guess the probable mortality outcome from a particular intervention. However, interestingly the ability to predict morbidity often deteriorates with the seniority of the clinician (Tables 1 and 2). To avoid these inaccuracies and to prevent

Table 1 Variation in Predictive Ability of Various Grades of Staff

Patient risk mortality (%)	10	30	70
First-year trainee (%)	9 (5–15)	28 (22–36)	65 (55–80)
Fifth-year trainee (%)	10 (5–15)	25 (20–35)	70 (60–80)
Consultant (%)	10 (5–15)	35 (25–40)	70 (60–80)

Note: Study based on three standardized patient histories with defined predicted outcomes of 10%, 30%, and 70% with regard to mortality using the POSSUM system. Fifty clinicians in each category were requested to assess the likely outcome as a percentage for each of the three patient histories. The median value and ranges are shown.

observer bias, many groups have designed and validated methods of assessment that use methodologies ranging from simple observational techniques up to more complex, mathematical scoring systems to predict surgical outcome. Some predictive models merely produce an assessment of high or low risk with various graduations between, whereas others produce a numerical prediction of mortality.

The most widely known and utilized method of identifying the risk of adverse outcome by apportioning a high or low risk is the ASA system (ASA scores 1 to 5, 1 normal and 5 expected post-operative death) (1). This is a quick and easy system to apply and can be readily communicated and understood by other clinicians and even nonclinicians. However, there can be problems in its application, particularly with ASA 2, where a systemic disease, even if very mild (e.g., rheumatoid arthritis only affecting one joint), can adversely affect the prediction; and in ASA 5, where the assessor almost self-selects the outcome. The system is, however, applicable over a wide range of surgical procedures, has been widely accepted in anesthetic circles, and provides an invaluable starting block for outcome prediction. Other similar systems (2–4) apportioning risk but without a numerical outcome prediction are applicable in certain settings, e.g., Shoemaker criteria (5). Other systems have been described, which deal specifically with particular types of complication (6).

Although such techniques have their value, particularly in inter-clinician communication and when dealing with large datasets, they are of little use when assessing an individual surgeon or an anesthetist practice. They are also of little benefit when auditing individual patient outcome. In this regard, more refined estimates of outcome prediction are needed. In critical care circles, the APACHE system, first designed in the 1980s (7) and then refined over the next 20 years, is probably the most widely known and utilized scoring system. Initially designed for the intensive care (ITU) setting, it has been applied to an increasing spectrum of non-ITU general surgical scenarios but with variable success (8–10). The technique requires observation over a 24-hour period, and the worst variables are applied to a mathematical formula

Table 2 Variation in Predictive Ability of Various Grades of Staff

Patient risk morbidity (%)	10	30	70
First-year trainee (%)	8 (5–20)	25 (20–40)	75 (50–80)
Fifth-year trainee (%)	9 (5–15)	28 (22–40)	70 (60–80)
Consultant (%)	5 (2–12)	20 (10–35)	50 (40–70)

Note: Study based on three standardized patient histories with defined predicted outcomes of 10%, 30%, and 70% with regard to morbidity using the POSSUM system. Fifty clinicians in each category were requested to assess the likely outcome as a percentage for each of the three patient histories. The median value and ranges are shown.

that has extensive correction weightings for individual disease conditions. In comparison with those methods discussed previously, it produces an individual numerical patient prediction for mortality; but, clearly, more variables are necessary, and the mathematics can be complex, usually requiring significant hardware and software support. These factors have limited its application in general surgery and in particular gastrointestinal surgery, where successful surgical intervention can have a major and immediate effect on physiological status (11).

In an attempt to overcome some of these difficulties, during the late 1980s general surgeons began to develop a methodology that would produce an individual patient prediction of both mortality and morbidity that utilized data that were regularly collected and easy to obtain. This led to the development of the POSSUM system (Fig. 2) (Table 3) (12), first published in 1991, which has now become one of the best known and widely applied methods for surgical audit. It has been validated in a wide range of surgical specialities, including vascular surgery (13,14), colorectal surgery (15,16), thoracic surgery (17), and general surgery (12,18–20). An orthopaedic POSSUM has been recently described and validated, in which the general equations are still utilized, but there are minor modifications to the operative severity score assessment (21). A modification of the POSSUM system has been devised, which is of particular use in individual patient prediction. The Portsmouth POSSUM (P-POSSUM) (22) system has proved to be particularly popular in vascular surgery (23–25). The same variables are assessed, but a linear rather than logistic

PHYSIOLOGICAL

SCORE	1	2	4	8
Age	<60	61 - 70	>71	
Cardiac signs		On Cardiac drugs or steroid	Oedema Warfarin	JVP
CXR	Normal		Border Cardio	Cardio megaly
Resp. signs		SOB Exertion	SOB stairs	SOB rest
CXR	Normal	Mild COAD	Mod COAD	Any other change
SYSTOLIC BP	110 - 130	131 - 170 / 100 - 109	>171 / 90 - 99	<89
Pulse	50 - 80	81 - 100 / 40 - 49	101 - 120	>121 / <39
Coma Score	15	12 - 14	9 - 11	<8
Urea	<7.5	7.6 - 10	10.1 - 15	>15.1
Na	>136	131 - 135	126 - 130	<125
K	3.5 - 5	3.2 - 3.4 / 5.1 - 5.3	2.9 - 3.1 / 5.4 - 5.9	<2.8 / >6
Hb	13 - 16	11.5 - 12.9 / 16.1 - 17	10 - 11.4 / 17.1 - 18	<9.9 / >18.1
WCC	4 - 10	10.1 - 20 / 3.1 - 3.9	>20.1 / <3	
ECG	Normal		AF (60 - 90)	Any other change

SURGICAL POSSUM

OPERATIVE SEVERITY

SCORE	1	2	4	8
Op	Minor	Inter	Major	Major +
No. of ops	1		2	>2
Blood loss	<100	101 - 500	501 - 999	>1000
Perin soiling	No	Serous blood (<250)	Local pus	Any other
Malignant	No	1o	Node mets	Distant mets
Time of op	Elec.		Emerg. resus	Emerg. no resus

Inter - Chole; TURP; Appendix
Major - Resection; Chole & duct; Amputation; Fem-pop
Major + APR; Pancreas; Liver; oesophagus; Aorta

Patient name:
Unit number:
DOB:
Consultant:
Operating surgeon: _____
Anaesthetist: _____
Operation date: _____
Date admitted: _____
Date discharged: _____

COMPLICATIONS

Haemorrhage
☐ Wound Deep
Infection
☐ Chest ☐ Septicaemia
☐ Wound ☐ PUO
☐ UTI ☐ Wound
☐ Deep ☐ dehiscence
Anastomotic leak
☐ Minor ☐ Major
Thrombosis
☐ DVT ☐ CVA
☐ PE ☐ MI
☐ Renal failure
☐ Resp. failure
☐ Cardiac failure
☐ Hypotension
☐ Any other

☐ DEATH
☐ NO COMPLICATIONS

Surgical Group (please tick)
☐ V = Vascular
☐ G = Gastrointestinal
☐ H = Hepatobiliary
☐ B = Breast / Endocine
☐ U = Urology
☐ M = Miscellaneous

Cl.Aud/Quality/surgical/RHxls/Mac3/July04

Figure 2 POSSUM Score Sheet. *Abbreviations*: CXR, chest X-ray; BP, blood pressure; Hb, hemoglobin; WCC, white cell count; ECG, electrocardiogram; PUO, unknown pyrexia; UTI, urinary infection; DVT, deep venous thrombosis; CVA, cerebrovascular accident; PE, pulmonary emboius; MI, myocardial infarction; JVP, raised jugulo-venous pressure; SOB, short of breath; COAD, chronic obstructive airways disease; NA, sodium; K, potassium.

Table 3 Operative Severity Score, Examples of Operative Magnitude

Operative classes
Minor
  Hernia
  Varicose veins
  Breast lumps
  Simple lumps
    Epididymal cysts
    Hydrocele
    Circumcision
Investigations: endoscopy (sigmoidoscopy, gastroscopy, cystoscopy)
Intermediate
  Cholecystectomy
  Transurethral resection of tumor
  Transurethral resection of prostate
  Prostatectomy
  Appendectomy
  Mastectomy
  Thyroidectomy
Major
  Cholecystectomy—exploration of common bile duct
  Colectomy
    Rt Hemicolectomy
    Lt Hemicolectomy
    Anterior resection
  Gastrectomy
  Bowel resection
  Any laparotomy
  Amputation
  Vascular: femoro-popliteal bypass
Major+
  Aortic aneurysm
  Aorto-bifem graft
  APR resection
  Esophago-gastrectomy
  Pancreatectomy
  Hepatectomy

model (Table 4) is used, making it an easier mathematical model to use and to self-design applicable software.

More recently, further refinements of the original POSSUM system have been described specifically for colorectal and oesophageal surgeons. Tekkis et al. have described both CR-POSSUM (Table 5), for colorectal surgeons, (26) and O-POSSUM (Table 6), for esophagogastric surgeons (27). These have the advantage of reducing the variables required for prediction and improving the accuracy for these particular fields

Table 4 POSSUM Equations for the Prediction of Adverse Outcomes (POSSUM and P-POSSUM Systems)

POSSUM mortality equation	Logit $R = \ln[R/(1 - R)] = -7.04 + (0.13 \times$ physiological score) $+$ $(0.16 \times$ operative severity score)
POSSUM morbidity equation	Logit $R = \ln[R/(1 - R)] = -5.91 + (0.16 \times$ physiological score) $+$ $(0.19 \times$ operative severity score)
P-POSSUM mortality equation	Logit $R = \ln[R/(1 - R)] = -9.065 + (0.16 \times$ physiological score) $+$ $(0.155 \times$ operative severity score)

Table 5 Colorectal POSSUM Scoring System

	Score				
	1	2	3	4	8
Physiological score					
Age	<60		61–70	71–80	>81
Cardiac failure	None or mild	Moderate	Severe		
Systolic blood pressure	100–170	>170 or 90–99	<90		
Pulse	40–100	101–120	>120 or <40		
Urea	<10	10.1–15.0	>15.1		
Hemoglobin	13–16	10–12.9 or 16.1–18	<10 or >18.1		
Operative severity score					
Operative severity	Minor		Intermediate	Major	Major complex
Peritoneal soiling	None or minor serous	Local pus	Free pus or feces		
Operative urgency	Elective		Urgent		Emergency
Cancer staging	None or Dukes A–B	Dukes C	Dukes D		
Colorectal POSSUM					

Note: The variables utilized follow the original POSSUM definitions.
Abbreviations: Dukes staging: A & B, confined to bowel wall; C, nodal spread; D, distant spread.
Source: From Ref. 26.

Table 6 The O-POSSUM Scoring System

Variable	Coefficient β
Age	0.055
POSSUM physiological score (Table 3)	0.080
POSSUM staging (x_1)	
No malignancy	0
Primary only	0.168
Nodal disease	0.365
Metastatic disease	1.042
Urgency of surgery (x_2)	
Elective	0
Emergency	0.678
Type of surgery (x_3)	
Esophagectomy	0
Total gastrectomy	0.283
Partial gastrectomy	−0.767
Palliative gastrojejunostomy	−0.366

Note: The coefficients β are inserted in the equation as indicated below. Logit $R = \ln[R/(1 - R)] = -7.566 + 0.055\,(\text{age in years}) + 0.080\,(\text{POSSUM physiological score}) + \text{POSSUM staging}\,(x_1) + \text{urgency of surgery}\,(x_2) + \text{type of surgery}\,(x_3)$.
Source: From Ref. 27.

of surgery. O-POSSUM is, however, somewhat complex and requires knowledge of individual variable coefficients similar to the APACHE systems. As yet, they have not been validated in other units, but the original estimation dataset was obtained from many differing sites across the United Kingdom. Because the variables and weightings are similar to the original POSSUM scoring system, it is likely that their accuracy will be confirmed by other observers. However, all these adaptations, unlike the original POSSUM system, have, as yet, no morbidity predictive model Cross speciality comparison is, of course, not possible.

USING PREDICTIVE MODELS OF SURGICAL OUTCOME

If one has the ability to assess and predict individual patient outcomes, how can this information be utilized?

The easiest and most widely utilized technique is as an audit aid when discussing adverse events. However, it soon became apparent that techniques of this sort could be used to assess individual surgeon/anesthetist and unit performance. The effects of extrinsic factors on surgical performance over time could then be assessed, and the effects of structure change and service provision on outcome could be estimated for the first time. Perhaps, the most uncomfortable of all these techniques could be applied as a "cost containment and quality assurance" issue—the so called "futility index." From a personal surgical perspective, their use as a guide to resuscitative measures would sit more comfortably with the Hippocratic Oath.

Finally, techniques of outcome prediction are a useful research tool when examining new methods of surgical and perioperative care, which involve a diverse mix of patients. The usual, double-blind controlled clinical trial methods are difficult to apply to these areas. The following section explores each of these techniques in more detail.

As an Audit Tool

Most clinical teams hold some form of mortality/morbidity meeting or review of critical evidence. It is an advantage when discussing an individual patient death or adverse event to have a numerical prediction for mortality to guide this review process. Systems such as POSSUM and APACHE, which produce such a prediction, have obvious advantages in this regard. Some authors have suggested that the p-POSSUM mathematical model has advantages in an individual case review, and this may well be the case in low-risk cases because both the POSSUM and APACHE models are logistic equations based on populations of patients rather than individuals. Certainly the P-POSSUM and POSSUM systems are the ones recommended by the Royal College of Surgeons of both England and Edinburgh and by National Confidential Enquiry into Peri-operative Deaths (NCEPOD), and are probably the methods of choice. The POSSUM system is the only system that produces a numerical prediction of morbidity across the surgical spectrum.

Clinical audit of adverse outcomes can be a particularly depressing affair. While it can be of great value to discuss cases where death occurs and predictive models indicate a risk of death of less than 20%, the opposite end of the spectrum (risk >80%) often yields little audit gain except to discuss whether the operation was indeed indicated. Predictive models of these types can produce a new audit spectrum, those patients whose risk exceeds a certain level (e.g., >50%) but who survive. Often, audit of these cases can identify best practice and produces changes in resuscitative protocols, which produce a sustained quality improvement. Such an approach has the added value of making clinical audit an uplifting rather than depressing experience.

Assessing Performance

Over the past 15 years, there has been increasing interest in the outcomes from an individual unit as well as an individual surgeon and anesthetist endeavor. Until recently, this was often based on anecdote rather than "hard" data. In the United States and the United Kingdom, some specialities (28–31) (in particular, cardiothoracic surgical units) have published their aggregated mortality rates for individual procedures as well as some forms of risk adjustment. Other European countries have followed suit, and most recently in England and Wales the Department of Health and later the Healthcare Commission have published 30-day mortality rates for emergency and elective general surgery as well as fractured neck of femur. As with all such rates, there must always be "winners" and "losers," and someone, by definition, must always lie outside the 95% confidence limits.

As any mathematician will point out, if you choose to take a radical stance and close the worst performing 5%, after ten years you will have closed 40% of units and probably still not improved overall care. Fortunately no country has chosen, to date, to take such a radical decision.

Mortality rates in isolation would appear to have little to recommend them and may indeed be hazardous. In the United States, where mortality rates are published, patient flows have been affected by patients traveling to the units with the lowest mortality rate who then choose the lowest-risk cases, returning the high-risk cases to other centers. This could become a self-fulfilling prophesy with the "best" units improving still further and the "worst" apparently deteriorating. Clearly, case mix and the range of procedures offered can have a radical effect on mortality rates.

A number of private companies in the United Kingdom (CHKS and Dr. Foster being the best known) now offer a range of methodologies for case mix adjustment that use Hospital Episode Statistic–based data. The case mix adjustment is usually based on age, mode of admission, speciality mix of the unit, and some comorbidity factors. However, none is free from bias, and all fail to address the fact that minor variations in the volume of high-risk cases (patients whose risk of death exceeds 20%) can have a radical effect on overall performance.

Methods that assess individual patient variables would appear to offer the best methodology for assessing surgeon and anesthetist performance. Table 7 illustrates the marked differences in outcome of surgeons with varying case mix. However, with the application of the POSSUM system, it is possible to predict the expected number of deaths; comparing this with the actual number yields a ratio (the observed to expected ratio, O/E ratio), which potentially produces a true quality measure (Tables 7 and 8) (32).

These techniques have now been widely validated, and, from personnel observations, it would appear that when performance deteriorates, it is in the management of patients whose risk lies between 10% and 80% that major differences in unit performance have been identified. Where O/E ratios are persistently above 1.00, examination of individual patient deaths and of the morbidity spectrum, when compared to similar clinician or unit spectra, can often identify the cause of poor performance. Local complications and wound-related problems are often surgeon related. Respiratory and cardiac problems are often anesthetist related. Renal and, to a lesser extent respiratory problems are often related to the availability of appropriate,

Table 7 Raw and Risk-Adjusted Outcome Measures for a 12-Month Period in One Unit

Surgeon and speciality	Mortality (%)	Morbidity (%)	O/E mortality	O/E morbidity
Vascular (Surgeon 1)	4.8	13.0	1.02	1.03
Hepatobiliary	2.6	10.0	0.96	0.96
Colorectal	2.9	15.1	1.00	0.99
Vascular (2)	3.5	13.6	0.98	0.98
Gastrointestinal	3.1	11.7	1.04	1.03
Urology (Surgeon 1)	0.3	2.1	0.5	0.75
Urology (2)	1.0	4.9	1.00	1.02

Note: Results apply to all nonday case surgery in seven individual surgical teams within one hospital. The O/E ratio indicates the observed number of adverse outcomes (O)/the predicted number of adverse outcomes (E).
Abbreviation: O/E, observed to expected ratio.

high-dependency facilities and to the overall quality of nursing services. While these may be oversimplifications, from a personal perspective, I have found them to be useful tools over the past 10 years when assessing both my own and other units (33).

Comparative data using the CR-POSSUM and O-POSSUM systems are at present awaited, but because the original derivation datasets were from multiple units there is little doubt that these methodologies will be applied to comparative audit.

To Assess the Effect of Extrinsic Factors and Service Provision and to Examine Changes Over Time

Anesthesia and surgery never stand still. New techniques continue to be introduced at an ever-increasing rate in an attempt to improve both overall outcomes and the range of patients offered surgery. Many patients once considered a poor operative risk are now offered surgical intervention. Mathematical modelling allows these factors to be assessed. As can be seen in Table 9, the volume of high-risk cases as assessed by the POSSUM system has steadily increased over the past 10 years. This has, however, been accompanied by a decrease in the number of patients whose risk of death following surgery exceeds 80%. This reduction does appear to coincide with the reports published by the NCEPOD and almost certainly represents a more rational and considered approach to patients in whom death will inevitably follow surgery (ASA4–5). While many clinicians may be uncomfortable with such an approach (section "As a Futility Index"), avoiding needless surgery in patients

Table 8 Use of the POSSUM System to Assess Hospital Performance Over Time

Year	Mortality (%)	Morbidity (%)	O/E ratio mortality	O/E ratio morbidity
1994	3.8	16.7	0.99	0.97
1995	3.7	15.5	1.01	1.00
1996	3.2	13.9	0.97	0.98
1997	3.8	13.9	0.97	0.98
1998	3.1	12.9	1.02	1.01
1999	3.4	14.2	0.98	0.95

Note: The hospital shown is a U.K. district general hospital providing emergency general surgery, noncardiac vascular surgery, and cancer surgery. All patients scored represent those undergoing nonday case surgery.
Abbreviation: O/E, observed to expected ratio.

Table 9 Variation in the Volume of High-Risk Patients Undergoing Surgery Over the Last 10 Years

	>20%	>40%	>80%
Change in volume during the period (1994–1999)	+16%	+5%	−5%
Change in volume during the period (1999–2004)	+31%	+11%	−35%

Note: Based on comparisons with the volume in the period 1989–1994. The hospital shown is a U.K. district general hospital providing emergency general surgery, noncardiac vascular surgery, and cancer surgery.

in extremis and in those with advanced terminal malignancy must surely be the correct clinical approach.

Despite these changes in case mix as well as surgical and anesthetic complexity, the overall outcomes from surgical intervention have appeared to have changed little over time. Recently, a number of papers have appeared in the literature, suggesting that outcomes do indeed appear to be improving. Boyd et al. (34) and Wilson et al. (35) have demonstrated that preoperative optimization can have a radical effect on overall survival. While there has been debate as to whether these improvements in predicted mortality are related to drug usage (e.g., dopexamine) or merely a reflection of fluid loading, there can be little doubt that optimization is to be encouraged (36,37). Many authors in the past, applying the APACHE and POSSUM systems, had demonstrated the beneficial effects of preoperative optimization, but it is only in recent years that this effect has been quantified (11). Wilson et al. demonstrated that mortality rates could be spectacularly improved as a result of dopexamine-assisted optimization. Such an approach does require, at the very least, high-dependency facilities with the appropriate intensive care nursing and medical support. Jones and de Cossart (8) and other authors (38) have demonstrated the effect of the lack of such facilities on outcomes (Table 10). Indeed a lack of available facilities in the United Kingdom with the attendant need to transfer acutely ill surgical patients may have a significant impact on outcome (Table 11). These factors may explain the apparent differences in outcome between British and American centers with similar case mix (39).

If we imagine a scenario in which major improvements in clinical management become widespread, the current models would become defunct. The advantage of outcome scoring systems with fixed variables is that improvements in care can be adapted into a new equation, allowing direct comparison over time (previous care using the old

Table 10 The Effect of Intensive Care Bed Availability on Risk-Adjusted Outcome from Operative Intervention in One Unit

Availability of intensive care beds (%)	Mortality O/E ratio	Morbidity O/E ratio
100	0.97	0.98
90	0.99	0.99
70	1.08	1.06
50	1.2	1.08

Note: The bed availability is expressed as a percentage of the total beds that should have been available at any one time. On occasions when beds were not available patients were transferred to neighboring units. In transferred patients the observed to expected ratios fell from 0.98 in resident patients to between 1.18 and 1.6 in transferred patients.
Abbreviation: O/E, observed to expected ratio.

Table 11 The Effect on Outcome of Transferring Patients Immediately Following Surgery to an Outside Intensive Care Unit

	Number	Resident following surgery	Transferred following surgery	O/E ratio resident	O/E ratio transferred
Study period (1999–2001)	163	148	15	0.97	1.6
Study period (2001–2003)	149	137	12	0.97	1.18

Note: The hospital shown is a United Kingdom district general hospital providing emergency general surgery, noncardiac vascular surgery, and cancer surgery.
Abbreviation: O/E, observed to expected ratio.

equation and future care using the new equation). Changing the goalposts and having them changed by others has always been part of a good clinician's remit.

It is not surprising that as methods for outcome prediction become more refined, they will be utilized to examine the impact of service provision. In this regard, examining the spectrum of patient risk in a clinical department can indicate the volume of high-dependency facilities required. As a rule, patients in whom the predicted risk exceeds 20% should be managed on an intensive care facility, and patients whose risk exceeds 10% a high-dependency or close-monitoring facility. In some countries the drop down from high dependency to general ward can be extreme, and some form of surgical, close-monitoring unit, which is ward-based, may be a useful adjunct, since it has the advantage of reduced costs over a high-dependency or intensive care unit.

As a Futility Index

In the past, surgeons and anesthetists have often approached outcome predictions from differing aspects. Let us examine the patient whose predictive model yields a mortality risk of 0.9. Anesthetists and intensivists might argue that this represented a 90% chance of fatality, whereas surgeons may only see a 10% survival. This differing philosophical approach resulted in many patients undergoing unnecessary surgery and was one of the initial observations made in the first NCEPOD reports. While this trend is decreasing it still remains a feature of later reports (40).

Using models as a futility index may sit uncomfortably with some clinicians, but they have been used in this way. APACHE has been used as a cost containment and quality assurance tool to identify who should and who should not be eligible for intensive care (41). Indeed, there is good evidence that cost containment has a major influence on the provision of surgical intensive care in Europe and the United Kingdom in particular (42,43), although this has only recently been examined using methods of risk adjustment (41).

Submitting an ASA 5 patient to surgery would seem at first glance pointless, but the interpretation as to whether the patient really is ASA 5 is often influenced by the clinician's skill, experience, and availability of backup facilities. APACHE and similar systems that have fixed variables and mathematical models allowing a numerical prediction avoid the problems with clinician insight and bias. Systems such as APACHE which allow a preoperative assessment are however open to potential abuse, and indeed some authors have questioned the application of APACHE to the general surgical patient since successful surgery can have a radical effect on patient physiology and thus outcome. In some ways POSSUM avoids this potential use since the total score variable is only available when the surgery has been completed. This anti-abuse facility does have some limitations since most experienced clinicians will be able to "fore guess" the operative findings in the majority of cases.

Rather than have a fixed approach to a futility index based on a single mortality prediction, a more holistic and multidisciplinary approach is to be preferred. Some units using the POSSUM system have applied criteria for referral for a more senior review. Some have adopted the three 8s rule (referral if three or more physiological variables score 8) and others a score cutoff of 33. Both methods achieve the same result by identifying the high-risk patient and allow a multidisciplinary discussion at high level as to the applicability of surgery and skill mix necessary to achieve a successful outcome. Clearly avoiding needless surgery in the moribund patient where surgery is unlikely to improve the patient's status, the patient with advanced untreatable malignancy, the patient with advanced irretrievable vascular disease, and the patient with advanced dementia are to be encouraged. Outcome predictive models can help in these cases but should form only part of the clinical discussion.

Predictive Models as a Research Tool

Finally, predictive outcome models could have a role, as yet unfulfilled, in research. One of the major problems with clinical trials, in particular, drug and treatment trials, has been the exclusion of patients who do not fit the norm. Most trials exclude patients with abnormal biochemical measurements and those with marked physiological disturbance. This often results in the selection of low-risk cases, which requires large patient numbers to achieve significance levels. Not only is this costly, both in time and monetary terms, to the pharmaceutical industry, it also could have theoretical clinical disadvantage of not identifying a useful treatment or intervention to the groups most in need. For example, if the administration of a drug to improve survival was only apparent in the patients at greatest risk (i.e., exceeding 20%), the inclusion of lower-risk patients may mask its effect. As the high-risk cases are nearly all emergency cases, these are the patients most often excluded from clinical trials.

Predictive models allowing a numerical prediction of outcome for individual patients with the ability to produce qualitative outcome measures could, in theory, be applied to clinical trials without the need for major exclusion criteria. This would reduce the numbers of patients required for statistical significance, improve the speed of data acquisition, and reduce the effect of unit differences in multinational and multisite trials.

As yet, few authors have used this approach, although some intensivists have applied this technology to trials using dopexamine as a preoperative optimizing agent (35). There is little doubt that such an approach could potentially have major benefits to patient care and allow the identification of interventions to help those patients most in need.

REFERENCES

1. Owens WD, Felts JA, Spitznagel EL. ASA physical status classifications: a study of consistency of ratings. Anesthesiology 1978; 49:239–243.
2. Mullen JL, Buzby GP, Waldman TG, et al. Prediction of operative morbidity and mortality by preoperative nutritional assessment. Surg Forum 1979; 30:80–82.

3. Greenberg AG, Saik RP, Pridham D. Influence of age on mortality of colon surgery. Am J Surg 1985; 150:65–70.

4. Pillai SB, van Rij AM, Williams S, et al. Complexity and risk-adjusted model for measuring surgical outcome. Br J Surg 1999; 86:1567–1572.

5. Shoemaker WC, Appel PL, Kram HB, et al. Prospective trial of supranormal values of survivors as therapeutic goals in high-risk surgical patients. Chest 1987; 94:1176–1186.

6. Goldman L, Caldera DL, Nussbaum SB, et al. Multifactorial index of cardiac risk in non-cardiac surgical procedures. N Engl J Med 1977; 297:845–850.

7. Knaus WA, Draper EA, Wagner DP, et al. Apache II: a severity of disease classification system. Crit Care Med 1985; 13:818–829.

8. Jones HJS, de Cossart L. Risk scoring in surgical patients. Br J Surg 1999; 86:149–157.

9. Edwards AT, Ng KJ, Shandall AA, et al. Experience with the APACHE II severity of disease scoring system in predicting outcome in a surgical intensive therapy unit. J R Coll Surg Edinb 1991; 36:37–40.

10. Lazarides MK, Arvanitis DP, Drista H, et al. POSSUM and APACHE II scores do not predict the outcome of ruptured infrarenal aortic aneurysm. Ann Vasc Surg 1997; 11:155–158.

11. McIlroy B, Miller A, Copeland GP, et al. Audit of emergency preoperative resuscitation. Br J Surg 1994; 81:1492–1494.

12. Copeland GP, Jones D, Walters M. POSSUM: a scoring system for surgical audit. Br J Surg 1991; 78:355–360.

13. Copeland GP, Jones D, Wilcox A, et al. Comparative vascular audit using the POSSUM scoring system. Ann R Coll Surg Engl 1993; 75:175–177.

14. Wijesinghe LD, Mahmood T, Scott DJA, et al. Comparison of POSSUM and the Portsmouth predictor equation for predicting death following vascular surgery. Br J Surg 1998; 85:209–212.

15. Sagar PM, Hartley MN, MacFie J, et al. Comparison of individual surgeon's performance. Dis Colon Rectum 1996; 38:654–658.

16. Tekkis PP, Kocher HM, Bentley AJ, et al. Operative mortality rates among surgeons: comparison of POSSUM and p-POSSUM scoring systems in gastrointestinal surgery. Dis Colon Rectum 2000; 43:1528–1532.

17. Brunelli A, Fianchini A, Xiume F, et al. Evaluation of the POSSUM scoring system in lung surgery. Thorac Cardiovasc Surg 1998; 46:141–146.

18. Wang TK, Tu HH. Colorectal perforation with barium enema in the elderly: case analysis with the POSSUM scoring system. J Gastroenterol 1998; 33(2):201–205.

19. Cajigas JC, Escalante CF, Ingelmo A. Application of the POSSUM system in bariatric surgery. Obesity Surg 1999; 9(3):279–281.

20. Gotonda N, Iwagaki H, Itano S. Can POSSUM, a scoring system for perioperative surgical risk, predict postoperative clinical course? Acta Med Okayama 1998; 52:325–329.

21. Mohamed K, Copeland GP, Boot DA, et al. An assessment of the POSSUM scoring system in orthopaedic surgery. J Bone Joint Surg Br 2002; 84(5):735–739.

22. Prytherch D, Whiteley MS, Higgins B, et al. POSSUM and Portsmouth POSSUM for predicting mortality. Br J Surg 1998; 85:1217–1220.

23. Midwinter MJ, Tytherleigh M, Ashley S. Estimation of mortality and morbidity risk in vascular surgery using POSSUM and the Portsmouth predictor equation. Br J Surg 1999; 86:471–474.

24. Prytherch DR, Ridler BM, Beard JD, et al. A model for national audit in vascular surgery. Eur J Vasc Endovasc Surg 2001; 21:477–483.

25. Prytherch DR, Sutton GL, Boyle JR. Portsmouth POSSUM models for abdominal aortic aneurysm surgery. Br J Surg 2001; 88:958–963.

26. Tekkis PP, Prytherch DR, Kocher HM, et al. Development of a dedicated risk-adjustment scoring system for colorectal surgery (colorectal POSSUM). Br J Surg 2004; 91:1174–1182.

27. Tekkis PP, McCulloch P, Poloniecki JD, et al. Risk adjusted operative mortality in oeso-phagogastric surgery: O-POSSUM scoring system. Br J Surg 2004; 91:288–295.
28. Poloniecki J, Valencia O, Treasure T, et al. Cumulative risk adjusted mortality chart for detecting changes in death rate: observational study of heart surgery. BMJ 1998; 316:1697–1700.
29. Lovegrove J, Valencia O, Treasure T, et al. Monitoring the results of cardiac surgery by variable life-adjusted display. Lancet 1997; 350:1128–1130.
30. Khuri SF, Daley J, Henderson W, et al. Risk adjustment of the postoperative mortality rate for the comparative assessment of the quality of surgical care: results of the National Veterans Affairs Surgical Risk Study. J Am Coll Surg 1997; 185:315–327.
31. Khuri SF, Daley J, Henderson W, et al. The National Veterans Administration Surgical Risk Study: risk adjustment for the comparative assessment of the quality of surgical care. J Am Coll Surg 1995; 180:519–531.
32. Copeland GP, Sagar P, Brennan J, et al. Risk adjusted analysis of surgeon performance. Br J Surg 1995; 82:408–411.
33. Copeland GP. Assessing the surgeon: 10 years experience with the POSSUM system. J Clin Excell 2000; 2:187–190.
34. Boyd O, Grounds RM, Bennett ED. A randomised clinical trial of the effect of deliberate perioperative increase of oxygen delivery on mortality in high risk surgical patients. J Am Med Assoc 1993; 270:2699–2707.
35. Wilson J, Woods I, Fawcett J, et al. Reducing the risk of major elective surgery: randomised controlled trial of preoperative optimisation of oxygen delivery. BMJ 1999; 318:1099–1103.
36. Davies SJ, Wilson RJT. Preoperative optimization of the high risk surgical patient. Br J Anaesth 2004; 93:121–128.
37. Ward N. Nutrition support to patients undergoing gastrointestinal surgery. Nutr J 2003; 2:18.
38. Copeland GP. The POSSUM system of surgical audit. Arch Surg 2002; 137:15–19.
39. Bennett-Guerrero E, Hyam JA, Shaefi S, et al. Comparison of p-POSSUM risk adjusted mortality rates after surgery between patients in the United States of America and the United Kingdom. Br J Surg 2003; 90:1593–1598.
40. National Confidential Enquiry into Perioperative Deaths. Then and Now: The 2000 Report into the National Confidential Enquiry into Perioperative Deaths (1st April 1998 to 31st March 1999). London: NCEPOD, 2000.
41. Civetta JM, Hudson-Civetta JA, Nelson LD. Evaluation of APACHE II for cost containment and quality assurance. Ann Surg 1990; 212:266–276.
42. Bion J. Cost containment: Europe. The United Kingdom. New Horiz 1994; 2:341–344.
43. Angus DC, Sirio CA, Clermont G, et al. International comparisons of critical care outcome and resource consumption. Crit Care Clin 1997; 13:389–407.

6

Reducing Morbidity After Colorectal Surgery: Surgical Perspectives

Anil Reddy, Vikram Garoud, and Robert Wilson
Department of Surgery, The James Cook University Hospital, Middlesbrough, U.K.

INTRODUCTION

Colorectal surgery has changed significantly over the last few years with a drift toward minimally invasive surgery and enhanced recovery programs or fast-track surgery. The aim is to reduce postoperative morbidity and recovery time. The vast majority of colonic resections in the United Kingdom at present are open resections, and the scope of our chapter is limited to major open intra-abdominal colorectal surgery.

A recent French prospective multicenter study (1) evaluating independent perioperative factors (patient factors, disease, and the operating surgeons) influencing morbidity and mortality in 1421 patients undergoing open or laparoscopic colonic resections for cancer and diverticular disease showed that the in-hospital death rate was 3.4%, and that the overall morbidity rate was 35%. Four independent preoperative risk factors of mortality were found: emergency surgery, old age (>70 years), weight loss greater than 10%, and neurological comorbidity (e.g., previous stroke, etc). Similarly independent risk factors associated with morbidity included old age (>70 years), neurological and cardiorespiratory comorbidity, hypoalbuminemia, prolonged operating time, and peritoneal contamination. Hence, knowledge about risk factors is vital to achieving a good outcome. In addition, preoperative optimization of the patient's cardiorespiratory and renal function is the cornerstone of good perioperative management (Chapters 7 and 8).

We have analyzed the available recent literature from databases such as Medline & Cochrane collaboration. This chapter does not cover fast track and minimally invasive surgery, but focuses on certain surgical issues pertaining to open colonic resections both in the elective and in the emergency setting. A brief description on preoperative optimization, followed by a description of methods used to monitor the patient and techniques to prevent and recognize postoperative complications, are included in this chapter. Specific issues that influence postoperative morbidity, where there is much debate between traditional and modern concepts [e.g., the use of mechanical bowel preparation (MBP) and nasogastric tubes, types of incisions, drains, fluid and nutritional support and the role of stomas] will be discussed.

This chapter also includes a brief description of well-established measures such as antibiotic prophylaxis, deep vein thrombosis (DVT), and prophylaxis and the use of regional anesthetic techniques.

PREOPERATIVE EVALUATION

Risk Assessment and Scoring Systems

Preoperative optimization of the various comorbid conditions and adequate control of physiological changes during the perioperative and postoperative period can lead to acceptable mortality and morbidity. The most commonly used method for risk assessment is the simple American Society of Anesthesiologists (ASA) score. Comorbid illness (organ system dysfunction and severity of functional impairment) serves as the basis for ASA classification and serves as a valuable tool, particularly in the elderly (2). This has been shown to accurately predict postoperative morbidity and mortality (3). Another commonly used method for the accurate assessment of the functional status of the patient, cognitive and physiological assessment, includes the scoring system Acute Physiology and Chronic Health Evaluation III score (4), which can identify subgroups of patients who have an increased probability of an adverse outcome in the perioperative period. This system includes factors such as age, physiologic parameters and chronic health status, and comorbid conditions and urgency of interventions for the prediction of mortality.

Another key issue in reducing the mortality associated with emergency surgery is the use of National Confidential Enquiry into Patient Outcome and Death (NCEPOD). This voluntary and confidential body (5) regularly reviews clinical practice relating to deaths that occur within 30 days of surgery, has made several recommendations as to how patient care can be improved, and specifically looks at both the surgical and the anesthetic aspects of patient care (6). Some of the key recommendations of NCEPOD have been the provision of adequate intensive therapy unit (ITU) and high dependency unit (HDU) and operating facilities in acute hospitals, provision of adequate monitoring facilities, optimization of high-risk patients prior to surgery, and involvement of senior grade personnel and categorization of operations to immediate, urgent, expedited, and elective so as to minimize surgery out of hours (NCEPOD report II 2003).

Preoperative nutritional assessment—especially in the elderly and malnourished patients and those who are likely to have major surgery—and its associated prolonged nutritional starvation status, (i.e., nil by mouth preoperatively and postoperatively), play a very important and predictable role in rapid recovery. Nutritional optimization gives an additional reserve to minimize postoperative complications and aids in wound healing.

Cardiorespiratory complications are a major source of morbidity and mortality associated with surgery in all age groups, but are particularly common among the elderly and those with a compromised reserve. Any underlying cardiorespiratory disease can exacerbate the normal physiologic decline and compound the risk of surgery. Accurate identification of both reversible and irreversible causes is critical prior to surgical intervention. The use of revised Goldman's criteria using six variables (7) for the assessment of cardiac risk, especially in the elderly, and the use of basic investigations to assess the cardiac and respiratory functional status can help identify those at risk and aid in adequate management.

Another important factor commonly seen is the delay in surgical intervention. This is particularly seen in the elderly age group due to a combination of various factors, such as the misdiagnosis (especially in the atypical presentations and delays in performing investigations). This can be particularly detrimental in acute emergencies.

PHYSIOLOGIC MONITORING OF SURGICAL PATIENTS

Monitoring physiological parameters provides advance warning of impending deterioration of one or more organ systems. These monitoring tools aid in both diagnostic evaluation and assessment of prognosis especially in critically ill patients. The ability to employ this knowledge to monitor and treat appropriately can be a critical determinant for patient outcomes. These encompass a spectrum of endeavors ranging in complexity from simple measurement of vital signs to oxidation status of mitochondrial enzyme cytochrome oxidase. A brief description of the commonly used methods has been made, although their description is beyond the scope of this chapter.

Methods used for physiological monitoring can be classified into simple standard methods, such as the vital signs, arterial blood pressure, and the electrocardiography and those specific to various organs. Monitoring of cardiac output and function is facilitated using central venous pressure (CVP) lines, pulmonary artery catheters, tissue capnometry, and thermodilution techniques. Minimally invasive alternatives for cardiac functional assessment include Doppler ultrasonography, impedance cardiography, transesophageal echocardiography, and pulse contour analysis. Monitoring of the respiratory function involves the use of arterial blood gases, pulse oximetry, and capnometry and the measurement of airway pressures during the respiratory cycle. These methods assess gas exchange status, neuromuscular activity, respiratory mechanics, and patient effort. In addition, they act as a guide toward optimization of tissue oxygenation, weaning from ventilator support, and to detect adverse events associated with respiratory failure and mechanical ventilation. Renal function has traditionally been monitored using urine output by the bedside in addition to the biochemical profile of measurement of blood and urinary electrolytes.

NUTRITIONAL AND METABOLIC SUPPORT

Basic principles in the management of the surgical patient include the maintenance of nutritional status. Several studies have been conducted to assess the role of optimizing nutrition prior to surgery. In a study conducted in patients undergoing hip surgery, preoperative oral carbohydrate treatment has been shown to attenuate postoperative insulin resistance, although no effect was seen on the nitrogen balance (8). These may play a role in the malnourished patients, although its role in routine colorectal surgery has not been proven. Numerous studies have been conducted on postoperative nutritional support. The use of total parenteral nutrition (TPN) perioperatively has been shown to benefit the malnourished, although there is no convincing data to support its benefit in healthy individuals undergoing major colorectal surgery, especially in those where the TPN is likely to be discontinued before 10 to 14 days. In addition, other problems have been associated with TPN use, including electrolyte disturbances, acid–base abnormalities, interference with anticoagulation, and CVP line–associated complications (i.e., pneumothorax, line sepsis, and DVT) (9). There is growing evidence to support the initiation of enteric feeding in the early postoperative period, prior to return of bowel function, because it can be well tolerated and was shown to be associated with fewer intestinal problems, such as prolonged ileus or constipation (10). Enteric feeding was also shown to be associated with minimal postoperative insulin resistance and nitrogen losses after major colorectal surgery (11). The role of enteric feeding in preference to TPN is further supported by the hypothesis of prevention of bacterial translocation in these subjects (12). In a controlled study conducted on animals, TPN was shown to cause global intestinal barrier failure, while elemental diet prevented barrier failure in the small intestine (13). They also showed that the addition of cellulose fiber to elemental diet could ameliorate further barrier failure in the ileum. Preoperative nutrition via the enteral route may provide better regulation of cytokine responses after surgery than parenteral nutrition (14). Certain considerations however have to be made to the nature of enteric nutritional support, because jejunal feeding tubes and small-bore nasogastric tubes are associated with a lower risk of aspiration pneumonia when compared with large-bore nasogastric tubes (15,16). In addition, patients who are enterally fed after a prolonged period are at risk of developing refeeding syndrome characterized by severe hypophosphatemia, electrolyte imbalances, and respiratory failure (17).

A prospective randomized controlled trial by Van Den Berghe et al. in 2001 demonstrated that tight glycemic control (insulin therapy) is associated with reduction in mortality and morbidity in the critical care setting in spite of limitations of the study (i.e., it included predominantly cardiac surgery patients) (18). Several studies have shown the importance of adequate glucocorticoid replacement during the perioperative period based on the length of surgery and the original steroid-deficient disease state (19–21). Other metabolic conditions, including adrenal and thyroid disease, need to be adequately assessed and replaced where appropriate (22) to prevent crisis states, such as adrenal insufficiency, thyrotoxicosis, hypothyroidism, or the "sick-euthyroid" syndrome.

THERMOREGULATION

Poor regulation in the core temperature [hypothermia ($<35°C$) and hyperthermia ($>38.6°C$)] have both been shown to affect the postoperative recovery. Hypothermia can induce a coagulopathic state through its effects on platelet and clotting cascade enzyme function. Other effects include cardiac arrhythmias, carbon dioxide retention and respiratory acidosis, paradoxical polyuria secondary to peripheral vasoconstriction and central shunting of blood, and deterioration in neurological function leading to coma. Systemic and local warming has been suggested to accelerate wound healing and minimize postoperative wound infection (23), although more research is needed to confirm this. The ongoing heat loss can be optimized using simple methods, such as maintaining a warm and dry environment, or active rewarming methods using heating blankets or heated intravenous fluids and intraperitoneal rewarming lavage during abdominal surgery; although alternate methods, such as vascular perfusion bypass and extracorporeal membrane oxygenation, have been described for other major surgical procedures (24,25). A recent United Kingdom–based pilot study demonstrated that perioperative administration of amino acid (vamin 18) increases the rate of recovery of body temperature, although the impact of this thermogenic effect on perioperative morbidity and mortality needs further evaluation (26).

Hyperthermia can be environmentally induced, medication induced (iatrogenic), endocrine induced (pheochromocytoma and thyroid storm), or neurologically induced (hypothalamic), and treated in a variety of ways (27). Prompt recognition of early warning signs prevents the mortality associated with hyperthermia. Withdrawal of the precipitant causes, control of manifest symptoms, and aggressive cooling methods, such as the use of fans, ice packs, and alcohol baths, have all been reported in the past as effective treatment measures.

PATIENT FACTORS

Age of the patient plays an important role both in disease presentation and in response to surgery, and can be a likely source of potential errors and complications. The most notable among these are the lack of physiologic reserve and the immune response in the extremes of age. Other important factors affecting these age groups include altered drug metabolism and clearance, and the ability to communicate, which thereby put them at high risk unless these issues are specifically addressed.

Another important patient factor is obesity and its associated higher risks, such as poor cardiorespiratory reserve and glycemic controls, DVT, sleep apnea, and gastroesophageal reflux disease. A recent study on patients undergoing elective gastric and colorectal surgery showed that body fat accumulation was independently associated with postoperative morbidity (28). They showed a statistically significant association between age ($\geq$70 years), lung dysfunction, cardiovascular dysfunction, and intra-abdominal fat with medical complications (pneumonitis or arrhythmia). Similarly, subcutaneous fat was shown to be independently associated with surgery-related complications (anastomotic leakage, intra-abdominal collections, or abdominal wound infection) postoperatively.

Preoperative optimization using dietary modification and exercise, adequate glycemic control in the perioperative period, and DVT prophylaxis and keeping the head of bed elevated at all times to improve functional residual capacity of the lungs have all been proven to be effective.

DEEP VEIN THROMBOSIS PROPHYLAXIS

DVT and pulmonary embolism (PE) are common postoperative complications that are associated with significant morbidity and mortality. A systematic review (29) supported a significant association between increased age, obesity, a past history of thromboembolism, varicose veins, the oral contraceptive pill, malignancy, Factor V Leiden gene mutation, general anesthesia, and orthopedic surgery with higher rates of postoperative DVT. A review of published reports with strict inclusion criteria (1966–2002) showed an incidence of DVT ranging from 3% to 28% in the Asian population and 28% to 44% in the Caucasian population, following general surgical operations (30).

Current evidence (30) supports the view that low-molecular-weight heparins (LMWH) are more effective than unfractionated heparin for the prevention of proximal DVT and better than oral anticoagulants for the prevention of in-hospital (mostly distal) venous thrombosis. A meta-analysis of the risk of DVT and PE after colorectal surgery (31) showed that heparin is better in preventing DVT and/or PE, although no difference was seen between unfractionated heparin and LMWH. A combination of graded compression stockings and heparin was shown to be better than heparin alone (odds ratio at 4.17; 95% confidence interval 1.37–12.70). A more recent review of all randomized controlled trials and meta-analyses (January 1980–July 2003) concluded that LMWH is the preferred choice in surgical prophylaxis (32). They also suggested that the new anticoagulant molecules fondaparinux and ximelagatran seem to have similar efficacy when compared with LMWH in the treatment of venous thromboembolism, and, in addition, have a twofold increase in efficacy in DVT prophylaxis.

ANTIBIOTIC PROPHYLAXIS

Postoperative wound infection is a health-care burden causing considerable morbidity because it increases the length of hospital stay, drains resources, and decreases productivity (33). Antibiotic prophylaxis has played a major role in reducing this morbidity and is well established in numerous surgical procedures. During the 1970s, studies revealed that antibiotic prophylaxis was inappropriate in more than half of all hospitalized patients (34,35). Song and Glenny, in their systematic review of antibiotic prophylaxis in colorectal surgery, summed up the general principles related to adverse effects of prolonged chemoprophylaxis, reminding surgeons that antibiotics are not a substitute for poor surgery (36). There is little disagreement with the fact that the medical fraternity administers antibiotics haphazardly, often ignoring evidence-based guidelines and disregarding the boundaries between prophylactic and therapeutic antibiotic administration. While the benefits of antibiotic prophylaxis include prevention of morbidity and mortality as well as reduction in duration and cost of hospitalization, inappropriate use of antibiotic prophylaxis can have disadvantages, such as the development of resistant strains (36). The necessary duration of postoperative antimicrobial prophylaxis is often unclear (37), although single-dose antibiotic administration has often been cited as sufficient to lower postoperative wound sepsis following elective colorectal surgery (38); this was essentially confirmed by Song and Glenny in their systematic review (36).

Antimicrobial prophylaxis for colorectal surgery is still controversial due to the identification of new risk factors, such as patient core temperature and tissue oxygenation, which can increase infection rate after colorectal surgery, indicating the need for further clinical trials (39).

NASOGASTRIC TUBES

Nasogastric tubes have been routinely used for several years on a prophylactic basis following major intra-abdominal surgery and on a therapeutic basis in intestinal obstruction. The perceived advantages of using nasogastric tubes included

- early return of bowel function
- provision of gastric decompression, thereby reducing the risk of aspiration and pulmonary complications
- protection against anastomotic leakage
- increased patient comfort
- reduced hospital stay
- reduced wound complications and incisional hernias
- enteric feeding

The prophylactic use of nasogastric tube has been questioned as patients find it uncomfortable, and studies have shown a greater frequency of pulmonary complications following its use (40). The best evidence for the usage of nasogastric tubes is contained in an excellent Cochrane review (41), wherein 28 randomized studies encompassing 4194 patients (with 2108 randomized to the routine tube use group and 2086 to the nonselective or selective use group) were evaluated to investigate the efficacy of nasogastric tube decompression. The authors showed that patients who did not have nasogastric tube had an earlier return of bowel function ($p < 0.00001$), an insignificant trend toward decrease in pulmonary complications ($p = 0.07$), and increased risk of wound infection ($p = 0.08$) and ventral hernia ($p = 0.09$). Anastomotic leak rates were no different between the two groups ($p = 0.70$). Patient comfort, nausea, vomiting, and length of stay seemed to favor the no-tube group, but heterogeneity encountered in these analyses made rigorous conclusions difficult. The authors concluded that routine nasogastric decompression does not achieve its intended goals and should be abandoned in favor of selective nasogastric tube usage. Evidence suggests that routine nasogastric tube usage is not justified, but certainly has a place in selected cases where patients develop troublesome gastric distension or repeated postoperative vomiting.

MECHANICAL BOWEL PREPARATION

To use or not to use! This is perhaps one of the most sensitive and controversial areas in colorectal surgery, and several studies have addressed this issue recently. The main reason for the popularity of MBP has been the belief that it reduces postoperative morbidity related to septic bowel content (42). Clinical experiences and observational studies have shown that mechanical removal of gross feces from the colon has been associated with decreased morbidity and mortality in patients undergoing operations of the colon (42).

A recent survey of members of the American Society of Colon and Rectal Surgeons showed that 99% of surgeons routinely used MBP with one-third using polyethylene glycol (PEG) exclusively (43). Adverse physiological changes after bowel preparation have been studied and include a significant decrease in exercise capacity and weight, increase in plasma osmolality, urea, and phosphate concentrations, and reduction in calcium and potassium concentrations (44). Moreover, traditionally patients are allowed only clear fluids a day prior to surgery along with the bowel preparation solution, which along with the multiple bowel actions needed makes the experience quite unpleasant. MBP appears to be going out of favor especially with the increasing interest in fast-track surgery, where omission of bowel preparation is one of the key elements (Chapter 22).

Certainly the vast majority of colorectal surgeons do not use bowel preparation in right colonic surgery, but its use in left-sided resections where the fecal bacterial load and anastomotic leak rates are higher is debatable. A more recent published randomized controlled trial evaluated the use of MBP prior to elective left-sided colonic surgery (43). This included 153 patients with 78 randomized to the MBP group (3 L of PEG in group 1 and 75 to the no MBP in group 2). The overall rate of abdominal infectious complications (anastomotic leak, intra-abdominal abscess, peritonitis, and wound infection) was 22% in group 1 and 8% in group 2 ($p = 0.028$); the anastomotic leak rate was 6% in group 1 and 1% in group 2 ($p = 0.021$); and extra-abdominal morbidity rates were 24% and 11%, respectively ($p = 0.034$).

The hospital stay was longer for group 1—mean (s.d) 14.9 (13.1) versus 9.9 (3.8) in group 2 ($p = 0.024$). They concluded that elective left-sided colorectal surgery is safe without MBP and is associated with reduced postoperative morbidity. Further evidence against MBP comes from a recent meta-analysis of seven randomized clinical trials of colorectal surgery with or without bowel preparation with PEG (45). They found significantly more anastomotic leakage after bowel preparation 5.6% than without 3.2% ($p = 0.032$), which was the primary outcome measure of this meta-analysis. Secondary outcomes such as abdominal septic complications (peritonitis, pelvic abscess, reoperation, wound abscess, wound dehiscence, and diarrhea), extra-abdominal septic complications (bronchopulmonary/urinary tract), and other nonseptic complications favored the no-preparation regimen, but the differences were not statistically significant. They concluded that MBP could safely be omitted before elective colorectal surgery.

The above meta-analysis also echoes the findings of a Cochrane database systematic review of MBP for elective colorectal surgery (46), wherein the overall anastomotic leak rate was significantly higher in the MBP group than the no-preparation group, but nonsignificant on stratification to leak rates in low-anterior resection or colonic surgery. Although there seems to be a fair amount of evidence against the use of MBP, it continues to be widely used. Most trials have incorporated PEG as the solution of choice and other agents such as sodium picosulphate and fleet phosphosoda, which are very popular in the United Kingdom. This practice needs to be evaluated in similar trials as above before one recommends against the use of bowel preparation, because it undoubtedly gives a clean operative field for the surgeon during performance of colonic anastomosis. (Anastomotic leakage is used as main outcome measure, but this depends on several factors, such as technique, vascularity of the bowel ends, tension on the anastomosis, etc.) In emergency situations, however, when there is a left-sided colonic obstruction/perforation, on-table antegrade colonic lavage via the appendicular stump (necessitating appendicectomy) is widely used because it facilitates performing an anastomosis at the same time as a single-stage procedure, thus avoiding a second laparotomy at a later date.

INCISIONS

There are several factors that are important in selecting the type of abdominal incision in colorectal surgery. The essential requirements of an incision are accessibility, ability to extend and preserve function, and the provision of a secure closure. Complications that can be prevented include pulmonary complications such as basal atelectasis and effusions, wound infections, burst abdomen, and incisional hernia, which add to the morbidity of the procedure. There are other important factors that need consideration, particularly the setting in which the operation is being performed (i.e., emergency or elective where speed of entry and certainty of diagnosis play a role). Cosmesis, presence of previous laparotomy scars, and body habitus are also important points to be considered. From the patient's perspective, control of postoperative pain and earlier return to normal function are vital.

Currently, open colorectal surgery remains still popular as reflected by a study (1998–2001) in England. Laparoscopic surgery constitutes only 0.1% of colorectal resections, but the usage is gradually increasing and can contribute to a great reduction in the postoperative morbidity (47). The recent interest in enhanced recovery programs underlines the importance of the debate that transverse incisions when compared to vertical incisions contribute to more rapid recovery (48).

A variety of incisions are available to gain access to the abdominal cavity, and it is important to consider the nerve and blood supply of the anterior abdominal wall to understand the effects of various incisions. The ones pertinent to colorectal surgery are discussed in this section. Median or midline incision through the linea alba has several advantages: it minimizes blood loss, avoids major nerves, and provides quick and easy access for exploration and for extending the incision if required. Making paramedian incisions, however, to the right or left of the midline has the advantage of avoiding major nerves, provides good access to the peritoneal cavity, and is associated with a lower risk of incisional hernia (49). Transverse incisions are made through the anterior rectus sheath and the rectus abdominis muscle divided. They have the advantages of low risk to neurovascular injury due to the segmental innervations and blood supply of the rectus and the ability to rejoin the muscular segments.

Ninety percent of all abdominal incisions for visceral surgery are vertical incisions (50). Midline and transverse incisions are the two commonest forms of incision used. There have been a number of studies that have compared these two incisions, but they have intrinsic drawbacks in the methodology used and one cannot derive any concrete conclusions from these. In a review encompassing 11 prospective and 7 retrospective trials, transverse incisions were shown to offer as good an access as vertical incision to most intra-abdominal structures, and resulted in significantly lower postoperative pain and pulmonary complication rates (51). They reported an increased risk of both burst abdomen and incisional hernia following midline incision when compared with transverse incisions. However, these reports need to be critically addressed because the technique of surgical closure plays an equally important role in preventing such complications.

The lack of clear evidence for superiority of transverse versus vertical incisions is the basis for currently ongoing POVATI trial—post surgical pain outcome of vertical and transverse abdominal incision trial (50).

ANASTOMOTIC TECHNIQUES

Anastomotic leakage contributes to significant morbidity and mortality after colorectal surgery. In addition to immediate morbidity, an increase in local recurrence of cancer has been shown in patients who leak after primary rectal anastomosis, although no significant difference in local recurrence or five-year survival was seen in a combined group of all curative colorectal cancer resections (52).

Several issues involved in this process need to be specifically addressed to minimize complications. Factors that play an important role include surgical techniques (suture technique and suture material), bowel integrity (anastomotic level, tension, blood supply, bowel obstruction, etc.), and surgical-tactical factors (primary anastomosis vs. discontinuity resection or formation of protective diverting stomas) (53,54). Anastomotic techniques are vital to ensure healthy bowel with adequate blood supply and are joined without undue tension. Anastomosis should be checked to ensure that they are patent and leak proof at the time of construction.

A recent review has suggested that various endogenous (diabetes, sepsis, infection, and malnutrition) and exogenous factors (steroids, radiation, and preoperative bowel preparation) play a role in anastomotic healing (54). A recent animal study has suggested that the use of local keratinocyte growth factor and insulin-like growth factor-I accelerates anastomotic healing and promotes mechanical stability (55), although further research is needed to identify similar factors. The traditional use of temporary defunctioning stomas, bowel preparation, antibiotic prophylaxis, and nutritional support are discussed in a different section of this chapter.

The use of stapling instruments has had a major impact on the practice of colorectal surgery. A stapling instrument facilitates the performance of anastomosis, particularly in regions with difficult anatomy (56). It may expedite a surgical procedure and is an adjunct to, and not a substitute for, meticulous surgical technique. Several randomized control trials in the past have shown no consistent difference in the rates of colonic anastomotic dehiscence between the suture and stapling techniques (57,58). However, one trial has shown an increase in the rate of local recurrence in the hand-sewn group (59). A recent study has suggested that hand-sewn colonic anastomoses (ileocolic, colocolic, and colorectal intraperitoneal anastomoses) with extramucosal one-layer continuous suture using synthetic slow absorbable monofilament should ideally be used in colorectal surgery (60). Complications related to the stapling technique are uncommon (56), although anastomotic stricture may be more frequent than when hand-sewn anastomosis is performed (61).

In conclusion, the choice of technique used is a matter of personal preference, but certainly all surgeons should have expertise in constructing hand-sewn anastomoses in case needed where staplers may not be available or are found to be faulty.

THE ROLE OF STOMAS

Stomas are constructed for several reasons in colorectal surgery and may be permanent [end colostomy after abdominoperineal resection for rectal cancer and end ileostomy after panproctocolectomy for inflammatory bowel disease or familial adenomatous polyposis (FAP)]. Stomas can be used to defunction temporarily a distal anastomosis or decompress the colon in a left-sided colonic obstruction where the choice lies between a loop ileostomy (incompetent ileocecal valve) and a transverse loop colostomy. Recently colonic stents have been used to relieve acute left colonic obstruction to either palliate the condition or to prepare the patient for elective surgery (62), thus avoiding the need for a stoma.

Stomas may add to the morbidity postoperatively. Several complications have been reported in literature (63), including necrosis, retraction, wound infection, and skin excoriation. Delayed complications include stenosis or prolapse of the stoma, parastomal herniation, and psychological impact on the patient. In addition, patients undergoing reversal of temporary stomas can develop other complications, such as wound infection, anastomotic leak, peritonitis, enterocutaneous fistulae, and intestinal obstruction. A recently conducted prospective study (64) showed a high complication rate (39.4%) following ileostomy, which included dermatitis (12.6%), erythema (7.1%), and stomal prolapse (3.1%). Similarly, closure of ileostomy was shown to be associated with a high-complication (33.1%) and mortality rates (0.9%) (64). Among these, wound infections (18.3%) and small-bowel obstruction (4.6%) were commonly seen. Anastomotic leak requiring surgery occurred in 2.8% and enterocutaneous fistula treated conservatively in 5.5%.

Traditionally, stoma teaching to patients starts postoperatively and this often delays discharge. Preoperative intensive community-based stoma teaching has been shown to result in shorter times to stoma proficiency, earlier discharge from the hospital, reduced stoma-related interventions in the community, and had no adverse effects on patient well-being (65). It is also imperative to mark the best site for the stoma preoperatively for the best results, so as to achieve a good functional result.

Anastomotic leakage is one of the most important factors influencing post-operative morbidity. The role of a protective stoma has been debated, including the choice of stoma (loop ileostomy versus loop colostomy). Loop ileostomy is generally preferred when compared with loop colostomy. A prospective controlled trial (66) showed that ileostomy was associated with significantly less odor ($p < 0.01$) and required less appliance changes ($p < 0.05$) and a reduced wound infection rate following closure.

The defunctioning stoma is essentially meant to prevent the disastrous consequences of anastomotic leaks rather than prevent the leak itself. A prospective multicenter study (67) showed no difference in the rate of anastomotic leaks; although significant leakage requiring surgery was significantly lower in the stoma group, thus indicating its benefit.

To conclude, stomas should be used whenever there is any element of uncertainty regarding a low rectal anastomosis or an ileoanal pouch/coloanal pouch, so as to avoid the ensuing complications of an anastomotic leak. Ileostomy is the preferred choice.

DRAINS AND COLORECTAL SURGERY

Intra-abdominal drains have traditionally been routinely used in major intra-abdominal colonic surgery, but their use has been questioned in recent times. There is a definite role for radiologically placed drains for drainage of post-operative intra-abdominal abscesses, but their prophylactic use at laparotomy is controversial. Complications related to drains include wound infections, incisional hernia, and intestinal obstruction, as well as erosion leading to fistulae and hemorrhage.

Abdominal drains have been shown to correlate with intra-abdominal bacterial contamination rather than infection (68). The perceived benefits of prophylactic drainage were stated to be prevention of intra-abdominal collections, monitoring of post-operative bleeding, prevention and recognition of anastomotic leaks, and possibly reduction of wound infection. Perhaps the most relevant outcome relating to postoperative morbidity is anastomotic leakage, which occurs in 3.4% to 6% of all colorectal cases (69). These are commonly associated with rectal anastomoses, being clinically significant in 2.9% to 15.3% of cases and a mortality risk of 6.0% to 39.3% (69).

A recent systematic review (68) evaluated six randomized control trials comparing drainage with nondrainage after anastomoses in elective colorectal surgery. A total of 1140 patients were enrolled in six trials with 573 allocated to the drainage group and 567 to nondrainage. Their outcome variables and results are shown in Table 1. They concluded that there is insufficient evidence to show that routine drainage after colorectal anastomoses prevents anastomotic and other complications. Two randomized multicenter controlled trials (70) comparing prophylactic abdominal drainage after colonic resection and suprapromontory anastomosis and pelvic drainage after elective rectal or anal anastomosis, respectively, have shown that drainage does not influence the severity of complications or improve the outcome. Current evidence supports that routine drainage is probably unnecessary for the vast majority of cases, but may play a role in the more difficult pelvic surgery where there is a likelihood of leakage or further blood loss that needs monitoring.

Table 1 Outcome Variables and Drainage

Outcome	Drainage ($N = 573$) (%)	No drainage ($N = 567$) (%)
Mortality	3	4
Clinical anastomotic dehiscence	2	1
Radiological anastomotic dehiscence	3	4
Wound infection	5	5
Reintervention	6	5
Extra-abdominal complications	7	6

PREVENTION OF POSTOPERATIVE ILEUS

Several factors may play a role in the development of ileus, including spinal–intestinal neural reflexes, local and systemic inflammatory mediators, generalized sympathetic hyperactivity, open intra-abdominal surgery, degree of bowel manipulation, and other exacerbating influences including exogenous and endogenous opiates and electrolyte abnormalities (71).

Previous studies have shown that laparoscopic approach reduces the duration of ileus by 27% to 40% in gastrointestinal (GI) surgery (72,73). Several methods have been described to restore the neural reflex action of the intestine. Postoperative early mobilization has been suggested to initiate a return of GI function, although no clear data supports the hypothesis (74,75). Epidural anesthesia (76–78) leading to a reduced perioperative narcotic use, limited use of nasogastric tubes (41,79) and early postoperative feeding (80,81), have all been shown to contribute significantly to the prevention of ileus.

Various drugs have been used, among which laxatives along with other therapies in multimode rehabilitation studies after abdominal surgery, showed promising results (82). Despite the theoretical promise of stimulating bowel function using metoclopramide and erythromycin, a consistent beneficial effect has not been shown in the randomized placebo-controlled trials conducted on patients with postoperative ileus (83,84). However, drugs such as neostigmine have been shown to be useful once colonic pseudoobstruction has set in (85), although larger randomized controlled trials are needed to support this. Studies on nonsteroidal anti-inflammatory drugs (NSAIDs) have shown some benefit in the prevention of ileus probably due to their anti-inflammatory action and opioid-sparing effect (86,87). Similarly a study on the use of opiate antagonists (ADL8-2698-Alvimopan) had a significant decrease in time to passage of flatus, bowel movement, and hospital discharge (88). Smaller studies on the cyclooxygenase-2 inhibitors (89) and chewing gum (90) have also shown some benefit, although larger-controlled trials are needed to support this.

PREVENTION OF POSTOPERATIVE ADHESIONS AND INTERNAL HERNIA

Adhesions (90% of cases) constitute the most common cause of early postoperative small-bowel obstruction; while internal and external hernias make up 7% of obstructions, the rest are secondary to infections/abscesses, etc. A recent cohort study has shown that the relative risks (RRs) of adhesion-related complications during the first four years of follow-up after open colorectal surgery ranged between 23.5% and 29.7% (91). The use of mucolytic enzymes such as hyaluronidase in the prevention of adhesions and subsequent bowel obstruction has produced conflicting results. No proven benefit has been seen in one study (92), whereas other studies have shown to prevent bowel obstructions (93,94). The technique of closing the mesenteric defects has been variably practiced among surgeons, although there is no convincing evidence to suggest that it prevents internal herniation.

PREVENTION OF GI BLEEDING

The most common intraoperative causes include a poorly tied suture, a technically poor staple line, or a missed injury (95,96). Bleeding from the upper GI tract (esophageal/gastric varices, duodenal ulcers, and gastric erosions) is the commonest cause of postoperative intestinal bleeding. Prompt endoscopy and treatment of the cause reduces its associated morbidity and mortality. The pathogenesis of stress ulceration is thought to be multifactorial and includes low gastric pH, mucosal ischemia due to hemorrhagic shock and sepsis (97), systemic acidosis (98), reduced bicarbonate secretion (99), and bile salt–induced disruption of the gastric mucosal permeability barrier (100).

Prevention of stress ulcers using proton pump inhibitors (PPI) and H_2 antagonists has been shown to be effective (101). A Cochrane database and MEDLINE systematic review of randomized controlled trials (January 1966–June 2002) suggested that misoprostol, PPI, and double-dose H_2 antagonists are effective in preventing chronic NSAID-related endoscopic gastric and duodenal ulcers, calthough misoprostol was associated with poor tolerance (102). Low-dose misoprostol (400 μg/day) reduced the risk of endoscopic gastric ulcers (RR = 0.39) as compared with H_2 antagonists at reducing the risk of endoscopic duodenal and gastric ulcers. Both double dose H_2 antagonists and PPIs were effective in reducing the risk of endoscopic duodenal and gastric ulcers and were better tolerated than misoprostol (102).

PREVENTION OF POSTOPERATIVE GI FISTULAE

Postoperative GI fistulae (both internal/external) are associated with extensive morbidity and mortality. The incidence of fistulae was low following in surgery on the lower GI tract, with the majority of studies reporting rates of 0% to 7% (56,103,104), although rates as high as 19% (105) have been found. In addition to the morbidity directly associated with the fistula, other complications can cause considerable psychological impact on the patient. These complications include fluid and electrolyte disturbances, abscess formation or local infection (e.g., urinary tract infection and bronchitis), general infection, multiorgan failure, sepsis, and bleeding. Furthermore, a postoperative fistula increases hospital stay, which obviously increases hospital costs. Common causes for fistula formation include the presence of distal obstruction, local inflammation or neoplastic disease, prior irradiation, poor nutritional status, poor anastomotic technique, and inappropriate use of drains and trauma (106–108). These can be prevented using simple precautionary measures, such as appropriate preoperative assessment and optimization of the patient, the use of contrast studies prior to surgery, and the use of appropriate surgical techniques.

POSTOPERATIVE CARE AND EARLY RECOGNITION
OF COMPLICATIONS

Postoperative care given to the patient plays an important role in the recovery of the patient. The cornerstones of postoperative management are adequate analgesia, maintenance of fluid and electrolyte balance, nutritional support, and early mobilization. Other factors that can ensure safe recovery of the patient include the appropriate management of urinary catheters, nasogastric tubes, and drains. Physiotherapy, if started early, can encourage early mobilization and prevent pulmonary complications. A coordinated team effort between the staff involved in the nursing, medical, and social care of the patient plays an integral part in the postoperative recovery. A high index of suspicion must be maintained to detect complications, such as anastomotic leaks, pneumonia, embolic events, and infections that have a considerable impact on the morbidity. Observation charts and vital parameters should be checked regularly, and daily abdominal and systemic examinations are vital.

Detection of Anastomotic Leaks

Early detection of anastomotic leaks after colorectal anastomosis is essential for adequate intervention to prevent peritonitis. The highest risks are in unprotected anastomoses less than 5 cm from the anal verge in men who smoke and/or drink excessively, particularly if they have received preoperative chemotherapy or chemoradiotherapy (109). The overall anastomotic leaks rate from resection of colonic tumors is about 4% (110), but subclinical leaks occur more frequently than clinically obvious leaks (111). Leaks are not always easy to identify, but the warning signs may include tachycardia, a leucocytosis, pyrexia, and abdominal pain and distension. Generalized peritonitis with septic shock may ensue, or some patients have localized peritoneal signs while others may develop a fecal fistula via the laparotomy wound. A high index of suspicion is required in detecting these early nonspecific signs of a leak and urgent surgical intervention may be required to avert a life-threatening situation. Prompt diagnosis and further laparotomy can reduce mortality following leakage. In addition to the clinical evaluation, the use of radiological investigations such as erect chest X rays, water-soluble contrast enema, and computed tomography (CT) scans can help in detecting these complications. A recent study has shown that measurement of endotoxin lipopolysaccharide (LPS) in the drain fluid and the total daily excreted LPS facilitates the early detection of anastomotic leaks, although further evaluation on a larger scale is needed (112).

Patients with generalized peritonitis need urgent surgery, although there is a place for conservative treatment in those with localized peritoneal signs. Supportive treatment with intravenous antibiotics and ultrasound- or CT-guided drainage of intra-abdominal collections may be necessary. Patients who develop fecal fistulae need nutritional support, skin protection, eradication of any sepsis, and further radiological investigations [CT/ultrasound (US) scans/contrast studies] to exclude associated collections, distal obstruction, and anastomotic integrity.

SPECIALIZATION IN COLORECTAL SURGERY

Among the factors that significantly influence the outcome include specialization, surgeon's caseload, supervision/training of a trainee, and the surgeon's learning curve (113). The individual surgeon has been shown as an independent prognostic factor for outcome in colorectal cancer surgery. This was supported by a further study on emergency left-sided colonic surgery, which showed that specialized colorectal surgeons were more likely to do a primary anastomosis and had reduced postoperative morbidity and mortality rates (14.5% and 10.4%) when compared to noncolorectal surgeons (24.3% and 17.4%). Trainees were also more likely to do a primary anastomosis when assisted by a colorectal specialist than when a noncolorectal consultant was present (72.1% vs. 47.5%) (114). Although most studies have shown that specialization in colorectal surgery reduces morbidity and improves primary anastomosis rates, a retrospective analysis on colonic resections by colorectal subspecialty-certified surgeons has shown no significant improvement in outcomes (115). The same report however suggested that increasing years of experience was associated with reduced mortality.

BLOOD TRANSFUSION

Blood transfusion in colorectal surgery has generated immense interest due to its associated risk of infective complications and recurrence in colorectal cancer. Preoperative iron supplementation for at least two weeks in anemic patients [hemoglobin (Hb) < 10 g/dL] undergoing colorectal cancer surgery has been shown to improve the hemoglobin and hematocrit levels prior to surgery and reduced the need for intraopertaive blood transfusion (116). Randomized controlled trials have shown that postoperative infectious complications in patients undergoing elective colorectal surgery and receiving buffy-coat poor blood were significantly higher than those who had no transfusion or were transfused with leukocyte-depleted blood. The specific infectious complications evaluated included wound infections: 12% versus 1% and 0%, respectively; intra-abdominal abscesses: 5% versus 0% and 0%, respectively; and postoperative pneumonia: 23% versus 3% and 3%, respectively; although no significant difference in mortality rates was seen between the three groups (117). They suggested that using leucocyte depletion with high-efficiency filters could reduce the undesirable effects of allogenic blood transfusion. A follow-up study by the same authors showed that after seven years follow-up, survival for those with leukocyte-depleted blood transfusion (41%) was not significantly different from transfusion of buffy-coat poor blood (45%) (118). A similar randomized controlled trial on 697 patients undergoing colorectal cancer surgery showed that survival rates in the nontransfusion group were significantly higher than the transfused group (72.9% vs. 59.6%) (118). However, there was no statistically significant difference in survival or recurrence rates between the packed cell and leukocyte-depleted groups or in recurrence rates between transfused and nontransfused groups. Local recurrences were more frequent in the transfused group, but were considered to be related to complicated surgery, especially for rectal cancer.

CONCLUSION

The outcome of colorectal surgery depends on the interplay of several factors and is tailored to the individual patient. Although an ideal patient, surgeon, surgery, etc. can be defined, every patient has to be evaluated individually, taking into account the criteria that reflect on the performance status, the underlying pathology, and the possible intervention to attain a good outcome. However, certain generalizations that can be applied to the entire group can be made, such as preoperative optimization, adequate peroperative and postoperative monitoring, use of antibiotics, DVT prophylaxis, and optimal fluid, electrolyte, and nutritional support where indicated. Studies have supported the use of transverse incisions where possible and selective use of nasogastric tubes and abdominal drains following colorectal surgery. Controversial topics include the use of bowel preparation and blood transfusion perioperatively. Specialization in colorectal surgery undoubtedly has a pivotal role in addition to the coordinated multidisciplinary teamwork between the various professionals involved in the pathway of patient care.

REFERENCES

1. Alves A, Panis Y, Slim K, Heyd B, Kwiatkowski F, Mantion G, et al. Postoperative mortality and morbidity in French patients undergoing colorectal surgery: results of a prospective multicenter study. Arch Surg 2005; 140(3):278–283, discussion 284.
2. Muravchick S. Preoperative assessment of the elderly patient. Anesthesiol Clin North Am 2000; 18(1):71–89, vi.
3. Cullen DJ, Apolone G, Greenfield S, Guadagnoli E, Cleary P, et al. ASA physical status and age predict morbidity after three surgical procedures. Ann Surg 1994; 220(1):3–9.
4. Knaus WA, Wagner DP, Draper EA, et al. The APACHE III prognostic system. Risk prediction of hospital mortality for critically ill hospitalized adults. Chest 1991; 100(6):1619–1636.
5. Hoile RW. The National Confidential Enquiry into peri-operative deaths (NCEPOD). Aust Clin Rev 1993; 13(1):11–15; discussion 15–16.
6. Gray A. United Kingdom national confidential enquiry into perioperative deaths. Minerva Anestesiol 2000; 66(5):288–292.
7. Wertheim WA, Perioperative risk. Review of two guidelines for assessing older adults. American College of Cardiology and American Heart Association. Geriatrics 2000; 55(7):61–66; quiz 69.
8. Soop M, Nygren J, Thorell A, et al. Preoperative oral carbohydrate treatment attenuates endogenous glucose release 3 days after surgery. Clin Nutr 2004; 23(4):733–741.
9. Btaiche IF, Khalidi N. Metabolic complications of parenteral nutrition in adults. Part 2. Am J Health Syst Pharm 2004; 61(19):2050–2057; quiz 2058–2059.
10. Kasparek MS, Mueller MH, Glatzle J, et al. Postoperative colonic motility increases after early food intake in patients undergoing colorectal surgery. Surgery 2004; 136(5): 1019–1127.
11. Soop M, Carlson GL, Hopkinson J, et al. Randomized clinical trial of the effects of immediate enteral nutrition on metabolic responses to major colorectal surgery in an enhanced recovery protocol. Br J Surg 2004; 91(9):1138–1145.
12. Wildhaber BE, Yang H, Spencer AU, Drongowski RA, Teitelbaum DH, et al. Lack of enteral nutrition—effects on the intestinal immune system. J Surg Res 2005; 123(1):8–16.
13. Mosenthal AC, Xu D, Deitch EA. Elemental and intravenous total parenteral nutrition diet-induced gut barrier failure is intestinal site specific and can be prevented by feeding nonfermentable fiber. Crit Care Med 2002; 30(2):396–402.
14. Lin MT, Saito H, Fukushima R, et al. Preoperative total parenteral nutrition influences postoperative systemic cytokine responses after colorectal surgery. Nutrition 1997; 13(1):8–12.
15. Davies AR, Bellomo R. Establishment of enteral nutrition: prokinetic agents and small bowel feeding tubes. Curr Opin Crit Care 2004; 10(2):156–161.

16. Ibanez J, Penafiel A, Marse P, Jorda R, Raurich JM, Mata F, et al. Incidence of gastro-esophageal reflux and aspiration in mechanically ventilated patients using small-bore nasogastric tubes. JPEN J Parenter Enteral Nutr 2000; 24(2):103–106.
17. Flesher ME, Archer KA, Leslie BD, McCollom RA, Martinka GP, et al. Assessing the metabolic and clinical consequences of early enteral feeding in the malnourished patient. JPEN J Parenter Enteral Nutr 2005; 29(2):108–117.
18. van den Berghe G, Wouters P, Weekers F, et al. Intensive insulin therapy in the critically ill patients. N Engl J Med 2001; 345(19):1359–1367.
19. Friedman RJ, Schiff CF, Bromberg JS. Use of supplemental steroids in patients having orthopaedic operations. J Bone Joint Surg Am 1995; 77(12):1801–1816.
20. Bromberg JS, Alfrey EJ, Barker CF, et al. Adrenal suppression and steroid supplementation in renal transplant recipients. Transplantation 1991; 51(2):385–390.
21. LaRochelle GE Jr., LaRochelle AG, Ratner RE, Borenstein DG, et al. Recovery of the hypothalamic-pituitary-adrenal (HPA) axis in patients with rheumatic diseases receiving low-dose prednisone. Am J Med 1993; 95(3):258–264.
22. Vincent JL, Abraham E, Annane D, Bernard G, Rivers E, Van den Berghe G, et al. Reducing mortality in sepsis: new directions. Crit Care 2002; 6(suppl 3):S1–S18.
23. MacFie CC, Melling AC, Leaper DJ. Effects of warming on healing. J Wound Care 2005; 14(3):133–136.
24. Bavaria JE, Pochettino A. Retrograde cerebral perfusion (RCP) in aortic arch surgery: efficacy and possible mechanisms of brain protection. Semin Thorac Cardiovasc Surg 1997; 9(3):222–232.
25. Azzam FJ, Fiore AC. Postoperative junctional ectopic tachycardia. Can J Anaesth 1998; 45(9):898–902.
26. Chandrasekaran TV, Morgan RN, Mason RA, Mangat PS, Watkins AJ, Carr ND, et al. Nutrient induced thermogenesis during major colorectal excision—a pilot study. Colorectal Dis 2005; 7(1):74–78.
27. O'Donnell J, Axelrod P, Fisher C, Lorber B, et al. Use and effectiveness of hypothermia blankets for febrile patients in the intensive care unit. Clin Infect Dis 1997; 24(6):1208–1213.
28. Tsukada K, Miyazaki T, Kato H, et al. Body fat accumulation and postoperative complications after abdominal surgery. Am Surg 2004; 70(4):347–351.
29. Edmonds MJ, Crichton TJ, Runciman WB, Pradhan M, et al. Evidence-based risk factors for postoperative deep vein thrombosis. ANZ J Surg 2004; 74(12):1082–1097.
30. Prandoni P, Sabbion P, Tanduo C, Errigo G, Zanon E, Bernardi E, et al. Prevention of venous thromboembolism in high-risk surgical and medical patients. Semin Vasc Med 2001; 1(1):61–70.
31. Wille-Jorgensen P, Rasmussen MS, Andersen BR, Borly L, et al. Heparins and mechanical methods for thromboprophylaxis in colorectal surgery. Cochrane Database Syst Rev 2003; 4:CD001217.
32. Gutt CN, Oniu T, Wolkener F, Mehrabi A, Mistry S, Buchler MW, et al. Prophylaxis and treatment of deep vein thrombosis in general surgery. Am J Surg 2005; 189(1):14–22.
33. Cruse PJ, Foord R. The epidemiology of wound infection. A 10-year prospective study of 62,939 wounds. Surg Clin North Am 1980; 60(1):27–40.
34. Roberts AW, Visconti JA. The rational and irrational use of systemic antimicrobial drugs. Am J Hosp Pharm 1972; 29(10):828–834.
35. Craig WA, Uman SJ, Shaw WR, Ramgopal V, Eagan LL, Leopold ET, et al. Hospital use of antimicrobial drugs. Survey at 19 hospitals and results of antimicrobial control program. Ann Intern Med 1978; 89(5 Pt 2 suppl):793–795.
36. Song F, Glenny AM. Antimicrobial prophylaxis in colorectal surgery: a systematic review of randomized controlled trials. Br J Surg 1998; 85(9):1232–1241.
37. Dellinger EP, Gross PA, Barrett TL, Krause PJ, Martone WJ, McGowan JE Jr., Sweet RL, et al. Quality standard for antimicrobial prophylaxis in surgical procedures. The Infectious Diseases Society of America. Infect Control Hosp Epidemiol 1994; 15(3): 182–188.

38. Rowe-Jones DC, Peel AL, Kingston RD, Shaw JF, Teasdale C, Cole DS, et al. Single dose cefotaxime plus metronidazole versus three dose cefuroxime plus metronidazole as prophylaxis against wound infection in colorectal surgery: multicentre prospective randomised study. BMJ 1990; 300(6716):18–22.

39. Jimenez JC, Wilson SE. Prophylaxis of infection for elective colorectal surgery. Surg Infect (Larchmt) 2003; 4(3):273–280.

40. Schwartz CI, Heyman AS, Rao AC. Prophylactic nasogastric tube decompression: is its use justified? South Med J 1995; 88(8):825–830.

41. Nelson R, Tse B, Edwards S. Systematic review of prophylactic nasogastric decompression after abdominal operations. Br J Surg 2005; 92(6):673–680.

42. Nichols RL, Condon RE. Preoperative preparation of the colon. Surg Gynecol Obstet 1971; 132(2):323–337.

43. Holte K, Nielsen KG, Madsen JL, Kehlet H, et al. Randomized clinical trial of mechanical bowel preparation versus no preparation before elective left-sided colorectal surgery. Br J Surg 2005; 92(4):409–414.

44. Bucher P, Gervaz P, Soravia C, Mermillod B, Erne M, Morel P, et al. Physiologic effects of bowel preparation. Dis Colon Rectum 2004; 47(8):1397–1402.

45. Slim K, Panis Y, Chipponi J. Mechanical colonic preparation for surgery or how surgeons fight the wrong battle. Gastroenterol Clin Biol 2002; 26(8–9):667–669.

46. Guenaga KF, Matos D, Castro AA, Atallah AN, Wille-Jorgensen P, et al. Mechanical bowel preparation for elective colorectal surgery. Cochrane Database Syst Rev 2005; 1:CD001544.

47. Sheldon TA, Cullum N, Dawson D, et al. What's the evidence that NICE guidance has been implemented? Results from a national evaluation using time series analysis, audit of patients' notes, and interviews. BMJ 2004; 329(7473):999.

48. Kehlet H, Dahl JB. Anaesthesia, surgery, and challenges in postoperative recovery. Lancet 2003; 362(9399):1921–1928.

49. Burger JW, van't Riet M, Jeekel J. Abdominal incisions: techniques and postoperative complications. Scand J Surg 2002; 91(4):315–321.

50. Reidel MA, Knaebel HP, Seiler CM, et al. Postsurgical pain outcome of vertical and transverse abdominal incision: design of a randomized controlled equivalence trial (ISRCTN60734227). BMC Surg 2003; 3(1):9.

51. Grantcharov TP, Rosenberg J. Vertical compared with transverse incisions in abdominal surgery. Eur J Surg 2001; 167(4):260–267.

52. Branagan G, Finnis D. Prognosis after anastomotic leakage in colorectal surgery. Dis Colon Rectum 2005; 48(5):1021–1026.

53. Testini M, Margari A, Amoruso M, Lissidini G, Bonomo GM, et al. The dehiscence of colorectal anastomoses: the risk factors. Ann Ital Chir 2000; 71(4):433–440.

54. Wagner OJ, Egger B. Influential factors in anastomosis healing. Swiss Surg 2003; 9(3):105–113.

55. Egger B, Inglin R, Zeeh J, Dirsch O, Huang Y, Buchler MW, et al. Insulin-like growth factor I and truncated keratinocyte growth factor accelerate healing of left-sided colonic anastomoses. Br J Surg 2001; 88(1):90–98.

56. Hansen O, Schwenk W, Hucke HP, Stock W, et al. Colorectal stapled anastomoses. Experiences and results. Dis Colon Rectum 1996; 39(1):30–36.

57. McGinn FP, Gartell PC, Clifford PC, Brunton FJ, et al. Staples or sutures for low colorectal anastomoses: a prospective randomized trial. Br J Surg 1985; 72(8):603–605.

58. Everett WG, Friend PJ, Forty J. Comparison of stapling and hand-suture for left-sided large bowel anastomosis. Br J Surg 1986; 73(5):345–348.

59. Docherty JG, McGregor JR, Akyol AM, Murray GD, Galloway DJ, et al. Comparison of manually constructed and stapled anastomoses in colorectal surgery. West of Scotland and Highland Anastomosis Study Group. Ann Surg 1995; 221(2):176–184.

60. Petitti T, Lippolis G, Ferrozzi L. Manual colonic anastomosis with continuous single layer suture. Our experience. G Chir 2003; 24(5):202–204.

61. Moran BJ. Stapling instruments for intestinal anastomosis in colorectal surgery. Br J Surg 1996; 83(7):902–909.
62. Morino M, Bertello A, Garbarini A, Rozzio G, Repici A, et al. Malignant colonic obstruction managed by endoscopic stent decompression followed by laparoscopic resections. Surg Endosc 2002; 16(10):1483–1487.
63. Shellito PC. Complications of abdominal stoma surgery. Dis Colon Rectum 1998; 41(12):1562–1572.
64. Garcia-Botello SA, Garcia-Armengol J, Garcia-Granero E, et al. A prospective audit of the complications of loop ileostomy construction and takedown. Dig Surg 2004; 21(5–6): 440–446.
65. Chaudhri S, Brown L, Hassan I, Horgan AF, et al. Preoperative intensive, community-based vs. traditional stoma education: a randomized, controlled trial. Dis Colon Rectum 2005; 48(3):504–509.
66. Williams NS, Nasmyth DG, Jones D, Smith AH, et al. De-functioning stomas: a prospective controlled trial comparing loop ileostomy with loop transverse colostomy. Br J Surg 1986; 73(7):566–570.
67. Marusch F, Koch A, Schmidt U, et al. Value of a protective stoma in low anterior resections for rectal cancer. Dis Colon Rectum 2002; 45(9):1164–1171.
68. Jesus EC, Karliczek A, Matos D, Castro AA, Atallah AN, et al. Prophylactic anastomotic drainage for colorectal surgery. Cochrane Database Syst Rev 2004; 4:CD002100.
69. Chambers WM, Mortensen NJ. Postoperative leakage and abscess formation after colorectal surgery. Best Pract Res Clin Gastroenterol 2004; 18(5):865–880.
70. Merad F, Hay JM, Fingerhut A, et al. Is prophylactic pelvic drainage useful after elective rectal or anal anastomosis? A multicenter controlled randomized trial. French Association for Surgical Research. Surgery 1999; 125(5):529–535.
71. Behm B, Stollman N. Postoperative ileus: etiologies and interventions. Clin Gastroenterol Hepatol 2003; 1(2):71–80.
72. Chen HH, Wexner SD, Iroatulam AJ, et al. Laparoscopic colectomy compares favorably with colectomy by laparotomy for reduction of postoperative ileus. Dis Colon Rectum 2000; 43(1):61–65.
73. KMochiki E, Nakabayashi Tamimura H, Haga N, Asao T, Kuwano H, et al. Gastrointestinal recovery and outcome after laparoscopy-assisted versus conventional open distal gastrectomy for early gastric cancer. World J Surg 2002; 26(9):1145–1149.
74. Waldhausen JH, Schirmer BD. The effect of ambulation on recovery from postoperative ileus. Ann Surg 1990; 212(6):671–677.
75. Kehlet H. Multimodal approach to control postoperative pathophysiology and rehabilitation. Br J Anaesth 1997; 78(5):606–617.
76. Liu SS, Carpenter RL, Mackey DC, et al. Effects of perioperative analgesic technique on rate of recovery after colon surgery. Anesthesiology 1995; 83(4):757–765.
77. Bredtmann RD, Herden HN, Teichmann W, et al. Epidural analgesia in colonic surgery: results of a randomized prospective study. Br J Surg 1990; 77(6):638–642.
78. Kanazi GE, Thompson JS, Boskovski NA. Effect of epidural analgesia on postoperative ileus after ileal pouch-anal anastomosis. Am Surg 1996; 62(6):499–502.
79. Cheatham ML, Chapman WC, Key SP, Sawyers JL, et al. A meta-analysis of selective versus routine nasogastric decompression after elective laparotomy. Ann Surg 1995; 221(5):469–476; discussion 476–478.
80. Hartsell PA, Frazee RC, Harrison JB, Smith RW, et al. Early postoperative feeding after elective colorectal surgery. Arch Surg 1997; 132(5):518–520; discussion 520–521.
81. Carr CS, Ling KD, Boulos P, Singer M, et al. Randomised trial of safety and efficacy of immediate postoperative enteral feeding in patients undergoing gastrointestinal resection. BMJ 1996; 312(7035):869–871.
82. Basse L, Raskov HH, Hjort Jakobsen D, et al. Accelerated postoperative recovery programme after colonic resection improves physical performance, pulmonary function and body composition. Br J Surg 2002; 89(4):446–453.

83. Cheape JD, Wexner SD, James K, Jagelman DG, et al. Does metoclopramide reduce the length of ileus after colorectal surgery? A prospective randomized trial. Dis Colon Rectum 1991; 34(6):437–441.
84. Smith AJ, Nissan A, Lanouette NM, et al. Prokinetic effect of erythromycin after colorectal surgery: randomized, placebo-controlled, double-blind study. Dis Colon Rectum 2000; 43(3):333–337.
85. Ponec RJ, Saunders MD, Kimmey MB. Neostigmine for the treatment of acute colonic pseudo-obstruction. N Engl J Med 1999; 341(3):137–141.
86. Kelley MC, Hocking MP, Marchand SD, Sninsky CA, et al. Ketorolac prevents postoperative small intestinal ileus in rats. Am J Surg 1993; 165(1):107–111; discussion 112.
87. Ferraz AA, Cowles VE, Condon RE, et al. Nonopioid analgesics shorten the duration of postoperative ileus. Am Surg 1995; 61(12):1079–1083.
88. Taguchi A, Sharma N, Saleem RM, et al. Selective postoperative inhibition of gastrointestinal opioid receptors. N Engl J Med 2001; 345(13):935–940.
89. Shafiq N, Malhotra S, Pandhi P. Effect of cyclooxygenase inhibitors in postoperative ileus: an experimental study. Methods Find Exp Clin Pharmacol 2002; 24(5):275–278.
90. Asao T, Kuwano H, Nakamura J, Morinaga N, Hirayama I, Ide M, et al. Gum chewing enhances early recovery from postoperative ileus after laparoscopic colectomy. J Am Coll Surg 2002; 195(1):30–32.
91. Parker MC, Wilson MS, Menzies D, et al. Colorectal surgery: the risk and burden of adhesion-related complications. Colorectal Dis 2004; 6(6):506–511.
92. Beck DE, Cohen Z, Fleshman JW, Kaufman HS, van Goor H, Wolff BG, et al. A prospective, randomized, multicenter, controlled study of the safety of Seprafilm adhesion barrier in abdominopelvic surgery of the intestine. Dis Colon Rectum 2003; 46(10): 1310–1319.
93. Tang CL, Seow-Choen F, Fook-Chong S, Eu KW, et al. Bioresorbable adhesion barrier facilitates early closure of the defunctioning ileostomy after rectal excision: a prospective, randomized trial. Dis Colon Rectum 2003; 46(9):1200–1207.
94. Kudo FA, Nishibe T, Miyazaki K, Murashita T, Nishibe M, Yasuda K, et al. Use of bioresorbable membrane to prevent postoperative small bowel obstruction in transabdominal aortic aneurysm surgery. Surg Today 2004; 34(8):648–651.
95. Smoot RL, Gostout CJ, Rajan E., et al, et al. Is early colonoscopy after admission for acute diverticular bleeding needed? Am J Gastroenterol 2003; 98(9):1996–1999.
96. Sorbi D, Gostout CJ, Peura D, et al. An assessment of the management of acute bleeding varices: a multicenter prospective member-based study. Am J Gastroenterol 2003; 98(11): 2424–2434.
97. Michida T, Kawano S, Masuda E, et al. Role of endothelin 1 in hemorrhagic shock-induced gastric mucosal injury in rats. Gastroenterology 1994; 106(4):988–993.
98. Cheung LY, Porterfield G. Protection of gastric mucosa against acute ulceration by intravenous infusion of sodium bicarbonate. Am J Surg 1979; 137(1):106–110.
99. Silen W, Merhav A, Simson JN. The pathophysiology of stress ulcer disease. World J Surg 1981; 5(2):165–174.
100. Ritchie WP Jr. Acute gastric mucosal damage induced by bile salts, acid, and ischemia. Gastroenterology 1975; 68(4 Pt 1):699–707.
101. Cash BD. Evidence-based medicine as it applies to acid suppression in the hospitalized patient. Crit Care Med 2002; 30(6 suppl):S373–S378.
102. Rostom A, Dube C, Wells G, et al. Prevention of NSAID-induced gastroduodenal ulcers. Cochrane Database Syst Rev 2002; 4:CD002296.
103. Torralba JA, Robles R, Parrilla P, et al. Subtotal colectomy vs. intraoperative colonic irrigation in the management of obstructed left colon carcinoma. Dis Colon Rectum 1998; 41(1):18–22.
104. Lee EC, Murray JJ, Coller JA, Roberts PL, Schoetz DJ Jr., et al. Intraoperative colonic lavage in nonelective surgery for diverticular disease. Dis Colon Rectum 1997; 40(6): 669–674.

105. Choen S, Tsunoda A, Nicholls RJ. Prospective randomized trial comparing anal function after hand sewn ileoanal anastomosis with mucosectomy versus stapled ileoanal anastomosis without mucosectomy in restorative proctocolectomy. Br J Surg 1991; 78(4): 430–434.
106. Fazio VW, Coutsoftides T, Steiger E. Factors influencing the outcome of treatment of small bowel cutaneous fistula. World J Surg 1983; 7(4):481–488.
107. Rubelowsky J, Machiedo GW. Reoperative versus conservative management for gastrointestinal fistulas. Surg Clin North Am 1991; 71(1):147–157.
108. Rolandelli R, Roslyn JJ. Surgical management and treatment of sepsis associated with gastrointestinal fistulas. Surg Clin North Am 1996; 76(5):1111–1122.
109. Alberts JC, Parvaiz A, Moran BJ. Predicting risk and diminishing the consequences of anastomotic dehiscence following rectal resection. Colorectal Dis 2003; 5(5):478–482.
110. Mella J, Biffin A, Radcliffe AG, Stamatakis JD, Steele RJ, et al. Population-based audit of colorectal cancer management in two UK health regions. Colorectal Cancer Working Group, Royal College of Surgeons of England Clinical Epidemiology and Audit Unit. Br J Surg 1997; 84(12):1731–1736.
111. Goligher JC, Graham NG, De Dombal FT. Anastomotic dehiscence after anterior resection of rectum and sigmoid. Br J Surg 1970; 57(2):109–118.
112. Junger W, Junger WG, Miller K, et al. Early detection of anastomotic leaks after colorectal surgery by measuring endotoxin in the drainage fluid. Hepatogastroenterology 1996; 43(12):1523–1529.
113. Renzulli P, Laffer UT. Learning curve: the surgeon as a prognostic factor in colorectal cancer surgery. Recent Results Cancer Res 2005; 165:86–104.
114. Zorcolo L, Covotta L, Carlomagno N, Bartolo DC, et al. Toward lowering morbidity, mortality, and stoma formation in emergency colorectal surgery: the role of specialization. Dis Colon Rectum 2003; 46(11):1461–1467; discussion 1467–1468.
115. Prystowsky JB, Bordage G, Feinglass JM. Patient outcomes for segmental colon resection according to surgeon's training, certification, and experience. Surgery 2002; 132(4): 663–670; discussion 670–672.
116. Okuyama M, Ikeda K, Shibata T, Tsukahara Y, Kitada M, Shimano T, et al. Preoperative iron supplementation and intraoperative transfusion during colorectal cancer surgery. Surg Today 2005; 35(1):36–40.
117. Jensen LS, Kissmeyer-Nielsen P, Wolff B, Qvist N, et al. Randomised comparison of leucocyte-depleted versus buffy-coat-poor blood transfusion and complications after colorectal surgery. Lancet 1996; 348(9031):841–845.
118. Jensen LS, Puho E, Pedersen L, Mortensen FV, Sorensen HT, et al. Long-term survival after colorectal surgery associated with buffy-coat-poor and leucocyte-depleted blood transfusion: a follow-up study. Lancet 2005; 365(9460):681–682.

7

Preoperative Assessment

Heinz E. Schulenburg, Stuart D. Murdoch, and Hamish A. McLure
Department of Anesthesia, St. James's University Hospital, Leeds, U.K.

INTRODUCTION

The preoperative visit is one of the cornerstones of good anesthetic practice. It gives the anesthetist an opportunity to assess the patient, optimize medical treatment, discuss anesthetic management, gain consent, and decide upon appropriate anesthetic equipment before the patient arrives in theater (Table 1). In the past, preoperative assessment was often performed in a haphazard fashion. Inexperienced junior members of the surgical team were tasked with organizing an assessment of fitness for surgery. A large number of investigations were ordered to satisfy "test-hungry" anesthetists and prevent cancellations. These tests were often unnecessary and frequently ignored. The lack of evidence for the benefits of these "routine" preoperative tests and their excessive cost led to the development of more structured assessment processes in the form of clinical guidelines (1). Many of these are dependent upon expert opinion and, even in the case of National Institute for Clinical Excellence (NICE) guidelines, consensus cannot always be reached. This confusion is the result of a dearth of well-constructed studies to enable evidence-based recommendations. Where studies into preoperative investigations have been conducted, they are usually aimed at risk stratification. While this information is clearly of benefit, there is little data on the ability of preoperative tests to change practice

Table 1 Goals of Preoperative Assessment

Identification of medical conditions
Initiation of further investigations
Optimization of medical treatment
Formulation of an anesthetic plan in terms of:
    Regional vs. general anesthesia, or both
    Premedication
    Monitoring
    Intravenous access
    Airway management
    Postoperative management
Discussion of risks and gaining informed consent

and improve outcome. Consequently, conflicting advice in preoperative assessment guidelines is widespread. This variation may be influenced by differences in the physiological and psychological characteristics of the local population, the medicolegal environment, and socioeconomic factors. In the guideline for cardiac assessment produced by the American College of Cardiology and American Heart Association, a much larger array of tests are recommended for patients with ischemic heart disease than would be expected in standard British practice (2).

The preoperative assessment should be performed in advance of surgery with enough time to allow for appropriate assessment, optimization, and consent. However, the shortage of beds in the British National Health Service has resulted in an increasing number of surgical patients being admitted to hospital on the day of surgery. Even patients with complex medical conditions, or those undergoing major surgery, may not appear till shortly before they are due in theater. In some centers, this problem has been tackled by the organization of preoperative assessment clinics, staffed by nurses, usually with the presence of, or access to senior anesthetists. Patients can be screened for medical problems, and investigations ordered according to predetermined guidelines. Anesthetic management issues can be introduced to the patient, setting the scene for a more informed discussion when the anesthetist, who is to give the anesthetic, meets the patient before the operation. It also provides an opportunity to identify those patients who would benefit from further assessment by an anesthetist before admission on the day of surgery. In one U.K. study, the use of nurse-led preoperative assessment for 2726 patients reduced the on-the-day cancellation rate from 11% to 5% (3). In a similar observational study in the Netherlands, over 20,000 patients were assessed in a preoperative assessment clinic (4). This resulted in a significant reduction in cancellation of patients from 2.0% to 0.9%.

Preoperative assessment should have a structured approach. This usually consists of a review of systems (centered on the cardiovascular and respiratory systems), a medication history (including allergies), and an anesthetic history. A physical examination, directed by the history, should be performed, with additional attention paid to consideration of airway anatomy and potential intubation difficulties. Where significant symptoms and signs are new, old and evolving, or severe, further investigations may be required.

SYSTEMS REVIEW

Cardiac Assessment

Assessment of the cardiovascular system aims to describe the patient's current cardiac status, how and if it can be improved, and what impact this morbidity may have on preoperative outcome. There has been a trend to offer surgery to patients with more severe morbidity, and to an increasingly elderly population of patients, in whom cardiac disease is more common (5). The first step in assessing the patient is to take a history for symptoms of chest pain, shortness of breath, orthopnea, ankle swelling, and palpitations, then perform an examination looking for evidence of cardiac disease (arrhythmias, failure, hypertension, murmurs, etc.). This will be sufficient for most patients. Simple bedside clinical data has been used by several authors to establish risk indexes. The first of these was by Goldman (6). Risk factors were analyzed by multivariate analysis to produce a table where points were awarded for different factors; these were then totaled to produce an overall score indicative of risk (Table 2). This system was modified by Detsky who added three further

Table 2 Goldman Risk Indices

Risk factor	Points
Third heart sound or jugular venous distension	11
Myocardial infarction in preceding 6 mo	10
Nonsinus rhythm	7
Abdominal, thoracic, or aortic operation	3
Age >70 yr	5
Significant aortic stenosis	3
Emergency operation	4
Poor patient condition	3

Note: Score 5 or less, cardiac mortality is 0.2%; score 6–25, cardiac mortality is 2%; score > 25 points, cardiac mortality is 56%.

variables, changed the point scoring system, and improved its accuracy in high-risk patients (Table 3) (7). A more recent scoring system is the "revised cardiac risk index," which was based on prospective data on over 4000 patients undergoing major noncardiac surgery (8). The authors identified six independent predictors of complications. This was validated in a second group of patients and proved to be more accurate than other published scores. Factors that have consistently proved to be a high risk for perioperative myocardial complications include recent myocardial infarction, residual ischemia after myocardial infarction, recent bypass graft or percutaneous transluminal coronary angioplasty (PTCA), angina class III–IV, clinical ischemia and congestive failure, and clinical ischemia with malignant arrhythmias (9).

Respiratory Assessment

The preoperative respiratory assessment is aimed at quantifying respiratory function in terms of gas exchange and ability to clear secretions. Anesthesia exerts multiple adverse effects upon the respiratory system. Inhalational anesthetic gases, opioids, and benzodiazepines are respiratory depressant agents, an effect that persists postoperatively (10). The induction of anesthesia produces a 20% reduction in functional residual capacity (FRC), which may last for several days after surgery (11). The

Table 3 Desky Scoring System

High-risk surgical procedures: intraperitoneal, intrathoracic, suprainguinal vascular
History of ischemic heart disease
History of congestive cardiac failure
History of cerebrovascular disease
Preoperative treatment with insulin
Raised serum creatinine

Note: Each factor was awarded one point if present. The score correlated with risk.

Points	Risk (%)
0	0.4
1	0.9
2	6.6
3 or more	11.0

reduced FRC encroaches on closing capacity leading to basal atelectasis. Atelectasis increases intrapulmonary shunting, worsening hypoxia. In addition, abdominal surgery has a significant effect on diaphragmatic movement, which reduces vital capacity (12). This is particularly marked in patients having upper abdominal surgery, where pain may be severe. Reduced lung volumes, shallow breathing, and the inability to cough lead to sputum retention and set the scene for infection. This effect is pronounced in smokers, the elderly, the obese, and in patients with underlying lung disease. In the immediate postoperative period, lung function will always be worse. So patients with little respiratory reserve may require respiratory support.

Respiratory assessment begins with eliciting a history of shortness of breath, wheeze, sputum production, smoking, and past symptoms of known lung disease, such as asthma, chronic obstructive pulmonary disease, recent chest infections, and previous hospital admissions with respiratory disease. Symptoms should be assessed for severity by asking about exercise tolerance and degree of dyspnea. Patients are usually good at evaluating their current status. Medical therapy and response to treatment are important, and specific enquiry should be made about the use of steroid therapy, because these patients may require perioperative steroid supplementation.

Past and present cigarette use should be documented. Cessation of smoking to reduce mucus secretions and allow recovery of airway mucociliary transport function is often advocated. To gain maximum benefit requires a period of abstinence of several weeks. Despite proven advantages, most units put little effort into reducing the level of smoking in their population because it is required at a time of intense psychological stress when success seems remote.

A thorough clinical respiratory examination is indicated if abnormalities are detected in the history, with vigilance for signs or complications of respiratory disease (e.g., right heart failure). An informal assessment of exercise tolerance, making the patient walk to the end of the ward and back, or climbing a flight of stairs can provide a reliable means of testing cardiorespiratory function and reserve. Where there is doubt, specific investigations should be performed.

Medication and Allergic History

The vast majority of surgical patients are regularly taking some form of medication. Most drugs have little bearing on anesthetic technique, but some exceptions may be important (Table 4). Drugs and dosages should be recorded along with an impression of compliance and the timing of recent drugs doses. It is interesting to note self-administered medication (e.g., herbal remedies) because they provide a useful insight into the personality of the patient, but they rarely impact on anesthetic management. In addition to current medication, it is important to note a history of allergy or other adverse reactions to previous medication, foodstuffs, or materials. Latex allergy is increasingly common and may produce a devastating reaction, which is characterised by a delayed onset of cardiovascular collapse. It is found more commonly in healthcare workers, and patients chronically exposed to latex (e.g., spina bifida) (13).

Medication and Allergic History

Probably the best indicator of future response to anesthesia is the response to previous anesthetics. If the patient has never been anesthetized, then a family history of problems should be sought, looking for malignant hyperthermia or pseudocholinesterase

Table 4 Significant Medication

Medication	Significance	Action
Steroids	Reduced adrenal response to stress resulting in perioperative hypotension	Perioperative steroid supplementation
Antiplatelet agents (e.g., aspirin, clopidogrel)	Hemorrhage	May need to be withheld for at least a week in some procedures (e.g., prostatectomy)
Antihypertensives	May exacerbate hypotensive effects of some agents	Risks of withholding higher than continuing, so maintain pre-op treatment
Heparin	Hemorrhage	Dosing interval may need to be adjusted prior to central regional blockade
Warfarin	Hemorrhage	May need to be stopped and substituted for heparin
Lithium	Increases sensitivity to muscle relaxants and may cause diabetes insipidus	Ideally withhold for 1 week prior to surgery
Tricyclic antidepressants	Block reuptake of norepinephrine and epinephrine. May predispose to arrhythmias	Avoid other arrhythmogenic anesthetic medication (e.g., halothane)
Monoamine oxidase inhibitors	Pethidine may cause hypotension and collapse, hyperthermia. Indirect acting sympathomimetics (e.g., ephedrine) may cause hypertensive crisis	Avoid pethidine. Carefully monitor use of morphine

deficiency. With luck, anesthetic charts will be available, supplying details of difficult cannulation, intubation, ventilation, response to drugs, and other adverse events. The patient should be asked about perioperative nausea and vomiting. In a patient with a difficult-looking airway, a history of severe sore throat following previous anesthetics may point toward difficulties with intubation. A description of pain intensity and duration following past surgery will help the anesthetist to formulate an analgesic plan tailored to the patient and their current operation.

Airway Assessment

Airway complications are the single most important cause of anesthetic-related morbidity and mortality. The incidence of difficult intubations is up to 5% (14). A careful history and examination, combined with bedside tests should give some indication of ease of intubation. Additional indicators of potential problems are cervical rheumatoid arthritis, airway malignancies, previous head and neck surgery, neck radiotherapy, diabetes, and syndromes associated with difficult airways (e.g., Downs syndrome, Pierre Robin syndrome, and Treacher Collins syndrome). When assessing the airway, the anesthetist should enquire about symptoms of reflux, as this will have a significant impact on the choice of airway device and the technique by which it is placed.

Bedside airway examination should include observing the patient for risk factors, such as a receding chin, protruding teeth, thickset neck, obesity, large breasts, beards, masses, limited gape, limited neck movement, and deviation of the trachea. A variety of tests have been devised for quickly assessing the patient's airway. These range from simple movement tests to more complex scoring systems.

Interincisor Gap

With the patient's mouth maximally open, the distance between the incisors is measured. If it is less than 4 cm or three-finger breaths, it is indicative of possible difficulties with airway management.

Calder Test

An inability to protrude the mandible in front of the upper incisors is associated with difficult laryngoscopy (15).

Thyromental Distance

This is a measurement between the top of the thyroid cartilage and the tip of the mandible, with the neck in full extension. Values less than 6.5 cm predict difficult intubation.

Modified Mallampati Score

This is the view obtained with the patient upright, head in neutral position, mouth maximally open, and protruding the tongue without phonating (16,17). It is graded I–IV, depending on the pharyngeal structures that are visible (Table 5). Class III (only the soft and hard palate is visible) and IV (only hard palate visible) are associated with difficult intubation. Despite its popularity, this test has a low sensitivity of around 60%.

Wilson Score

Five factors (obesity, reduced head and neck movement, reduced jaw opening, presence of buck teeth, or a receding mandible) are given 0 to 2 points, to a maximum of 10 points (18). A score of more than two predicts 75% of difficult intubations.

Although appealing, these bedside airway-screening tests have only moderate discriminative power for identifying patients with potentially difficult airways. Each test alone has a sensitivity of 20% to 62%, and specificity of 80% to 97%. Combining two or three tests adds incremental diagnostic value. When used together, the Modified Mallampati, thyromental distance, and interincisor gap yield a sensitivity and specificity of up to 85% and 95%, respectively (19). Despite these impressive figures, the usefulness of these tests remains controversial. However, they play an important

Table 5 Modified Mallampati Score

Grade	View at laryngoscopy
I	Uvula, faucial pillars, soft palate visible
II	Faucial pillars and soft palate visible
III	Only soft palate visible
IV	Only hard palate visible

safety role by directing the anesthetist toward thinking about a plan of action in case of failure to intubate.

INVESTIGATIONS

The routine ordering of "baseline" tests such as a full blood count, electrolyte screen, blood glucose, electrocardiogram (ECG), and chest X ray (CXR) has largely been abandoned. NICE has produced a comprehensive document suggesting appropriate investigations in virtually all clinical scenarios. The type of surgery is graded into minor, moderate, and major. Patients are then stratified by age with investigation tables in sections depending on specific system pathology. To find the recommended investigations, the pathology section is found first. The patient's age is selected and then the type of surgery is decided upon. Armed with this information, the clinician can select appropriate investigations. A summary handbook has been produced, but to access the full document, the clinician must have access to the NICE web site. "Routine" tests are still recommended in certain circumstances, although the supporting evidence is often weak.

Full Blood Count, Electrolytes, and Blood Glucose

A full blood count is often requested for female patients, those with a history of cardiorespiratory symptoms, Asians, and those with a history of bleeding. Abnormal results are relatively common. Up to 5% of patients have a hemoglobin level, which is lower than 10 to 10.5 g/dL (20). However, this leads to a change in management in only 0.1% to 2.7% of patients (20). As the tolerance to anemia increases, it is likely that the number of management changes will be reduced even further. Routine clotting examination is performed less often, but again, there is little evidence that they change management and, even less, that they affect outcome. Abnormalities of routine electrolyte testing are found in only 1.4% to 2.5% of patients (20). Management is very rarely altered as a result.

Electrocardiogram

The use of a preoperative ECG is recommended for a wide range of patients according to NICE guidance. It is inexpensive, noninvasive, easy to obtain, and safe. The incidence of ECG abnormalities increases with age and American Society of Anesthesiologists (ASA) status. Many units have a policy in which patients have an ECG if they are between the ages of 50 and 60, or 40 if they are diabetic, if they have a history of cardiovascular disease, or have an electrolyte imbalance. However, when the evidence for the use of a preoperative ECG was analyzed by NICE and Munro, they both reported that abnormal ECG results altered management in only 5.8% and 2.2%, respectively (20).

Chest X Ray

Preoperative CXRs are often ordered, but are rarely useful. Munro estimated that the CXR is abnormal in 2.5% to 37%, but affects clinical management in only 0% to 2.1% (20). In 1979, a working party from the Royal College of Radiologists produced guidelines on preoperative CXR indications, which reduced the number of tests that were performed (21). They recommended performing a preoperative CXR in patients with acute respiratory symptoms, those with possible metastases, those with cardiorespiratory disease who have not been imaged in the last year, and recent immigrants from countries where tuberculosis is endemic. The NICE guidelines are even more restrictive with preoperative CXRs performed only in patients with worsening respiratory disease and those with severe cardiovascular disease and renal disease with hypertension.

Blood Gases

A baseline arterial blood gas is useful in patients with severe respiratory disease. A $PaCO_2$ more than 6.0 kPa is indicative of progressive respiratory failure and is predictive of postoperative complications. Blood gases analysis should be done on any patient who is breathless at rest or with minimal exertion.

Peak Flow

The peak expiratory flow rate (PEFR) is not reliable as an isolated reading, but it can provide important information on responsiveness to bronchodilator treatment in patients with asthma or chronic obstructive pulmonary disease (COPD). The current status may be assessed if the patient has kept a peak flow diary. Values of less than 200 L/min predict a significantly reduced ability to expectorate effectively postoperatively.

Spirometry

Forced vital capacity (FVC), forced expiratory volume in one second (FEV_1), and the ratio of FEV_1/FVC may be assessed. Values greater than 70% for the FEV_1/FVC ratio is seen as within normal limits. A FEV_1 of less than 1 L suggests that effective coughing and clearance of sputum may be impaired postoperatively, and that a period of intensive care therapy may be indicated. Spirometry has been used to assess risk in patients with significant respiratory disease. However, there is some evidence that suggests that spirometry is not of significant predictive value for respiratory complications, even in patients with severe respiratory disease (22). It is helpful in patients with limited mobility where the patient's functional ability (e.g., walking up and down the ward or climbing stairs) cannot be tested. Spirometry may help in selecting patients who will benefit from preoperative efforts to improve pulmonary function (e.g., bronchodilation therapy, physiotherapy, and deep-breathing exercises).

Echocardiography

A cardiac echo can reveal important information about the heart, including left ventricular function, valvular anatomy, and pressures within the cardiopulmonary system. Detection of significant stenosis, particularly aortic stenosis, or regurgitation in the valves can alter management and significantly reduce perioperative mortality. An assessment of left ventricular function is useful in patients with cardiac failure, although it tends to predict further episodes of ventricular dysfunction rather than ischaemic complications. The authors of a large study examining the benefit of routine echocardiography in a population with known or suspected heart disease, concluded that echocardiography had limited additional prognostic value in identifying complications (23). However, in isolation, a low ejection fraction did identify patients at risk of congestive cardiac failure and ventricular tachycardia.

Exercise Electrocardiogram/Stress Echo

In patients with an abnormal ECG or echocardiography, where cardiac symptoms are severe or when surgery is likely to place high demands on the cardiovascular system, additional tests may be performed to identify individuals at higher risk of cardiac complications. An exercise ECG may be performed to reveal signs of ischemia in patients whose resting ECG is normal, but who have symptoms suggestive of cardiac disease. In patients who are unable to exercise, pharmacological agents such as dobutamine may be administered to stress the heart, and echocardiography used to assess cardiac functional reserve. The appearance of wall-motion abnormalities at low stress levels has been shown to predict an increased risk for perioperative events.

Chest Computer Tomography

Chest CT is more often performed by the surgical team to identify the extent of neoplastic disease, but it may provide useful information for the anesthetist in patients with tracheal distortion, or with mediastinal masses whose lungs may be difficult to ventilate due to outflow obstruction.

SPECIFIC MEDICAL CONDITIONS

Hypertension

The management of preoperative hypertension is contentious. In the medical setting, hypertension is clearly related to an increase in cardiovascular events and death (24). The significance of hypertension in the perioperative period is unclear. Prys-Roberts demonstrated an increase in blood pressure lability and myocardial ischemia in patients defined as hypertensive, but with no difference in outcome (25). This led to the recommendation that blood pressure should be treated prior to surgery, and patients should be delayed until blood pressure control had been achieved. However, many of the patients in this study had very severe hypertension, with systolic blood pressure greater than 200 mmHg (even the control group had systolic blood pressure, which would now be considered pathological). Since then, many further studies have examined the relationship between hypertension and perioperative outcome. Howell performed a meta-analysis reviewing hypertension and perioperative events (26). He concluded that while there was a small increase in perioperative risk associated with hypertension, this might be due to an end-organ damage rather than hypertension. In terms of a patient presenting with raised blood pressure at the time of surgery, if systolic blood pressure is less than 180 mmHg and diastolic blood pressure below 110 mmHg, surgery should proceed. This is in line with the recommendations of the American Heart Association/American College of Cardiologists. In patients with blood pressure in excess of this limit, the American guidelines advocate a delay in surgery while the blood pressure is treated. Howell et al. highlight the scarcity of data supporting this and suggest that if the patient is otherwise fit for surgery, then it should proceed but with vigilance with regard to blood pressure control, aiming to maintain it at near normal levels (26). This seems especially apt in patients with malignant disease where delay may be detrimental to the patient.

Recent Myocardial Infarction

Traditionally, a six-month interval between myocardial infarction and anesthesia was recommended to reduce cardiovascular risk—a plateau level that could not be substantially further reduced (27). More recently, this advice has changed and consideration is now made of the size and nature of the infarct, its effect on the patient, and the treatment received at time of infarction (28). This means that patients who have a small infarct with no other physiological change in their condition may be considered for surgery within six weeks, although risk may still be increased up to three months. In patients with a more extensive infarction, the risk is increased for a longer duration and, if further infarction occurs, may be permanently increased. As the use of antithrombotic drugs (e.g., clopidogrel) increases, care must be taken in managing the needs of hemostasis for surgery and thrombosis prevention for the heart.

Valvular Heart Disease

Valvular heart disease may have a significant effect during anesthesia. The most important lesion from an anesthetic perspective is aortic stenosis, which was identified by Goldman and the National Confidential Enquiry into Patient Outcome and Death (NCEPOD) report as a major cause of perioperative cardiac complications and death in elderly patients. Aortic stenosis is most commonly caused by degenerative changes to a normal aortic valve, leading to progressive fibrosis and calcification. This process leads to a gradual decrease in the area of the aortic outlet. The outflow obstruction is initially compensated for by ventricular hypertrophy. As the stenosis worsens or coronary artery disease is added, patients may decompensate and experience angina, syncope, and dyspnea on exertion. On examination, patients with aortic stenosis have a slow rising, low volume pulse. On auscultation, an ejection systolic murmur may be heard in the aortic area radiating to the carotids. The suggestion of aortic stenosis should warrant an echocardiography prior to anesthesia. Invasive monitoring of the cardiovascular system is usually performed to allow early intervention and treatment of cardiovascular instability. Coronary artery filling depends upon maintaining an adequate filling time and pressure. The anesthetic technique should avoid tachycardia, vasodilation, and hypotension because this will result in myocardial ischemia and a downward spiral of further hypotension. The use of epidurals in this group of patients is controversial, due to the reduction in systemic vascular resistance. However, with judicious use of vasoconstrictors and incremental epidural dosing, safe satisfactory anesthesia may be achievable.

Asthma

Asthma is characterized by reversible airway obstruction, airway inflammation, mucus hypersecretion, and airway hyperreactivity. Preoperative assessment should be directed at determining the recent course and control of the disease. Resolution of recent exacerbations should be confirmed. Specific triggers, especially the response to nonsteroidal anti-inflammatory drugs (NSAIDS), should be inquired about. The number of recent hospitalizations will give an indication of the severity of the patient's condition. Exercise tolerance should be assessed. PEFR measurement can be helpful, but serial measurements (Peak flow diary) are more informative. Normal values exceed $200\,L/min$. FEV_1/FVC should normally be greater than 70%. A FEV_1, FEV_1/FVC, or a PEFR less than 50% of the predicted normal for that patient indicates moderate-to-severe asthma. An increase of greater than 15% in FEV_1 postbronchodilator therapy is considered clinically significant and an indication of poor control. Inhaled bronchodilators may need to be changed to nebulized bronchodilators during the period of admission. Benzodiazepine and nebulized bronchodilator are useful premedicants. Patients on long-term steroid therapy should receive supplemental doses, preoperatively and postoperatively.

Chronic Obstructive Pulmonary Disease

Chronic obstructive pulmonary disease (COPD) is characterized by airflow obstruction that is generally progressive, and may be accompanied by partially reversible airway hyperreactivity and increased sputum production. The majority of patients are minimally symptomatic. Many patients have some evidence of reversibility of airway obstruction. With advanced COPD, there is maldistribution of ventilation and perfusion resulting in larger areas of intrapulmonary shunting. Hypoxemia is common, leading to pulmonary hypertension and right-heart failure. As with asthma, the emphasis in assessment is on determining current status. Enquiry should be made about recent exacerbations or respiratory tract infections and hospitalizations. Recent changes in dyspnea, wheezing, coughing, and sputum production should be noted. A careful cardiovascular evaluation should be performed to elicit cardiac complications of respiratory disease. It is important to determine whether there is any evidence of reversibility of airway obstruction, because these patients might benefit from preoperative bronchodilator therapy. Patients with a change in sputum should be considered for preoperative chest physiotherapy as well as antibiotics to reduce secretions. Nebulized bronchodilators should be prescribed for patients with evidence of reversibility. Oxygen therapy may be indicated in patients with pulmonary hypertension.

Obesity

Marked obesity produces a restrictive pulmonary pattern. Oxygen consumption is increased and desaturation occurs rapidly in the apnoeic obese patient. FRC is reduced in awake obese patients, and decreases significantly with general anesthesia, rapidly encroaching on closing capacity. Spirometric values and, especially, vital capacity are reduced in relation to the body mass index (BMI). With progressive obesity, the Obesity Hypoventilation Syndrome (OHS) may develop. OHS is characterized by hypoxemia, pulmonary hypertension, polycythemia, and obstructive sleep apnea with loss of carbon dioxide respiratory drive. Preassessment should concentrate on the degree of respiratory impairment and the cardiorespiratory reserve.

Obstructive sleep apnoea is defined as more than five episodes of apnoea per hour of sleep. Apnoea is characterized by the cessation of airflow for longer than 10 seconds. During these periods of apnoea, the PaO_2 decreases and $PaCO_2$ rises, leading to arousal. Obstructive sleep apnea (OSA) is graded in severity by the apnoea/hypopnoea index (AHI). Patients with OSA experience sleep fragmentation and daytime somnolence. Severe OSA, AHI > 30, can result in chronic night time hypoxemia, with pulmonary hypertension and cor pulmonale as possible consequences. Obesity is a major risk factor for OSA, although neck circumference greater than 42 cm correlates better with OSA than obesity itself.

During preassessment, a high degree of suspicion is required to diagnose OSA. The history is of utmost importance because OSA can be diagnosed based on history alone. Inquiry should be made about snoring, daytime sleepiness, restless sleep, and the partner, particularly should be asked about breath holding at night. If suspected, the patient should be referred for overnight polysomnography and continuous positive airway pressure (CPAP) initiated if appropriate. The degree of cardiac involvement should be assessed (i.e., right-heart failure). Blood gas analysis is indicated in severe OSA to determine the patient's baseline PaO_2 and to assess whether there is hypercapnia. Patients with severe OSA treated with nighttime CPAP should have their CPAP continued during their period of hospitalization, and CPAP should be available on recovery. Sedative premedicants should be avoided.

PREMEDICATION

The advent of more potent, less irritant anesthetic induction agents has reduced the need for premedication. However, there is still a role aimed at targeting specific problems (e.g., anxiety, acid aspiration prophylaxis, bronchospasm, prevention of allergic reactions, nausea and vomiting), and as an antisialogue prior to airway manipulation. Admission on the day of surgery may hamper appropriate timing of premedication, requiring list-order changes, although this introduces further risks.

Sedative premedication used to be widely prescribed. However, it is now usually reserved for the pathologically anxious who were not adequately calmed by the preoperative visit, or to reduce myocardial workload in those patients with poorly controlled hypertension or those with significant ischemic heart disease. It is often difficult to guess the correct dose and timing for individual patients, so inadequate anxiolysis or prolonged awakening are relatively common in patients who have received sedative premedication. Benzodiazepines (temazepam, diazepam, and lorazepam) are rapidly absorbed after oral administration. However, the response is highly variable and may precipitate respiratory failure in elderly or infirm patients. Zopiclone is not a benzodiazepine, but acts on the benzodiazepine receptor and has a similar sedative action. It is also well absorbed after oral administration, but may leave patients with an unpleasant taste in their mouth. Opioids (e.g., morphine, and pethidine) used to be part of the standard premedication cocktail. Long-acting agents were given preemptively as a vital part of the analgesic technique. However, although they reduced the quantity of anaesthetic agent administered, they increased the incidence of nausea and vomiting and had little advantage over opioids given intraoperatively. Antihistamines may be surprisingly sedating, have an antiemetic function and may be useful if allergic reactions occur.

Prophylaxis is used in patients at risk of acid aspiration. Acid reflux is reduced by administering an H_2-receptor blocker, preferably several hours before surgery (e.g., oral ranitidine: 150 mg), or a proton pump inhibitor (e.g., oral omeprazole: 20 mg) to decrease gastric fluid volume and increase gastric fluid pH. In addition, prokinetic drugs (e.g., oral metoclopramide: 10 mg) may be given to increase gastric emptying followed by an antacid (such as sodium citrate), immediately prior to anesthesia.

Antibiotic prophylaxis is recommended to prevent deep infection in patients with congenital heart lesions, those who have a prosthetic heart valve, or those at risk of endocarditis. This usually consists of penicillin, sometimes in combination with an aminoglycoside. The procedures at highest risk are those that produce a significant bacteremia, such as gastrointestinal, urological, or dental surgery. Low-risk procedures such as ophthalmic surgery do not require antibiotic prophylaxis unless the airway is to be instrumented. In operations where prosthetic joints, arterial grafts, or mesh hernia repairs, the surgeons often prescribe antibiotics as premedication or to be given at induction of anesthesia.

Patients with a history of bronchospasm may benefit from bronchodilator therapy immediately prior to anesthesia. In patients with severe disease, steroids and antihistamines may also prove beneficial. A similar cocktail of steroids and both H_1- and H_2-blocking antihistamines may be used in patients with a history of allergic reactions. In patients with a history of severe nausea and vomiting, antiemetics may be added to the premedication cocktail. Antisialogues (atropine, glycopyrolate, and hyoscine) may be useful in patients with suspected difficulties with intubation, where airway manipulations (e.g., fibreoptic intubation) are anticipated.

CONSENT

The well-publicized abuse of patients' trust by a minority of doctors has eroded public confidence in medical self-regulation. Palpable public cynicism toward doctors, the wide availability of medical information in the media and on the internet, and an increasingly demanding and litigious public has changed the medicolegal climate in the United Kingdom. In an attempt to win back public favor and avoid imposition of restrictive policing by the state, the medical profession has attempted culture change, moving to a system where doctors' work is transparent and accountable. One area where this is most evident is consent to medical treatment. Over the last decade, the issue of consent has changed from a box-ticking exercise to a major hurdle of public relations in daily clinical practice, in audit, and in research. Processes must be seen to be in place to allow patients to be fully involved in decisions about their care. The path to these decisions, including information about risks and side effects, which have been explained, must be documented.

In 1999, the Association of Anaesthetists of Great Britain and Ireland (AAGBI) produced an advisory document on Information and Consent for Anaesthesia (29). This set out the circumstances in which consent must be sought, and guidelines for action when obtaining consent was impossible (e.g., children and mentally ill or comatose adults). The document recommended that for competent patients, consent must be obtained, orally or in writing, for any procedure that carries a material risk. The Department of Health (DOH) had previously stated that written consent should be obtained for general anesthesia. However, the AAGBI felt that this was unnecessary as written consent is not a requirement for local or regional anesthesia (30). Although a signature on an anesthetic consent form is not required, the anesthetist should document details of anesthetic techniques that have been discussed and agreed to, and list material risks that have been explained. A checklist of risks for the anesthetic chart was not recommended as it was thought this could distract the anesthetist from exercising clinical judgment about what to discuss with individual patients.

The problem for the anesthetist is to decide what constitutes a material risk and how that information should be presented to each patient. Failure to provide sufficient information could be seen as a breach of duties if the patient subsequently comes to harm and claims that they would not have undergone the procedure if they had been told about all the risks. Material risks are defined as those that a reasonable person in the patient's position would be likely to attach significance. A legal principle known as the Bolam test used to be the standard against which a doctor's performance would be measured (31). In this setting, application of the Bolam principle would suggest that a practitioner could avoid prosecution if they had provided a similar amount of information to that which would have been provided by a reasonably competent practitioner in a similar position. However, the courts are placing greater importance on evidence-based practice, such that the Bolam principle alone may not provide an adequate defense. Accordingly, health-care providers are adopting a more defensive medicolegal strategy. Patients are being told, or given comprehensive preoperative patient information leaflets, which detail all risks. Although this may improve the legal defense, not all patients are reassured by this deluge of information, and some patients may prefer not to be told about unpleasant aspects or complications (32). Unfortunately, for the nervous patient, an anesthetist is unlikely to be successfully sued for giving too much information to the patient as part of the consent process.

SUMMARY

Preoperative assessment is an important part of the surgical pathway. The anesthetist must develop skills in assessing patients, understand the demands that anesthesia and surgery are likely to have on an individual patient, and should have the current medical knowledge to know when there are opportunities for the patient's condition to be optimized. They should be able to communicate problems to other members of the perioperative team and should know what information should be given to the patient and document that these discussions have occurred. Without these skills, the patient may not achieve the best possible outcome, and the anesthetist may find themselves under close scrutiny in a court.

REFERENCES

1. NCCAC. Preoperative Tests, The Use of routine Preoperative Tests for Elective Surgery-Evidence, Methods and Guidance. London: NICE, 2003.
2. Eagle K, Berger P, Calkins. Guideline update for perioperative cardiovascular evaluation for non-cardiac surgery-executive summary: a report of the American College of Cardiology/American Heart Association Task Force on Practice Guidelines. J Am Coll Cardiol 2002; 39:542–553.
3. Rai M, Pandit J. Day of surgery cancellations after nurse-led pre-assessment in an elective surgical centre: the first 2 years. Anaesthesia 2003; 58:692–699.
4. Van Klei W, Moons K, Rutten C. The effect of Outpatient Preoperative Evaluation of hospital inpatients on cancellation of surgery and length of hospital stay. Anesth Analg 2002; 94:644–649.
5. Mangano D. Perioperative cardiac morbidity. Anesthesiology 1990; 72:153–184.
6. Goldman L, Caldera D, Nussbaum S. Multifactorial index of cardiac risk in noncardiac surgical procedures. N Eng J Med 1977; 297:845–850.
7. Detsky A, Abrams H, McLaughlin J. Predicting cardiac complications in patients undergoing non-cardiac surgery. J Gen Intern Med 1986; 1:211–219.
8. Lee T, Marcantonio E, Mangione C. Derivation and prospective validation of a simple index for prediction of cardiac risk of major noncardiac surgery. Circulation 1999; 100: 1043–1049.
9. Chassot P, Delabays A, Spahn D. Preoperative evaluation of patients with, or at risk of, coronary artery disease undergoing non-cardiac surgery. Br J Anaesth 2002; 89:747–759.
10. Jones J, Sapsford D, Wheatley R. Postoperative hypoxaemia: mechanisms and time course. Anaesthesia 1990; 45:566–573.
11. Wahba R. Perioperative functional residual capacity. Can J Anaesth 1991; 38:384–400.
12. Ford G, Whitelaw W, Rosenal T, et al. Diaphragm function after upper abdominal surgery in humans. Am Rev Respir Dis 1983; 127:431–436.
13. Dakin M, Yentis S. Latex allergy: a strategy for management. Anaesthesia 1998; 53: 774–781.

14. Shiga T, Wajima Z, Inoue T, Sakamoto A. Predicting difficult intubation in apparently normal patients: a meta-analysis of bedside screening tests performance. Anesthesiology 2005; 103:429–437.
15. Calder I. Predicting difficult intubation. Anaesthesia 1992; 47:528–530.
16. Samsoon G, Young J. Difficult tracheal intubation: a retrospective study. Anaesthesia 1987; 42:487–490.
17. Mallampati S, Gatt S, Gugino L, et al. A clinical sign to predict difficult tracheal intubation: a prospective study. Can Anaesth Soc J 1985; 32:429–434.
18. Wilson M, Spiegelhalter D, Robertson J, Lesser P. Predicting difficult intubation. Br J Anaesth 1988; 61:211–216.
19. Merah N, Wong D, Ffoulkes-Crabbe D, et al. Modified Mallampati test, thyromental distance and inter-incisor gap are the best predictors of difficult laryngoscopy in West Africans. Can J Anaesth 2005; 52:291–296.
20. Munro J, Booth A, Nicholl J. Routine preoperative testing: a systematic review of the evidence. Health Technol Assess 1997; 1:1–62.
21. Fowkes F, Davies E, Evans K, et al. Multicentre trial of four strategies to reduce use of a radiological test. Lancet 1986; 1:367–370.
22. Upchurch GJ, Proctor M, Henke P, et al. Predictors of severe morbidity and death after elective abdominal aortic aneurysmectomy in patients with chronic obstructive pulmonary disease. J Vasc Surg 2003; 2003.
23. Halm E, Browner W, Tubau J, et al. Echocardiography for assessing cardiac risk in patients having noncardiac surgery. Study of Perioperative Ischemia Research Group. Ann Intern Med 1996; 15:433–441.
24. Stamler J, Stamler R, Neaton J. Blood pressure, systolic and diastolic, and cardiovascular risks. U.S. population data. Arch Intern Med 1993; 153:598–615.
25. Prys-Roberts C, Meloche R, Foex P. Studies of anaesthesia in relation to hypertension. I. Cardiovascular responses of treated and untreated patients. Br J Anaesth 1971; 43: 122–137.
26. Howell S, Sear J, Foex P. Hypertension, hypertensive heart disease and perioperative cardiac risk. Br J Anaesth 2004; 92:570–583.
27. Rao T, Jacobs K, El-Etr A. Reinfarction following anaesthesia in patients with myocardial infarction. Anesthesiology 1983; 59:499–505.
28. Tuman K. Perioperative cardiovascular risk: assessment and management. Anesth Analg 2001; 92:1451–1454.
29. Information and consent for anaesthesia. London: The Association of Anaesthetists of Great Britain and Ireland, 1999.
30. A guide to consent for examination and treatment. London: Department of Health, 1990.
31. Bolam v Friern Hospital Management Committee, 1957.
32. Farnill D, Inglis S. Patients' desire for information about anaesthesia: Australian attitudes. Anaesthesia 1994; 49:162–164.

8

Perioperative Fluid Management and Optimization

Korat Farooq and R. Jonathan T. Wilson
Department of Anesthesia, York Hospital, York, U.K.

INTRODUCTION

Perioperative fluid management is a major component of anesthetic practice for abdominal compartment surgery. Achieving an optimal fluid status in the surgical patient is not simply a matter of fluid loss replacement, but also requires an assessment of the patient needs, and an understanding of the pathophysiology of the perioperative period.

The aim of fluid administration is to maintain an effective circulating volume, augment cardiac output (CO), and provide adequate tissue perfusion for oxygen and nutrient delivery. Failure to optimize fluid therapy throughout the perioperative period can lead to tissue hypoperfusion and impaired oxygen delivery. This can lead to organ dysfunction, increasing the likelihood of postoperative morbidity and mortality.

The choice of intravenous fluid for replacement requires an understanding of the fluid composition, fluid compartment homeostasis, and their effects on intravascular volume expansion. The first part of this chapter reviews the physiology of perioperative fluid management. The second part reviews how maximizing cardiac function and oxygen delivery through carefully monitored use of fluids and inotrope can significantly affect outcome in the high-risk patient undergoing abdominal surgery.

FLUID COMPARTMENT HOMEOSTASIS

A 70-kg adult contains approximately 42 L of water. Body water is divided into further compartments (Fig. 1). The intracellular and extracellular compartments are separated by cell membranes that are freely permeable to water but relatively impermeable to ionized particles, such as sodium and potassium ions. Na^+/K^+ adenosine triphosphate (ATP)–dependent pumps in cell membranes extrude Na^+ and Cl^+ ions to maintain a sodium gradient across the cell wall. The extracellular fluid (ECF) volume is determined by the amount of sodium and water that are present. Sodium excretion is in turn governed by the activity of the renin-angiotensin-aldosterone system, the sympathetic nervous system, and atrial natriuretic peptide secretion.

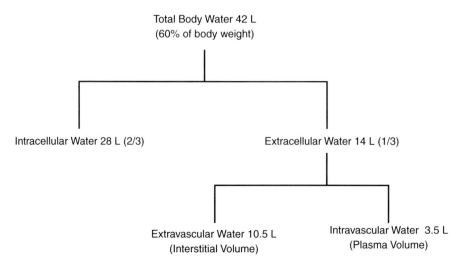

Figure 1   Body water distribution in a 70-kg man.

Capillary endothelium and arterial and venous walls separate the intravascular and extravascular compartment. Water and small ions move freely through these compartments. The intravascular compartment contains water, ions, plasma proteins, red blood cells, white bloods cells, and platelets. The capillary endothelium is rather impermeable to larger molecules, such as albumin, and synthetic colloids suspensions, such as dextrans, gelatins, and starches. These larger molecules should, in theory, remain in the intravascular compartment, and therefore have implications for acute fluid resuscitation.

Fluid transportation across compartments is governed by the Starling equilibrium:

$$Jv = K[(P_c - P_i) - \sigma(\pi_c - \pi_i)] \tag{1}$$

where Jv is the rate of outward fluid movement across capillary bed; K, ultrafiltration coefficient; P_c, hydrostatic pressure in the capillary; P_i, hydrostatic pressure in the interstitium; σ, reflection coefficient; π_c, oncotic pressure in the capillary; and π_i, oncotic pressure in the interstitium.

The transcapillary fluid movement is dependent on the difference in the capillary and interstitium hydrostatic and colloid osmotic pressures, and relevant capillary bed permeability coefficients.

The reflection coefficient is a measure of capillary permeability to albumin. If the capillary endothelium is totally impermeable to albumin, then σ equals 1. However, if the endothelium is completely permeable to albumin and no gradient exists, then σ equals 0. The reflection coefficient of a capillary bed varies in range from 0 (liver) to 0.9 (brain) (1). In cases of increased capillary permeability, such as that seen in sepsis, trauma, burns, or indeed major surgery, the reflection coefficient will reduce toward zero, favoring fluid sequestration from the intravascular space into the interstitium, third spaces, and tissues.

In health, the net intracapillary pressures supersede the pressures in the interstitial compartment, resulting in a continuous capillary leak called tissue fluid, which in turn drains back into the systemic circulation via the lymphatic system.

INTRAVENOUS REPLACEMENT FLUIDS

Commercially available intravenous replacement fluids vary according to their constituents, indications for use, and limitations. They can be conveniently classified into crystalloids and colloids. They differ in their chemical, physical, and physiological properties, summarized in Tables 1 and 2.

Crystalloids

Crystalloids contain inorganic ions (e.g., Na^+), small organic molecules (e.g., glucose), or both, dissolved in water. The resulting solution may be hypotonic, isotonic, or hypertonic with respect to plasma, and is capable of passage through a semipermeable membrane.

Crystalloids provide a short-term expansion of the circulating volume before rapid distribution occurs throughout the various fluid compartments.

In a solution of dextrose, the glucose molecules are rapidly metabolized and, effectively, an infusion of 1 L of 5% dextrose is equivalent to giving 1 L of water. After infusion, less than 10% remains intravascularly, because water is equally distributed across all compartments (Fig. 1). Hence intravascular resuscitation will be minimal. When the total body water is depleted, such as in dehydration, 5% dextrose is a means of giving free water and is an appropriate solution for resuscitation of the intracellular compartment. Hypertonic glucose solutions (e.g., 40% Dextrose) are reserved for providing metabolic substrate or reversing hypoglycemia.

When 1 L of an isotonic balanced salt solution (BSS) such as NaCl 0.9% or Ringers Lactate is infused, approximately 25% will remain intravascular (Fig. 1), because the distribution of these crystalloids are limited to the ECF with little movement intracellularly. Hence within the ECF compartment, 1 L of a BSS will distribute between the interstitial fluid (three-fourths) and plasma volume (one-fourth). Hence in the case of resuscitation with crystalloid, following a 1 L drop in the circulating volume, 4 L of a BSS crystalloid solution would be required to restore the circulating volume. Such large crystalloid volumes could lead to tissue edema in susceptible tissues.

Colloids

A colloid is a suspension of finely divided particles of large molecular weight dispersed in a continuous medium. They can be either semisynthetic (gelatins, dextrans, and starches), or naturally occurring plasma derivatives (albumin, fresh frozen plasma,

Table 1 Composition of Commonly Used Crystalloid Solutions

Solution	Osmolarity (mosm/L)	Na^+ (mmol/L)	Cl^- (mmol/L)	K^+ (mmol/L)	Ca^{2+} (mmol/L)	$HCO3^-$ (mmol/L)	Glucose (mg/L)	Lactate (mmol/L)
NaCl 0.9%	308	154	154	–	–	–	–	–
Dextrose 4% saline 0.15%	264	30	30	–	–	–	40	–
Dextrose 5%	252	–	–	–	–	–	50	–
Hartmann's	278	131	111	5	2	–	–	29
Na HCO3 8.4%	2000	1000	1000	–	–	–	–	–

Table 2 Composition of Commonly Used Colloids

Solution	Molecule	Average molecular weight (Da)	Na$^+$ (mmol/L)	Cl$^-$ (mmol/L)	K$^+$ (mmol/L)	Ca^{2+} (mmol/L)
Gelofusine^{TM}	Gelatin	30,000	154	125	<0.4	<0.4
Haemaccel^{TM}	Polygeline	35,000	145	145	5	6.25
Dextran 40	Dextran	40,000	154	154	–	–
Dextran 70	Dextran	70,000	154	154	–	–
Voluven	Tetrastarch	130,000	154	154	–	–
HAES-steril	Pentastarch	264,000	154	154	–	–
Hespan	Hetastarch	450,000	150	150	–	–
Albumin 4.5%	Albumin	69,000	<160	136	<2	–

and immunoglobulins). Colloid molecules are usually suspended in saline. They normally remain in the intravascular compartment due to their large molecular weight.

Gelatins

Gelatin-based colloids are manufactured from hydrolysis of bovine collagen, and have an effective half-life of up to two hours within the circulation before being excreted. There is a small risk of anaphylaxis with gelatin use. Due to their short duration of action, their use as plasma expanders is limited.

Starches

Starch solutions consist of amylopectin etherified with hydroxyethyl groups, and vary considerably with respect to molecular weight and the ratio of substituted to nonsubstituted glucose molecules. They remain in the circulation for much longer, having an intravascular half-life of up to 24 hours. Clearance of the larger starch molecules occurs via the reticuloendothelial system. Traditionally, the dose of starch used has been limited by side effects, such as impaired clotting, renal dysfunction, and pruritus. But the recent trend has been to produce lower molecular weight starches with less substitution, and these can be used in larger doses because side effects are reduced.

Other Colloids

Dextrans consist of polysaccharides, classified according to their molecular weight. They have an intravascular half-life of three hours. They may precipitate allergic reactions and interfere with clotting mechanisms. Human albumin solution (HAS) is derived from pooled human plasma. It has an intravascular half-life of 24 hours, but if it crosses damaged cerebral and pulmonary capillaries, tissue edema can ensue. Prion disease transmission through HAS use is an uncertainty.

Colloids as Plasma Expanders. Unless capillary permeability is altered, most of an administered dose of colloid will remain in the intravascular compartment, and cause a degree of plasma volume expansion (PVE), which is useful when circulating volume is depleted. The degree of PVE of an infused colloid is dependent on the solute content and particle size. In the plasma, colloids exert oncotic pressure and thus retain fluid in the circulating volume. PVE following colloid administration occurs due to the movement of water along osmotic gradients toward a higher concentration of solute to achieve intravascular isotonicity. The duration of PVE is dependent on the rate of colloid loss from the intravascular compartment due to metabolism, glomerular filtration, and passage through the capillary endothelium. Resistance to intravascular metabolism is dependent on the chemical properties of the molecule. One liter of gelatin produces a PVE of 0.2l after 90 minutes, whereas dextran and hetastarch both produce a similar PVE of 0.7l over a similar period (2). In addition to intravascular expansion, improved blood capillary flow through reduced viscosity may enhance tissue oxygen delivery.

Fluid replacement therefore must be directed toward the compartment that is fluid depleted. In acute blood loss where intravascular volume is reduced, a colloid or suitable crystalloid will replete this compartment and restore the circulating volume. If there is continued gastrointestinal (GI) tract fluid losses (containing water and electrolytes) an isotonic BSS such as Ringers Lactate can be administered to replete the ECF, unless losses are profound and the circulating volume is compromised requiring colloid resuscitation.

FLUID HOMEOSTASIS AND MAJOR SURGERY

The integrity of the capillary endothelial beds is disturbed during disease, trauma, or major surgical procedures. Major surgery elicits a stress response of combined endocrine and inflammatory that can lead to capillary endothelial cell dysfunction, promoting increased capillary permeability. Increased vascular permeability causes interstitial edema, increased fluid sequestration, and intravascular volume depletion. Such losses are difficult to quantify due to their movement to nonspecific anatomical areas. Furthermore, sequestered fluid, although physically present, does not contribute to fluid homeostasis in the acute phase. If the area of involvement is sufficiently large, such as in colorectal resection or retroperitoneal exploration, intravascular volume repletion may be significant.

Perioperative Fluid Losses

Preoperative Period

Abdominal surgery causes major fluid and electrolyte shifts (Table 3).

Fasting and Bowel Preparation. All elective patients presenting to theater have an element of fluid deficit due to a preoperative starvation period, but this should not lead to major fluid compartment shifts or obvious hypovolemia. Neuroendocrine compensatory mechanisms via anti-diuretic hormone (ADH) release, renin-angiotensin-aldosterone, atrial natriuretic peptide (ANP) release, and increased sympathetic activity all act to maintain the intravascular volume during starvation. Fluid deficit constitutes the hourly fluid requirement multiplied by the hours since "nil by mouth" plus any external and third-space losses. If hypovolemia is present, preoperative fluid administration is required to restore cardiovascular stability and circulating volume.

Preoperative fluid deficit may be more substantial in patients who present with diarrhea, vomiting, excessive body temperature, polyuria due to diuretic therapy, or an increased nasogastric output associated with an ileus or obstructive bowel pathology. Similar dehydration is observed in patients receiving preoperative bowel preparation. This can lead to significant water and electrolyte rich fluid loss from the GI tract. Patients receiving bowel preparation without fluid replacement have been shown to have postural hypotension, reduced body weight, increased creatinine,

Table 3 Causes of Perioperative Fluid Losses

Preoperative	Intraoperative	Postoperative
Starvation	Insensible losses (evaporation	Surgical drains
Diarrhea	from wound, respiratory	Third-space losses (paralytic ileus,
Vomiting	tract, etc.)	sequestered interstitial fluid)
Bowel preparation	Hemorrhage	Nasogastric loss
Nasogastric loss	Third-space loss	Hemorrhage
Pyrexia		
Gastrin accurate		
intestinal hemorrhage		

and reduced urine output (3). Fluid deficits in excess of 4 L may occur, adversely affecting perioperative outcome (4,5).

Losses arising from nasogastric tubes or urine output can be accurately measured while losses due to pyrexia or increased ambient temperatures can be estimated. Diarrhea may contain a high potassium content (20–40 mmol/L), while vomit has a high chloride content (80–100 mmol/L). Patients taking diuretic therapy may lose 50 to 70 mmol of K^+/L of urine. Hence such measurable losses of water and electrolytes can be replaced accurately. Insensible losses in the pyrexial patient from sweating and respiration increase by up to 10% for each degree rise in body temperature (6). This can be compensated for by an increase in the normal water, Na^+ and K^+ intake of 15% for each degree centigrade above normothermia.

Simple dehydration should be corrected with the administration of a balanced isotonic crystalloid, with supplemental potassium to reverse any associated and electrolyte abnormality.

Anemia. Certain carcinomas, particularly right-sided colonic and gastric tumors, customarily present with iron-deficiency anemia from chronic microscopic blood loss. The anemia can be severe enough to cause new-onset angina or dyspnea. In such cases, preparation prior to surgery should include a blood transfusion to increase the red cell mass and restore the oxygen-carrying capacity. This is particularly important in the elderly patient with limited cardiorespiratory reserve. Borderline anemia may become significant during surgery because administration of intravenous replacement fluids can cause further hemodilution.

Intraoperative Period

Fluid replacement during surgery must accommodate the preoperative deficit, maintenance fluid, hemorrhage, and the insensible, evaporative, and third-space losses. Fluid hemodynamics are also affected by regional anesthesia techniques.

Blood Loss. Estimation of blood loss during surgery is readily achieved by measuring suction reservoirs, weighing swabs, and monitoring hemoglobin decline. Maintenance of adequate oxygen delivery (DO_2) should be the aim rather than simply replacing lost blood:

$$DO_2 = cardiac\ output\ (L/min) \times arterial\ O_2\ content\ (CaO_2)$$

$$Arterial\ O_2\ content = hemoglobin\ (g/L) \times 1.34 \times arterial\ oxygen\ saturation \quad (2)$$

A patient with a "normal" CO of 5 L/min, arterial oxygen saturation of 99%, and hemoglobin of 145 g/L generates an oxygen delivery of 1000 mL/min. Intraoperative reductions in arterial oxygen content generally occur through reductions in hemoglobin from blood loss. Maintenance of oxygen delivery requires a compensatory increase in CO. In an elderly patient with a history of cardiac disease, a compensatory increase in CO may be difficult to achieve, and these patients are particularly at risk of inadequate tissue perfusion leading to multiorgan dysfunction.

Blood volume depletion can be augmented with crystalloid/colloid where oxygen delivery is not compromised, thereby avoiding potential transfusion complications. Unfortunately, determining the adequacy of oxygen-carrying capacity during the intraoperative phase is not simple. The use of a minimum hemoglobin level or hematocrit as a transfusion threshold has limitations based on the potential variability from patient to patient regarding individual oxygen requirements. It is generally recommended that the majority of patients will only require transfusion if hemoglobin levels fall below 80 g/L. However, patients with cardiac dysfunction may require a higher hemoglobin concentration to compensate for an inability to increase their CO appropriately.

Insensible Losses. Insensible and evaporative water loss during abdominal surgery occurs due to lengthy peritoneal exposure time. Loss due to evaporation is difficult to quantify and is usually not significant; however, additional fluid may be required in longer procedures. Humidification of the operative theater and covering exposed bowel loops help minimize such losses. In addition, humidification of anhydrous anesthetic gases minimizes respiratory water loss.

It is customary to replace insensible losses with a balanced crystalloid solution at rates of 5 to 10 mL/kg/hr. However, recent work has suggested that a degree of fluid restriction may be beneficial in patients undergoing abdominal surgery. These studies looked at relatively fit patients, but demonstrated reductions in postoperative complication rates, time to return of gut function, and length of hospital stay (7).

Regional Anesthesia. Regional anesthesia is often the preferred choice of analgesia for major abdominal surgery. A variable degree of sympathetic blockade results, leading to reduced stress response to surgery and mechanical ventilation. The loss of sympathetic tone causes peripheral vasodilatation and venous pooling, leading to a drop in the effective circulating volume. Upper thoracic epidural blockade is associated with a significant reduction in preload and impaired cardiac sympathetic drive, resulting in a reduction in CO and hypotension (8). Sufficient fluid must be administered to maintain venous return, blood pressure, and CO. Vasopressors with sympathomimetic activity can restore the CO without excessive fluid administration. A fit and healthy subject can tolerate this sympathectomy well, particularly with a prior fluid load. Elderly patients however, many of whom take antihypertensives or diuretics, or have cardiac disease, may not be able to mount an adequate compensatory response, and are more likely to need support with vasoactive drugs.

Third-Space Losses. Third-space loss refers to fluid that leaks out of the interstitium and pools into transcellular fluid spaces. Functionally, it is not available to the intravascular space, and if not accounted for, can lead to significant hypovolemia. Fluid can accumulate in the pleural and peritoneal cavities and the bowel lumen. Such potential spaces normally contain small volumes of fluid, but following major surgery, there is extensive tissue damage and circulating inflammatory mediators, leading to cellular endothelial dysfunction and increased fluid leakage. Third-space losses are variable, but during the course of a lengthy laparotomy through a large abdominal incision, such losses can exceed 10 mL/kg/hr (9). Such losses have been quantified using segmental bioelectrical impedance analysis (10). The composition of third-space loss fluid is equivalent to ECF in electrolyte concentration. Therefore replacement of such fluid is best with an isotonic BSS, such as Ringers Lactate. Estimating fluid losses in bowel obstruction is particularly difficult because large volumes of fluid can be retained within the bowel lumen where it cannot be measured. Obstruction associated with ischemic bowel injury will have some degree of bowel wall edema and fluid sequestration into the peritoneal cavity, amounting to large third-space losses. Fluid replacement goals here should aim to replete both the intravascular and interstitial volumes, correction of electrolyte deficits, and optimize tissue perfusion and oxygen delivery. The fluid lost to bowel and third spaces such as ascites is similar to plasma in electrolyte composition, so a BSS is a suitable first choice for intravascular repletion. If crystalloid is given too rapidly, greatly increasing filling and capillary hydrostatic pressures, tissue edema may ensue, further encouraged by an associated hypoalbuminemia that is often present in this patient group.

Postoperative Period

Measurable fluid losses in the postoperative period may occur from intra-abdominal surgical drains, vomiting, nasogastric tube drainage, and stoma and urine outputs. If the patient is unable to take oral fluid, these losses should be replaced intravenously. Electrolytes and hemoglobin levels should be repeated at regular intervals until the patient is in a stable position.

MONITORING THE CIRCULATION

Electrocardiogram

Hypovolemia may present as tachycardia, although this can be masked by drugs such as beta-blockers or angiotensin converting enzyme (ACE) inhibitors. Hypokalemia or hypomagnesemia can cause dysrhythmias, usually atrial fibrillation, while hyperkalemia can cause elevation of T-waves. S-T segment analysis can detect myocardial ischemia, which can be provoked by hypotension, causing reduced coronary perfusion pressure, or by a fall in hemoglobin concentration in the susceptible patient.

Blood Pressure

Blood pressure reflects systemic vascular resistance (SVR) and CO. During anesthesia for abdominal surgery, SVR may decrease from the vasodilatory effects of the anesthetic agents used, or from regional blockade. In itself it is not an accurate guide to intravascular volume status.

Direct measurement of blood pressure using arterial cannulation is of value in the high-risk patient with decreased cardiorespiratory reserve, preferably sited before induction of anesthesia. Arterial blood gases can be used to record base deficit or lactate levels, which can be considered as surrogate markers of the adequacy of tissue perfusion and oxygen delivery.

Urine Output

Patients should be catheterized prior to the procedure, and a urine output of greater than 0.5 to 1.0 mL/kg/hr generally indicates adequate renal perfusion and circulating volume.

Central Venous Pressure

Central venous pressure (CVP) is a useful guide to intravascular fluid status and can be used in the postoperative period as well as during surgery in the higher-risk patient. The absolute CVP figure is not by itself a useful guide to circulating volume status. The CVP should be "challenged" with a fluid bolus (200 mL colloid over 15 minutes), and changes noted. If there is a less than 3 cmH$_2$O rise in CVP, even transiently, the challenge should be repeated until CVP rises greater than 3 cmH$_2$O, and stays up. At this point, the patient can be considered adequately filled, and CVP should then be observed at regular intervals to note (and treat) any downward trends indicating ongoing fluid loss.

A central venous oxygen saturation measure can be a useful guide to the adequacy of oxygen delivery. A figure less than 70% would suggest increased tissue oxygen extraction in the face of decreasing oxygen delivery.

Stroke Volume/Cardiac Output Monitoring

For the patient at increased risk of complications, optimizing the circulation and oxygen delivery can improve outcome. To do this accurately, a measure of CO or stroke volume is required. This is discussed in further detail below.

OPTIMIZING OXYGEN DELIVERY IN THE HIGH-RISK PATIENT

Major body-cavity surgery causes a strong inflammatory response, which in turn causes a marked increase in oxygen requirements. To match the demand, a patient will have to be able to elevate their CO accordingly. The high-risk patient is one who cannot spontaneously elevate their CO to the required level, and is at risk of inadequate tissue perfusion and consequent multiorgan dysfunction (11).

Best outcomes in the high-risk surgical patient require stroke volume and cardiac index (CI) monitoring to ensure the patient's circulation is optimally filled. Once optimal filling has been achieved, it is logical to measure indices of tissue perfusion and oxygen demand, such as base deficit, lactate levels, mixed venous oxygen saturation, or GI mucosal pHi. If these variables indicate persistent tissue hypoperfusion, it is likely that the CI and oxygen delivery at the point of optimal filling are still inadequate, and will need to be improved with inotropic support.

The Importance of Adequate Oxygen Delivery

In patients undergoing major surgery, commonly monitored physiological parameters, such as heart rate, systemic blood pressure, CVP, temperature, and hemoglobin are poor predictors of complications after surgery. Less commonly measured parameters, such as CO, oxygen delivery, and gastric mucosal pH (pHi) have been shown to be better predictors of postoperative outcome (12,13).

Survivors of major surgery tend to have a higher CI (the CO divided by body surface area), oxygen delivery (DO$_2$), and oxygen consumption (VO$_2$) than non-survivors (12). Moreover, normal values of these parameters are not necessarily predictive of survival, because 76% of patients who die following critical illness have achieved normal values (14).

The presence of an oxygen debt can be demonstrated despite normal hemodynamic and oxygen transport parameters in both postoperative and critically ill patients. An observational study from Bland and Shoemaker showed that increases in CO leading to a "supranormal" oxygen delivery of greater than $600\,mL/min/m^2$ was associated with greater survival than those whose postoperative oxygen delivery was less than $600\,mL/min/m^2$, but still within an acceptable range (12). In a further study, it was demonstrated that the magnitude and duration of oxygen deficit was greatest in nonsurvivors, slightly less in survivors with organ failure, and least in survivors without organ failure (15).

Oxygen delivery is dependent on an adequate CO, which, in turn, is optimal if the stroke volume is maximized. Poeze et al. showed that patients with lower stroke volumes after cardiac surgery, as measured by esophageal Doppler, were more likely to have complications (16). The reduced cardiac performance seen in nonsurvivors suggests that the ability to increase cardiac work, and hence oxygen delivery, sufficiently to meet the increased metabolic need of the postoperative phase is associated with increased survival.

There have been numerous attempts to extrapolate these observational findings to interventional studies. While those in the setting of established critical illness have been largely unsuccessful, prophylactic application of this approach (e.g., in the high-risk surgical patient) has consistently yielded positive results.

The Role of the Gut in Postoperative Complications

In recent years, much interest has been directed toward the role of the gut in the pathogenesis of postoperative morbidity and mortality. Low GI mucosal pH (pHi) and increased gastric luminal carbon dioxide tension are highly predictive of postoperative complications. It can be shown that with increasing global oxygen delivery, splanchnic oxygen delivery increases, and a parallel change is seen in splanchnic oxygen consumption, suggesting that improved systemic oxygen delivery improves splanchnic oxygen delivery and hence pHi (17).

Gastric pHi has been shown to be a good predictor of outcome after major surgery, and in critically ill patients. Optimizing stroke volume during cardiac surgery using esophageal Doppler–guided fluid therapy improved gastric pHi, reduced complications, and shortened intensive care unit and hospital stay (18).

Optimization of Oxygen Delivery

In patients who are at high risk of complications or death, a deliberate attempt to elevate DO_2 to supranormal levels prior to surgery reduces mortality and morbidity (19–21). These studies have been relatively small in size, but do show a consistent outcome benefit in the highest-risk patients. The techniques have relied on CO monitoring, generally using pulmonary artery catheter inserted preoperatively on intensive care. Despite the requirement for intensive care preoperatively, this technique has been found to be highly cost-effective because of the prevention of complications after surgery that prolonged hospital stay. A health economics study concluded that preoperative optimization of oxygen delivery had a 93% probability of being a cost-effective intervention compared to standard practice (22). However, because of the invasive nature of pulmonary artery catheterization and other logistical problems, this approach is not universally accepted.

Because of the relationships between stroke volume, CI, and oxygen delivery, elevation of stroke volume will also have the effect of increasing CI and oxygen delivery. Noninvasive, intraoperative measurement of stroke volume is possible using an esophageal Doppler probe, inserted after induction of anesthesia. Optimizing the stroke volume using this technique has been shown to reduce postoperative mortality, morbidity, and length of hospital stay compared to standard care in patients undergoing abdominal surgery, cardiac surgery, and trauma surgery (4,18,23).

Although timings of interventions and monitoring may differ, the principle of hemodynamic optimization is the same, and collectively these strategies may be known as "goal-directed therapies." In contrast, studies of preoperative hemodynamic intervention, using invasive monitoring, which do not target supra-normal values of DO_2 or do not study the highest-risk groups of patients, have not demonstrated clear benefits in outcome (24,25).

GOAL-DIRECTED THERAPY IN PRACTICE

These goals are achieved using titrated fluids and inotrope. Various techniques for measuring CO are available, and their various advantages and disadvantages are summarized in Table 4.

In modern practice, after basic preoperative resuscitation, most surgical patients can have their circulation optimized intraoperatively, using measurements of stroke volume from esophageal Doppler, or other noninvasive or semi-invasive techniques.

Although some patients will achieve target DO_2 with volume resuscitation alone, a variable but significant proportion will require inotropic support to obtain the predefined hemodynamic goals. Optimal filling is achieved when further fluid challenges fail to produce any further increase in stroke volume or CO. At this point, the patient will be on the plateau of their "Starling" curve where myocardial

Table 4 Some Available Technology for Measuring Cardiac Output in the Surgical Patient

	Advantages	Disadvantages
Pulmonary artery catheter	Can be used in awake and asleep patients	Invasive: requires central venous catheterization
	Continuous measurements available	Can cause rare but serious complications
Lithium dilution (LiDCO™)	Highly accurate measurements	Invasive: requires arterial cannulation
	Can be used in awake and asleep patients	Not continuous, limited to 20 measurements per day
Pulse contour analysis (PulseCo™)	Provides continuous measurements	Requires regular calibration if major shifts in systemic vascular resistance occur
	Can be used in awake and asleep patients	
Esophageal Doppler	Noninvasive	Difficult to use in the awake patient
	Provides continuous signal after focusing	May require frequent re-focusing before measurements
Pulse contour analysis (PiCCO™)	Provides continuous measurements	Invasive: requires cannulation of femoral artery which may be difficult in patients under going abdominal/vascular surgery
	Can be used in awake and asleep patients	

contractility, and hence CO, is maximized through the well-filled ventricle causing optimum tension in the muscle fibers. However, for some patients, optimal filling will not by itself be adequate to ensure optimal oxygen delivery, and indices of tissue perfusion such as urine output, base deficit, lactate levels, mixed venous oxygen saturation, or gastric pHi should be measured. If tissue hypoperfusion persists, it is likely that the CI and DO_2 at the point of optimal filling is still inadequate and will need to be improved with inotropic support. The effect of inotrope is to elevate the position of the "Starling" curve through enhanced myocardial contractility, hence increasing CO, oxygen delivery, and tissue perfusion to the desired level.

After surgery the high-risk patient should be nursed in a location where indices of tissue perfusion, and hence oxygen delivery, can be monitored closely. Usually this requires high-dependency care. Optimization strategies should be continued for 24 hours after surgery, or until all monitored parameters are stable and satisfactory.

The Role of Fluids and Inotrope in the Optimization of Oxygen Delivery

Although some patients achieve target oxygen delivery with volume resuscitation alone, a proportion requires inotropic support to obtain hemodynamic goals. The use of inotrope is not without consequence, because they may alter regional blood flow and cause tissue hypoxia and myocardial oxygen supply; and demand requirements can be mismatched with the potential to cause myocardial ischemia, and increased systemic oxygen consumption can occur. There appears to be a difference in outcome when different inotropes are used: in the Wilson study, mortality was reduced in both groups that received fluid and an inotrope (dopexamine or adrenaline), but there was a marked reduction in complications and hospital length of stay only in the dopexamine group. Dopexamine has been shown to preserve gut barrier function, improve gastric intramucosal pH and therefore splanchnic oxygen delivery, and to reduce inflammatory changes in the GI mucosa after major abdominal surgery (26,27).

The role of inotrope in optimization of the high-risk surgical patients may encompass other factors apart from an increase in oxygen transport variables. Catecholamines inhibit tumor necrosis factor and alter the interleukin (IL)-6 to IL-10 ratio, and this modulation of the cytokine response may be a mechanism that influences the decreased morbidity and mortality seen in the optimization trials.

CONCLUSION

The patient having major abdominal surgery faces considerable fluid shifts during the perioperative period. By having an understanding of the different types of losses that are occurring at different stages, the anesthetist will be able to correct them with the most appropriate fluid.

Patients with limited cardiorespiratory reserve are at an increased risk of mortality and morbidity; to successfully manage these high-risk patients, it is appropriate to monitor stroke volume and CI, and to use these parameters to ensure that the patient's circulation is optimally filled. Once optimal filling has been achieved, it is logical to measure indices of tissue perfusion and oxygen demand, such as base deficit, lactate levels, mixed venous oxygen saturation, or GI mucosal pHi. If these variables indicate persistent tissue hypoperfusion, it is likely that the CI and oxygen delivery at the point of optimal filling is still inadequate, and will need to be improved with inotropic support.

REFERENCES

1. McGough K, Kirby R. Fluid, electrolytes, blood, and blood substitutes. In: Kirby R, Gravenstein N, eds. Clinical Anesthesia Practice. 2d ed. Philadelphia: Saunders, 2002:770–790.
2. Lamke LO, Liljedahl SO. Plasma volume changes after infusion of various plasma expanders. Resusitation 1976; 5:93–102.
3. Sanders G, Mercer SJ, Saeb-Parsey K, et al. Randomised clinical trial of intravenous fluid replacement during bowel preparation for surgery. Br J Surg 2001; 88:1363–1365.
4. Gan TJ, Soppitt A, Maroof M, et al. Goal-directed intraoperative fluid administration reduces length of hospital stay after major surgery. Anesthesiology 2002; 97:820–826.
5. Mythen MG, Webb AR. Intraoperative gut mucosal hypoperfusion is associated with increased post-operative complications and cost. Intensive Care Med 1994; 20:99–104.
6. Perioperative fluid management http://www.qeqmh.demon.co.uk/guides/fluids.html (accessed May 2005).
7. Nisanevich V, Felenstein I, Almogy G, et al. Effect of intraoperative fluid management on outcome after intraabdominal surgery. Anesthesiology 2005; 103:25–32.
8. Sharrock NE, Mineo R, Urquhart B, et al. Hemodynamic response to low-dose epinephrine infusion during hypotensive epidural anesthesia for hip replacement. Reg Anesth 1990; 15:295–299.
9. Grocott MPW, Mythen MG, Gan TJ. Perioperative fluid management and clinical outcome in adults. Anaesth Analg 2005; 100:1093–1106.
10. Tatara T, Tsuzaki K. Measurement of extracellular water volume by bioelectrical impedance analysis during perioperative period of esophageal resection. Masui 1999; 48:1194–1201.
11. Davies SJ, Wilson RJT. Preoperative optimization of the high-risk surgical patient. Br J Anaesth 2004; 93(1):121–128.
12. Bland RD, Shoemaker WC, Abraham E, et al. Hemodynamic and oxygen transport patterns in surviving and nonsurviving postoperative patients. Crit Care Med 1985; 13: 85–90.
13. Poeze M, Takala J, Greve JW, et al. Preoperative tonometry is predictive for mortality and morbidity in high-risk surgical patients. Intensive Care Med 2000; 26:1272–1281.
14. Bland RD, Shoemaker WC, Shabot MM. Physiologic monitoring goals for the critically ill patient. Surg Gynecol Obstet 1978; 147:833–841.
15. Shoemaker WC, Appel PL, Kram HB. Role of oxygen debt in the development of organ failure sepsis, and death in high-risk surgical patients. Chest 1992; 102:208–215.
16. Poeze M, Ramsay G, Greve JW, et al. Prediction of postoperative cardiac surgical morbidity and organ failure within 4 hours of intensive care unit admission using esophageal Doppler ultrasonography. Crit Care Med 1999; 27:769–776.
17. Uusaro A, Ruokenen E, Takala J. Splanchnic oxygen transport after cardiac surgery: evidence for inadequate tissue perfusion after stabilization of hemodynamics. Intensive Care Med 1996; 22:26–33.
18. Mythen MG, Webb AR. Perioperative plasma volume expansion reduces the incidence of gut mucosal hypoperfusion during cardiac surgery. Arch Surg 1995; 130:423–429.
19. Shoemaker WC, Appel PL, Kram HB, et al. Prospective trial of supranormal values of survivors as therapeutic goals in high-risk surgical patients. Chest 1988; 94:1176–1186.
20. Boyd O, Grounds RM, Bennett ED. A randomized clinical trial of the effect of deliberate perioperative increase of oxygen delivery on mortality in high-risk surgical patients. JAMA 1993; 270:2699–2707.
21. Wilson J, Woods I, Fawcett J, et al. Reducing the risk of major elective surgery: randomised controlled trial of preoperative optimisation of oxygen delivery. BMJ 1999; 318: 1099–1103.
22. Fenwick E, Wilson J, Sculpher M, et al. Pre-operative optimisation employing dopexamine or adrenaline for patients undergoing major elective surgery: a cost-effectiveness analysis. Intensive Care Med 2002; 28(5):599–608.

23. Sinclair S, James S, Singer M. Intraoperative intravascular volume optimisation and length of hospital stay after repair of proximal femoral fracture: randomised controlled trial. BMJ 1997; 315:909–912.
24. Sandham JD, Hull RD, Brant RF, et al. A randomized, controlled trial of the use of pulmonary artery catheters in high-risk surgical patients. N Engl J Med 2003; 348:5–14.
25. Takala J, Meier-Hellman A, Eddleston J, et al. Effect of dopexamine on outcome after major abdominal surgery: a prospective, randomized, controlled multicenter study. European Multicenter Study Group on Dopexamine in Major Abdominal Surgery. Crit Care Med 2000; 28:3417–3423.
26. Smithies M, Yee TH, Jackson L. Protecting the gut and the liver in the critically ill: effects of dopexamine. Crit Care Med 1994; 22:789–795.
27. Byers RJ, Eddleston JM, Pearson RC, et al. Dopexamine reduces the incidence of acute inflammation in the gut mucosa after abdominal surgery in high-risk patients. Crit Care Med 1999; 27:1787–1793.

9
Regional Anesthesia in Abdominal Surgery

Timothy Jackson and Frank Loughnane
Department of Anesthesia, St. James's University Hospital, Leeds, U.K.

INTRODUCTION

The introduction of regional anesthetic techniques into mainstream medical practice in the late 19th and early 20th centuries brought with it the promise of a new era in which surgery could be performed in a safer and more comfortable fashion. While regional techniques were almost universally adopted in the field of ophthalmology at an early stage, it was not until World War I that, building on Koller's work, techniques were developed that allowed major abdominal surgery to proceed. Gaston Labat was recruited to bring these techniques to the Mayo Clinic, Rochester, Minnesota in 1921. Until then, deep ether anesthesia was required to provide adequate muscle relaxation, and, in turn, was associated with a high incidence of complications, especially atelectasis and pulmonary infection, in all but the most skilled of hands. Labat's preferred anesthetic technique for abdominal surgery was multiple, bilateral paravertebral nerve blockade. The short duration of spinal and epidural anesthesia was a limiting factor until the introduction of epidural catheters in the 1940s. The further developments in and improved safety of general anesthesia through the 20th century served to obscure the early promise of regional anesthesia for much of that time. More latterly, however, a number of randomized control studies and meta-analyses have reawakened interest in these techniques, and it could now be said that regional anesthesia is undergoing a renaissance and earning its place at the forefront of perioperative care.

CENTRAL NEURAXIAL TECHNIQUES

Epidural Anesthesia

Epidural anesthesia, although developed in the late 19th century (1), has only recently come to form a core element of the perioperative management of patients undergoing abdominal surgery.

The main advantages of epidural anesthesia are that it can be performed safely (2), and, with an indwelling catheter as standard, it allows us to take maximum advantage of the physiological benefits of the technique. Characteristics desired of any anesthetic technique for abdominal surgery are that it be able to optimize splanchnic vascular flow and bowel peristalsis, and attenuate the stress response to surgery (3).

It seems therefore reasonable to expect that epidural anesthesia be adopted as part of a wider perioperative strategy, which also includes standardized mobilization and feeding protocols, and shows evidence of reduced hospital stay in patients undergoing gastrointestinal surgery (4–6).

Although epidurals have been shown to influence homeostasis in a variety of different ways, its clinical outcome shall be reviewed in this chapter. The basic pharmacology and anatomy pertinent to optimal epidural utilization will be assumed here.

Influence of Epidural Anesthesia on Surgical Factors

Ileus. The development of postoperative ileus is multifactorial in nature with the pain response, bowel handling, electrolyte disturbances, and systemic opioid use (7–10) all contributing. A balance exists between parasympathetic innervation, which increases motility, and sympathetic inhibition, which is usually the controlling factor (11). During epidural anesthesia, sympathetic stimulation can be inhibited at the thoracolumbar level, while the parasympathetic tone (predominantly from the vagus) remains unaffected. The net effect is a tendency toward increased motility and the resolution of postoperative ileus.

Postoperative ileus may be assessed in various ways with most methods relying on surrogate clinical markers of a return to normal peristaltic function (e.g., time to passage of feces). The majority of studies have shown a reduction in the duration of ileus, but some showed no difference (Table 1). A Cochrane review has concluded that epidural usage reduces postoperative ileus by 36 hours (24) on average, although there was faster return of bowel function when local anesthetic regimes alone were compared to opioid-based regimes. Further studies have also demonstrated that thoracic epidural is superior to lumbar in limiting ileus (23).

Anastomotic Leakage. There is some evidence to suggest that epidural anesthesia may provide some protection against anastomotic breakdown or leakage (25). Sympathetic blockade results in an increase in splanchnic blood flow, which may aid healing at the anastomotic site (26). However, animal studies have shown no difference in anastomotic bursting pressure when epidural is compared to general anesthesia (26), and randomized controlled trials either show no significant difference (13,14) or produce contrary results (18,27). A meta-analysis of randomized trials with 562 patients did not detect a difference in anastomotic leakage rates when epidural local anesthetic–based regimes were compared to systemic opioids or epidural opioids (Table 2) (28).

Blood Loss. Despite suggestions that blood loss might be reduced due to reductions in splanchnic arterial and venous blood pressure, several randomized controlled trials have not demonstrated a difference in blood loss or transfusion requirement (12,13,18,28).

Coagulation. There is encouraging evidence that epidural anesthesia reduces the incidence of thromboembolism in orthopedic patients when compared with general anesthesia alone (29). In the postoperative period, a relatively hypercoagulable state exists and both an improvement in lower limb blood flow (30) and a reduction in prothrombotic plasminogen activator inhibitor 1 (31,32) have been demonstrated with epidural anesthesia. However, this benefit may not extend to thoracic epidural (31) because changes in lower limb blood flow are less pronounced.

Table 1 Effect of Epidural Analgesia on Duration of Postoperative Ileus After Gastrointestinal Surgery

References	Year	No. of patients	Study type	Outcome	P
Liu et al. (12)	1995	54	RCT	Earlier flatus with epidural	<0.005
Bredtmann et al. (13)	1990	116	RCT	Earlier feces with epidural	<0.001
Ahn et al. (14)	1988	30	RCT	Earlier flatus and feces with epidural	<0.001
Scheinin et al. (15)	1987	60	RCT	Earlier feces with epidural	<0.05
Jayr et al. (16)	1993	153	RCT	Earlier flatus with epidural	<0.05
Carli et al. (17)	2001	42	RCT	Earlier flatus with epidural	0.001
				Earlier feces with epidural	0.005
Carli et al. (18)	2002	64	RCT	Earlier flatus and feces with epidural	<0.01
Wallin et al. (19)	1986	30	RCT	No difference in transit time of radio-opaque markers	>0.05
Welch et al. (20)	1998	59	RCT	No difference in time to first feces	0.97
Neudecker et al. (21)	1999	20	RCT	No difference in time to first feces	0.8
Hjortso et al. (22)	1985	100	RCT	No difference in time to first feces	>0.4
				No difference in time to first flatus	>0.8
Scott et al. (23)	1996	179	RCS	Greater stool output with epidural	<0.05

Abbreviations: RCT, randomized clinical trial; RCS, retrospective case-note study.
Source: Adapted from Ref. 3.

Wound Healing. Postoperative wound oxygen tension has been postulated to correlate with the incidence of wound infection (33). Because epidural anesthesia causes vasodilatation and blockade of sympathetic responses, several studies have looked at the association between epidural anesthesia and wound oxygenation and shown a positive correlation (34,35). There is as yet, however, no proven relationship between epidural usage and lower wound infection rates.

Stress Response. The stress response to surgery is a multifaceted neuro-humoral response to a surgical insult, and may be associated with considerable morbidity, including the systemic inflammatory response syndrome. Its magnitude can be assessed using various surrogate markers, including circulating adrenaline and noradrenaline, oxygen consumption, and various other circulating adrenal hormones. All of these elements of the response are suppressed by epidural administration of both opioids and local anesthetics (36–38), although to varying degrees, suggesting that pain-mediated pathways may only be partly responsible (39).

Table 2   Effect of Epidural Analgesia on Anastomotic Dehiscence After Gastrointestinal Surgery

| References | Year | No. of patients | Study type | Patients with anastomotic breakdown (%) | | P |
				Epidural	General	
Bredtmann et al. (13)	1990	116	RCT	8.7	5.0	n.s.
Ahn et al. (14)	1988	30	RCT	0	0	n.s.
Carli et al. (18)	2002	64	RCT	3	7	>0.05
Ryan et al. (27)	1992	80	RCT	9	3	>0.05

Abbreviations: RCT, randomized clinical trial; n.s., not significant.
Source: Adapted from Ref. 3.

Influence of Epidural Anesthesia on Comorbidity

Cardiac Function.   When assessing the effects of an epidural on the cardiac function of a patient undergoing abdominal surgery, it should be borne in mind that the effects on the cardiovascular system are complex and variable. They depend on multiple factors, including the resultant autonomic effects, the pharmacological effects of any absorbed local anesthetic, and the hemodynamic status of a patient who is fasted and likely to have received bowel preparation.

The direct physiological effects of epidurals depend upon the anatomical level of insertion. Higher levels are associated with direct effects on the heart and baroreceptor reflexes, whereas lower levels result in a sympathetic block of the lower limbs with consequent effects on the vascular resistance and blood pressure.

Physiologically, the heart rate is influenced by the balance between the sympathetic and parasympathetic tones, and so a high thoracic epidural affecting T1–T4 can block the sympathetically mediated cardiac accelerator fibers. Studies have demonstrated this by showing a blunting of the bradycardia response associated with blood pressure changes in humans (40). Goertz et al. also found that tachycardic responses to reductions in blood pressure were affected in anesthetized humans (41), suggesting that sympathetic integrity is central to baroreceptor responses. Nevertheless, a high thoracic epidural leaves some sympathetic fibers unblocked, because the response to hypercapnia is not totally abolished (42).

Studies investigating the effects of thoracic epidural on ventricular function have demonstrated somewhat equivocal results, with some showing reductions in stroke volume or contractility (43,44) and others not showing such reductions (45,46). This difference in results can be explained by variations in the anesthetic technique and variations in the particular thoracic segments blocked.

It has been shown that thoracic epidural anesthesia favorably affects the myocardial oxygen supply–demand relationship in artificially infarcted dogs (47–49), and also reduces the incidence of ischemia-induced arrhythmias in rats (50). This picture in animals of a cardioprotective effect on coronary ischemia has been reproduced in humans (51,52).

Nevertheless, little influence on postoperative cardiac morbidity has been shown (53). Various studies have shown improvements in surrogate markers, such as cardiac failure (54), intensive therapy unit (ITU) length of stay (55), and episodes of tachyarrhythmia in the first 24 hours (56). Meta-analyses of 1173 general and vascular surgical patients did show a reduction in myocardial infarction rates (57,58). The conclusion is that, overall, the evidence for a cardioprotective role for thoracic epidural anesthesia is more disappointing than one would expect. Possible reasons for this may be that the study periods are of too short a duration to pick up many cardiac events, and are not selective enough for the most high risk patients, who may well show the greatest benefit (3,59–62).

Pulmonary Function. The lungs are innervated by the sympathetic system (T2–T7) and from the parasympathetic system via the vagus (63). In healthy subjects, the effects of epidural blockade of motor nerves in impairing respiration are more noticeable than any effects on the autonomic nervous system.

Of more relevance here is the impact of epidural anesthesia upon patients with high levels of respiratory comorbidity, where experimental data could be misleading. High thoracic epidural certainly may have disadvantageous effects on respiratory function. However, in clinical practice, the ability to block the pain-related inability to cough and deep breathe outweigh any minor reductions in lung volumes or forced expiratory volume in one second.

Although there is some evidence that thoracic epidural anesthesia can reduce the ventilatory response to CO_2 (64), there is no effect on hypoxic drive (65) and, therefore, this is a safe method of analgesic management in patients who habitually retain CO_2.

In cases of bronchospasm, thoracic epidural does not affect airway resistance, suggesting that such bronchospasm is unrelated to sympathetic blockade (66).

Diaphragmatic dysfunction is an important factor in the development of postoperative respiratory complications, and several human studies have demonstrated different responses of the diaphragm both in terms of direct muscle function and electromyograph (EMG) signals (67–69), the explanation for which is complex and likely to involve unblocked phrenic innervation. There is some evidence that the overall effect is toward an improvement in diaphragmatic function under thoracic epidural anesthesia, with subsequent avoidance of respiratory complications (68,70,71).

The results of a meta-analysis by Ballantyne et al. are a welcome addition to the literature and help to clarify the situation. It shows clear benefits in terms of postoperative pulmonary complications when epidural anesthesia is extended into the perioperative period, both for opioid-based (reduced atelectasis and infection) and local anesthetic-based regimes (increased S_pO_2 and reduced infections) (72). Criticism can be made, however, of the level of analgesia attained, and attention may need to focus on better "dynamic pain control" (permitting pain-free movement, coughing, etc.) (73) in order to see differences in postoperative respiratory function indices, which have so far been lacking (74).

Postoperative Pain Control. This is one area where the literature is clear. A number of randomized controlled trials have shown a clear reduction in pain scores with epidural anesthesia when compared with either intramuscular opioids or patient-controlled intravenous opioids. Bias has been a factor in some such studies (12,19), because failure to provide adequate analgesia for technical reasons caused exclusion of the patient from the analysis groups; hence we include only those that displayed an intention-to-treat analysis (13,17,18). Although some trials failed to clearly specify their intention to treat (16,75–78), the overall result, however, was that all the above trials showed reduced pain scores in the epidural study groups. A meta-analysis of studies published between 1966 and 2002 demonstrated that epidural analgesia provided better quality pain relief than parenteral opioids. This was significant for every type of surgery except for pain at rest following thoracic surgery (79).

Patient Factors and Technical Issues

Complications.   Drugs commonly used are either opioids or local anesthetics. Opioids can display differing complications depending on their epidural-related site of action. For instance, highly lipophilic drugs (e.g., fentanyl) penetrate the spinal cord more quickly, whereas less lipophilic drugs (e.g., morphine) remain in the cerebrospinal fluid and can therefore distribute more widely, with various side effects, including dizziness, nausea, and respiratory depression (80). Also urinary retention can occur in a significant number of patients, necessitating urinary catheterization (81).

Local anesthetic drugs are responsible for the hemodynamic changes commonly seen, including hypotension, bradycardia, and alterations in cardiac output. Higher concentrations can lead to significant degrees of motor blockade. Procedure-related complications range from those that might be classified as minor, such as catheter migration resulting in unacceptable analgesia or unilateral blockade, to serious, such as permanent neurological injury. Fortunately, the technique is relatively safe with the incidence of serious complications being 0.52 per 10,000 procedures (82), half of which include neurological injury, and the remainder include toxic reactions, opioid overdose, and bacterial infection.

A matter of ongoing debate in the anesthetic community is the relative safety of inserting an epidural in the awake versus anesthetized patient. Many anesthetists cite the ability of an awake patient to identify sensations that may herald impending neurological trauma; however, many also continue to insert epidurals in anesthetized patients (83), despite the devastating effects of intraspinal insertion.

Contraindications.   As with other procedures, these can be classified into absolute and relative. Absolute contraindications include patient refusal, which in one study was recorded as 17% of patients offered epidural management (84), the explanations for this being varied. Other contraindications are coagulopathy and sepsis. Both are frequently seen in patients who present for emergency surgery (85), who may be elderly and have a number of comorbidities, which would make epidural anesthesia attractive. The decision may not be straightforward in such a clinical setting. Although simple analysis would suggest that epidural anesthesia is contraindicated in these circumstances, the literature is not conclusive. Coagulopathy is a complex concept at the bedside, and involves a variety of clinical diagnoses. Laboratory tests are becoming increasingly sophisticated in their ability to predict actual clotting environments in the context of epidural (and spinal) anesthesia (86), and, therefore, there has been some debate on the topic. Other factors to bear in mind are the concomitant administration of drugs that may affect platelet function while not affecting routine hematology (87), prophylactic heparin, which can be associated with epidural hematoma formation (88,89), and even the surgical procedure itself (e.g., splenectomy and effects on platelets) (90). Most countries now have protocols for the appropriate timing of regional anesthetic insertion and removal relative to administration of perioperative thromboprophylaxis.

Cardiac pathology, of which aortic stenosis is the classic example, is a relative contraindication to epidural anesthesia, and it must be remembered that cardiovascular collapse may occur if the sympathetic block exceeds the cardiac system's ability to compensate.

Patient and Organizational Outcomes

Much of the clinical evidence mentioned so far concentrates on information gathered over a limited period of postoperative time, and is designed to answer a relatively specific question. Of greater importance to the patient, and increasingly to the clinicians involved, is whether an intervention makes any difference to the overall outcome.

The most persuasive argument in this matter was put forward in a meta-analysis in 2000 of 9559 patients, in 141 trials, including all forms of surgery (although the majority of trials involved general, gynecology, urology, and vascular surgery). The authors concluded there was approximately a 30% reduction in overall mortality, and significant reductions in deep venous thrombosis, pulmonary embolus formation, transfusion requirements, pneumonia, and respiratory depression (91). Their caveat was that the extent of some of these benefits was unclear and that the relationship between regional anesthesia and general anesthesia was complex.

Further randomized controlled trials have been performed since the Rodgers meta-analysis, which tend to disagree with the original findings in overall outcomes, showing no difference in mortality (92,93). But some reduction again was shown in respiratory complications (93).

In terms of cost and resource outcomes, it has been difficult to show a reduction in these with perioperative epidural anesthesia (12,13,16–18,20,21,78), although shortened stay has been reported in centers where aggressive multimodal rehabilitation programs are established (4–6).

Spinal Anesthesia

Spinal anesthesia also has a place, albeit more limited, in abdominal surgery. The dense block afforded by intrathecal injection of a relatively small dose of local anesthetic makes it an attractive technique for lower abdominal surgery. There would seem to be little benefit over general anesthesia for major abdominal surgery, because the necessity to control respiration for appropriate access to the abdominal cavity, and difficulty in titrating precise levels of anesthesia to upper abdominal dermatomal levels make this technique largely the province of obstetric (94), gynecological (95), and urological (96) procedures, where a more limited block is appropriate to the surgical field.

Spinal anesthesia is intended to stray more cephalad only in a limited numbers of patients undergoing abdominal surgery, usually in response to unacceptable cardiorespiratory comorbidity, or when adverse airway pathology necessitates maintenance of consciousness. By their very nature, such situations are uncommon, and the literature concerning them by no means forms a sound evidence base (97,98).

Physiologically, spinal anesthesia has similar effects to those of epidural techniques, although the sympathetic blockade is more profound and may be a particular problem in the elderly, who are more likely to be in the position of requiring regional anesthesia as the sole anesthetic technique (99,100).

There are, however, other areas related to abdominal surgery where spinal anesthesia may be considered a more standard approach. It has been considered as an appropriate technique for groin hernia surgery, although there is a wealth of evidence to support local anesthetic/field block techniques (101,102). Spinal anesthesia may have a place in bilateral surgery, and in the evolving laparoscopic techniques (103).

DISCRETE NERVE BLOCKS

Paravertebral Nerve Blocks

Paravertebral injections are now commonly performed as a treatment for post-thoracotomy pain. Their reported benefit is that, due to closer proximity to the sympathetic chain, they offer the most profound sympathetic blockade (because at the same time, there is a block of sensory impulses as they enter the intervertebral foraminae) (104). By blocking several levels at once the technique provides excellent analgesia. Because this block is normally employed in a unilateral fashion, the hemodynamic effects of the sympathetic blockade are usually minor; however, it provides arguably the most profound inhibition of surgical stress response.

Of relevance to abdominal surgery, such blocks are commonly performed to augment analgesia for unilateral procedures and have been described for surgery to gallbladder and kidney, and even inguinal hernia repair (105). One should remember, however, that Gaston Labat's original thesis described bilateral paravertebral blockade as allowing ideal conditions for major abdominal surgery.

Intercostal Nerve Block and Interpleural Block

Although mainly associated with thoracic surgery (106–108), intercostals block has also been used to provide analgesia for unilateral upper abdominal procedures (109,110). Such analgesia is short lived because absorption from this site is rapid.

The cholecystectomy model has been studied to compare interpleural and intercostal block (111,112) with reasonable results on pain control, although it must be remembered that the potential complications of pneumothorax and rapid absorption of local anesthetic agent by the vascular pleura occur. Nevertheless, these form a useful adjunct for surgery to gallbladder, liver, and kidney when other more central techniques may be contraindicated.

Rectus Sheath Block

Although considered an outdated technique by many (113), this can be used to provide analgesia to midline incisions, either as an alternative to epidural analgesia postlaparotomy, or even in the setting of conscious surgery in the high-risk patient.

Inguinal Field Block

This is a well-described technique, and is now the standard mode of anesthesia for day-case hernia repair. It offers benefits in terms of faster recovery and superior patient satisfaction (114). This block also comprises ilioinguinal nerve blockade, which can also be used for such procedures as appendectomy.

Miscellaneous Nerve Blocks

By their very nature, these blocks form a heterogeneous group. There are descriptions of various techniques to augment general anesthesia, examples of which include pouch of Douglas block (115), hypogastric nerve block (116), and mesosalpinx block (117) for gynecological laparoscopic procedures. Clearly, the use of such techniques does not carry with it the weight of large subject number investigations, but they remain interesting adjuncts to the conduct of balanced anesthesia.

SPECIAL PATIENT GROUPS

Children

In principle, any anesthetic technique that is applied to adults can also be applied to the pediatric population, with the appropriate consideration of anatomical and physiological differences. Both central neuraxial techniques and peripheral nerve blocks are performed in pediatric anesthesia; however, one technique not mentioned previously takes on greater significance in the management of anesthesia for abdominal surgery—caudal epidural.

Owing to the anatomical differences of the epidural space, and its contents being much more loosely arranged in young children, the spread of local anesthetic solutions is more easily obtained. Thus, catheter techniques can be employed via a caudal access point; with increasing volumes of local anesthetic solution, sufficient dermatomal anesthesia can be obtained to cover abdominal surgery (118). A full description of caudal anesthesia is beyond the scope of this text.

The Pregnant Woman

This is a situation in which regional anesthesia assumes great importance. In early pregnancy, risks of general anesthesia are probably similar to the risks in the non-pregnant state, but by the second trimester, intra-abdominal pressure begins to rise and lower esophageal tone is already reduced, so regurgitation risk is high (119).

The benefits of regional anesthesia are the maintenance of spontaneous respiration and airway, and minimal drug challenge to the fetus. Risks of regional anesthesia in the heavily pregnant woman are the usual generic risks, apart from an exaggerated hypotensive response to sympathetic block. Beyond the 20th week of pregnancy, left lateral tilt should be employed, and the requirement for vasopressors expected.

The Elderly Patient

Most of the issues pertaining to regional anesthesia have been discussed earlier; however, the salient points bear reiteration. Elderly patients are more likely to have comorbidity affecting cardiovascular and respiratory reserve. This makes them simultaneously more likely to receive greater benefit from a regional technique, and more susceptible to the consequences of regional block, such as hemodynamic instability, temperature regulation, development of pressure sores in sensory-blocked areas, and urinary retention. Due to the higher incidence of cognitive and sensory impairments, the elderly patient undergoing a solely regional anesthetic may require greater preparation and monitoring throughout the procedure.

SUMMARY

Regional anesthesia has a significant role to play in abdominal surgery. The central role of epidural anesthesia is underpinned by various favorable physiological effects (cardiovascular and respiratory), as well as attenuating the surgical stress response. True outcome data are not as positive as initially hoped for, although there are clear benefits, particularly, in terms of respiratory complications, analgesia, and reduced postoperative ileus. There are no greatly demonstrated benefits in terms of cardiac outcomes, and equivocal results in terms of overall mortality.

However, there are still benefits for the patient who is considered "high-risk" from a cardiorespiratory point of view, and together with aggressive rehabilitation programs, epidural anesthesia can reduce hospital stay; so there is still much to offer selected individuals.

REFERENCES

1. Tuffier TH. Anesthesie medullaire chirurgicale par injection sous-arachno lombaire de coca; technique et resultants. La Semaine Medicale 1900; 20:167–169.
2. Tanaka K, Watanabe R, Harada T, Dan K. Extensive application of epidural anesthesia and analgesia in a university hospital: incidence of complications related to technique. Reg Anesth 1993; 18:34–38.
3. Fotiadis RJ, Badvie S, Weston MD, et al. Epidural analgesia in gastrointestinal surgery. Br J Surg 2004; 91:828–841.
4. Bradshaw BG, Liu SS, Thirlby RC. Standardised perioperative care protocols and reduced length of stay after colon surgery. JAMA 1998; 186:501–506.
5. Kehlet H, Morgensen T. Hospital stay of 2 days after sigmoidectomy with a multimodal rehabilitation programme. Br J Surg 1999; 86:227–230.
6. Basse L, Hjort-Jakobsen D, Billesbolle P, et al. A clinical pathway to accelerate recovery after colonic resection. Ann Surg 2000; 232:51–57.
7. Yukioka H, Bogod DG, Rosen M. Recovery of bowel motility after surgery. Detection of time to first flatus from carbon dioxide concentration and patient estimate after nalbuphine and placebo. Br J Anaesth 1987; 59:581–584.
8. Wilder-Smith CH, Hill L, Wilkins J, et al. Effects of morphine and tramadol on somatic and visceral sensory function and gastrointestinal motility after abdominal surgery. Anesthesiology 1999; 91:639–647.
9. Ingram DM, Sheiner HJ. Postoperative gastric emptying. Br J Surg 1981; 68:572–576.
10. Nimmo WS, Heading RC, Wilson, et al. Inhibition of gastric emptying and drug absorption by narcotic analgesics. Br J Clin Pharm 1975; 2:509–513.
11. Steinbrook RA. Epidural anesthesia and gastrointestinal motility. Anesth Analg 1997; 86:837–844.
12. Liu SS, Carpenter RL, Mackey DC, et al. Effects of postoperative analgesia technique on rate of recovery after colon surgery. Anesthesiology 1995; 83:757–765.
13. Bredtmann RD, Herden HN, Teichmann W, et al. Epidural analgesia in colonic surgery: results of a randomized prospective study. Br J Surg 1990; 77:638–642.
14. Ahn H, Bronge A, Johansson K, et al. Effects of continuous postoperative epidural analgesia on intestinal motility. Br J Surg 1988; 75:1176–1178.
15. Scheinin B, Asantila R, Orko R. The effect of bupivacaine and morphine on pain and bowel function after colonic surgery. Acta Anesthesiol Scand 1987; 31:161–164.
16. Jayr C, Thomas H, Rey A, et al. Postoperative pulmonary complications. Epidural analgesia using bupivacaine and opioids versus parenteral opioids. Anesthesiology 1993; 78:666–676.
17. Carli F, Trudel JL, Belliveau P. The effect of intraoperative thoracic epidural anesthesia and postoperative analgesia on bowel function after colorectal surgery: a prospective, randomized trial. Dis Colon Rectum 2001; 44:1083–1089.
18. Carli F, Mayo N, Klubien K, et al. Epidural analgesia enhances functional exercise capacity and health-related quality of life after colonic surgery: results of a randomized trial. Anesthesiology 2002; 97:540–54.
19. Wallin G, Cassuto J, Hogstrom S, et al. Failure of epidural anesthesia to prevent postoperative ileus. Anesthesiology 1986; 65:292–297.
20. Welch JP, Cohen JL, Vignati PV, et al. Pain control following elective gastrointestinal surgery; is epidural anaesthesia warranted. Conn Med 1998; 62:461–464.
21. Neudecker J, Schwenk W, Junghans T, et al. Randomized controlled trial to examine the influence of thoracic epidural analgesia on postoperative ileus after laparoscopic sigmoid resection. Br J Surg 1999; 86:1292–1295.
22. Hjortso NC, Neumann P, Frosig F, et al. A controlled study on the effect of epidural analgesia with local anaesthetics and morphine on morbidity after abdominal surgery. Acta Anaesthesiol Scand 1985; 29:790–796.

23. Scott AM, Starling JR, Ruscher AE, et al. Thoracic versus lumbar epidural effect on pain control and ileus resolution after restorative proctocolectomy. Surg 1996; 120:688–695.
24. Jorgensen H, Wetterslev J, Moiniche S, et al. Epidural local anesthetic versus opioid-based analgesic regimens on postoperative gastrointestinal paralysis, PONV and pain after abdominal surgery. Cochrane Database Syst Rev 2000; 4:CD001893.
25. Sala C, Garcia-Granero E, Molina MJ, et al. Effect of epidural anesthesia on colorectal anastomosis: a tonometric study. Dis Colon Rectum 1997; 40:958–961.
26. Schnitzler M, Kilbride MJ, Senagore A. Effect of epidural analgesia on colorectal anastomotic healing and colonic motility. Reg Anesth 1992; 17:143–147.
27. Ryan P, Schweitzer SA, Woods RJ. Effects of epidural and general anesthesia compared with general anesthesia alone in large bowel anastomosis. A prospective study. Eur J Surg 1992; 158:45–49.
28. Holte K, Kehlet H. Epidural analgesia and risk of anastomotic leakage. Reg Anesth Pain Med 2001; 26:111–117.
29. Modig J, Borg T, Karlstrom G, et al. Thromboembolism after total hip replacement: role of epidural and general anesthesia. Anesth Analg 1983; 62:174–180.
30. Modig J, Malmberg P, Karlstrom G. Effect of epidural versus general anesthesia on calf blood flow. Acta Anesthesiol Scand 1980; 24:305–309.
31. Mellbring G, Dahlgren S, Reiz S, et al. Thromboembolic complications after major abdominal surgery; effect of thoracic epidural analgesia. Acta Chir Scand 1983; 149: 263–268.
32. Modig J, Borg T, Bagge I, et al. Role of extradural and general anaesthesia in fibrinolysis and coagulation after total hip replacement. Br J Anaesth 1983; 55:625–629.
33. Hopf HW, Hunt TK, West JM. Wound tissue oxygen tension predicts the risk of wound infection in surgical patients. Arch Surg 1997; 152:997–1005.
34. Buggy DJ, Doherty WL, Hart EM, et al. Postoperative wound oxygen tension with epidural or intravenous analgesia: a prospective, randomized, single blind clinical trial. Anesthesiology 2002; 97:952–958.
35. Kabon B, Fleischmann E, Treschan T, et al. Thoracic epidural anesthesia increases tissue oxygenation during major abdominal surgery. Anesth Analg 2003; 97:1812–1817.
36. Kehlet H. Surgical stress, the role of pain and analgesia. Br J Anaesth 1989; 63:189–195.
37. Carli F, Webster J, Pearson M, et al. Protein metabolism after abdominal surgery: effect of 24 hour extradural block with local anaesthetic. Br J Anaesth 1991; 67:729–734.
38. Kouraklis G, Glinavou A, Raftopoulos L, et al. Epidural analgesia attenuates the systemic response to upper abdominal surgery: a randomized trial. Int Surg 2000; 85: 353–357.
39. Christensen P, Brandt MR, Rem J, et al. Influence of extradural morphine on the adrenocortical and hypoglycaemic response to surgery. Br J Anaesth 1982; 54:23–27.
40. Takeshima R, Dohi S. Circulatory response to baroreflexes, valsalva maneuver, coughing, swallowing and nasal stimulation during acute cardiac sympathectomy by epidural blockade in awake humans. Anesthesiology 1989; 3:418–424.
41. Goertz A, Heinrich H, Seeling W. Baroreflex control of heart rate during high thoracic epidural anesthesia. Anaesthesiology 1992; 97:984–987.
42. Sundberg A, Wattwil M. Circulatory effects of short-term hypercapnia during high thoracic epidural in elderly patients. Acta Anesthesiol Scand 1987; 31:81–86.
43. Reiz S. Circulatory effects of epidural anesthesia in patients with cardiac disease. Acta Anesthesiol Belg 1988; 39(suppl 2):22–27.
44. Goertz AW, Seeling W, Heinrich H, et al. Influence of high thoracic epidural anesthesia on left ventricular contractility assessed using end-systolic pressure-length relationship. Acta Anesthesiol Scand 1993; 37:38–44.
45. Tanaka K, Harada T, Dan K. Low dose thoracic epidural anesthesia induces discrete thoracic analgesia without reduction in cardiac output. Reg Anesth 1991; 16:318–321.

46. Niimi Y, Ichiose F, Saegusa H, et al. Echocardiographic evaluation of global left ventricular function during high thoracic epidural anesthesia. J Clin Anesth 1997; 9: 118–124.
47. Davis RF, DeBoer LWV, Maroko PR. Thoracic epidural anesthesia reduces myocardial infarct size after coronary occlusion in dogs. Anesth Analg 1986; 65:711–717.
48. Klassen GA, Bramwell RS, Bromage PR, et al. The effect of acute sympathectomy by epidural anesthesia on the canine coronary circulation. Anesthesiology 1980; 52:8–15.
49. Rolf N, Van der Welde M, Wouters PF, et al. Thoracic epidural anesthesia improves functional recovery from myocardial stunning in conscious dogs. Anesth Analg 1996; 83:935–940.
50. Blomberg S, Ricksten SE. Thoracic epidural anesthesia decreases the incidence of ventricular arrhythmias during acute myocardial ischaemia in anaesthetised rats. Acta Anaesthesiol Scand 1988; 32:173–178.
51. Blomberg S, Curelaru I, Emanuelsson H, et al. Thoracic epidural anaesthesia in patients with unstable angina pectoris. Eur Heart J 1989; 10:437–444.
52. Blomberg S, Emanuelsson H, Ricksten SE. Thoracic epidural anaesthesia and central hemodynamics in patients with unstable angina pectoris. Anesth Analg 1986; 69: 558–562.
53. Tuman KJ, McCarthy RJ, Speiss BD, et al. Does choice of anesthetic agent significantly alter outcome after coronary artery surgery? Anesthesiology 1989; 70:189–198.
54. Yeager MP, Glass DD, Neff RK, et al. Epidural anesthesia in high risk surgical patients. Anesthesiology 1987; 66:729–736.
55. de Leon-Casasola OA, Parker BM, Lema MJ, et al. Epidural analgesia versus intravenous patient-controlled analgesia: differences in the postoperative course of cancer patients. Reg Anesth 1994; 19:307–315.
56. Beattie WS, Buckley DN, Forrest JB. Epidural morphine reduces the risk of postoperative myocardial ischaemia in patients with cardiac risk factors. Can J Anesth 1993; 40:532–541.
57. Beattie WS, Badner NH, Choi P. Epidural analgesia reduces postoperative myocardial infarction: a meta-analysis. Anesth Analg 2001; 93:853–858.
58. Beattie WS, Badner NH, Choi PT. Meta-analysis demonstrates statistically significant reduction in postoperative myocardial infarction with the use of thoracic epidural analgesia. Anesth Analg 2003; 97:919–920.
59. Mangano DT, Browner WS, Hollenberg M, et al. Association of perioperative myocardial ischaemia with cardiac morbidity and mortality in men undergoing noncardiac surgery. The Study of Perioperative Ischaemia Research Group. N Eng J Med 1990; 323:1781–1788.
60. Mangano DT, Siliciano D, Hollenberg M, et al. Postoperative myocardial ischemia. Therapeutic trials using intensive analgesia following surgery. The Study of Perioperative Ischemia (SPI) Research Group. Anesthesiology 1992; 76:342–353.
61. Plumlee JE, Boettner RB. Myocardial infarction during and following anesthesia and operation. South Med J 1972; 65:886–889.
62. Tarhan S, Moffit EA, Taylor WF, et al. Myocardial infarction after general anesthesia. JAMA 1972; 220:1451–1454.
63. Veering BT, Cousins MJ. Cardiovascular and pulmonary effects of epidural anaesthesia. Anaesth Intensive Care 2000; 28:620.
64. Kochi T, Sako S, Nishiro T, et al. Effect of high thoracic epidural anaesthesia on ventilatory response to hypercapnia in normal volunteers. Br J Anaesth 1989; 62:362–367.
65. Sakura S, Saito Y, Kosaka Y. Effect of epidural anaesthesia on the ventilatory response to hypoxaemia. Anaesth 1993; 48:205–209.
66. Groeben H, Schwalen A, Irsfeld S, et al. High thoracic epidural does not alter airway resistance and attenuates the response to an inhalational provocation test in patients with bronchial hyper reactivity. Anesthesiology 1993; 81:868–874.

67. Mankikian B, Cantineau JP, Bertrand M, et al. Improvement of diaphragmatic function by a thoracic extradural block after upper abdominal surgery. Anesthesiology 1988; 68:379–386.
68. Pansard JL, Mankikian B, Bertrand M, et al. Effects of thoracic extradural block on diaphragmatic electrical activity and contractility after upper abdominal surgery. Anesthesiology 1993; 78:63–71.
69. Fratacicilli MD, Kimball WR, Wain JC, et al. Diaphragmatic shortening after thoracic surgery in humans. Effects of mechanical ventilation and thoracic epidural anesthesia. Anesthesiology 1993; 79:654–665.
70. Rademaker BM, Ringers J, Odoom JA, et al. Pulmonary function and stress response after laparoscopic cholecystectomy: comparison with subcostal incision and influence of thoracic epidural analgesia. Anesth Analg 1992; 75:381–385.
71. Spence AA, Smith G. Postoperative analgesia and lung function: a comparison of morphine with extradural block. Br J Anaesth 1971; 43:144–148.
72. Ballantyne JC, Carr DB, deFerranti S, et al. The comparative effects of postoperative analgesic therapies on pulmonary outcome: cumulative meta-analyses of randomized controlled trials. Anesth Analg 1998; 86:598–612.
73. Bell SD. The correlation between pulmonary function and resting and dynamic pain scores in post aortic surgery patients. Reg Anesth 1991; 16(suppl).
74. Flisberg P, Tornebrandt K, Walther B, et al. Pain relief after esophagectomy. Thoracic epidural analgesia is better than parenteral opioids. J Cardiothoracic Vasc Anesth 2001; 15:282–287.
75. Kilbride MJ, Senagore AJ, Mazier WP, et al. Epidural analgesia. Surg Gynecol Obstet 1992; 174:137–140.
76. George KA, Wright PM, Chisakuta AM, et al. Thoracic epidural analgesia compared with patient controlled intravenous morphine after upper abdominal surgery. Acta Anaesthesiol Scand 1994; 38:808–812.
77. Madej TH, Wheatley RG, Jackson IJB, et al. Hypoxemia and pain relief after lower abdominal surgery: comparison of extradural and patient-controlled analgesia. Br J Anaesth 1992; 69:554–557.
78. Senagore AJ, Delaney CP, Mekhail N, et al. Randomized clinical trial comparing epidural anaesthesia and patient-controlled analgesia after laparoscopic segmental colectomy. Br J Surg 2003; 90:1195–1199.
79. Block BM, Liu SS, Rowlingson AJ, et al. Efficacy of postoperative epidural analgesia: a meta-analysis. JAMA 2003; 290:2455–2463.
80. Davies GK, Tolhurst-Cleaver CL, James TL. Respiratory depression after intrathecal narcotics. Anaesth 1980; 35:1080–1083.
81. Rawal N, Mollefors K, Axelsson K, et al. An experimental study of urodynamics of morphine and naloxone reversal. Anesth Analg 1983; 62:641–647.
82. Aromaa U, Lahdensuu M, Cozanitis DA. Severe complications associated with epidural and spinal anaesthesias in Finland 1987–1993. A study based on patient insurance claims. Acta Anaesthesiol Scand 1997; 41:445–452.
83. Romer HC, Russell GN. A survey of the practice of thoracic epidural analgesia in the United Kingdom. Anaesthesiology 1998; 53:1016–1022.
84. Loo CC, Thomas E, Tan HM, et al. Sedation for the conduct of lumbar epidural anaesthesia: a study using subanaesthetic doses of ketamine in combination with midazolam. Ann Acad Med Singapore 1997; 26:200–204.
85. Gallimore SC, Hoile RW, Ingram GS, et al. The Report of the National Confidential Enquiry into Perioperative Deaths. HMSO: London, 1994–1995.
86. Kassis J, Fugere F, Dube S. The safe use of epidural anesthesia after subcutaneous injection of low dose heparin in general abdominal surgery. Can J Surg 2000; 43:289–294.
87. Heller AR, Litz RJ. Why do orthopedic patients have a higher incidence of complications after central neuraxial blockade–correspondence. Anesthesiology 2005; 102:1286.

88. Vandermeulen E, Van Aken H, Vermylen J. Anticoagulants and spinal-epidural anesthesia. Anesth Analg 1994; 79:1165–1177.
89. Horlocker TT, Wedel DJ. Neuraxial block and low molecular weight heparin: balancing perioperative analgesia and thromboprophylaxis. Reg Anesth Pain Med 1998; 23(suppl 2): 164–177.
90. McLure HA, Trenfield S, Quereshi A, et al. Post-splenectomy thrombocytopenia: implications for regional analgesia. Anaesthesiology 2003; 58:1106–1110.
91. Rodgers A, Walker N, Schug S, et al. Reduction of postoperative mortality and morbidity with epidural or spinal anaesthesia: results from overview of randomized trials. Br Med J 2000; 321:1493.
92. Allen G. Epidural anesthesia and analgesia did not reduce most comorbid outcomes in high-risk patients having major abdominal surgery. ACP J Club 2002; 137:84.
93. Rigg J, Jamrozik K, Myles P, et al. Epidural anaesthesia and analgesia and outcome of major surgery: a randomized trial. Lancet 2002; 359:1276.
94. Burns SM, Cowan CM. Spinal anaesthesia for caesarean section: current clinical practice. Hosp Med 2000; 61:855–858.
95. Ghiardinii G, Baraldi R, Bertellini C, et al. Advantages of spinal anaesthesia in abdominal gynaecologic surgery. Clin Exp Ob Gynaecol 1998; 25:105–106.
96. Hatch PD. Surgical and anaesthetic considerations in transurethral resection of the prostate. Anaesth Intensive Care 1987; 15:203–211.
97. Tran QH, Kaufman I, Schricker T. Spinal anaesthesia for a patient with type I sialidosis undergoing abdominal surgery. Acta Anaesthesiol Scand 2005; 45:919–921.
98. Varela A, Yuste A, Villazala R, et al. Spinal anesthesia for emergency abdominal surgery in uncontrolled hyperthyroidism. Acta Anaesthesiol Scand 2005; 49:100–103.
99. Carpenter RL, Caplan RA, Brown DL, et al. Incidence and risk factors for side effects of spinal anesthesia. Anesthesiology 1992; 76:906–916.
100. Arndt JO, Bomer W, Krauth J, et al. Incidence and time course of cardiovascular side effects during spinal anesthesia after prophylactic administration of intravenous fluids or vasopressor. Anesth Analg 1998; 87:347–354.
101. Song D, Greilich N, White P, et al. Recovery profiles and costs of anesthesia for outpatient unilateral inguinal herniorrhaphy. Anesth Analg 2000; 91:876–881.
102. Nordin P, Hernell H, Unosson M, et al. Type of anesthetic and patient acceptance in groin hernia repair: a multicentre randomized trial. Hernia 2004; 8:220–225.
103. Cartagena J, Vicenta JP, Moreno-Egea A, et al. Regional anaesthesia in the outpatient treatment of bilateral inguinal hernias using totally extraperitoneal laparoscopy. J Ambulatory Surg 2003; 10:55–59.
104. Richardson J, Jones J, Atkinson R. The effect of thoracic paravertebral blockade on intercostals somatosensory evoked potentials. Anesth Analg 1998; 87:373–376.
105. Weltz C, Klein S, Arbo J, et al. Paravertebral block anesthesia for inguinal hernia repair. World J Surg 2003; 27:425–429.
106. Sabanathan S, Mearns AJ, Bickford Smith PJ, et al. Efficacy of continuous extrapleural intercostals nerve block on post thoracotomy pain and pulmonary mechanics. Br J Surg 1990; 77:221–225.
107. Taylor R, Massey S, Stuart-Smith K. Postoperative analgesia in video-assisted thoracoscopy, the role of intercostals blockade. J Cardiothoracic Vasc Anesth 2004; 18: 317–321.
108. Concha M, Daguino J, Cariaga M, et al. Analgesia after thoracotomy: epidural fentanyl/ bupivacaine compared with intercostals nerve block plus intravenous morphine. J Cardiothoracic Vasc Surg 2004; 18:322–326.
109. Knowles P, Hancox D, Letheren M, et al. An evaluation of intercostals nerve block for analgesia following renal transplantation. Eur J Anaesth 1998; 15:457–461.
110. Carbonell AM, Harold KL, Mahmutovich AJ, et al. Local injection for the treatment of suture site pain after laparoscopic ventral hernia repair. Am Surg 2003; 69:688–691.

111. Blake DW, Donnan G, Novella J. Interpleural administration of bupivacaine after cholecystectomy: a comparison with intercostals nerve block. Anaesth Intensive Care 1989;
17:269–274.
112. van Kleef JW, Burm AGL, Vletter AA. Single dose interpleural versus intercostals blockade. Nerve block characteristics and plasma concentration profiles after administration
of 0.5% bupivacaine with epinephrine. Anesth Analg 1990; 70:484–488.
113. Muir J, Ferguson S. The rectus sheath block–well worth remembering. Anaesthesiology
1996; 51:893–894.
114. Aasbo V, Thuen A, Raeder J. Improved long-lasting postoperative analgesia, recovery
function and patient satisfaction after inguinal hernia repair with inguinal field block
compared with general anesthesia. Acta Anesthesiol Scand 2002; 46:674–678.
115. Haldane G, Stott S, McMenemin I. Pouch of Douglas block for laparoscopic sterilisation.
Anaesthesiology 1998; 53:598.
116. Whitlow BJ, Lovell D, Maher R, et al. A double blind trial of hypogastric nerve block for
postoperative pain relief following laparoscopic excision of endometriosis. Gynecol Surg
2005; 2:5–6.
117. Moiniche S, Jorgensen H, Wetterslev J, et al. Local anesthetic infiltration for postoperative pain relief after laparoscopy: a qualitative and quantitative systematic review of
intraperitoneal, port site infiltration and mesosalpinx block. Anesth Analg 2000;
90:899–912.
118. Eck JB, Ross AK. Paediatric regional anaesthesia–what makes a difference? Best Pract
Res Clin Anaesthesiol 2002; 16:159–174.
119. Vanner RG. Gastro-oesophageal reflux and regurgitation during general anaesthesia for
termination of pregnancy. Int J Obs Anaesth 1992; 1:123–128.

10

Sedation for Endoscopic Procedures

Udvitha C. Nandasoma and Mervyn H. Davies
Liver Unit, St. James's University Hospital, Leeds, U.K.

HISTORICAL BACKGROUND

Endoscopy using bamboo or hollow reeds illuminated with candles was described in both ancient Egypt and Greece (1). The development of electric light sources toward the end of the 19th century rekindled interest in the practical application of endoscopy. The invention of optical fibers allowing efficient transmission of light along fine glass fibers allowed the development of flexible endoscopes and led to the adoption of endoscopy as a routine diagnostic and therapeutic tool.

Conscious sedation has been used to facilitate endoscopy from its inception and has been routinely administered by the endoscopist. The perception of many endoscopic procedures as inherently low-risk minor procedures has meant that sedation practice in gastrointestinal (GI) endoscopy has often lagged behind current standards of care in anesthesiology. Guidelines from national bodies setting minimum standards of care and monitoring for patients having endoscopic procedures under sedation should help improve clinical practice (2). The evidence base with regard to sedation in endoscopy remains limited. Many clinical trials have lacked the power to identify important clinical correlates of observations, such as hypoxia and cardiac rhythm disturbance frequently seen during endoscopy. Similarly, real clinical benefit for interventions, such as monitoring with pulse oximetry or supplemental oxygen, has been hard to demonstrate. Even assessing the effect of sedation on a patient's experience and tolerance of endoscopy is made difficult by the fact that individuals recruited to such trials appear to be significantly different in their characteristics from those who decline to participate (3).

ENDOSCOPIC PROCEDURES AND THEIR ASSOCIATED RISK FACTORS

Complications from diagnostic endoscopy remain rare. Therapeutic procedures, such as percutaneous endoscopic gastrostomy (PEG), endoscopic retrograde cholangiopancreatography (ERCP), and therapy for GI bleeding are associated with significant morbidity and mortality. The 2004 report of the U.K. National Confidential Enquiry into Patient Outcome and Death reported 30-day mortalities of 6%, 2%, and 5%

for PEG, ERCP, and therapeutic upper GI endoscopy following an audit of 136,000 upper GI endoscopic procedures (1). Interpretation of these mortality statistics is complicated by the difficulty in separating mortality specific to endoscopy and that due to the underlying comorbidities of many patients undergoing endoscopic procedures.

Percutaneous Endoscopic Gastrostomy

PEG insertion is used increasingly in the long-term management of nutritional failure in chronic neurological disease, stroke-related dysphagia, and head and neck malignancy.

Therefore, patients undergoing this procedure often have significant cardiovascular comorbidity, malignancy, and established or developing nutritional failure. They may be at intrinsically higher risk of aspiration, due to either a defect in the swallowing mechanism or mechanical obstruction. In addition to this, the procedure is performed with the patient supine.

Endoscopic Retrograde Cholangio-Pancreatography

Due to the advent of magnetic resonance cholangio-pancreatography, most patients undergo ERCP for biliary intervention. The procedure itself is associated with complications of pancreatitis, postsphincterotomy bleeding, duodenal perforation, and sepsis. Many patients have obstructive jaundice with its inherent complications and underlying biliary sepsis or even preexisting gallstone-related acute pancreatitis.

Gastrointestinal Bleeding

Patients presenting with significant GI blood loss tend to be older and often have significant associated comorbidity. Variceal bleeding related to decompensated chronic liver disease represents an increasingly frequent cause for acute GI hemorrhage. Hypovolemic shock is common and under-resuscitation of patients prior to endoscopy is commonly reported. The procedure is often performed as an emergency, and the patient may have a significant gastric content placing them at risk of aspiration.

Esophageal Dilatation

Esophageal dilatation is indicated for a wide variety of conditions causing esophageal obstruction. It is associated with an esophageal perforation rate of 2% with an overall mortality rate of 1% (4). Patients with dysphagia, especially in association with achalasia, may have considerable food residue or retained secretions within the esophagus and be at risk of pulmonary aspiration.

Colonoscopy

Colonoscopy is associated with a risk of colonic perforation. Approximately 1% of procedures are complicated by bradycardia or hypotension, though these events rarely have clinically significant sequelae. It should be remembered that the process of bowel cleansing–required precolonoscopy can be associated with a range of electrolyte disturbances. Elderly patients taking diuretics and antagonists of the renin–angiotensin system appear most at risk, and hyperphosphatemia and hypocalcemia can be particular problems associated with sodium phosphate–containing cathartics. It is suggested that offending drugs should be discontinued if possible prior to administration of the preparation, and consideration given to inpatient preparation and electrolyte monitoring of especially vulnerable patients (5).

SPECIAL PATIENT GROUPS

Postmyocardial Infarction

Endoscopic procedures increase myocardial stress and can be associated with transient dysrhythmias. It is suggested that elective procedures are delayed 10 to 12 weeks from the acute event; however, endoscopy and colonoscopy have been safely performed in stable patients and should be considered when the procedure is strongly indicated (6–10).

Pregnancy

Data on the safety of all endoscopic procedures during pregnancy are limited (11). It is generally recommended that procedures be undertaken only when strongly indicated. The fetus is sensitive to maternal hypoxia and this could be generated by the procedure, associated sedation, or inferior vena caval compression and decreased uterine blood flow from maternal positioning. Additionally, third-trimester patients may be at theoretical risk of acid aspiration, although data are lacking in this area.

Uteroplacental transfer of drugs is also a theoretical risk, particularly during early gestation when there is greatest risk of fetal malformation. At all stages of pregnancy, sedative drugs have the potential to influence placental blood flow and to interfere with smooth muscle reactivity.

Of the drugs used to facilitate endoscopy, midazolam, pethidine, naloxone, and propofol are preferred on the basis of limited data. Flumazenil is little studied in pregnancy but has been associated with behavioral changes in male rats exposed in utero. The recent guidelines from the American Society for Gastrointestinal Endoscopy provide useful advice (12).

Difficult-to-Sedate Patients

A history of prior difficulty with conscious sedation, benzodiazepine use, and heavy alcohol use are predictors of difficulty with sedation. Problems may be experienced in up to 30% of such patients and paradoxical agitation with benzodiazepines has been described.

UNSEDATED ENDOSCOPY

Endoscopy without sedation reduces the risks of respiratory depression and also reduces the procedural recovery time and cost of endoscopic procedures. Many endoscopic procedures such as flexible sigmoidoscopy and diagnostic upper GI endoscopy can be performed without sedation. The additional time and resource implications of practicing conscious sedation has led to much interest in identifying patients who can undergo such procedures in a satisfactory fashion without sedation.

Many patients experience significant anxiety prior to an endoscopic procedure. Concerns about the procedure and the underlying diagnosis both contribute significantly to this. In patient surveys, younger age and male sex are associated with lower rates of preferring sedation, though factors such as age of more than 75 years and reduced pharyngeal sensitivity are most predictive of an adequate endoscopic study without sedation. Individual variability means that the clinical utility of these predictors remains limited (13). In a randomized controlled study comparing sedation to placebo in a group of Canadian patients, the use of sedation was the most predictive factor in a multivariate analysis for successful endoscopy (14). However, predicting an individual's tolerance of an endoscopic procedure is difficult and an individualized approach to patient care should be taken.

CARDIORESPIRATORY CHANGES DURING ENDOSCOPY

Arterial hypoxemia, tachycardia, and increased systolic blood pressure are all associated with endoscopic procedures (15). These changes are in part due to the activation of a classic endocrine stress response with elevated cortisol and catecholamine levels (15). Up to half of endoscopic procedures may be associated with a degree of hypoxemia (16). This is also reported in procedures not involving sedation and observed to be most profound in the minutes immediately following endoscope insertion.

In nonsedated patients, factors predictive of hypoxemia have been found to be a basal oxygen saturation that is less than 95%, preexisting respiratory disease, multiple attempts at intubation, emergency procedures, and an American Society of Anesthesiologists (ASA) score of III or IV (17). Operator inexperience, longer procedural time, and dwelling of the endoscope in the pharynx have also been correlated with a greater risk of procedure-related desaturation. Sedation will tend to exacerbate hypoxemia in these situations.

Safe and effective therapeutic and diagnostic endoscopy can be performed in appropriately selected patients at the extremes of age (18). However, even with dose adjustment, the elderly remain more prone to oxygen desaturation with sedative drugs (19).

Upper GI endoscopy, ERCP, and colonoscopy may be associated with myocardial stress. In healthy unsedated volunteers, there is a significant increase in cardiac stress as measured by the myocardial rate pressure product (20). Patients with stable coronary disease may experience silent periods of ischemia during endoscopy, though this is rarely symptomatic. The significance of this is unclear in terms of patient morbidity or mortality. The incidence of ST segment depression is reduced by the use of supplemental oxygen. In some studies endoscopy carried out in patients with coronary disease using sedation has been associated with reduced procedure-related tachycardia and myocardial stress, though other studies show no effect (21). An excess of ventricular extrasystoles, though with no sustained arrhythmias or morbidity, was described. Colonoscopy is also associated with hypoxemia in up to 41% of patients (22); this is also associated with measurable myocardial stress.

Hypoxia is common during both sedated and unsedated endoscopic procedures. Although high-risk patients can be identified, the predictors of desaturation are not sensitive or specific enough to identify subgroups at particular risk. Although definite adverse effects from these cardiorespiratory changes seen at endoscopy have not been defined, it should be realized that the studies were limited in their power to exclude clinically important effects. Supplemental oxygen can certainly correct the hypoxia observed during endoscopy and also appears to abrogate the myocardial ischemia that can result from procedure-related tachycardia in vulnerable patients. In addition to this, reports and papers continue to catalogue "not infrequent" oxygen desaturation to less than 85% (23), a figure considered unacceptable and dangerous in anesthetic practice. This could largely be prevented by appropriate use of supplemental oxygen and arterial oxygen saturation monitoring with pulse oximetry.

Monitoring

It is recommended that all patients undergoing GI procedures should be assessed continuously during the procedure in terms of their conscious level, hemodynamic status, and respiratory status. Clinical observation is augmented by the use of electronic blood pressure monitoring and pulse oximetry for patients undergoing endoscopic procedures under sedation or with preexisting respiratory or cardiac disease. Capnography has been suggested to be superior to clinical observation and pulse oximetry in detecting early respiratory depression (24).

There has been much interest in the utility of the electroencephalogram (EEG) as a measure of depth of sedation to augment clinical observation. The most widely studied device is the bispectral monitor. It relies on the phenomenon that the EEG becomes slower and more regular as sedation or anesthesia deepens. Monitoring of the EEG and complex mathematical manipulation generates a dimensionless number, termed the bispectral index, reflecting the patient's state of sedation. The bispectral index has shown some utility in the tracking of benzodiazepine- and opiate-induced sedation (25,26). In anesthetic practice, EEG-based approaches have been shown to be useful in reducing consumption of anesthetic drugs, recovery time, and complications related to anesthesia. The utility of the bispectral probe in titrating propofol dosage for conscious sedation during endoscopic procedures had not yet been established, and some studies have shown a significant lag between the onset of moderate sedation and change in the bispectral index (27).

TOPICAL PHARYNGEAL ANESTHESIA

Topical anesthetic sprays are often used in unsedated upper GI endoscopy to suppress the gag reflex and improve patient tolerance of upper GI endoscopy. Satisfactory endoscopy can be carried out using this method, and the practicality of many dyspepsia services is dependent upon this approach. The data are conflicting as to whether pharyngeal anesthesia, in fact, improves patient tolerance. Small, randomized trials have suggested that topical anesthesia improves tolerance of endoscopy (28,29), but other data suggests that it has no effect on patient tolerance but does make intubation easier when compared with midazolam-sedated and unsedated patients (30). Complications are uncommon but there have been a number of reports of methemoglobinemia (31) and of cardiovascular collapse in elderly patients or when the agent had been administered by gargle rather than by metered dose device. There appears to be no clear advantage to the administration of pharyngeal anesthesia in combination with intravenous sedation (32), and the recent U.K. endoscopy National Confidential Enquiry into Patient Outcome and Death (NCEPOD) report noted that pulmonary aspiration was consistently associated with the use of combined intravenous sedation and topical anesthesia (1).

INTRAVENOUS SEDATION

Intravenous sedation has been consistently shown to improve the tolerability and success of endoscopic procedures. The commonest approach is to use an intravenous benzodiazepine, either alone (e.g., in diagnostic upper GI endoscopy) or in combination with an opiate (e.g., in therapeutic endoscopy, ERCP, and colonoscopy). This approach has limitations in prolonged or difficult procedures, and more recently, there has been interest in endoscopist- or nurse-administered propofol as a sedative agent.

CHOICE OF AGENTS

Benzodiazepines

Midazolam and diazepam remain the most commonly used benzodiazepine agents. Midazolam is termed an "ultra-short" half-life benzodiazepine and is metabolized rapidly by hydroxylation. The resulting α-hydroxylated compound is eliminated with a half-life of one hour after conjugation with glucuronic acid. Nevertheless, accumulation of midazolam metabolites has been described in patients, especially in cases where the drug is given by continuous infusion. Diazepam has a longer half-life and produces the active metabolite nordiazepam that has an elimination half-life in excess of 24 hours. Benzodiazepines increase heart rate and lower blood pressure; in normal subjects, this effect is minor. Respiratory depression is the most important side effect of concern when benzodiazepines are used. Arterial oxygen desaturation is common during both sedated and unsedated endoscopy. It appears clear that sedation, especially in the elderly or those with preexisting pulmonary disease, does increase the frequency of desaturation episodes (33). However, with oxygen therapy and appropriate monitoring, dose-adjusted sedation can be safely administered to most groups (34). The half-life of most benzodiazepines, including midazolam, is increased in the elderly, and a significantly lower dose is required to achieve satisfactory sedation (35–37).

There is little evidence as to the typical dose of benzodiazepine required for a particular procedure or indeed which of the commonly used agents is most suitable for use in the setting of GI endoscopy. A small study did, however, suggest that low-dose intravenous midazolam ($35\,\mu g/kg$) was as effective in improving procedure tolerability and was associated with less postprocedural inconvenience and fewer episodes of procedure-associated desaturation events than a dose of $70\,\mu g/kg$. These doses equate to 2.5 and 5 mg in a 70-kg patient. The mean dose of midazolam used in clinical practice also appears to have decreased over time (38).

Due to its shorter half-life, midazolam is the benzodiazepine of choice for endoscopic sedation in many centers. It does appear to achieve procedural amnesia in more patients than diazepam, but some studies suggest that it may confer no advantage in terms of rapidity of recovery or postprocedural course over diazepam (39). Midazolam appears to be significantly more potent and associated with more carbon dioxide retention than diazepam (40).

It is recommended that the dose of a benzodiazepine should be titrated gradually to achieve the desired level of sedation. The overriding principle is that the patient should experience anxiolysis and relaxation but without loss of verbal contact or airway control. Slurring of speech and eye closing are the most commonly used indicators of adequate sedation. It has been common endoscopic practice to give sedative benzodiazepines as a bolus injection rather than by titration. A number of large case series suggest that this approach is safe in most patients (41). A U.K. audit suggested that lower doses of midazolam should be used when given as a bolus, patients less than 70 years of age requiring a mean midazolam dose of 4.65 mg and those above 70, a mean dose of 1.89 mg to achieve adequate sedation (35). This audit was conducted at a time where much higher doses than these were not uncommon; however, the trend in current clinical practice suggests that adequate sedation can be achieved with even lower doses. Patients with cirrhosis and portal hypertension are, in general, more sensitive to the effects of sedative medication, including benzodiazepines, and may experience a prolonged recovery period (42) or hepatic encephalopathy. Benzodiazepines demonstrate significant synergy when given with opiates (43). It is therefore recommended that the opiate is given first as a bolus and the dose of benzodiazepine is titrated gradually to achieve the desired level of sedation.

Reversal of benzodiazepine-induced sedation can be achieved with flumazenil, which acts as an antagonist at benzodiazepine receptors. This agent is effective and generally safe. It does, however, have a shorter half-life than the benzodiazepines and so resedation after its initial administration is possible. Some have suggested that routine use of flumazenil can allow more rapid discharge and more efficient use of time within the endoscopy department for routine cases. Due to the wide range of patients opting for outpatient endoscopy and the fact that most patients are discharged home rather than to a medically supervised environment, this approach has yet to gain widespread acceptance.

Some patients develop paradoxical agitation in response to the administration of midazolam; this also appears to respond to flumazenil (44). Benzodiazepine dosage and administration, therefore, needs to be carefully considered for each individual patient, the dose required will be determined by patient age and comorbidities, including cardiorespiratory, renal, and hepatic dysfunction.

Opiates

Opiate drugs are used in endoscopic practice for procedures such as colonoscopy and ERCP, usually in combination with a benzodiazepine. Fentanyl and pethidine are the most commonly used agents. Fentanyl, a synthetic opioid, has theoretical advantages over pethidine in that it has a shorter duration of action, and the respiratory depression seen with fentanyl is of shorter duration. Direct comparative data is, however, scarce. Respiratory depression seen with either of these agents can be reversed by the use of naloxone. The combination of pethidine and midazolam has been shown to improve patient tolerance during colonoscopy (45). A study in pediatric patients demonstrated no significant difference in safety or efficacy between fentanyl and pethidine drugs (46).

Pethidine has traditionally been preferred for biliary procedures due to its relaxant effect on the sphincter of Oddi; however, sphincter spasm in response to fentanyl appears to be rare (47).

Propofol

There has been increasing interest in the use of propofol for endoscopic procedures, including ERCP and colonoscopy (48). Propofol is a lipophilic compound unrelated to other intravenous anesthetic agents. It has been used widely in anesthetics and intensive care since its introduction in 1989. It has a rapid onset of action, producing sedation within 30 to 60 seconds and having a very short plasma half-life of the order of a few minutes. Its pharmacokinetics is little different in patients with cirrhosis or renal dysfunction, though clearance is slower in the elderly (48). Propofol has been safely administered by endoscopists or nurse assistants (49) or used in the context of a patient-controlled sedation system (50). Propofol generally produced a more rapid onset of sedation and a greater depth of sedation, and patients receiving propofol recovered more quickly. Not all trials, however, associated this with increased levels of patient satisfaction (50,51). The use of propofol has a number of limitations; it has little or no analgesic effect and achieving moderate sedation can be difficult because of its narrow therapeutic window. Due to the ingredients of its emulsion preparation, propofol cannot be administered to those with a soya bean or egg allergy. It should not be used for awake sedation in pregnancy, and lactating women must be advised to discard breast milk for 24 hours following administration.

Although propofol can be given safely in the context of the endoscopy department, it is a potent drug and its use must be governed by the implementation of training, monitoring, and care protocols that recognize this.

CONCLUSIONS

Traditionally, endoscopists have administered sedation for endoscopy. The practice shows considerable variation between centers and between countries. This, in part, is due to differences in patient expectation, but is also due to the unstructured way in which training in sedation practice has been delivered to endoscopists. Endoscopy is a procedure performed so commonly that even a low complication rate will result in many patients suffering harm. For some time, developments in endoscopic practice far out paced the development of sedation techniques appropriate to these new procedures. National guidelines and the investigation of new methods of monitoring and delivering sedation are beginning to improve patient care and safety.

REFERENCES

1. Cullinane M, Hargraves CMK, Lucas S, et al. "Scoping our Practice", the 2004 Report of the National Confidential Enquiry into Patient Outcome and Death. London, England: HMSO, 2004.
2. Waring JP, Baron TH, Hirota WK, et al. Guidelines for conscious sedation and monitoring during gastrointestinal endoscopy. Gastrointest Endosc 2003; 58(3):317–322.
3. Abraham NS, Wieczorek P, Huang J, et al. Assessing clinical generalizability in sedation studies of upper GI endoscopy. Gastrointest Endosc 2004; 60(1):28–33.
4. Quine MA, Bell GD, McCloy RF, et al. Prospective audit of upper gastrointestinal endoscopy in two regions of England: safety, staffing, and sedation methods. Gut 1995; 36(3):462–467.
5. Ainley EJ, Winwood PJ, Begley JP. Measurement of serum electrolytes and phosphate after sodium phosphate colonoscopy bowel preparation: an evaluation. Dig Dis Sci 2005; 50(7):1319–1323.
6. Cappell MS. Safety and efficacy of colonoscopy after myocardial infarction: an analysis of 100 study patients and 100 control patients at two tertiary cardiac referral hospitals. Gastrointest Endosc 2004; 60(6):901–909.
7. Cappell MS. Safety of push enteroscopy after recent myocardial infarction. Dig Dis Sci 2004; 49(3):509–513.
8. Cappell MS. Risks versus benefits of flexible sigmoidoscopy after myocardial infarction: an analysis of 78 patients at three medical centers. Am J Med 2004; 116(10):707–710.

9. Cappell MS. Gastrointestinal endoscopy in high-risk patients. Dig Dis Sci 1996; 14(4): 228–244.

10. Cappell MS. Safety and clinical efficacy of flexible sigmoidoscopy and colonoscopy for gastrointestinal bleeding after myocardial infarction. A six-year study of 18 consecutive lower endoscopies at two university teaching hospitals. Dig Dis Sci 1994; 39(3): 473–480.

11. Cappell MS. The fetal safety and clinical efficacy of gastrointestinal endoscopy during pregnancy. Gastroenterol Clin North Am 2003; 32(1):123–179.

12. Qureshi WA, Rajan E, Adler DG, et al. ASGE guideline: guidelines for endoscopy in pregnant and lactating women. Gastrointest Endosc 2005; 61(3):357–362.

13. Abraham N, Barkun A, Larocque M, et al. Predicting which patients can undergo upper endoscopy comfortably without conscious sedation. Gastrointest Endosc 2002; 56(2): 180–189.

14. Abraham NS, Fallone CA, Mayrand S, et al. Sedation versus no sedation in the performance of diagnostic upper gastrointestinal endoscopy: a Canadian randomized controlled cost-outcome study. Am J Gastroenterol 2004; 99(9):1692–1699.

15. Tonnesen H, Puggaard L, Braagaard J, et al. Stress response to endoscopy. Scand J Gastroenterol 1999; 34(6):629–631.

16. Dark DS, Campbell DR, Wesselius LJ. Arterial oxygen desaturation during gastrointestinal endoscopy. Am J Gastroenterol 1990; 85(10):1317–1321.

17. Alcain G, Guillen P, Escolar A, et al. Predictive factors of oxygen desaturation during upper gastrointestinal endoscopy in nonsedated patients. Gastrointest Endosc 1998; 48(2):143–147.

18. Clarke GA, Jacobson BC, Hammett RJ, et al. The indications, utilization and safety of gastrointestinal endoscopy in an extremely elderly patient cohort. Endoscopy 2001; 33(7):580–584.

19. Yano H, Iishi H, Tatsuta M, et al. Oxygen desaturation during sedation for colonoscopy in elderly patients. Hepatogastroenterology 1998; 45(24):2138–2141.

20. Adachi W, Yazawa K, Owa M, et al. Quantification of cardiac stress during EGD without sedation. Gastrointest Endosc 2002; 55(1):58–64.

21. Yazawa K, Adachi W, Owa M, et al. Can sedation reduce the cardiac stress during gastrointestinal endoscopy? A study with non-invasive automated cardiac flow measurement by color Doppler echocardiography. Scand J Gastroenterol 2002; 37(5):602–607.

22. Bilotta JJ, Floyd JL, Waye JD. Arterial oxygen desaturation during ambulatory colonoscopy: predictability, incidence, and clinical insignificance. Gastrointest Endosc 1990; 36(suppl 3):S5–S8.

23. Bell GD. Premedication, preparation, and surveillance. Endoscopy 2002; 34(1):2–12.

24. Vargo JJ, Zuccaro G Jr., Dumot JA, et al. Automated graphic assessment of respiratory activity is superior to pulse oximetry and visual assessment for the detection of early respiratory depression during therapeutic upper endoscopy. Gastrointest Endosc 2002; 55(7):826–831.

25. Bower AL, Ripepi A, Dilger J, et al. Bispectral index monitoring of sedation during endoscopy. Gastrointest Endosc 2000; 52(2):192–196.

26. Leslie K, Absalom A, Kenny GN. Closed loop control of sedation for colonoscopy using the Bispectral Index. Anaesthesia 2002; 57(7):693–697.

27. Chen SC, Rex DK. An initial investigation of bispectral monitoring as an adjunct to nurse-administered propofol sedation for colonoscopy. Am J Gastroenterol 2004; 99(6):1081–1086.

28. Campo R, Brullet E, Montserrat A, et al. Topical pharyngeal anesthesia improves tolerance of upper gastrointestinal endoscopy: a randomized double-blind study. Endoscopy 1995; 27(9):659–664.

29. Mulcahy HE, Greaves RR, Ballinger A, et al. A double-blind randomized trial of low-dose versus high-dose topical anaesthesia in unsedated upper gastrointestinal endoscopy. Aliment Pharmacol Ther 1996; 10(6):975–979.

30. Ristikankare M, Hartikainen J, Heikkinen M, et al. Is routine sedation or topical pharyngeal anesthesia beneficial during upper endoscopy? Gastrointest Endosc 2004; 60(5): 686–694.
31. Kuschner WG, Chitkara RK, Canfield J Jr., et al. Benzocaine-associated methemoglobinemia following bronchoscopy in a healthy research participant. Respir Care 2000; 45(8): 953–956.
32. Davis DE, Jones MP, Kubik CM. Topical pharyngeal anesthesia does not improve upper gastrointestinal endoscopy in conscious sedated patients. Am J Gastroenterol 1999; 94(7):1853–1856.
33. Freeman ML, Hennessy JT, Cass OW, et al. Carbon dioxide retention and oxygen desaturation during gastrointestinal endoscopy. Gastroenterology 1993; 105(2):331–339.
34. Christe C, Janssens JP, Armenian B, et al. Midazolam sedation for upper gastrointestinal endoscopy in older persons: a randomized, double-blind, placebo-controlled study. J Am Geriatr Soc 2000; 48(11):1398–1403.
35. Smith MR, Bell GD, Quine MA, et al. Small bolus injections of intravenous midazolam for upper gastrointestinal endoscopy: a study of 788 consecutive cases. Br J Clin Pharmacol 1993; 36(6):573–578.
36. Smith MT, Heazlewood V, Eadie MJ, et al. Pharmacokinetics of midazolam in the aged. Eur J Clin Pharmacol 1984; 26(3):381–388.
37. Bell GD, Spickett GP, Reeve PA, et al. Intravenous midazolam for upper gastrointestinal endoscopy: a study of 800 consecutive cases relating dose to age and sex of patient. Br J Clin Pharmacol 1987; 23(2):241–243.
38. Mulcahy HE, Hennessy E, Connor P, et al. Changing patterns of sedation use for routine out-patient diagnostic gastroscopy between 1989 and 1998. Aliment Pharmacol Ther 2001; 15(2):217–220.
39. Bell GD, Morden A, Coady T, et al. A comparison of diazepam and midazolam as endoscopy premedication assessing changes in ventilation and oxygen saturation. Br J Clin Pharmacol 1988; 26(5):595–600.
40. Zakko SF, Seifert HA, Gross JB. A comparison of midazolam and diazepam for conscious sedation during colonoscopy in a prospective double-blind study. Gastrointest Endosc 1999; 49(6):684–689.
41. Simon IB, Lewis RJ, Satava RM. A safe method for sedating and monitoring patients for upper and lower gastrointestinal endoscopy. Am Surg 1991; 57(4):219–221.
42. Hamdy NA, Kennedy HJ, Nicholl J, et al. Sedation for gastroscopy: a comparative study of midazolam and Diazemuls in patients with and without cirrhosis. Br J Clin Pharmacol 1986; 22(6):643–647.
43. Ben Shlomo I, abd-el-Khalim H, Ezry J, et al. Midazolam acts synergistically with fentanyl for induction of anaesthesia. Br J Anaesth 1990; 64(1):45–47.
44. Weinbroum AA, Szold O, Ogorek D, et al. The midazolam-induced paradox phenomenon is reversible by flumazenil. Epidemiology, patient characteristics and review of the literature. Eur J Anaesthesiol 2001; (12):789–797.
45. Radaelli F, Meucci G, Terruzzi V, et al. Single bolus of midazolam versus bolus midazolam plus meperidine for colonoscopy: a prospective, randomized, double-blind trial. Gastrointest Endosc 2003; 57(3):329–335.
46. Ali S, Davidson DL, Gremse DA. Comparison of fentanyl versus meperidine for analgesia in pediatric gastrointestinal endoscopy. Dig Dis Sci 2004; 49(5):888–891.
47. Jones RM, Detmer M, Hill AB, et al. Incidence of choledochoduodenal sphincter spasm during fentanyl-supplemented anesthesia. Anesth Analg 1981; 60(9):638–640.
48. Chen SC, Rex DK. Review article: registered nurse-administered propofol sedation for endoscopy. Aliment Pharmacol Ther 2004; 19(2):147–155.
49. Rex DK, Overley C, Kinser K, et al. Safety of propofol administered by registered nurses with gastroenterologist supervision in 2000 endoscopic cases. Am J Gastroenterol 2002; 97(5):1159–1163.

50. Bright E, Roseveare C, Dalgleish D, et al. Patient-controlled sedation for colonoscopy: a randomized trial comparing patient-controlled administration of propofol and alfentanil with physician-administered midazolam and pethidine. Endoscopy 2003; 35(8): 683–687.
51. Ulmer BJ, Hansen JJ, Overley CA, et al. Propofol versus midazolam/fentanyl for outpatient colonoscopy: administration by nurses supervised by endoscopists. Clin Gastroenterol Hepatol 2003; 1(6):425–432.

11

Anesthesia for Esophagogastric Surgery

Ian H. Shaw
*Department of Anesthesia and Intensive Care, Newcastle General Hospital,
Newcastle upon Tyne, U.K.*

INTRODUCTION

Mediastinal surgery is a major undertaking and challenging to both the anesthetist and the surgeon. Esophageal surgery can involve manipulation of the contents of two major body cavities, the thorax and the abdomen, with consequences for the cardio-respiratory and gastrointestinal systems. The management of these patients is often lengthy and multidisciplinary, and the anesthetist has a pivotal role in achieving a successful outcome from any surgical intervention (1). Sherry (2) has identified pulmonary and cardiovascular dysfunction and anastomotic leaks as postoperative complications that might be directly influenced by anesthetic management. Published evidence supports the recommendation that anesthesia and surgery for esophagogastric disease should only be conducted in specialist centers with a minimum level of activity (3,4).

DISEASES OF THE ESOPHAGUS

The esophagus is susceptible to several pathological insults (Table 1), many of which are beyond the scope of this chapter. Of particular note is the progressive increase in the incidence of esophagogastric cancer recorded in the United Kingdom over the past decade.

Esophageal Carcinoma

There is a marked geographical and ethnic distribution of esophageal cancer. Recent decades have seen a progressive increase in the incidence of adenocarcinoma of the esophagus and gastric cardia such that it now accounts for 65% of all esophageal cancers (5) in the Western world. The typical patient is male, middle aged or elderly, with a predisposing history of hiatus hernia, reflux, and obesity. Chronic reflux generates metaplastic change in the distal esophagus (Barrett's esophagitis), which can subsequently undergo malignant transformation in susceptible individuals. Patients with Barrett's esophagitis have a 40-fold increased risk of developing esophageal cancer (6) compared to the general population.

Table 1 Typical Esophageal Lesions, Which May Necessitate Surgical Intervention

Tumors	Squamous carcinoma
	Adenocarcinoma
Lower esophageal sphincter incompetence	
Benign strictures	Secondary to reflux esophagitis
	Caustic ingestion
Perforation	Traumatic rupture
	Persistent vomiting
	Iatrogenic
Foreign body	Dentures, coins, food, microbatteries, etc.
Diverticulum	
Esophageal varices	
Tracheoesophageal fistula	Congenital
	Acquired

Squamous carcinoma of the esophagus is more common worldwide, especially in the Far East, and can be predisposed by achalasia, strictures, Plummer-Vinson syndrome, diverticulae, and esophagitis. There is also a correlation between smoking and chronic excess alcohol ingestion (7). Although the tumor can arise at any level, the majority of squamous tumors are found in the middle-third of the esophagus. Submucosal infiltration of the adjacent adventitial tissue is not uncommon at presentation. Regional lymph-node involvement carries a poor prognosis. The lung and liver are the common sites of metastatic deposits in disseminated disease.

Whichever tumor type exists, correct staging of the tumor is the most important prognostic variable (8). The pattern of tumor infiltration and spread is determined by the site of the primary tumor. Diagnosis and staging involve endoscopy, spiral computed tomography scanning, endoscopic ultrasound, and bronchoscopy. Diagnostic laparoscopy may be necessary, where there are doubts about the extent of any subdiaphragmatic disease. Typically esophageal carcinoma presents with progressive dysphagia and may be associated with discomfort, nutritional impairment, and weight loss. Dysphagia correlates with a poorer prognosis. The increasing availability of open-access endoscopy services and the screening of susceptible patients can also result in the early detection of carcinoma in patients in whom systemic changes are minimal. Patients in this latter group have a much improved prognosis with 95% survival after five years (5).

SURGERY FOR ESOPHAGOGASTRIC CANCER

Only one-third of patients presenting with esophageal cancer are suitable for surgical resection (5,9,10). Over 40% are inoperable at presentation and a further 25% are unfit for surgery (9). Esophagogastric cancer is one of the most challenging pathological conditions confronting a surgeon on account of the magnitude of the surgical resection and reconstruction. In specialist centers, the 30-day operative mortality can be as low as 4%. Worldwide, the five-year survival after surgery is 10% (11). Curative surgical resection of esophageal malignancy is based on the principle that if all malignant tissue is removed, then resection with reconstruction will lead to survival and possible cure (12). This assumes that operative mortality is low and the patient has sufficient cardiopulmonary reserve to withstand the procedure.

Before assigning a particular surgical approach, the nature, position, and stage of the esophageal tumor, as well as an assessment of the individual patient's cardio-respiratory reserve, must be taken into account.

Surgical Approach to Esophageal Carcinoma

As esophageal cancer spreads longitudinally in the submucosal lymphatics, adequate tumor resection on either side of the palpable tumor is critical to a successful outcome, as is comprehensive abdominal and mediastinal lymphadenectomy. Generous access to the esophagus and adjacent tissues must be provided. The anesthetist has a key role to play in this respect. As the esophagus is related to many important anatomical structures during its passage through the mediastinum (Table 2), per-operative difficulties can arise for the anesthetist.

The position of the esophageal tumor is the major determinant in dictating the most appropriate surgical approach. The majority of tumors arise in the distal two-thirds of the esophagus. The surgical approach to middle- and lower-third esophageal cancers are given in Table 3.

The transhiatal approach, while avoiding a thoracotomy, remains controversial, because the access is restricted and only true esophagogastric junction tumors can be operated on. Anastomotic disruption and recurrent laryngeal nerve (RLN) injury are more common after transhiatal surgery (10,13). One comparative study failed to show any cardiopulmonary benefit of the transhiatal route when compared to a transthoracic approach (14). The left thoracoabdominal approach, popular in the past, was largely undertaken for palliative reasons. Wide resection margins and worthwhile lymphadenectomy are impossible due to limited access.

For curative surgery, the two-stage Ivor-Lewis laparotomy and subsequent right thoracotomy are now the accepted approach to the thoracic esophagus and mediastinal lymph nodes (5). The first stage involves gastric mobilization at laparotomy. The

Table 2 Relative Anatomy of the Esophagus

Anterior relations	Recurrent laryngeal nerves
	Trachea
	Left bronchus
	Right pulmonary artery
	Aortic arch
	Left atrium
	Pericardium
Lateral relations	Common carotid artery
	Subclavian artery
	Descending aorta
	Thoracic duct
	Mediastinal pleura
	Lung
Posterior relations	Vertebral column
	Cervical and prevertebral fascia
	Posterior intercostal arteries

Note: The esophagus originates in the neck at the caudal border of the cricoid cartilage opposite C6 and descends through the superior and posterior mediastinum before passing through the diaphragm at T10, terminating at the gastric cardia, a distance of 25 cm. The esophagus is closely related to the vagus nerves throughout its entire length.

Table 3 Surgical Approach to Esophageal Carcinoma

Transhiatal
Left thoraco-abdominal
Two-stage Ivor-Lewis
Two-team Ivor-Lewis
Endoscopically assisted esophageal resection

Note: The position of the esophageal tumor is the major determinant in dictating the surgical approach, the nature of which the anesthetist must be familiar with before inducing anesthesia.

second stage involves generous resection of the tumor and lymph nodes, delivering the stomach into the posterior mediastinum and fashioning an anastomosis in the chest. A synchronous two-team approach, in which the laparotomy and thoracotomy proceed simultaneously, although of shorter duration, is associated with more complications in Western patients (15). Some surgeons favor percutaneous feeding jejunostomy for early postoperative nutritional support, especially, in high-risk patients.

The 10% of tumors arising in the upper-third of the esophagus are invariably inoperable. Surgery, when indicated, involves a three-stage technique, with the esophageal remnant delivered up into the left neck. Cervical incisions are associated with a higher incidence of RLN injury (13).

Several reports have appeared in the literature describing endoscopically assisted esophageal resection. Preliminary results do not as yet show any definitive advantage. In one series, mortality was reduced, but major morbidity was reported in 32% of the patients (16); one possible factor for this is the prohibitive length of the operation.

NONOPERATIVE TREATMENT

Nonoperative treatment of esophageal cancer involves neoadjuvant chemoradiotherapy. Palliative treatment, such as stenting and laser therapy, is directed primarily at relieving dysphagia.

ANESTHESIA FOR ESOPHAGEAL SURGERY

Preoperative Preparation

Although esophageal surgery is still associated with significant mortality, improved surgical techniques, anesthesia, and intensive care are all attributable to the improved outcome, when compared with past decades (1). Meticulous preoperative evaluation, risk stratification, patient selection, and optimization are a prerequisite to successful surgical outcome after esophageal surgery (17,18).

A critical discussion of preanesthetic assessment and optimization is included in Chapters 7 and 8 and elsewhere (19–21). Only those aspects with specific relevance to anesthesia for esophageal surgery will be discussed below.

Coexisting Disease

Patients presenting for esophageal surgery have a high incidence of coexisting disease (18). The incidence of organ dysfunction and coexisting medical conditions increases with old age. Increasing age has been identified as one risk factor in relation to

Table 4 Risk Factors Identified at Preoperative Assessment, Which Have Been Reported to Correlate with the Incidence of Postoperative Respiratory Complications After Esophagectomy[a]

Increasing age (18,22–25,30)
Increasing ASA grade (25)
Impaired performance status (24,31,32)
Impaired cardiac function (7,31)
Impaired respiratory function (18,25,30,33–37)
Decreased PaO_2 (7,18,31,36)
Decreased vital capacity/closing volume (31,36)
Smoking (11,34,38)
Low BMI (25)
Low albumin (36,39,40)
Impaired hepatic function (7,18,25,36)
Diabetes mellitus (35)
Tumor stage and location (25,36)
Preoperative chemoradiotherapy (30,41–43)

[a]No single predictive risk factor has been identified as superior. Many patients will have more than one risk factor.
Abbreviations: BMI, body mass index; ASA, American Society of Anesthesiologists.

postoperative complications following esophageal surgery (22–25). Specialist centers have reported that, with appropriate case selection and intensive perioperative management, elderly patients can have a satisfactory surgical outcome (9,26–28).

No single parameter has been shown to directly correlate with outcome after esophageal surgery. Physiological and operative severity scoring systems such as POSSUM (*P*hysiological and *O*utcome *S*everity *S*core for en*U*meration of *M*ortality and *M*orbidity) are unreliable in predicting mortality and morbidity after esophagectomy (29). Regardless, a number of preoperative factors have been implicated as being associated with an increased mortality and morbidity (Table 4).

Preoperative pulmonary and hepatic function has been reported as significantly more impaired in patients presenting with squamous cell carcinoma (7,25). By contrast, those with adenocarcinoma had a higher incidence of obesity and cardiac dysfunction. Hyperfibrinogenemia, a common finding preoperatively, positively correlates with the stage of the esophageal disease (44).

Cardiopulmonary Reserve

The preoperative assessment of organ function as a predictor of postoperative morbidity and mortality following esophageal surgery remains a contentious issue. Patients with esophageal disease often have a higher incidence of cardiovascular and chronic respiratory disease. The view that suboptimal preoperative cardiorespiratory function is associated with a higher incidence of complications is undisputed (7,18,25,30,31,33,35,36). Cardiovascular and chronic respiratory disease should be optimized during the preoperative staging period in consultation with specialist physicians if necessary. Patient cooperation is crucial.

The majority of patients undergoing upper gastrointestinal surgery only require basic preoperative investigations (Table 5). Preoperative assessment is discussed in Chapter 7 and elsewhere in relation to esophagogastric surgery (17). Only those investigations with particular implications for esophageal surgery are discussed below.

Table 5 Routine Preoperative Investigations for Esophagogastric Surgery

Hematological	Hemoglobin
	Coagulation screen
	Blood cross-match (4 units)
Biochemical	Urea and electrolytes
	Liver function tests
	Blood glucose
	Arterial blood gases on air
Electrocardiogram	Resting 12 lead ECG
Radiology	PA chest X ray
Pulmonary function tests	Pre- and postbronchodilation
Exercise test	Stair climb (Pulse, BP, and SpO_2)
Supplementary	Fiberoptic bronchoscopy
	Echocardiography
	Lung diffusion capacity

Abbreviations: ECG, electrocardiogram; BP, blood pressure; PA, posterior-anterior.

Exercise Tolerance

Cardiopulmonary reserve can initially be assessed by taking a careful history regarding a patient's physical activities. Although subjective, exercise tolerance can provide a measure of cardiorespiratory reserve. Any patient who remains asymptomatic after climbing several flights of stairs, walking up a steep hill, running a short distance, cycling, swimming, or performing heavy physical work should tolerate the rigors of esophageal surgery. In the absence of cardiac monitoring, an apparent ability to perform these activities does not conclusively exclude cardiorespiratory disease.

In recent years, there has been a growing interest in exercise testing (Chapter 21) as a means of assessing a patient's cardiopulmonary reserve (45). One means of quantifying exercise tolerance is to invite the patient to climb several flights of stairs (46–48). The appeal of stair climbing is its simplicity and the patient's familiarity with the task. Patients with musculoskeletal disorders, peripheral vascular disease, and obesity may be unable to complete any form of dynamic exercise testing. Patients unable to climb two flights of stairs were found to have a higher incidence of coexisting cardiopulmonary disease, higher ASA grade, and more perioperative complications (49). Anesthesia for oncological surgery involving a thoracotomy lasting over eight hours duration has been identified as a particular risk in exercise-limited patients. Patients with unlimited exercise tolerance have fewer serious complications (45).

Dynamic respiratory exercise testing involving expired gas analysis may be, however, more discriminating. Nagamatsu et al. (32) found a correlation with postoperative complications following esophagectomy and maximum oxygen uptake during exercise. Arterial oxygen desaturation during exercise appears to have some predictive value as regards to postoperative complications in patients undergoing a pneumonectomy. Exercise-induced hypotension is an ominous sign and may indicate ventricular impairment secondary to coronary artery disease (50).

Arterial Blood Gases

Hypercarbia alone, in the absence of impaired exercise tolerance, does not appear to be a good predictor of postoperative complications following esophagectomy. Preoperative hypoxia at rest on air, suggesting a preexisting intrapulmonary shunt, correlates with hypoxemia following thoracotomy for nonpulmonary surgery (51) and with a higher incidence of pulmonary morbidity and mortality following esophagec-tomy (22,31,52). Hypoxic patients who were also symptomatic at rest required more postoperative ventilatory support (53), the hypoxia persisting for up to four days postoperatively (51). A significant preexisting intrapulmonary shunt may preclude any subsequent one-lung anesthesia (OLA). In one study, the PaO_2/FiO_2 ratio clearly differentiated survivors from nonsurvivors, as did the level of procalcitonin 24 hours after surgery (37).

Pulmonary Function Tests

It is accepted that static pulmonary function tests alone cannot reliably predict which patients will tolerate esophageal surgery. Much of the published evidence relating pulmonary function testing to outcome after thoracotomy concerns lung reduction surgery. Esophageal surgery, during which a lung is temporarily collapsed to facilitate surgical access, is, however, associated with postoperative pulmonary compromise (54,55). Pulmonary function tests must be considered in conjunction with the arterial blood gases and the patient's exercise tolerance. Where a reversible component is observed, this must be optimized, if necessary, in consultation with a respiratory physician.

It is to be expected that significantly impaired pulmonary function tests will result in difficulties in maintaining adequate oxygenation during OLA and during the postoperative period. Nagawa et al. (32) reported that FVC (forced vital capa-city) was the most reliable predictor of postoperative pulmonary complications after esophagectomy. An FEV_1 (forced expired volume in one second) <1.2 L or an FEV_1/FVC ratio of $<75\%$ has been identified as an important precursor to pulmon-ary complications following noncardiothoracic surgery (56). Suboptimal pulmonary function tests in the presence of hypoxemia are also of particular significance (31). Reduced preoperative FEV_1 and FVC were associated with greater mortality and morbidity following esophagectomy (33,34). Although there are always exceptions, patients whose pulmonary function tests are less than 50% predicted can be expected to tolerant thoracotomy and OLA poorly. Persistently altered pulmonary function tests have been noted six months after recovery from esophageal surgery (57).

Smoking

It has long been established that smoking correlates with an increase in complica-tions following anesthesia and surgery (38,49). Nonsmokers have a much lower mortality following esophagectomy (11). Wetterslev et al. (38) reported a positive correlation with years of smoking and late postoperative hypoxemia and complica-tions after upper abdominal surgery in patients with no previous cardiorespiratory symptoms. Smoking has also been identified as a predisposing factor in the etiology of postoperative adult respiratory distress syndrome, following esophagectomy (54,58). Every effort should be made to encourage smokers to stop smoking preoperatively, ideally for eight weeks or more.

Nutritional Status

Esophageal cancers can affect the ability of the patient to eat and drink. Gross malnu-trition invariably indicates inoperable disease (12). In patients with early tumors, weight loss may be minimal or absent. A body mass index of less than $20 \, kg/m^2$ has been identified as a predictor of pulmonary complications following esophagectomy (23), as has hypoalbuminemia (36,39,53). Malnourished patients have a lower exercise tolerance and are susceptible to pulmonary infections and delayed wound healing (59). A preoperative period of nutritional optimization under dietetic advice may be indicated, although evidence that preoperative nutritional support improves outcome remains elusive (10). Obese patients are prone to pulmonary complications, particularly if associated with smoking and chronic obstructive pulmonary disease (59).

Conduct of Anesthesia

There is no consensus as to the best anesthetic technique for esophageal surgery. From the published literature, a technique combining general anesthesia, neuromuscular paralysis, peroperative ventilation, and epidural analgesia seems to be the most popular. General anesthesia can be achieved with a volatile agent or by target-controlled total intravenous anesthesia (TIVA). Unlike TIVA, volatile anesthetic agents obtund the pulmonary vasoconstrictor response. In reality, at normal MAC (mean alveolar concentration) values, this is probably of little clinical significance. Opiate infusions such as remifentanil also have their advocates. Patients with preoperative dysphagia may have food debris trapped in their proximal esophagus and be at risk of regurgitation and aspiration.

The perioperative monitoring of patients undergoing esophageal surgery requires urinary catheterization, invasive blood pressure, and central venous pressure monitoring. This allows instantaneous detection of any cardiovascular instability associated with surgical manipulation of mediastinal and hiatal structures. A nasogastric tube facilitates gastric decompression.

Surgical operative time for an esophagectomy, excluding dedicated anesthetic time, is on average six to eight hours (15,40,60). Core temperature must be monitored, and measures to minimize heat loss adopted.

Patients undergoing esophageal cancer surgery are at risk of thromboembolic complications. Low-dose heparin together with thromboembolic deterrent (TED) stockings should be provided preoperatively and intermittent pneumatic calf compression peroperatively. Patients with a previous history of thromboembolic phenomenon may require preoperative vena caval filter insertion.

The prophylactic administration of antibiotics decreases morbidity and shortens hospital stay. In patients undergoing esophageal surgery, cefuroxime and metronidazole continued into the postoperative period have been shown to be the most efficacious (61).

Peroperative Management

Although esophageal surgery can be performed with two-lung ventilation (62), unilateral lung deflation allows greater surgical access and facilitates extensive lymphadenectomy, the latter being a prerequisite for curative surgery. Anesthesia for esophageal surgery should only be undertaken by anesthetists familiar with double lumen tubes (DLT) and the complexities of one-lung ventilation (2,63).

A detailed discussion of the practice and physiology of OLA during esophageal surgery is beyond the scope of this chapter, and readers are advised to consult another publication (64). An Ivor-Lewis esophagectomy requires the placement of a left DLT. Malposition of the endobronchial limb is excluded by auscultation of the chest, demonstrating that both lung fields can be isolated and ventilated adequately. Confirmatory fiberoptic bronchoscopy has been shown to significantly reduce the incidence of misplaced DLTs and peroperative hypoxia. When presented with a patient who is difficult to intubate, DLTs can be unforgiving. Modern fiberoptically guided bronchial blockers, passed through the lumen of a normal endotracheal tube, have been used successfully for esophageal surgery (65).

The anesthetic management of the first stage of a two-stage esophagectomy is similar to the management of an abdominal gastrectomy (Chapter 12). The serious problems for the anesthetist, namely hypoxia and cardiovascular instability, arise from the need for a thoracotomy and OLA during the second stage of the operation.

Hypoxia during OLA for nonpulmonary esophageal surgery can be of greater magnitude than during lung-reduction surgery. The more normal the preoperative lung function, the greater the peroperative shunt. Having excluded DLT displacement during mediastinal dissection and manipulation, recruitment maneuvers such as continuous positive airway pressure (CPAP) to the nondependent lung and PEEP (positive end expiratory pressure) to the dependent lung have been described (64), as have various ventilatory strategies (66). The choice of ventilatory strategy may be important in the etiology of postoperative acute lung injury (ALI) (55). A significant increase in PaO_2 during OLA has been achieved by intermittent compression of the nondependent lung (67).

Surgical manipulation of the hiatus and mediastinum can be associated with sudden cardiovascular instability. Delivering the mobilized stomach through the hiatus into the chest is especially hazardous in this respect. Inadvertent surgical compression of the inferior vena cava or the right atrium can precipitate a sudden reduction in cardiac output with deleterious effects. If this cardiovascular instability is concurrent with a period of relative hypoxia during OLA and or hypovolemia, the situation can become potentially life threatening if left uncorrected. Good communication between the surgeon and the anesthetist is therefore mandatory.

Perioperative fluid management in gastrointestinal surgery remains a contentious issue (68). Traditionally, intravenous fluids are given in sufficient volume to maintain an adequate CVP, cardiac output, and urine production, and losses are replaced with crystalloid or colloid. Blood is only considered when the hematocrit falls below 0.25.

Excessive fluid resuscitation can be deleterious, leading to edema of the gastrointestinal tract and decreased gut motility with subsequent malabsorption. Kita et al. (40) found that a regimen of strict fluid restriction during esophagectomy reduced postoperative pulmonary complications and shortened the hospital stay. No adverse circulatory disturbances were noted. A reduction in postoperative complications as a result of perioperative intravenous fluid restriction has also been reported by others (60,69,70).

As the average reported blood loss during an esophagectomy ranges from 175 to 700 mL (60,71,72), transfusion is not normally necessary. Optimization of the preoperative hemoglobin is usually a prerequisite. An adequate hemoglobin concentration must be maintained for oxygen transport and anastomotic preservation. Tissue oxygenation does not appear to be compromised at a hematocrit between 0.25 and 0.30, provided normovolemia is maintained, and that there are no contraindications to hemodilution.

The literature cites increasing evidence that patients with esophageal carcinoma, who received autologous blood, have a less favorable surgical outcome (22,25,72,73). Transfusions greater than three units have been reported to have an adverse effect on late survival after oncological esophageal resection (72). In one study, patients who had been given blood appeared to be more prone to infection (39), especially if other risk factors were present.

Immunosuppressant effects of autologous blood increase with the volume transfused as well as postoperative complications (11). The latter observation may, however, simply reflect the circumstances that necessitated a large blood transfusion rather than any specific immunosuppressive effect. In one series, a preoperative blood loss of over 1000 mL was predictive of death (11).

In the past, it was a common practice to provide ventilatory support after esophageal surgery, often for up to 24 hours or more (40,74). This was felt to be advantageous in allowing vital functions to be optimized, to aid lung expansion and for efficient endobronchial suction and physiotherapy in a group of patients at acknowledged risk from respiratory morbidity. Current evidence supports early or immediate extubation after esophagectomy (11,75–77). This has largely been facilitated by the use of established intraoperative epidural analgesia.

Analgesia

Most published evidence to date suggests that adequate analgesia following esophageal surgery is a prerequisite if a reduction in postoperative cardiopulmonary complications is to be achieved (11,78–82). Thoracic epidural analgesia may need to be employed postoperatively for five days before any beneficial effect is observed on the complication rate (81).

Epidural anesthesia, using a continuous infusion of opiate, local anesthetic, or a combination of both, appears to be the most popular and efficacious. An established sensory block to T4 prior to the induction of general anesthesia is said to improve the immediate outcome following esophagectomy when compared to an epidural used only in the postoperative period.

Opiate patient-controlled analgesia (PCA) has also been used effectively following esophagectomy (5,80,81). When compared with epidural analgesia, not all studies have demonstrated epidural analgesia's superiority (83). Whether the long-term surgical outcome is improved by the choice of analgesic technique remains to be established.

Discomfort can also arise from sites unrelated to surgery. The inability to move around freely in the immediate postoperative period, shoulder pain arising from an unfamiliar posture during thoracotomy, difficulties with micturition, gastrointestinal distension, and hypothermia can all exacerbate existing discomfort. Provided there are no contraindications to their use, supplementation with nonsteroidal anti-inflammatory (NSAIF) drugs is often sufficient. Postoperative analgesia for upper gastrointestinal surgery, including epidural analgesia, is discussed fully in Chapter 25.

POSTOPERATIVE CARE

If the skills of the anesthetist and surgeon are to be consolidated, the postoperative care must be of a high standard in an environment that can provide cardio-respiratory monitoring and experienced dedicated nursing care. This may be in an intensive care or high dependency unit depending on the individual patient's needs (Chapter 27). Patients are most at risk of developing serious complications in the first three to four days following esophageal resection. Several complications are potentially fatal (Table 6).

Cardiopulmonary compromise and anastomotic leaks are of particular concern. Early diagnosis and prompt intervention are crucial.

Table 6 Postoperative Complications in 228 Patients Following Ivor-Lewis Esophagectomy in the Northern Esophagogastric Cancer Unit, Royal Victoria Infirmary, Newcastle upon Tyne, a Specialist Referral Center in the United Kingdom

	Numbers
Medical complications	
Major	
Bronchopneumonia	34
Respiratory failure; ADRS	4
Myocardial infarction; unstable angina	5
Cardiac failure	2
Thromboembolism	3
Minor	
Arrhythmias	6
Psychiatric	4
Infective diarrhea	3
Urinary tract infection	2
Surgical complications	
Major	
Anastomotic leaks	4
Gastrotomy leaks	2
Gastric necrosis	3
Thoracic bleed	6
Chyle leaks	2
Gastrointestinal bleed	1
Pancreatitis	1
Gastrobronchial fistula	1
Laryngeal nerve palsy	1
Empyema lung	1
Minor	
Wound infection	15
Persistent effusion	9
Minor pneumothorax	8
Epistaxis	2

Note: 30-day mortality was 2%, rising to 4% for in-hospital mortality.
Abbreviation: ADRS, acute respiratory disease syndrome.
Source: From Ref. 34.

Cardiovascular Complications

Between 5% and 10% of patients who have undergone an esophagectomy will experience cardiovascular complications (34). Cardiac dysrhythmias are not infrequent following esophagectomy. Postoperative atrial fibrillation (AF), which has been reported to occur in 22% of patients (84), must be investigated promptly because it may be a systemic manifestation of some serious underlying complication. The predictive variables of AF include age, history of cardiac disease, increased intraoperative blood loss, and extensive high thoracic dissection. Mediastinitis secondary to an anastomotic leak, surgical sepsis, and misplaced chest drains have all been implicated (13,17). AF associated with sepsis typically starts after day 3, whereas the earlier onset of AF appears to be less sinister (84). Patients who experience AF postoperatively have more pulmonary complications and a threefold increase in postoperative mortality (84), particularly in the presence of other complications (13). There is no evidence that prophylactic digitalization is of any value in patients who have undergone an esophagectomy (13). Whether alternative antiarrhythmic drugs will offer some protection against AF and other dysrhythmias following esophageal surgery has yet to be established.

Pulmonary Complications

Pulmonary complications such as pneumonia, ALI, and acute respiratory distress syndrome (ARDS) after esophageal surgery are the principal causes of morbidity and mortality (11,52). Between 25% and 64% of patients will experience some impairment of pulmonary function (11,25,57,85,86). A variety of coexisting medical conditions have been implicated as precursors, making some patients more susceptible to such complications (Table 4). The patients with impaired preoperative cardiopulmonary function and exercise tolerance are at increased risk. The transposition of a distensible stomach into the chest may further embarrass respiratory function.

Upper abdominal and thoracic incisions are detrimental to ventilatory mechanisms and gas exchange. An obtunded cough reflex and RLN injury increase the risk of pulmonary aspiration (13). Postoperative hypoxia, lasting for several days, is a common sequela to esophageal surgery. Sputum retention and inability to clear secretions predispose to basal atelectasis. All patients must receive humidified oxygen and regular physiotherapy appropriate to their needs in the postoperative period, and its efficacy must be monitored.

Several postoperative strategies have been advocated to minimize pulmonary morbidity and mortality following esophageal surgery. In this respect, effective analgesia has consistently been identified as the most beneficial (11,79–81,83). Postoperative CPAP has been reported as superior to breathing exercises in preventing respiratory distress in postesophagectomy patients (86). Prolonged ventilation is associated with a higher mortality (87). Whooley et al. (11) identified their aggressive use of postoperative bronchoscopy for bronchial toilet and aspiration as correlating with a reduction in mortality.

The pathophysiology of ALI after esophagectomy is similar to that of classic ARDS (55). The incidence of ARDS, which is a major cause of morbidity and mortality after esophagectomy, is quoted as 14% to 33% (54). Lung injury after OLA may reflect ischemia-reperfusion and ventilator-induced injury (55). Proinflammatory cytokines, which precede lung injury, are released during OLA and esophageal surgery (88). The lungs become permeable to protein, mediated by an increase in cytokines, interleukin (IL)-6 and IL-8, arachidonic acid, and thromboxane B_2 (55).

The degree of intraoperative hypotension and hypoxemia during OLA correlates with postoperative lung injury after esophagectomy. Prolonged OLA time, particularly if associated with cardiovascular instability, increases the risk of developing postoperative ARDS (54).

In one study, patients given a low-dose infusion of the pulmonary vasodilator prostaglandin E_1 (PGE_1) during esophageal surgery had improved oxygenation in the early postoperative period (89). It was postulated that PGE_1, by inhibiting proinflammatory cytokine IL-6 production, attenuated the inflammatory response within the lung.

Anastomotic Leaks

Impaired healing can result in mediastinal anastomotic leaks in 10% to 15% of patients (1), and may account for up to 50% of postoperative deaths (62) as a result of mediastinitis, systemic sepsis, and ARDS. Cervical anastomoses are at greater risk of leakage than intrathoracic anastomoses. Severe malnutrition is associated with an increased anastomotic leak rate as has prolonged manipulation of the tissues during surgery (90). During intra-abdominal mobilization, perfusion through the site of the potential anastomosis falls by 55% (91), and oxygen tension in the gastric fundus decreases by 50% (92). An attempt to enhance gastrointestinal mucosal perfusion following esophagectomy, using dopexamine, failed to demonstrate any improvement (93). Inadequate oxygen delivery in the immediate postoperative period correlates with subsequent anastomotic leakage (74). It is imperative that the surgical anastomoses are protected from hypoperfusion and ischemia.

ANESTHESIA IN PATIENT WITH PREVIOUS ESOPHAGECTOMY

Esophagectomy involves the removal of the lower esophageal sphincter and unavoidable truncal vagotomy, especially of the gastric antrum. Gastric peristalsis and pyloric coordination are disrupted (94), and the thoracic gastric remnant reacts poorly to food ingestion. Reflux after esophagectomy appears to be influenced by the negative pressure environment within the chest relative to the positive pressure that exists in the abdomen (94). Despite modern surgical techniques, patients who have previously undergone an esophagectomy are at significant risk of regurgitation and aspiration during any subsequent anesthesia (95). Gastroduodenal reflux also occurs. The risk of aspiration may be further compounded by coexisting RLN damage. Vocal cord paralysis is a commonly recognized source of morbidity (cervical dissection) following esophageal surgery (13). Consequently, laryngeal surface electrodes activated by transcutaneous nerve stimulation have been advocated as a means of reducing the vulnerability of the RLN during OLA in esophageal surgery (96). Patients with RLN injury have a 10-fold increase in postoperative pulmonary complications and a much poorer quality of life (97).

Any subsequent general anesthesia in such patients should involve a rapid sequence induction.

ANESTHESIA FOR NONMALIGNANT ESOPHAGEAL SURGERY

The anesthetic management for surgical intervention in nonmalignant conditions of the esophagus is essentially identical to that discussed above. A detailed discussion of these conditions is beyond the scope of this chapter and standard texts should be consulted.

Foreign Bodies

The esophagus is the narrowest region of the gastrointestinal tract except for the appendix. The normal esophagus is not uniform in diameter. Relative constrictions occur at the level of the cricopharyngeus 15 cm from the incisor teeth, where it crosses the aortic arch at 22.5 cm and the left main bronchus at 27.5 cm and as it pierces the diaphragm at 40 cm. Ingested foreign body impaction is predominantly a pediatric phenomenon, the cervical esophagus being the commonest site. Adults tend to impact dentures, meat, and bones. Food impaction is more common in the distal-third of the esophagus and is invariably associated with underlying pathology. An ingested foreign body is unlikely to cause subsequent problems, provided it passes safely through the lower esophageal sphincter (98).

About 20% of ingested foreign bodies will require prompt flexible or rigid endoscopic removal (99). The latter, although necessitating general anesthesia, is preferred by some for the superior therapeutic access it provides to the cervical esophagus. Esophageal trauma can result during attempts to recover impacted foreign bodies. Surgery is rarely indicated.

Of special note is the ingestion and impaction of button batteries, almost exclusively by toddlers and small children. Leakage of the alkaline corrosive contents can rapidly give rise to local necrosis, stricture formation, esophageal perforation, and acquired tracheoesophageal fistula (TOF). Urgent extraction is always indicated, and anesthesia should not be delayed.

Esophageal Rupture and Perforation

The etiology of esophageal perforation can be spontaneous, iatrogenic, traumatic, or due to ingestion of corrosive substances (98). As the esophagus lacks a serosal layer, thoracic perforation can readily result in mediastinal contamination, causing potentially fatal mediastinitis. Esophageal trauma requires specialist care.

Spontaneous lower longitudinal esophageal rupture has been reported, following a sudden rise in intraesophageal pressure during vomiting, weight lifting, defecation, or the Heimlich maneuver. Rarely, conservative management is indicated; thoracotomy and surgical intervention are preferred when significant mediastinal contamination is evident. Surgery can involve primary repair, esophageal resection, T-tube drainage of a partially repaired rupture, and esophageal exclusion and diversion. The rationale of the latter approach is to protect the esophageal injury from further damage by gastric secretions.

Iatrogenic esophageal injury is a well-recognized phenomenon of endoscopy and dilatation and accounts for 33% to 73% of all esophageal perforations (98). Proximal perforation is more common if the esophagus is normal, whereas the more distal perforations tend to be associated with underlying pathology. Endoprosthesis insertion for palliation of inoperable carcinoma has a perforation rate of 5%. Other precipitating causes include endotracheal intubation and longstanding nasogastric tubes. It is too early as yet to say whether the increasing popularity of transesophageal echocardiography (TOE) will be associated with an increase in iatrogenic esophageal injury.

Traumatic perforation of the esophagus is rare and usually secondary to penetrating injuries such as stab or gunshot wounds, particularly in the cervical region where it is more vulnerable. Such injuries are often life threatening because adjacent vital structures are involved. Subcutaneous surgical emphysema should raise suspicions of esophageal rupture. The surgical approach will depend on the site of the perforation. Mortality for patients with penetrating injuries of the esophagus is 15% to 27%. Time from injury to management is critical if complications are to be avoided (100). Blunt trauma of the esophagus is extremely rare and mostly the result of blast injuries.

The ingestion of caustic substances can cause catastrophic upper gastrointestinal injuries and may be accompanied by pulmonary aspiration and facial injuries. Children predominate in accidental ingestion and adults attempting suicide when ingestion is intentional. The severity of the injury depends on the corrosiveness of the substance and the quantity ingested. Strong alkaline injuries are the more common, reflecting the availability of such corrosives. Alkali ingestion is especially harmful to the esophagus, although the acid environment does offer some degree of protection (98).

Anesthetic management involves establishing a patent airway and endotracheal intubation, as necessary, antisecretory medication, antibiotics, analgesia, and rehydration. Nasojejunal enteral nutrition is often necessary. Steroid therapy has not been shown to improve outcome (101). Emergency esophagogastrectomy may be indicated when serve burns give rise to esophageal necrosis and the risk of life-threatening mediastinitis. The mortality in this latter group is high; those who survive and develop strictures may require regular dilatation.

Acquired Tracheoesophageal Fistula in Adults

The formation of an acquired TOF is a rare but serious complication of malignancy and trauma. A tract from the gastrointestinal tract to the airway bypasses the normal protection of the larynx. Iatrogenicity, malignancy, and trauma account for the majority of acquired TOFs. Over 50% of acquired TOFs are secondary to mediastinal malignancy—in particular, esophageal and bronchial carcinoma. Endotracheal cuff–related trauma is the commonest nonmalignant cause.

Preoperative management is directed at optimizing the patient's physical status before undertaking a definitive surgical repair by minimizing further pulmonary aspiration and infection.

The anesthetic management of acquired TOF can be complex and has been reviewed recently (102).

Gastroesophageal Reflux

The anesthetic management of patients presenting for antireflux surgery of the lower esophageal sphincter is discussed fully in Chapter 14.

CONCLUSION

Anesthesia for surgical resection of the esophagus for carcinoma is increasing in frequency. Prior to any esophageal surgery, a meticulous assessment of the patient's preoperative health status is mandatory. Patients with impaired cardiopulmonary reserve tolerate esophageal surgery poorly. Coexisting remediable risk factors should be identified early and optimized in the preoperative period. No single preoperative test can reliably predict postoperative outcome. Effective postoperative analgesia correlates with an improved outcome. A high standard of postoperative care is necessary to consolidate the peroperative skills of the anesthetist and surgeon.

REFERENCES

1. Muller JM, Erasmi H, Stelzner M, et al. Surgical therapy of oesophageal carcinoma. Br J Surg 1991; 77:845–857.
2. Sherry KM. How can we improve the outcome of oesophagectomy? Br J Anaesth 1991; 77:612–613.

3. Swisher SG, DeFord L, Merriman KW, et al. Effect of operative volume on morbidity, mortality, and hospital use after esophagectomy for cancer. J Thorac Cardiovasc Surg 2000; 119:1126–1134.

4. Guidance on Commissioning Cancer Services. Improving Outcomes in Upper Gastrointestinal Cancers: The Manual. London: NHS Executive, Department of Health, 2001.

5. Griffin SM. Carcinoma of the oesophagus. Surgery 2000; 18:194–197.

6. Dildey P, Bennett MK. Pathology of benign, malignant and premalignant oesophageal and gastric tumours. In: Griffin SM, Raimes SA, eds. Upper Gastrointestinal Surgery. 3rd ed. London: W.B. Saunders Company, 2001:1–31.

7. Bollschweiler E, Schroder W, Holscher AH, et al. Preoperative risk analysis in patients with adenocarcinoma or squamous cell carcinoma of the oesophagus. Br J Surg 2000; 87:1106–1110.

8. Thomas P, Doddoli C, Lienne P, et al. Changing patterns and surgical results in adenocarcinoma of the oesophagus. Br J Surg 1997; 38:477–478.

9. Dresner SM, Wayman J, Shenfine J, et al. Presentation, management and outcome of oesophageal malignancy in patients aged over 75 years. Br J Surg 1999; 86:421–422.

10. Sherry KM, Smith FG. Anaesthesia for oesophagectomy. Continuing education in anaesthesia. Crit Care Pain 2003; 3:87–90.

11. Whooley BP, Law S, Murthy SC, et al. Analysis of reduced death and complication rates after esophageal resection. Ann Surg 2001; 233:338–344.

12. Griffin SM. Surgery for cancer of the oesophagus. In: Griffin SM, Raimes SA, eds. Upper Gastrointestinal Surgery. 2d ed. London: W.B. Saunders Company, 2001: 121–154.

13. Force S. Complications following esophagectomy: atrial fibrillation, recurrent laryngeal nerve injury, chylothorax and pulmonary complications. Semin Thorac Cardiovasc Surg 2004; 16:117–123.

14. Jacobi CA, Zieren HU, Muller JM, et al. Surgical therapy of esophageal carcinoma: the influence of surgical approach and esophageal resection on cardiopulmonary function. Eur J Cardiothorac Surg 1997; 11:32–37.

15. Hayes N, Shaw IH, Raimes SA, et al. Comparison of conventional Lewis Tanner two stage oesophagectomy with synchronous two team approach. Brit J Surg 1995; 82:95–97.

16. Schuchert MJ, Luketich JD, Fernando HC. Complications of minimally invasive esophagectomy. Semin Thorac Cardiovasc Surg 2004; 16:133–141.

17. Shaw IH. Anaesthetic aspects and case selection for oesophageal and gastric cancer surgery. In: Griffin SM, Raimes SA, eds. Upper Gastrointestinal Surgery. 3rd ed. London: W.B. Saunders Company, 2006:81–103.

18. Kuwano H, Sumiyoshi K, Sonoda K, et al. Relationship between preoperative assessment of organ function and postoperative morbidity in patients with oesophageal cancer. Eur J Surg 1998; 164:581–586.

19. Eagle KA, Brundage BH, Chaitman BR, et al. Guidelines for perioperative cardiovascular evaluation for non-cardiac surgery. J Am Coll Cardiol 1996l; 27:910–948.

20. American Society of Anesthesiologists Task Force. Practice advisory for preanesthesia evaulation. Anesthesiolgy 2002; 96:485–496.

21. Sonneveld JPC, Ligtenberg JJM, Wierda JMKH, et al. Preoperative optimisation of high risk patients. Int J Intensive Care 1999; 6:54–59.

22. Tsutsui S, Moriguchi S, Morita M, et al. Multivariate analysis of postoperative complications after esophageal resection. Ann Thorac Surg 1992; 53:1052–1056.

23. Alexiou C, Beggs D, Salama FD, et al. Surgery for oesophageal cancer in elderly patients: the view from Nottingham. J Thorac Cardiovasc Surg 1998; 116:545–553.

24. Ferguson MK, Martin TR, Reeder LB. Mortality after oesophagectomy: risk factor analysis. World J Surg 1997; 21:599–603.

25. Gockel I, Exner C, Junginger T. Morbidity and mortality after esophagectomy for esophageal carcinoma: a risk analysis. World J Surg Oncol 2005; 3:37–44.

26. Poon RTP, Law SYK, Chu KM, et al. Esophagectomy for carcinoma of the esophagus in the elderly. Ann Surg 1998; 227:357–364.
27. Kinugasa S, Tachibana M, Yoshimura H, et al. Esophageal resection in elderly patients: improvement in postoperative complications. Ann Thorac Surg 2001; 71:414–418.
28. Jin F, Chung F. Minimising perioperative adverse events in the elderly. Br J Anaesth 2001; 87:608–624.
29. Zafirellis KD, Fountolakis A, Dolan K, et [...] in patients with oesophageal cancer undergoing resection. [...] 5.
30. Avendano CE, Flume PA, Silvestri GA, e[...] ons after esopha-gectomy. Ann Thorac Surg 2002; 73:922–9[...]
31. Bartels H, Stein HJ, Siewert JR. Preoperati[...] ative mortality of oesophagectomy for resectable oesophage[...] 5:840–844.
32. Nagamatsu Y, Shima I, Yamana H, et a[...] f cadiopulmonary reserve with the use of expired gas analysi[...] patients with carci-noma of the thoracic oesophagus. J Thor[...] 21:1064–1068.
33. Abunasra H, Lewis S, Beggs L, et al. Predictors of operative death after oesophagectomy for carcinoma. Br J Surg 2005; 92:1029–1033.
34. Griffin SM, Shaw IH, Dresner SM. Early complications after Ivor-Lewis subtotal eso-phagectomy with two field lymphandectomy. Risk factors and management. J Am Coll Surg 2002; 194:285–297.
35. Zhang GH, Fujita H, Yamana H, et al. Preoperative prediction of mortality following surgery for esophageal cancer. Kurume Med J 1992; 39:159–165.
36. Nagawa H, Kobori O, Muto T. Prediction of pulmonary complications after transtho-racic oesophagectomy. Br J Surg 1994; 81:860–862.
37. Szakmany T, Marton S, Koszegi T, et al. Clinical and biochemical parameters in predict-ing mortality in the early postoperative period following oesophagectomy. Br J Anaesth 2002; 89:25–26.
38. Wetterslev J, Hansen EG, Kamp-Jensen M, et al. PaO2 during anaesthesia and years of smoking predict late postoperative hypxaemic complications after upper abdominal surgery in patients without preoperative cardiopulmonary dysfunction. Acta Anaesthe-siol Scand 2000; 44:9–16.
39. Imperatori A, Rovera F, Dominioni L, et al. Infection after oesophagectomy: the role of blood transfusion and of other risk factors. Br J Surg 1999; 86:837.
40. Kita T, Mammoto T, Kishi Y. Fluid management and postoperative respiratory distur-bances in patients with transthoracic esophagectomy for carcinoma. J Clin Anesth 2002; 14:252–256.
41. Dupart G, Chalaoui J, Sylvestre J, et al. Pulmonary complications of multimodal therapy for esophageal carcinoma. Can Assoc Radiol J 1987; 38:27–31.
42. Jawde RMA, Mekhail T, Adelstein D, et al. The impact of induction chemoradiotherapy for esophageal cancer on pulmonary function tests. Correlation with postoperative acute respiratory complications. Chest 2002; 122:101S.
43. Liedman B, Johnsson E, Merke C, et al. Preoperative adjuvant radiochemotherapy may increase the risk in patients undergoing thoracoabdominal esophageal resections. Dig Surg 2001; 18:169–175.
44. Wayman J, O'Hanlon D, Hayes N, et al. Fibrinogen levels correlate with stage of disease in patients with oesophageal cancer. Br J Surg 1997; 84:185–188.
45. Biccard BM. Relationship between the inability to climb two flights of stairs and out-come after major non-cardiac surgery: implications for the pre-operative assessment of functional capacity. Anaesth 2005; 60:588–593.
46. Bolton JWR, Weiman DS, Haynes JL, et al. Stair climbing as an indicator of pulmonary function. Chest 1987; 92:783–788.
47. Pollock M, Roa J, Benditt J, et al. Estimation of ventilatory reserve by stair climbing. Chest 1993; 104:1378–1383.

48. Girish M, Trainer E, Dammann O, et al. Symptom limited stair climbing as a predictor of postoperative cardiopulmonary complications after high-risk surgery. Chest 2001; 120:1147–1151.

49. Reilly DF, McNeely MJ, Doerner D, et al. Self-reported exercise tolerance and the risk of serious perioperative complications. Arch Intern Med 1999; 159:2185–2192.

50. Fletcher GF, Balady G, Froelicher VF, et al. Exercise standards. Circulation 1995; 91:580–615.

51. Entwhistle MD, Roe PG, Sapsford DJ, et al. Patterns of oxygenation after thoracotomy. Br J Anaesth 1991; 67:704–711.

52. Fan ST, Lau WY, Yip WC, et al. Prediction of postoperative pulmonary complications in oesophagogastric surgery. Br J Surg 1987; 74:408–410.

53. Nunn JF, Milledge JS, Chen D, et al. Respiratory criteria of fitness for surgery and anaesthesia. Anaesth 1988; 43:543–551.

54. Tandon S, Batchelor A, Bullock R, et al. Perioperative risk factors for acute lung injury after elective oesophagectomy. Br J Anaesth 2001; 86:633–638.

55. Baudouin SV. Lung injury after thoracotomy. Br J Anaesth 2003; 91:132–142.

56. Wong DH, Weber EC, Schell MJ, et al. Factors associated with postoperative pulmonary complications in patients with severe chronic obstructive pulmonary disease. Anaesth Analg 1995; 80:276–284.

57. Crozier TA, Sydow M, Siewert JR, et al. Postoperative pulmonary complication rate and long-term changes in respiratory function following esophagectomy with oesophagogastrectomy. Acta Anaesthesiol Scand 1992; 36:10–15.

58. Warner D, Warner M, Offord K, et al. Airway obstruction and perioperative complications in smokers undergoing abdominal surgery. Anesthesiology 1999; 90:372–379.

59. Kempainen RR, Benditt JO. Evaluation and management of patients with pulmonary disease before thoracic and cardiovascular surgery. Semin Thorac Cardiothorac Surg 2001; 13:105–115.

60. Neal JM, Wilcox RT, Allen HW. Near-total esophagectomy: the influence of standardized multimodal management and intraoperative fluid restriction. Reg Anesth Pain Med 2003; 28:328–334.

61. Sharpe DA, Renwick P, Mathews KH, et al. Antibiotic prophylaxis in oesophageal surgery. Eur J Cardiothorac Surg 1992; 6:561–564.

62. Tachibana M, Abe S, Tabara H, et al. One lung or two lung ventilation during transthoracic oesohagectomy? Can J Anaesth 1994; 41:710–715.

63. Report of the National Confidential Enquiry into Perioperative Deaths 1996/1997. London: NCEPOD, 1998.

64. Slinger PD. Management of one-lung anesthesia: international anaesthetic research society review course lectures. Anesth Analg 2005; 100(suppl); 89–94.

65. Vanner R. Arndt endobronchial blocker during oesophagectomy. Anaesth 2005; 60: 295–296.

66. Tsui SL, Chan CS, Chan AS, et al. A comparison of two-lung high frequency positive pressure ventilation and one-lung ventilation plus 5 cmH$_2$0 non-ventilated lung CPAP in patients undergoing anaesthesia for oesophagectomy. Anaesth Inten Care 1991; 19:205–212.

67. Ishikawa S, Nakazawa K, Makita K. Progressive changes in arterial oxygenation during one-lung anaesthesia are related to the response to compression of the non-dependent lung. Br J Anaesth 2003; 90:21–26.

68. Joshi GP. Intraoperative fluid restriction improves outcome after major elective gastrointestinal surgery. Anesth Analg 2005; 101:601–605.

69. Brodner G, Pogatzki E, Van Aken H, et al. A multimodal approach to control postoperative pathophysiology and rehabilitation in patients undergoing abdominothoracic oesophagectomy. Anaesth Analg 1998; 86:228–234.

70. Brandstrup B, Tonnesen H, Beier-Holgersen R, et al. Effects of intravenous fluid restriction on postoperative complications: comparison of two perioperative fluid regimens. Ann Surg 2003; 238:641–648.

71. Craig SR, Adam DJ, Yap PL, et al. Effect of blood transfusion on survival after esophagectomy for carcinoma. Ann Thorac Surg 1998; 66:356–361.
72. Langley SM, Alexiou C, Bailey DH, et al. The influence of perioperative blood transfusion on survival after esophageal resection for carcinoma. Ann Thorac Surg 2002; 73:1704–1709.
73. Karl RC, Schreiber R, Boulware D, et al. Factors affecting morbidity, mortality and urvival in patients undergoing Ivor-Lewis esophagectomy. Ann Surg 2000; 23:635–643.
74. Kusano C, Baba M, Tako S, et al. Oxygen delivery as a factor in the development of fatal postoperative complications after oesophagectomy. Br J Surg 1997; 84:252–257.
75. Caldwell MTP, Murphy PG, Page R, et al. Timing of extubation after oesophagectomy. Br J Surg 1993; 80:1537–1539.
76. Yukioka H. Earlier extubation after esophagectomy is successfully performed with thoracic epidural bupivicaine combined with thoracic and lumbar epidural morphine. Anesth Analg 1999; 89:1592.
77. Chandrarashekar MV, Irving M, Wayman J, et al. Immediate extubation and epidural analgesia allow safe management in a high dependency unit after two-stage oesophagectomy. Br J Anaesth 2003; 90:474–449.
78. Terai T, Yukioka H, Fujimori M. Administration of epidural bupivicaine combined with epidural morphine after oesophageal surgery. Surgery 1997; 121:359–365.
79. Watson A, Allen PR. Influence of thoracic epidural analgesia on outcome after resection for oesophageal cancer. Surgery 1994; 115:429–432.
80. Tsui SL, Law S, Fok M, et al. Postoperative analgesia reduces mortality and morbidity after esophagectomy. Am J Surg 1997; 173:472–477.
81. Flisberg P, Tornebrandt K, Lundberg J. Pain relief after esophagectomy: thoracic epidural is better than parentral opiods. J Cardiothorac Vasc Anaesth 2001; 15:279–281.
82. Fotiadia RJ, Badvie SI, Weston MD, et al. Epidural analgesia in gastrointestinal surgery. Br J Surg 2004; 91:828–841.
83. Peyton P, Myles PS, Silbert B, et al. Perioperative epidural analgesia and outcome after major abdominal surgery in high risk patients. Anaesth Analg 2003; 96:548–554.
84. Murthy SC, Law S, Whooley BP, et al. Atrial fibrillation after oesophagectomy is a marker for postoperative morbidity and mortality. J Thorac Cardiovasc Surg 2003; 126:1162–1167.
85. Dumont P, Wihlm JM, Hentz JG, et al. Respiratory complications after surgical treatment of esophageal cancer. A study of 309 patients according to the type of resection. Eur J Cardiothorac Surg 1995; 9:539–543.
86. Olsen MF, Wennberg E, Johnsson E, et al. Randomised clinical study of the prevention of pulmonary complications after thoracoabdominal resection by two different breathing techniques. Br J Surg 2002; 89:1228–1234.
87. Ferguson MK, Durkin AE. Preoperative prediction of the risk of pulmonary complications after oesophgagectomy. J Thorac Cardiovasc Surg 2002; 123:661–668.
88. Cree RT, Warnell IH, Staunton M, et al. Alvelolar and plasma concentrations of interleukin-8 and vascular endothelium growth factor following oesophagectomy. Anesthesiology 2004; 59:867–871.
89. Nakazawa K, Narumi Y, Ishikawa S, et al. Effect of prostaglandin E_1 on inflammatory responses and gas exchange in patients undergoing surgery for oesophageal cancer. Br J Anaesth 2004; 92:199–203.
90. Cassivi SD. Leaks, strictures and necrosis: a review of anastomotic complications following esophagectomy. Semin Thorac Cardiovasc Surg 2004; 16:124–132.
91. Boyle NH, Pearce A, Hunter D, et al. Scanning laser Doppler flowmetry and intraluminal recirculating gas tonometry in the assessment of gastric and jejunal perfusion during esophageal resection. Br J Surg 1998; 85:1407–1411.
92. Cooper GJ, Sherry KM, Thorpe JA, et al. Changes in gastric tissue oxygenation during mobilisation for oesophageal replacement. Eur J Cardiovasc Thorac Surg 1988; 45:451–452.

93. Boyle NH, Roberts PC, McLuckie A, et al. Dopexamine does not improve jejunal or gastric tube mucosal perfusion following oesophageal resection. Crit Care 1999; 3(suppl 1):161–162.
94. Burrows WM. Gastrointestinal function and related problems following esophagectomy. Semin Thorac Cardiovasc Surg 2004; 16:142–151.
95. Aly M, Jamieson GG. Reflux after oesophagectomy. Br J Surg 2004; 91:137–141.
96. Hemmerling TH, Schmidt J, Jacobi KE, et al. Intraoperative monitoring of the recurrent laryngeal nerve during single lung ventilation in esophagectomy. Anesth Analg 2001; 92:662–664.
97. Hulscher JB, van Sanick JW, Devriese PP, et al. Vocal cord paralysis after subtotal oesophagectomy. Br J Surg 1999; 86:1583–1587.
98. Dresner SM, Griffin SM. Oesophageal emergencies. In: Griffin SM, Raimes SA, eds. Upper Gastrointestinal Surgery. 2d ed. London: W.B. Saunders Company, 2001: 393–429.
99. Webb WA. Management of foreign bodies in the upper gastrointestinal tract. Gastrointest Endosc 1995; 41:39–51.
100. Smakman N, Nicol AJ, Walther G. Factors affecting outcome in penetrating oesophageal trauma. Br J Surg 2004; 91:1513–1519.
101. Anderson KD, Rouse TM, Randolph JG. Controlled trial of corticosteroids in children with corrosive injury of the esophagus. New Engl J Med 1990; 323(10):637–640.
102. Raman D, Shaw IH. Aquired tracheo-oesophageal fistula in adults. Continuing education in anaesthesia. Crit Care Pain 2006; 6:105–108.

12
Anesthesia for Gastric Surgery

Ian H. Shaw and Ian H. Warnell
Department of Anesthesia and Intensive Care, Newcastle General Hospital, Newcastle upon Tyne, U.K.

INTRODUCTION

Upper gastrointestinal (GI) surgery is a major surgery which impinges on both the cardiovascular and the respiratory systems. Satisfactory anesthesia for gastric surgery requires the anesthetist to be familiar with both gastric physiology and pathology.

Two of the most common conditions that an anesthetist may be called upon to exercise their skills are in the management of gastric carcinoma and gastric hemorrhage. By necessity, only those aspects pertinent to the understanding of these conditions and anesthetic care will be discussed. Preoperative assessment and preparation of patients undergoing GI surgery are critical to outcome (Chapter 7).

ANATOMY OF THE STOMACH

The stomach is a mobile muscular sac capable of great variation in size and fixed at either end. It has a short lesser curve and a longer greater curve, and consists of a fundus, body, pyloric antrum, and pylorus. The fundus, which is invariably full of gas, is in contact with the left dome of the diaphragm. A significant proportion of the stomach lies beneath the lower ribs. The upper part of the lesser curve is overlapped by the left lobe of the liver and the convexity of the greater curve lying in contact with the transverse colon. Attached to the greater curve is the greater gastrocolic omentum. Other relationships of the stomach include the spleen, left kidney, and adrenal. The pylorus lies in close proximity to the head of the pancreas. Consequently, any of these major adjacent structures can be involved in gastric disease.

The stomach wall is composed of an outer serous coat, then a mucosal coat of three layers of smooth involuntary muscle, an underlying submucosal coat containing the lymphatics, neural, and vascular plexus, and, finally, the mucous coat. The latter is separated from the stomach contents by a layer of mucus. The stomach is a poor absorptive area on account of it lacking the extensive villus structure seen in other parts of the GI tract.

The lymphatic drainage of the stomach is important because it has a major influence on the outcome of surgery for gastric carcinoma. The lymphatic drainage from the stomach is zonal. Lymph drains to the nodes in close proximity to these zones and is ultimately transported to the hepatic, splenic, aortic, and, in particular, the celiac nodes.

The arterial blood supply to the stomach is derived from the left gastric, hepatic, and splenic arteries. The vessels pass through the greater omentum and ramify throughout the submucosa forming an extremely rich anastomotic arterial network. Hence, gastric hemorrhage can be catastrophic. The venous drainage of the stomach mirrors the arterial supply. The major veins are the left and right gastric and gastroepiploic veins, which all untimely drain directly or indirectly into the portal vein.

The nerve supply to the stomach is entirely autonomic, the parasympathetic supply arising from the anterior and posterior vagal trunks.

Sympathetic innervation, which runs alongside the major arteries, is almost entirely derived from the celiac plexus. Division of these autonomic nerves at surgery can have implications for any subsequent anesthesia. For a more detailed description of the anatomy of the stomach, the reader should consult the recent review by Daniels and Allum (1).

LOWER ESOPHAGEAL SPHINCTER

A detailed discussion of the physiology of the GI tract and stomach is discussed in Chapter 1. The stomach, which stores and processes food for digestion, secretes about 2.5 L of acidic gastric juice daily. Gastric juice has a pH of 1.0 to 3.5. Situations in which gastric emptying is delayed or impossible have major implications for the conduct of anesthesia. The acidity of gastric juice is also significant in the etiology of peptic ulceration of the stomach.

The lower esophageal sphincter (LOS) forms the border between the stomach and the esophagus. The LOS is the main determinant in preventing retrograde reflux of gastric contents. The left margin of the lower esophagus forms an acute angle with the gastric fundus, and the right crus of the diaphragm forms a sling around the abdominal esophagus (2). The competency of the LOS is affected by physiological and extraneous factors, many of which influence the conduct of anesthesia.

The tendency to regurgitation of gastric contents is brought about by a difference between the LOS pressure and the intragastric pressure (the barrier pressure). Typically, a pressure of 10 to 30 mmHg at the end of expiration is observed with a normal intragastric pressure of 7 mmHg or more. Although regurgitation can occur in the presence of a normal LOS pressure, more typically regurgitation is a result of a transient relaxation of the LOS tone (3,4). LOS pressure can be affected by coexisting local and systemic pathology and nasogastric intubation (5). Medication, including many drugs used in anesthetic practice, can also affect the competency of the LOS (Table 1) (2,5–7).

Cricoid pressure has been demonstrated to decrease LOS pressure (2), possibly as a result of stimulation of cricoid cartilage mechanoreceptors. The absence of esophageal peristalsis in achalasia can raise the LOS pressure, allowing food trapping in the esophagus with the risk of subsequent regurgitation. Large meals, pregnancy, supine posture, and gastric outflow obstruction predisposes to the LOS barrier being overcome (5).

The major concern, to the anesthetist, of regurgitation of gastric contents is the high risk of contamination of the airway and lungs, a potentially fatal complication.

Table 1 Effect of Drugs Used in Anesthesia on the Lower Esophageal Sphincter Tone

Increase	Decrease	No change
Metoclopramide	Atropine	Propranolol
Cyclizine	Glycopyrrolate	Cimetidine
Neostigmine	Dopamine	Ranitidine
Suxamethonium	Thiopentone	Atracurium
Pancuronium	Tricyclic antidepressants	
Alpha-adrenergic agonists	Beta-adrenergic agonists	
Antacids	Enflurane	
Cisapride	Halothane	
Ergometrine	Opiates	
Cholinergics	Propofol (transient)	

Source: From Ref. 8. Copyright of The Board of Management and Trustees of the British Journal of Anaesthesia. Reproduced by permission of Oxford University Press/British Journal of Anaesthesia.

GASTRIC ASPIRATION

Pulmonary pneumonitis, secondary to aspiration, is uncommon during anesthesia, but can result in mortality and significant morbidity. The incidence of aspiration during anesthesia is between 0.7 and 4.7 per 10,000 (2,9), with a mortality of 3.8% to 4.6% (10,11). The risk of pulmonary aspiration is an important consideration in planning anesthesia for patients with gastric pathology. Several studies have identified both elective and emergency abdominal surgery, a recent meal, delayed gastric emptying, obesity, autonomic neuropathy, diabetes, known gastroesophageal disease, and pain as contributory factors to pulmonary aspiration (2,5,12,13). For a comprehensive discussion of gastric emptying in relation to anesthesia, Petring and Blake (13) should be consulted.

In an attempt to minimize the risk of aspiration, preoperative starvation is mandatory where possible. Preanesthetic pharmacoprophylaxis to reduce acidity and volume of gastric contents includes the administration of acid antagonists such as sodium citrate, H_2-blockers (rantidine and cimetidine), proton pump inhibitors, (omeprazole and lansoprazole), and gastrokinetics (metoclopramide). However the efficacy of such pharmacological interventions in the prevention of pulmonary aspiration has been questioned (9,14,15).

GASTRIC CARCINOMA

Over 90% of gastric tumors are adenocarcinomas arising from dysplasia in the lining of the gastric mucosa and typically present late in their natural history. The remaining 10% of tumors are malignant lymphomas or smooth muscle tumors. Even rarer are oat cell carcinomas, carcinoid, and mesodermally derived tumors.

Gastric adenocarcinoma is the sixth most commonly occurring cancer in the United Kingdom, accounting for over 7500 deaths per annum. Although the overall incidence of gastric cancer has been falling in recent decades, it remains one of the commonest worldwide cancers, particularly in the Far East and South America (16,17). A relative change in tumor epidemiology has been reported. The incidence of proximal gastric cardia tumors has increased significantly, as have tumors of the lower-third of the esophagus. This has led to the postulation that they may share a common etiology with an associated environmental influence.

Precursors of gastric carcinoma include chronic gastritis, gastric metaplasia and dysplasia, polyps, previous gastric cancer surgery under the age of 40, and pernicious anemia. Chronic peptic gastric ulceration is not thought to be a major precursor to carcinoma. Carcinoma is more commonly seen in those with a high-carbohydrate or salt-rich diet.

In recent years, *Helicobacter pylori* infection has been identified as a predisposing cofactor in the etiology of gastric carcinoma (18). The frequency of *H. pylori* infection of gastric mucosa in adults, in the United Kingdom, is estimated to be in the range of 15% to 40%. The damage caused by *H. pylori* alone is not regarded as sufficient to induce gastric carcinoma, but thought to rely on coexisting dietary, environmental, and predisposing immunological cofactors. Although 70% of patients with gastric ulcers are infected with *H. pylori*, not all patients who develop gastric carcinoma are *H. pylori* positive, nor do all patients with *H. pylori* develop gastric carcinoma (15). Regardless, this has opened the way to prophylactic eradicative therapy with antibacterial and antisecretory drugs.

Mortality from gastric cancer is falling and may in part be due to elective screening detecting cancers at an earlier treatable stage. Open-access endoscopic screening programs have been established for those at risk.

Early Gastric Cancer

Early tumors are those malignant tumors limited to the gastric mucosa or submucosa and independent of lymph-node involvement. They are typically found in the lower two-thirds of the stomach. Detection is often during routine-check endoscopy in susceptible patients or in those with anemia. Many are asymptomatic. Early detection of such tumors has considerable implications for the patient's long-term survival, 95% being alive after five years. Predictably, submucosal invasion is associated with worsening long-term survival.

Advanced Gastric Cancer

Advanced gastric neoplasms are often diffuse in nature and are particularly common at the esophagogastric junction. These aggressive, late-presenting tumors carry a poor prognosis, in that they are often large, exhibit early submucosal invasion, extend into the esophagus, and are spread readily by the lymphatic system. Distal tumors can spread into the duodenum, causing outflow obstruction. Serosal involvement implies a five-year survival of only 7% and correlates with the number of lymph nodes involved (17).

Gastric Polyps

Seven percent of patients over 80 years of age have gastric polyps. The most common form are hyperplastic polyps found in the antrum and invariably, although not exclusively, remain benign. Of greater concern are antral adenomas, 40% of which have the capacity for malignant transformation. Polyps detected in younger patients are uncommon, but exhibit more frequent malignant transformation.

Gastrointestinal Stromal Tumors

Over three-quarters of GI stromal tumors, which are derived from stromal fibroblasts, are benign and found mainly in the middle-third of the stomach. They can be bulky and have the potential for metastatic spread into adjacent structures such as the spleen and pancreas.

Gastric Lymphomas

In the United Kingdom, the stomach is the commonest site for GI lymphomas. Lymphomas can be classified as either being derived from T-cells or B-cells. B-cell lymphomas are often multiple, more common in the elderly, and associated with local disease.

Gastric Carcinoid

Gastric carcinoids represent less than 0.5% of gastric tumors. Although invasive, they tend to be limited to the submucosa, and metastases are confined to the local lymph nodes. Gastric carcinoids are derived from endocrine cells, which proliferate due to hypergastrinemia, such as can occur in Zollinger–Ellison Syndrome or in association with multiple endocrine neoplasia (MEN) type 1.

SURGERY FOR GASTRIC CANCER

The surgical approach to gastric cancer is dictated by the site and extent of the tumor, the patient's age, and physical status. Surgery usually involves total or partial gastric resection of the primary lesion and associated lymphadenectomy. If the tumor has breached the submucosa, there may be extensive lateral spread requiring more radical surgery, such as splenectomy, distal pancreatectomy, and extended wide resection (19). Patients in the latter group are invariably presented for palliative surgery. Good communication between the surgical and anesthetic teams is essential before undertaking anesthesia, because the extent of the surgery can have major implications for the conduct of the anesthetic.

For tumors of the distal-third of the stomach, a subtotal gastrectomy is usually performed. Approximately 80% of the stomach is resected along with the first part of the duodenum. Cardia tumors can be particularly difficult and may require a transhiatal approach. Middle-third cancers usually necessitate a total gastrectomy. For proximal-third cancers, which are often more advanced at surgery, a choice exists between a proximal subtotal or total gastrectomy. Anastomosis of the distal stomach to the esophagus can produce a poor functional result, added to which is the increased frequency of nutritional problems in such patients. Whichever approach is adopted, sufficiently wide resection margins are essential if recurrence is to be avoided.

Lymph-node metastasis is a common mode of spread of gastric cancer and can occur in the absence of hematogenous spread, resulting in a localized, albeit, malignant tumor. This is the rationale behind extensive curative lymphadenectomy. For the anesthetist, this has a number of implications. Operating time will be longer, and surgical manipulation of the major adjacent structures could affect the patient's operative well being.

The more extensive the surgery, the greater the reserves required of the patient during the postoperative recovery period. Mortality and morbidity after gastric surgery is higher when the spleen and distal pancreas have been resected. This is further exacerbated by increasing age and suboptimal physical status. Splenectomy may increase the incidence of septic and thromboembolic complications after gastrectomy (20). The resultant modulation of the immune response, in theory, could influence long-term survival after gastric cancer surgery. Consequently, many surgeons will avoid splenectomy where at all possible.

Of no doubt, however, is the increased morbidity and mortality following gastrectomy and distal pancreatectomy. Pancreatic leakage, abscess formation, fistulae, acute pancreatitis, and diabetes have all been reported. More extensive surgery is associated with greater blood loss, possibly necessitating blood transfusion.

Conscious of the greater complications associated with the more extensive surgical options, limited gastric resection in elderly and compromised patients may suffice. While recognizing the chance of a cure is reduced, this is compensated by a shorter operation and anesthetic, less mortality and morbidity, and a lower incidence of subsequent nutritional difficulties.

The normal stomach plays an important role in regulating the rate at which ingested food enters the small intestine, facilitating adequate mixing with pancreatic juices and bile. Failure to do this will overwhelm the digestive and absorptive capacity of the small intestine. Following gastric resection, some form of anatomical reconstruction is necessary to accommodate these demands and maintain the patient's nutritional status. The most commonly adopted reconstruction is a Roux-en-Y technique with duodenal bypass, and the intention is to prevent reflux of the duodenal contents into the gastric remnant or esophagus. A less popular alternative approach is to suture the gastric remnant to the duodenal stump, having interposed a segment of jejunum.

Where a patient is felt to be at a particular risk of postoperative debility, a feeding jejunostomy may be established. Alternatively, a long, narrow-bore feeding tube is placed distally into the small intestine.

ANESTHESIA FOR GASTRIC CANCER SURGERY

Postoperative mortality and morbidity after gastric cancer surgery depends to a large degree on the preoperative physiological status of the patient. Any benefit derived from surgery will depend not only on the stage of the gastric disease but also on the fitness of the patient to withstand anesthesia and surgery (21). Without sufficient physiological reserve, the demands of the immediate postoperative period will not be well tolerated. This is particularly true of upper GI surgery, which impinges on the patient's cardiorespiratory system.

Preassessment

A full discussion of preoperative assessment, investigation, and optimization is discussed elsewhere (Chapters 7 and 8). Careful preoperative assessment is essential before assigning the patient to a particular therapeutic option. As patient optimization may be a multidisciplinary process, early communication between the surgical and anesthetic teams is essential.

The literature has repeatedly failed to identify a specific preoperative risk factor that reliably predicts the outcome after gastric surgery. The preponderance of cardiorespiratory complications following gastric surgery (22) makes the evaluation of the cardiovascular and respiratory systems the main focus of any preoperative assessment and optimization. Numerous studies agree that in major abdominal surgery, coexisting medical conditions and increasing age, all carry an increased perioperative risk (23,24). Preexisting ischemic heart disease, poorly controlled hypertension, and pulmonary dysfunction are all associated with increased operative morbidity after gastric surgery (23). Worthy of special note in patients presenting for gastric surgery is nutritional status, smoking, anemia, and previous chemotherapy.

Nutritional Status

Weight loss of more than 10% is associated with a higher rate of complications and mortality after abdominal surgery (25). Significant weight loss in association with hypoalbuminemia may indicate malnutrition and advanced gastric disease. Malnourished patients are more prone to pulmonary infections, delayed wound healing (26), and complications following upper GI surgery (25). Serum iron, calcium, and essential trace elements should be measured and corrected, if necessary, by a period of enteral feeding in consultation with a dietician. After a laparotomy, small-bowel motility usually recovers before gastric motility. The small intestine may be able to absorb nutrients as early as the first postoperative day, whereas the stomach can exhibit delayed emptying for several days.

Smoking

Smoking is common in patients presenting for gastric surgery and merits specific mention. A sixfold increase in postoperative pulmonary complications has been reported in patients who continue to smoke (27,28). Even in patients with no known preoperative cardiorespiratory dysfunction, postoperative hypoxemia following upper abdominal surgery has been shown to correlate with the length of time and the quantity of cigarettes a patient has smoked (28). All attempts should be made to encourage the patient to cease smoking in the immediate preoperative period. Cessation for one month or less does not appear to improve outcome (28).

ANEMIA AND BLOOD TRANSFUSION IN GASTRIC SURGERY

Anemia (defined by the World Health Organization as a hemoglobin concentration less than 13 g/dL in men and 12 g/dL in women) is common in patients who need gastric surgery. Patients with gastric cancer can present with anemia of multifactorial etiology (Table 2). Neoplasms presenting with anemia tend to have a poorer outcome. We summarize some features of anemia below, but for an in-depth description, the reader should cousult Weiss and Goodnough (29).

Table 2 Etiology of Anemia in the Patient with Gastric Cancer

Iron-deficiency anemia	Blood loss from tumor and peptic ulceration
	Malnourishment
Anemia of chronic disease	Chronic disease induces the release of interleukins, cytokines, and hepcidin (an acute phase protein), which reduces duodenal iron absorption. Iron is also diverted from the circulation to ferritin stores in the liver and reticuloendothelial system. Red cell proliferation is impaired, and the erythropoietin response blunted (29)
Bone marrow suppression	Secondary to neoadjuvant radiotherapy/chemotherapy
	Tumor infiltration of bone marrow
Intraoperative blood loss	Loss of red blood cell mass during surgery

Pathophysiology of Anemia in Gastric Disease

Hemoglobin concentration in a patient with gastric cancer can fall significantly without ill-effect as normal oxygen delivery is approximately four times the oxygen demand. However, when hemoglobin concentration decreases below a critical threshold, oxygen consumption and delivery falls.

Compensatory sympathetic stimulation increases stroke volume and heart rate. In normovolemic patients who are anesthetized or taking adrenergic β-blockers, stroke volume increases in preference to the heart rate. A decrease in blood viscosity leads to an increase in venous return and a reduction in systemic vascular resistance with a concomitant increase in cardiac output. The oxygen dissociation curve shifts to the right [2,3-diphosphoglycerate (DPG) increases], facilitating oxygen release in the tissues, and blood flow is preferentially diverted to vital organs. Capillary recruitment facilitates increased oxygen extraction. If these mechanisms fail to satisfy oxygen demand, hypoxia ensues.

Clinical Effects of Anemia

There are many published reports of surgical patients surviving severe anemia, but generally hemoglobin concentrations less than 5 g/dL carry a significant mortality (30). Mortality and morbidity increases as pre- and postoperative hemoglobin concentrations fall below 10 g/dL, but most noticeably below 7 g/dL (31,32).

Anemia reduces blood viscosity and may increase coronary blood flow and cardiac output. In a patient with heart disease, a common coexisting condition in gastric cancer, the hemoglobin concentration may be critical because of the high myocardial oxygen extraction ratio and the possibility of impaired myocardial blood supply. Although the optimal hemoglobin concentration in such a patient remains equivocal (33), the current literature suggests that moderate anemia (10 g/dL and above) is well tolerated in patients with coronary artery disease, whether they are β-blocked or not (34,35).

Heart disease, coexisting with a preoperative hemoglobin concentration of less than 10 g/dL (31) and postoperative hemoglobin level less than 6 g/dL, is associated with an increased postoperative mortality. Perioperative reversible electrocardiographic changes have been observed in human volunteers (36) and elderly patients subject to isovolemic hemodilution to 5 g/dL (37).

Acute anemia (below 7 g/dL) can produce a reversible impairment of cognitive function (38), and treating anemia has been associated with improved quality of life in patients on chemotherapy (39). These observations may be relevant when considering appropriate hemoglobin concentrations in the elderly gastric patient with cerebrovascular disease.

Preoperative Treatment of Anemia

Patients with gastric cancer may present with the symptoms of anemia or it may be an incidental finding during preassessment and tumor staging. Where indicated, the preoperative staging period should be utilized to optimize the patient's preoperative hemoglobin. Identifying the correct etiology of the anemia is important for subsequent treatment.

Iron-Deficiency Anemia

Iron deficiency results in a hypochromic microcytic anemia. Total body iron stores are depleted with reduced serum iron and ferritin (an iron-storage protein) concentrations and commonly increased transferrin (an iron-transporting protein) and decreased transferrin saturation. Treatment is with oral iron preparations, if the ferritin concentration is less than 30 ng/mL. With values greater than 50 ng/mL, iron absorption is likely to be low, and treatment ineffective.

Anemia of Chronic Disease

Chronic disease generates a normochromic normocytic anemia and is differentiated from iron-deficiency anemia by normal or raised ferritin levels. Normal levels of soluble transferrin receptor can be used to differentiate anemia of chronic disease from iron deficiency. Iron therapy is not generally recommended in anemia of chronic illness, unless there is concomitant iron deficiency, because of an increased risk of acute cardiac events in the presence of long-term immune activation (29). A low ratio of soluble transferrin receptor concentration to the log of the ferritin concentration may be helpful in differentiating anemia of chronic disease from iron deficiency.

Preoperative Erythropoietin

Erythropoietin can reduce perioperative transfusion requirements (40), but is an expensive option. There is also some controversy over its use in cancer patients, because some tumors have erythropoietin receptors, which, if stimulated, may influence tumor growth. Erythropoietin receptor activity has been identified in some gastric cancers (41).

Blood Transfusion

Allogeneic blood has become more scarce and expensive. When considering allogeneic blood transfusion, it is important to balance the risks of transfusion with the benefits of treating the anemia. These issues have been comprehensively reviewed recently (42,43).

Transfusion Trigger Levels. From the published evidence, it is reasonable, assuming normovolemia that red blood cells should be given for hemoglobin concentrations below 7 g/dL. Blood transfusion is rarely required if the hemoglobin is greater than 10 g/dL, unless there are any coexisting risk factors. If the hemoglobin concentration is between 7 and 10 g/dL, transfusion may be still beneficial if any of the following physiological triggers are observed (Table 3).

In patients at risk of myocardial ischemia, new electrocardiographic ST depression of greater than 0.1 mV or elevation of greater than 0.2 mV for more than one minute, or new myocardial wall motion abnormalities detected by transesophageal echocardiography, should prompt serious consideration for red blood cell transfusion.

Table 3 Summary of Nonhemoglobin-Based Triggers Which May Aid Transfusion Decisions

Clinical triggers	Relative tachycardia (HR > 120–130% of baseline or >110–130/min)
	Relative hypotension (mean arterial pressure <60 mmHg depending on age, heart disease, hypertension)
Physiological triggers	$PvO_2 < 32$ mmHg
	$O_2ER > 50\%$
	Decrease in $VO_2 > 10\%$
Evidence of myocardial ischemia	ST changes (new ST depression >0.1 mV or ST elevation >0.2 mV)

Abbreviations: HR, heart rate; O_2ER, oxygen extraction ratio; VO_2, oxygen consumption.
Source: From Ref. 43.

The decision to transfuse a patient with gastric cancer should be made on each patient's individual clinical circumstances. The above discussion may help to rationalize which patients will benefit from red cell transfusion. Useful and practical guidelines can be found in various sources, for example, the Scottish Intercollegiate Guidelines Network (44).

Efficacy of Red Cell Transfusion. Efficacy of blood transfusion for anemia has yet to be clearly demonstrated. Increasing hemoglobin concentration should improve oxygen delivery and, therefore, oxygen consumption. However, results of clinical studies are contradictory. Some studies fail to show a measured increase in oxygen delivery, and most show no increase in oxygen consumption. It is possible that many anemic patients have no oxygen "debt" and do not need red cells. Another explanation for these findings may be that oxygen storage and release by transfused red cells are impaired by changes, which occur during storage, such as a decrease in 2,3-DPG, adenosine triphosphate (ATP) and the release of proinflammatory mediators. This may explain some of the clinical findings associated with the use of older blood, for instance, the association with splanchnic ischemia (45) and reduced survival in sepsis, and an increased incidence of postoperative pneumonia (46) in coronary artery by-pass graft (CABG) patients.

Observational studies in critical care patients failed to show any reduction in morbidity or mortality, if blood had been transfused (47,48). Generally, it is the sicker patients who receive blood transfusions, a situation that complicates meaningful interpretation of the published data. The largest randomized controlled trial examining the efficacy of blood transfusion in critical care patients (49) failed to show any advantage in maintaining the hemoglobin concentration between 10 and 12 g/dL rather than 7 to 9 g/dL.

Transfusion-Related Immunomodulation. Of particular interest and controversy is the possible effect of allogeneic transfusion on upper GI tumor recurrence. Allogeneic blood transfusion contains soluble and cell-associated antigens, which may result in transfusion-related immune modulation (TRIM). The proposed mechanism of TRIM has not been clarified, but may involve allogeneic plasma or changes due to blood storage; the favored hypothesis is a leucocyte-mediated effect. With leucodepletion of donor blood in the United Kingdom, this may be irrelevant.

Many observational cohort studies have demonstrated an association between allogeneic blood transfusion and tumor recurrence and tumor-related mortality. Many of these, including several studies of gastric cancer, have been reviewed in depth by Vamvakas and Blajchman (50).

The results are frequently conflicting. Important problems include the failure to account for possible confounding variables such as clinical stage of malignancy, perioperative blood loss, and coexisting chronic illness. The lack of randomization in observational studies may also allow, as yet, unidentified confounding variables to influence the results. The large variation between the results and differences between study designs have made meta-analysis difficult and open to criticism. Neither observational nor randomized studies to date support a conclusive clinical effect.

ANESTHETIC CONSIDERATION

Anesthesia and Neoadjuvant Therapy

Neoadjuvant therapy is a chemotherapy, a radiotherapy, or a combination of both given before surgery to "downstage" a tumor. The aim is to facilitate surgical resection and to improve surgical outcome. A combination of cisplatin, epirubicin, and 5-fluorouracil is the most likely neoadjuvant regime, which will be encountered in patients undergoing gastrectomy. The therapy is given in three three-weekly cycles preoperatively and then again postoperatively.

Although still the subject of ongoing clinical trails, this chemotherapeutic regime has been shown to effectively "downstage" gastric tumors. Whether long-term survival is improved when compared to surgery alone has yet to be established (51,52). Each of these agents belongs to a different pharmacological drug group and has its own side effects and toxicity profile (Table 4).

The toxicity of these adjuvant therapies might suggest that they could contribute to an already established perioperative morbidity and mortality associated with gastrectomy. Most evidence concerning chemotherapy and perioperative mortality has been recorded for esophageal cancer rather than stomach cancer. Although there are reports of increased complication rates following chemotherapy, these are mainly from small studies. Generally, the larger and randomized studies have been unable to record an increase in morbidity or 30-day mortality (52–55). However, a recent meta-analysis of randomized trials of over 700 patients concluded that combined chemotherapy and radiotherapy regimes produce a higher 90-day perioperative mortality for esophagectomy, although long-term survival was improved (56).

While anticancer chemotherapy is associated with a number of unwanted side effects, of interest to the anesthetist are the persistent reports of acute lung injury (ALI). Bleomycin was one of the first drugs reported to be associated with ALI, a situation thought to be exacerbated by high-inspired oxygen concentrations. Subsequently, many other chemotherapeutic agents have been implicated (57). The patient can become symptomatic (typically, a nonproductive cough) during or even some weeks after completion of a course of chemotherapy.

Drug-induced ALI takes the form of diffuse interstitial pneumonitis and fibrosis, with pulmonary function tests showing a restrictive ventilatory defect, impaired diffusing capacity, and often hypoxemia. Cessation of therapy does not always resolve the situation. The lungs are more susceptible to infection. This has major implications for the postoperative care of gastric cancer patients who have undergone chemotherapy. Lung diffusion capacity has been shown to decrease in patients receiving chemoradiotherapy for esophageal cancer. This decrease was dose related, and the patients were subsequently more prone to postoperative acute respiratory complications (58).

Table 4 Chemotherapeutic Agents Used as Part of Neoadjuvant Chemotherapy in Gastric Cancer

Agent	Profile
5-Fluorouracil	The most active agent for upper gastrointestinal tumors. An antimetabolite, which interferes with cell division, is given as a continuous infusion. Toxicity is unusual, but may cause myelosuppression, mucositis, or a cerebellar syndrome
Epirubicin	A cytotoxic anthracycline antibiotic. This group of drugs may be cardiotoxic, and cause a cardiomyopathy and heart failure
Cisplatinum	A platinum compound which can cause nephrotoxicity, ototoxicity, peripheral neuropathy, hypomagnesemia, myelosuppression, and anemia of chronic illness
Etoposide	Occasionally used and can cause myelosuppression, alopecia, and nausea and vomiting

Patients with neoplastic disease who require mechanical ventilation for respiratory failure, independent of surgery, have a mortality rate in excess of 70% (59–61). Upper abdominal surgery for gastric cancer is associated with an increased postoperative risk of pulmonary infection, which can only exacerbate any drug-induced pulmonary injury.

Pulmonary infections, particularly of *Pneumocystis carinii* and *Mycoplasma pneumoniae*, are common in patients receiving chemotherapy (61). It is imperative that patients are free from infection when presenting for gastric surgery.

Patients can also present for incidental surgery unrelated to the cancer during a course of treatment when consideration has to be given to potential complications that could arise (62). Any postchemotherapy residual effects, such as bone marrow suppression, may have implications for the conduct of the anesthetic.

Immunosuppression, Surgery, and Anesthesia

Surgical manipulation of the intestinal muscularis releases inflammatory mediators, such as cytokines, interleukins, tumor necrosis factor, and cyclooxygenase-2 (63). Peritoneal macrophages also offer local host defense against intraperitoneal infection. Mediator release is in proportion to the surgical insult (64), being less if a laparoscopic technique is used (63). The intestinal inflammatory response triggers an intraperitoneal and systemic immune response as well as depressing gut motility. Major surgery markedly suppresses cell-mediated immunity (CMI) and peritoneal phagocyte activity.

Anesthesia also has the potential to modulate the immune system. Immunosuppressive properties of anesthetics have been reported, although their significance in relation to anesthesia for gastric cancer surgery remains unclear (65). Lymphocyte mobilization is known to be impaired in patients with advanced cancer (66). Even after successful surgical resection, there is a risk of residual tumor cells remaining. Because neoplastic cells act antigenically, any factors causing depression of CMI could lead to tumor recurrence. In this respect, the choice of anesthetic technique could theoretically be important.

Many of the observed effects relate to in vitro observations. Thiopentone and propofol inhibit both monocyte and neutrophil function (67). Volatile anesthetics demonstrate a time- and dose-dependent deleterious effect on neutrophil and lymphocyte function as well as increasing proinflammatory cytokines (68). In vivo studies, although contradictory, suggest that anesthetics may modulate the immune system directly or by affecting the stress response. The anesthesia technique does appear to influence proinflammatory cytokine response (69,70). Opiates have been observed to have dose-dependent immunosuppressive properties.

Of great interest is the observation that epidural anesthesia blocks the stress-induced changes in lymphocyte subpopulation in patients undergoing gastrectomy. B-cells, total T-cells, and inducer T-cells decreased, and suppressor T-cells increased in those patients who did not have an epidural (a combination associated with suppression of immunity). Patients with an effective epidural showed no significant change in lymphocyte subpopulation (71).

Conduct of Anesthesia

The literature does not support one particular anesthetic technique over another. Consequently, the selected technique is largely a matter of individual personal choice, while taking into account the clinical condition of the patient. There are, however, several important issues to consider, which are especially important in gastric surgery.

Distal and antral tumors, which are often extensive at presentation, may be associated with gastric outflow obstruction with the concomitant risk of regurgitation and aspiration on induction of anesthesia. Patients with proximal tumors may also have a predisposition to esophageal reflux. It is therefore important to consider whether to include H_2 antagonists or proton pump inhibitors with premedication. It is also important to consider whether a "rapid sequence induction" would be appropriate.

Patients who have undergone previous gastric or gastroesophageal surgery, particularly for peptic ulcer disease, can present specific difficulties for the anesthetist. Gastroesophageal reflux is common after gastric surgery and can be neutral, acid, or alkaline. Surgery involving truncal vagotomy is associated with acid reflux. Neutral or alkaline reflux is more common following gastrectomy when it is invariably accompanied by bile reflux. Precautions against aspiration should be taken, if these patients present for subsequent anesthesia. Other complications following gastric surgery include dumping, reactive hypoglycemia, and malabsorption (72) (which can give rise to anemia). After vagotomy, diarrhea can be especially problematic and may cause electrolyte abnormalities.

The usual anesthetic technique for gastric surgery is endotracheal intubation, facilitated by muscle relaxants, and intermittent positive pressure ventilation. Maintenance is usually with volatile agents aided by intravenous opiates [either long acting, such as morphine, or short acting such as an infusion (e.g., remifentanil)] or epidural anesthesia. This popular technique has a number of advantages, particularly in the postoperative period (Chapters 9 and 25).

Gastric surgery is frequently lengthy. It is therefore important to take special care with the associated problems. Heat and evaporative losses can be considerable. Almost half of all patients undergoing gastric surgery will become hypothermic unless adequate precautions are taken (73). Heat loss must be monitored, and appropriate airway humidification and warming blankets must be utilized to maintain normothermia (73). Postoperative hypothermia can lead to shivering and exacerbate any coexisting symptoms of nausea and pain.

Measures to prevent thromboembolism and pressure area injury must also be taken. If a procedure is lengthy, or tumor resection is extensive, consideration should be given to invasive monitoring. The patient should be nursed postoperatively in facilities appropriate to the patient's individual needs and the extent of the surgery.

Nasogastric intubation is necessary to protect the anastomosis and avoid GI distension in the postoperative period, a potentially serious complication. Innocuous gastric distension has been shown to reduce blood flow in the coronary, splenic, renal, and iliac vascular beds in pigs via a sympathetically mediated mechanism (74). Preservation of the anastomotic blood supply is critical to operative success and survival, and in this respect the anesthetist has a major role to play.

ANTITHROMBOEMBOLIC PROPHYLAXIS

Patients with carcinoma are at greater risk of thromboembolic complications (61). Several factors increase the risk of thromboembolic phenomenon in patients with gastric neoplasia, including intrinsic tumor procoagulant activity, chemotherapeutic and hormonal agents, surgery, immobility, and central venous catheters (75). The risk can be minimized by prophylactic low-dose heparin therapy, fitting thromboembolic deterrent (TED) stockings, and peroperative intermittent pneumatic calf compression. Thromboembolic therapy would have to be coordinated with any proposed extradural analgesia.

High-risk patients or those with a previous history of deep vein thrombosis or pulmonary embolism may require preoperative placement of an inferior vena cava filter. Although their efficacy has been favorably reported (76), this still requires careful consideration as placement is not without complications and their efficacy has been questioned by some authors (77).

PROPHYLACTIC ANTIBIOTIC THERAPY

There is good evidence that prophylactic broad-spectrum antibiotic therapy, in the absence of infection, can decrease morbidity, shorten hospital stay, and reduce infection-related costs (78). Many patients with malignant disease are immunosuppressed and prone to infection, particularly by atypical microorganisms. This is further exacerbated by any previous chemo- or radiotherapy.

Preincision prophylactic antibiotics are most effective at preventing wound infections rather than postoperative pulmonary or urinary infections and intra-abdominal abscesses. The principal source of bacteria is the GI flora, of which *Escherichia coli* and *Bacteroides fragilis* predominate. The most commonly used antibiotics for this purpose are cephalosporin and metronidazole (78).

The reduction in gastric acid production, sometimes seen in gastric cancer, can promote the colonization of the stomach by opportunistic bacteria and fungi. Consequently, there is a risk of peritoneal cavity or systemic sepsis at surgery.

STAGING LAPAROSCOPY IN GASTRIC SURGERY

In recent years, laparoscopy has become a popular technique to establish accurate staging of gastric tumors in patients for whom surgery is being considered. Intra-abdominal tumor deposits in lymph nodes, the liver, and peritoneal surfaces, which have been missed by noninterventional imaging, can be identified sparing the patient an unnecessary laparotomy (79). Interestingly, there is some published evidence to show that laparoscopy may suppress the immune response (80) in a similar way to laparotomy. This has given rise to the concern that laparoscopy may promote favorable conditions for metastatic growth, a major concern if the patient is found to have operable disease at laparoscopy (81). In one study of staging laparoscopy, the procedure was tolerated by compromised patients so badly that major surgery was abandoned for more conservative treatment (79). In consequence, the current recommendation is that staging laparoscopy should be limited to those patients in whom resectability is uncertain following radiological and ultrasound staging, or if intra-abdominal metastases are suspected (81).

ANALGESIA FOLLOWING GASTRIC SURGERY

Pain after gastric surgery can be appreciable. The evidence to date suggests that effective postoperative analgesia is a prerequisite if a reduction in cardiopulmonary complications is to be achieved (82). The choice of analgesia can also influence regional blood flow and GI function (83,84). This critical aspect of anesthetic care is discussed in Chapter 25.

GASTROINTESTINAL HEMORRHAGE

Upper GI hemorrhage is a common and potentially life-threatening emergency. App-roximately one-third of all upper GI hemorrhages originate in the stomach (Table 5).

Although surgical intervention requiring anesthesia is now much less common, the anesthetist may be called upon to assist in the resuscitation and management of compromised patients. Surgical intervention is indicated when therapeutic endo-scopy has failed and the hemorrhage is recurrent. Patients in intensive care are also susceptible to upper GI hemorrhage.

Erosive Gastritis

It is estimated that up to 20% of patients taking nonsteroidal anti-inflammatory drugs (NSAIDs) will develop gastric or duodenal ulcers (85). Fortunately major gas-tric hemorrhage or perforation is rare, occurring in about 1.5% of patients taking NSAIDs (86). Most bleeding ulcers will stop spontaneously.

Peptic ulceration appears to be more common in those infected with *H. pylori*. Although eradicative antibiotic therapy has been shown to reduce the incidence of ulceration, the evidence currently available suggests that eradication neither protects the patients from nor promotes the healing of ulcers associated with NSAID therapy. In this respect, proton pump inhibitor therapy may be more beneficial. Patients who have experienced a previous gastric hemorrhage as a result of ulcer disease are at a sixfold risk of further gastric hemorrhage should they ingest NSAIDs, regardless or eradicative therapy.

Long-term low-dose prophylactic aspirin therapy has become popular in the past decade. Low-dose aspirin is less likely to cause gastric hemorrhage than NSAIDs (87). However, as with NSAID therapy, in the presence of *H. pylori* infec-tion, there is a five-fold increase of hemorrhagic risk. History of previous ulceration exacerbates the risk 15-fold (88).

Erosive Stress Ulceration

Multiple superficial stress ulceration, the etiology of which is multifactorial, has long been recognized as a complication in seriously ill patients in intensive care (89). Pep-tic ulceration and erosive gastritis account for 25% and 13%, respectively, of all GI

Table 5 Causes of Upper Gastrointestinal Hemorrhage Arising from the Stomach

Erosive gastritis	NSAIDs, aspirin
Erosive stress ulceration	
Gastric erosion	Peptic ulceration
	Smoking
	Acute or chronic alcohol excess
	Steroid therapy
Carcinoma	
Mallory Weiss tear	
Gastric varices	
Foreign body	

Abbreviation: NSAIDs, non-steroidal anti-inflammatory drugs.

Table 6 Factors Predisposing to Erosive Stress Ulceration in the
Critically Ill

Burns	Respiratory failure (acute respiratory
Severe sepsis	distress syndrome)
Head injury	Renal failure
Multiple trauma	Hepatic failure
Multiorgan failure	Coagulopathy

bleeding in intensive care unit patients (90). Hemorrhagic gastritis secondary to impaired mucosal blood flow often accompanies the physiological stress associated with major pathological insults (Table 6). Local ischemia results in acid-pepsin destruction of the mucosa, leading to gastric ulceration and hemorrhage. Consequently, maintaining splanchnic oxygenation and perfusion in the critically ill is thought to be important in helping to preserve the gastric mucosa.

Prophylactic measures also include H_2-blockade to reduce the gastric pH, or, alternatively, providing mucosal protection with sucralfate, a combination of aluminum hydroxide and sulfated sucrose. The reduction in gastric pH must be offset against the risk of bacterial overgrowth with its deleterious consequences. Antacid prophylaxis alone does not prevent upper GI bleeding in high-risk critically ill patients (91). More recently, enteral feeding alone has been identified as beneficial in maintaining mucosal integrity. For a fuller discussion on the prophylaxis of stress ulceration in the critically ill, the reader should consult Maier et al. (92).

Gastric Erosion

Peptic ulceration is the commonest cause of upper GI bleeding. The magnitude of the bleed is dependent on the size of the vessel eroded. Over 70% of bleeding peptic ulcers usually stop spontaneously by the time diagnostic endoscopy is performed. The risk of further bleeding can be predicted from characteristic clinical and endoscopic features (Table 7) (93).

In the past, a bleeding gastric ulcer mandated a partial gastrectomy. An often effective and less traumatic alternative was to underrun the ulcer with a suture via a small gastrotomy. While most gastric bleeding can now be managed endoscopically,

Table 7 Clinical and Endoscopic Features Associated with a
Higher Risk of Peptic Ulcer Rebleeding

Clinical features
  Rapid bleeding with hemodynamic instability
  Anemia on admission
  Ongoing transfusion requirement
  Hematemesis (fresh blood)
  Fresh blood per rectum
  Increasing age and coexisting disease
Endoscopic features
  Pulsatile bleeding
  Visible vessel (of which over 50% will rebleed)
  Clot in ulcer crater
  Ulcer near the left gastric artery high on lesser curve
  Ulcers near the gastroduodenal artery

an exception is often large ulcers on the lesser curve. Ulcers in this position can involve the adjacent left gastric and splenic arteries with the risk of massive hemorrhage.

Endoscopic therapeutic laser photocoagulation, bipolar diathermy, sclerotherapy, and adrenaline injection (94) under sedation all carry the risk of aspiration of gastric blood and cardiovascular collapse should the patient be inadequately resuscitated. Surgery is still the preferred option where the bleeding is recurrent or impossible to stop endoscopically. From the anesthetic perspective, it is important that such patients are carefully assessed as to the adequacy of the resuscitation prior to induction. A rapid sequence induction is mandatory on account of the stomach being contaminated with blood.

Although duodenal perforation is more common, gastric ulcers can also erode and perforate the stomach wall. The incidence of perforated gastric ulcers has fallen due to modern antiulcer medication. When perforation occurs, the ulcers tend to be large, especially on the lesser curve. In this instance, surgery may be indicated. Patients with a history of chronic symptomatic ulceration are most at risk. Blood loss from ulcerated gastric carcinoma is invariably occult. Acute hemorrhage is rare.

Mallory Weiss Tear

Almost 90% of Mallory Weiss tears are located on the gastric side of the gastroesophageal junction. Excessive alcohol ingestion can lead to severe vomiting and retching, resulting in a linear tear of the gastric mucosa. Although initially brisk, the bleeding invariably stops spontaneously. Occasionally therapeutic endoscopic intervention is required.

Gastric Varices

Variceal bleeding accounts for 4% of all upper GI hemorrhage (94). Gastroesophageal varices, secondary to portal hypertension, are present in about 50% of patients with hepatic cirrhosis. Almost 30% of these patients will experience an episode of variceal hemorrhage. Having bled, the risk of further hemorrhage is high. Bleeding is associated with an appreciable mortality.

Foreign Body

Injuries to the stomach following the ingestion of foreign bodies (FBs) are uncommon and rarely require anesthetic intervention. Provided a FB passes freely through the LOS, its passage through the GI tract is usually uneventful (95).

ANESTHESIA AND MASSIVE GASTRIC HEMORRHAGE

Most gastric hemorrhages are managed either conservatively or by therapeutic endoscopic intervention. Where the hemorrhage is persistent or severe, and requires surgery, then the involvement of an anesthetist is inevitable. The primary anesthetic goal in a patient compromised by severe gastric hemorrhage is to facilitate rapid surgical access in order to isolate the site of bleeding, while simultaneously resuscitating the patient and maintaining tissue oxygenation and perfusion. The rate of blood loss will dictate the time available for resuscitation. Depending on the circumstances, it may be pertinent to admit the patient preoperatively to a critical care facility for assessment, monitoring, and preoptimization. Surgery must not be delayed unnecessarily and a degree of urgency should prevail.

The etiology of the hemorrhage should be considered. Variceal bleeding is invariably associated with hepatic impairment, which will influence the conduct of anesthesia. It is also important to note any comorbidity. The elderly and patients with significant coexisting disease have a higher mortality following massive GI bleeding (96).

The initial anesthetic management is identical to that for any bleeding patient. The patient should be given high-flow oxygen via a nonrebreathing system, and intravenous access should be achieved with large-bore cannula or a central venous line. A urine output should be monitored following bladder catheterization. The degree of impaired perfusion and cardiovascular compromise will dictate the intravenous fluid and blood requirements. An intravenous fluid pressure infuser and an adequate supply of blood should be available. Severe life-threatening hemorrhage may necessitate O-negative blood transfusion.

Anesthesia will require a rapid sequence induction in a slightly head up position, if tolerated. Regurgitation of blood is a significant risk. Shocked patients cool quickly, and every attempt should be made to maintain normothermia. All intravenous infusions should be warmed. Having achieved surgical hemostasis, the circulating volume and hemoglobin can then be optimized in the immediate postoperative period. Where a patient is nursed postoperatively will be dependent upon the needs of an individual patient.

CONCLUSION

Anesthesia for gastric surgery can present the anesthetist with several challenges. Knowledge of gastric anatomy, physiology, and pathology all contribute to the understanding of the patient's predicament, as well as being fundamental in the delivery of safe and appropriate anesthetic care.

REFERENCES

1. Daniels IR, Allum WH. The anatomy and physiology of the stomach. In: Fielding JWL, Hallissey MT, eds. Upper Gastrointestinal Surgery. London: Springer-Verlag, 2004: 17–37.
2. Ng A, Smith G. Gastroesophageal reflux and aspiration of gastric contents in anaesthetic practice. Anesth Analg 2001; 93:494–513.
3. Schoemann MN, Tippett MD, Akkermans LM, et al. Mechanisms of gastroesophageal reflux in ambulant healthy human subjects. Gastroenterol 1995; 108:289–291.
4. Dent J, Holloway RH, Toouli J, et al. Mechanisms of lower oesophageal sphincter incompetence in patients with symptomatic gastroesophageal reflux. Gut 1998; 29:1020–1028.
5. Feneck RO. Pre-anaesthetic preparation of the emergency patient. Bailliere's Clin Anaesthesiol 1998; 12:433–450.
6. Aitkenhead AR. Anaesthesia and the gastro-intestinal tract. Eur J Anaesthesiol 1988; 5:73–112.
7. Brock-Utne JG, Downing JW. The lower oesophageal sphincter and the anaesthetist. S Afr Med J 1986; 70:170–171.
8. Cotton BR, Smith G. The lower oesophageal sphincter and anaesthesia. Br J Anaesth 1984; 56(1):37–46.

9. List WF, Prause G. Pre-anaesthetic fasting and aspiration. Bailliere's Clin Anaesthesiol 1998; 12:497–450.

10. Kluger MT, Short TG. Aspiration during anaesthesia: a review of 133 cases from the Australian Anaesthetic Incident Monitoring Study (AIMS). Anaesthesia 1999; 54: 19–26.

11. Warner MA, Warner ME, Weber JG, et al. Clinical significance of pulmonary aspiration during the perioperative period. Anesthesiology 1993; 78:56–62.

12. Sia RL. Aspiration during anaesthetic induction: a hazard in elective abdominal surgery. Anesth Analg 1974; 53:479–480.

13. Petring OU, Blake DW. Gastric emptying in adults: an overview related to anaesthesia. Anaesth Intensive Care 1993; 21:774–781.

14. Smith G, Ng A. Gastric reflux and pulmonary aspiration in anaesthesia. Miner Anesthesiol 2003; 69:402–406.

15. Pisegna JR, Martindale RG. Acid suppression in the perioperative period. J Clin Gastroenterol 2005; 39:10–16.

16. Neugut AI, Hayek M, Howe G. Epidemiology of gastric cancer. Semin Oncol 1996; 23:281–291.

17. Bennet MK. Pathology of malignant and premalignant oesophageal and gastric cancers. In: Griffin SM, Raimes SA, eds. Upper Gastrointestinal Surgery. 1st ed. London: W.B. Saunders Company, 1997:1–34.

18. Parsonnet J, Freidman CD, Vandersyteen DP, et al. Helicobacter infection and the risk of gastric carcinoma. N Engl J Med 1991; 325:1127–1131.

19. Raimes SA. Surgery for cancer of the stomach. In: Griffin SM, Raimes SA, eds. Upper Gastrointestinal Surgery. 1st ed. London: W.B. Saunders Company, 2001:155–202.

20. Otsuji E, Yamaguchi T, Sawai K, et al. Total gastrectomy with simultaneous pancreaticosplenectomy or splenectomy in patients with advanced cancer. Br J Cancer 1999; 79:1789–1793.

21. Shaw IH. Anaesthetic assessment and perioperative care. In: Griffin SM, Raimes SA, eds. Upper Gastrointestinal Surgery London. 2nd ed. London: W.B. Saunders Company, 2001:93–120.

22. Xue FS, Li BW, Zhang GS, et al. The influence of surgical site on early postoperative hypoxemia in adults undergoing elective surgery. Anesth Analg 1998; 88:213–219.

23. Dick WF. Preoperative screening for elective surgery. Bailliere's Clin Anaesthiol 1998; 12:349–371.

24. Doyle RL. Assessing and modifying the risk of postoperative pulmonary complications. Chest 1999; 115:77S–81S.

25. McClave SA, Snider HL, Spain DA. Peroperative issues in clinical nutrition. Chest 1999; 115:64S–76S.

26. Kempainen RR, Bennett JO. Evaluation and management of patients with pulmonary disease before and thoracic and cardiovascular surgery. Sem Thor Cardiothor Surg 2001; 13:105–115.

27. Rodrigo C. The effects of cigarette smoking on anaesthesia. Anesth Prog 2000; 47: 143–150.

28. Wetterslev J, Hansen EG, Kamp-Jensen M, Roikjaer O, Kanstrup IL. PaO$_2$ during anaesthesia and years of smoking predict late postoperative hypxaemic complications after upper abdominal surgery in patients without preoperative cardiopulmonary dysfunction. Acta Anaesthesiol Scand 2000; 44:9–16.

29. Weiss G, Goodnough LT. Anaemia of Chronic disease. N Engl J Med 2005; 352(10): 1011.

30. Viele M, Weiskopf RB. What can we learn about the need for transfusion from patients who refuse blood? The experience with Jehovah's Witnesses. Transfusion (Paris) 1994; 34:396–401.

31. Carson JL, Duff A, Poses RM, et al. Effect of anaemia and cardiovascular disease on surgical mortality and morbidity. Lancet 1996; 348:1055–1060.

32. Carson J, Noveck H, Berlin JE, et al. Mortality and morbidity inpatients with very low postoperative Hb levels who decline blood transfusion. Transfusion (Paris) 2002; 42:812–818.
33. Spahn DR, Dettori N. Transfusion in the cardiac patient. In: Hebert PC, Hebert CHL, eds. Critical Care Clinics. Saunders, 2004:269–279.
34. Spahn DR, Schmid ER, et al. Hemodilution tolerance in patients with coronary artery disease who are receiving chronic beta-adrenergic blocker therapy. Anesth Analg 1996; 82:687–684.
35. Spahn DR, Seifert B, et al. Effects of chronic beta blockade on compensatory mechanisms in patients with coronary artery disease. Br J Anaesth 1997; 78:381–385.
36. Leung JM, Weiskopf RB, Feiner J. Electrocardiographic ST-segment changes during acute, severe isovolemic hemodilution in humans. Anesthesiology 2000; 93:1004–1010.
37. Hogue CW, Goodnough LT, Monk TG. Perioperative myocardial ischemic episodes are related to hematocrit level in patients undergoing radical prostatectomy. Transfusion (Paris) 1998; 38:924–931.
38. Weiskopf R, Kramer JH, Viele M, et al. Acute severe isovolaemic anemia impairs cognitive function and memory in humans. Anesthesiology 2000; 92(6):1646–1652.
39. Littlewood TJ, Bajetta E. Effects of epoetin alfa on hematologic parameters and quality of life in cancer patients receiving nonplatinum chemotherapy; results of a randomized, double-blind, placebo-controlled trial. J Clin Oncol 2001; 19(11):2865–2874.
40. Laupacis A, Fergusson D. Erythropoietin to minimise blood transfusion: a systematic review of randomised trials. The International Study of Peri-operative Transfusion (ISPOT) Investigators. Transfus Med 1998; 8:309–317.
41. Ribatti D, Marzullo A, Nico B, et al. Erythropoietin as an angiogenic factor in gastric carcinoma. Histopathology 2003; 42(3):246.
42. Madjdpour C, Spahn DR. Allogeneic red blood cell transfusions: efficacy, risks, alternatives and indications. Br J Anaesth 2005; 95(1):33–42.
43. Marcucci C, Madjdpour C. Allogeneic blood transfusions: benefit, risks and clinical indications in countries with a low or high human development index. Br Med Bull 2004; 70:15–28.
44. www.sign.ac.uk.
45. Marik PE, Sibbald WJ. Effect of stored blood transfusion on oxygen delivery in patients with sepsis. JAMA 1993; 269:3024–3029.
46. Leal-Noval SR, Jara-Lopez I, Garcia-Garmendia JL, et al. Influence of erythrocyte concentrate storage time on postsurgical morbidity in cardiac surgery patients. Anesthesiology 2003; 98:815–822.
47. Corwin HL, Gettinger A, Pearl RG, et al. The CRIT study: anaemia and blood transfusion in the critically ill-current clinical practice in the United States. Crit Care Med 2004; 32:39–52.
48. Vincent JL, Baron JF, Reinhart K, et al. Anaemia and blood transfusion in critically ill patients. JAMA 2002; 288:1499–1507.
49. Hebert PC, Wells G, Blajchman MA. A multicenter, randomized, controlled clinical trial of transfusion requirements in critical care. N Engl J Med 1999; 340:409–417.
50. Vamvakas EC, Blajchman MA. Deleterious clinical effects of transfusion-associated immunomodulation: fact or fiction? Blood 2001; 97(5):1180–1195.
51. Allum WH, Griffin SM, et al. Guidelines in the management of oesophageal and gastric cancer. Gut 2002; 5(suppl 5):1–23.
52. Cunningham D, Allum D, Weeden S. Perioperative chemotherapy in operable gastric cancer and lower oesophageal cancer: a randomised controlled trail of UK NCRI Upper GI Clinical Studies Group. Eur J Cancer Suppl 2003; 1:S18.
53. Medical Research Council Working Party on oesophageal cancer. Surgical resection with or without preoperative chemotherapy in oesophageal cancer: a randomised controlled trial. Lancet 2002; 359:1727–1733.
54. Marcus SG, Cohen D, et al. Complications of gastrectomy following CPT-11 based neoadjuvant chemotherapy for gastric cancer. J Gastrointest Surg 2003; 7:1015–1023.

55. Kelley S, Coppola ST, et al. Neoadjuvant chemotherapy is not associated with a higher complication rate versus surgery alone in patients undergoing oesophagectomy. J Gastrointest Surg 2004; 8:227–232.

56. Fiorica F, Di Bona D, Schepis F, et al. Perioperative chemotherapy for oesophageal cancer: a systematic review and meta-analysis. Gut 2004; 53:925–930.

57. Twohig KJ, Matthay RA. Pulmonary effects of cytotoxic agents other than bleomycin. Clin Chest Med 1990; 11:31–54.

58. Jawde RM, Mekhail T, Adelstein D, et al. The impact of induction chemotherapy for esophageal cancer on pulmonary function tests: correlation with postoperative acute respiratory complications. Chest 2002; 122:101S.

59. Snow R, Miller W, Rice D, et al. Respiratory failure in cancer patients. JAMA 1979; 241:2039–2042.

60. Schapria DV, Studnicki J, Bradham DD, et al. Intensive care, survival, and expense of treating critically ill cancer patients. JAMA 1993; 269:783–786.

61. Pastores SM. Acute respiratory failure in critically ill patients with cancer. Crit Care Clin 2001; 17:623–646.

62. Kvolik S, Glavas-Obrovac L, Sakic K, et al. Anaesthetic implications of anticancer chemotherapy. Eur J Anaesthesiol 2003; 20:859–871.

63. Sido B, Teklote JR, Friess H, et al. Inflammatory response after abdominal surgery. Best Pract Res Clin Anaesthesiol 2004; 18:439–454.

64. Lennard TW, Shenton BK, Borzotta A, et al. The influence of surgical operations on components of the human immune system. Br J Surg 1985; 72:771–776.

65. Shakhar G, Ben-Eliyahu S. Potential prophylactic measures against postoperative immunosuppression: could they reduce recurrence rates in oncological patients? Ann Surg Oncol 2003; 10:972–992.

66. Grzelak I, Olszewski WL, Engest A. Influence of surgery on the responsiveness of blood lymphocytes in patients with advanced cancer. J Surg Oncol 1988; 37:73–79.

67. Schneemilch CE, Schilling T. Effects of general anaesthesia on inflammation. Best Pract Res Clin Anaesth 2004; 18:493–507.

68. Kotani N, Takahashi S, Sessler DI, et al. Volatile anaesthetics augment expression of proinflammatory cytokines in rat alveolar macrophages during mechanical ventilation. Anesthesiology 1975; 43:563–569.

69. Crozier TA, Muller JE, Quittkat D, et al. Effect of anaesthesia on the cytokine responses to abdominal surgery. Br J Anaesth 1994; 72:280–285.

70. Sheeran P, Hall G. Cytokines in anaesthesia. Br J Anaesth 1997; 78:201–219.

71. Hashimoto T, Hashimoto S, Hori Y, et al. Epidural anaesthesia blocks changes in peripheral lymphocyte subpopulations during gastrectomy. Acta Anaesthesiol Scand 1995; 39:294–298.

72. Anderson JR. Treatment of the complications of previous upper GI surgery. In: Griffin SM, Raimes SA, eds. Upper Gastrointestinal Surgery. 2nd ed. London: W.B. Saunders Company, 2001:367–390.

73. Nguyen NT, Fleming NW, Singh A, et al. Evaluation of core temperature during laparoscopic and open gastric bypass. Obes Surg 2001; 5:570–575.

74. Vacca GM, Battaglia A, Grossini E, et al. The effect of distension of the stomach on peripheral blood flow in anaesthetised pigs. Exp Physiol 1996; 81:385–396.

75. Green KB, Silverstein RL. Hypercoagualability in cancer. Hematol Oncol Clin North Am 1996; 10:499–770.

76. Schwartz RE, Marrera AM, Conlon KC, et al. Inferior vena cava filters in cancer patients: indications and outcome. J Clin Oncol 1996; 14:652–657.

77. Cohen JR, Ventura F, Foccoli P, et al. Greenfield filter as primary therapy for deep venous thrombosis and/or pulmonary embolism in patients with cancer. Surgery 1991; 109:12–15.

78. Mazuski J, Sawyer RG, Nathens AB, et al. The surgical infection society guidelines on antimicrobial therapy for intra abdominal infections. Surg Infect 2002; 3:161–173.

79. Molloy RG, McCourtney JS, Anderson JR. Laparoscopy in the management of patients with cancer of the gastric cardia and oesophagus. Br J Surg 1995; 82:352–354.
80. Volz J, Volz-Koster S, Kanis S, et al. Modulation of tumour-induced lethality after pneumoperitoneum in a mouse model. Cancer 2000; 89:262–266.
81. Lehnert T, Rudek P, Kienle K, et al. Impact of diagnostic laparoscopy on the management of gastric cancer: a prospective study of 120 consecutive patients with primary gastric adenocarcinoma. Br J Surg 2002; 89:471–475.
82. Tsui SL, Law S, Fok M, et al. Postoperative analgesia reduces mortality and morbidity after esophagectomy. Am J Surg 1997; 173:472–477.
83. Tweedle D, Nightingale P. Anaesthesia and the gastrointestinal surgery. Acta Chir Scandinavica 1989; 550(suppl):131–139.
84. Lydon AM, Cooke T, Duggan F, et al. Delayed postoperative gastric emptying following intrathecal morphine and intrathecal bupivicaine. Can J Anaesth 1999; 46:544–599.
85. Elta G, Behler E, Nostrant T, et al. Endoscopic diagnosis of gastritis: causative factors in 100 patients. South Med J 1987; 80:1087–1090.
86. Laine L. Proton pump inhibitor co-therapy with non-steroidal anti-inflammatory drugs. Rev Gastroenterol 2000; 4:S33–S41.
87. Sorensen HT, Mellernkjaar L, Blot WJ, et al. Risk of upper gastrointestinal bleeding associated with low-dose aspirin. Am J Gastroenterol 2000; 95:2218–2224.
88. Drug and Therapeutics Bulletin. *Helicobacter pylori* eradication in non-steroidal antiflammatory drug (NSAID) associated ulcers. Drug Ther Bull 2005; 42:37–40.
89. MacDonald AS, Pyne DA, Freeman AN, et al. Upper gastrointestinal bleeding in the intensive care unit. Can J Surg 1978; 21:81–84.
90. Hills KS, Westaby D. Management of severe non-variceal upper gastrointestinal bleeding. In: Garradr G, Foex P, eds. Principles and Practice of Critical Care. Oxford: Blackwells, 1997.
91. Pinilla JC, Oleniuk FH, Reed D, et al. Does antacid prophylaxis prevent upper gastrointestinal bleeding in critically ill patients? Crit Care Med 1985; 13:646–650.
92. Maier RV, Mitchel D, Gentilello L. Optimal therapy for stress gastritis. Ann Surg 1994; 220:353–360.
93. NIH Consensus Development Conference. Therapeutic endoscopy and bleeding ulcers. JAMA 1989; 262:1369–1372.
94. Steele RJC. The treatment of non-variceal upper gastrointestinal bleeding. In: Griffin SM, Raimes SA, eds. Upper Gastrointestinal Surgery. 1st ed. London: W.B. Saunders Company, 1997:361–390.
95. Webb WA. Management of foreign bodies of the upper gastrointestinal tract. Gastrointest Endosc 1995; 41:39–51.
96. Darle N, Haglund U, Medegard A, et al. Management of massive gastroduodenal haemorrhage. Acta Chir Scandinavica 1980; 146:277–282.

13
Anesthesia for Bariatric Surgery

Robert Thomas and Mark Bellamy
Intensive Care Unit, St. James's University Hospital, Leeds, U.K.

INTRODUCTION

According to the World Health Organization, more than one billion adults are over-weight (1). The most widely accepted definition of obesity is the Body Mass Index (BMI). It is calculated as the weight in kilograms divided by square of height in meters.

$$\text{BMI} = \frac{\text{Weight(kg)}}{\text{Height(m}^2)}$$

The healthy BMI range is considered to be between 20 and 24 kg/m². Obesity is classified as between 25 and 30 kg/m² and morbid obesity as greater than 40 or 35 kg/m² in the presence of obesity-related comorbidity. An adult mean BMI of 22 to 23 kg/m² is found in Africa and Asia, while values of 25 to 27 kg/m² are prevalent across North America and Europe, and in some Latin American, North African, and Pacific Island countries.

The prevalence of obesity has tripled since the 1980s in the developed world; however, it is not just limited to these societies. For example, Samoa has an incidence of more than 75% in its population. The current epidemic of obesity is a result of a global increase in the consumption of energy dense foods combined with reduced physical activity as societies become more urbanized. Furthermore, there has been increased attention focusing on the genetic and endocrine influences responsible for predisposing a person to obesity.

This chapter will discuss the current theories of the causes of obesity, the associated comorbidities, treatment options available, anesthetic assessment of the morbidly obese patient, and the perioperative management of the patient undergoing bariatric surgery.

PHYSIOLOGY OF ENERGY METABOLISM

The control of energy intake and expenditure is coordinated by a system with central and peripheral components (2). The hypothalamus is the primary central organ that receives inputs from the gastrointestinal system, endocrine system, central and peripheral nervous systems, and adipose tissue. Multiple chemical mediators are involved in this system. The main chemical mediators include insulin, cholecystokinin, norepinephrine, dopamine, serotonin, and leptin.

Cholecystokinin is a peptide that consists of subtypes A and B. Type A is found in the gastrointestinal system and type B is found centrally, particularly in the nucleus tractus solitarius and area postrema. Stimulation of these receptors results in the sensation of satiety (3).

Insulin acts centrally and peripherally. Its role in the neurophysiology of feeding is to inhibit the production of neuropeptide Y, inhibit the reuptake of norepinephrine, and amplify the effects of cholecystokinin (4).

Neuropeptide Y is an appetite stimulant that is produced by the hypothalamus and is transported axonally to the paraventricular nucleus. Its production is increased by insulin and glucocorticoids and is inhibited by leptin and estrogen (5). The role of neuropeptide Y receptor agonists in the medical management of obesity was recently reviewed; however, results to date in studies on rats have been equivocal.

Leptin is produced by adipose tissue and is thought to inhibit the production of neuropeptide Y. Low levels are thought to be important in signalling inadequate energy stores sufficient for reproduction and growth. This results in increased intake by the individual (6). Research to date has focused on plasma leptin concentrations in obese subjects and the hypothesis of leptin resistance. However, its exact role in obesity has not been fully elucidated.

Genetic Effects

Apart from specific disorders such as Prader–Willi, Alstrom, and Cohen syndromes that have a single gene mutation responsible for obesity, the majority of obesity disorders may be considered multifactorial (7). Teleologically, the ability to store energy in the form of adipose tissue conferred a survival advantage. However, in modern day society, factors, such as lower socioeconomic class, lifestyle choices, westernized diet, and multiple genetic factors, may all be partly responsible for predisposition to obesity (7). Studies to date have focused on the genes responsible for leptin and carboxypeptidase E, but there is no one particular gene or sequence that is considered to be solely responsible for the majority of cases (8–10).

Comorbidities associated with obesity include hypertension, dyslipidemia, ischemic heart disease, diabetes mellitus, osteoarthritis, and obstructive sleep apnea (OSA) (11). These conditions need to be considered when assessing a patient for bariatric surgery.

To date, there are three main options in treating obesity. These are behavioral, medical, and surgical (12). Behavioral approaches include a dedicated medical team, including a dietician and psychologist, and focus on diet modification, exercise, and behavioral strategies (13).

Drug therapy to date includes sympathomimetic, serotonin-reuptake inhibitors, and drugs with combined sympathomimetic and serotonin-reuptake inhibitor properties (Table 1).

The first agents used in the medical management were fenfluramine and phentermine. These acted by increasing the release of catecholamines (14). The major draw back with these combined drugs was the association with valvular heart disease and pulmonary hypertension (15–17). The manufacturer of the combined agent of phentermine and fenfluramine (Phen-fen) voluntarily withdrew it from the market in 1997 (18).

Table 1 Drug Classes Used in the Management of Obesity

Sympathomimetics	Phentermine, phenmetrazine, phendimetrazine, diethylproprion, phyenylpropanolamine	Increase adrenergic activity or increase brain catecholamine concentration. Not suitable in ischemic heart disease
Serotonin-reuptake inhibitors	Fenfluramine	Advantages—does not increase blood pressure, increased metabolic rate well tolerated
Combined sympathomimetic and serotonin-reuptake inhibitor	Sibutramine	Inhibits the reuptake of serotonin, norepinephrine, and dopamine
Leptin		Protein responsible for relaying the sensation of satiety to the hypothalamus. Thought to be deficient in some morbidly obese patients

Sibutramine acts centrally by inhibiting the reuptake of serotonin, norepinephrine, and dopamine, and increases satiety via its action on the hypothalamus (19,20). Compared to older agents, such as phentermine and fenfluramine, sibutramine has not been associated with cardiac valve lesions (21).

Significant side effects of sibutramine include hypertension and cardiac arrhythmias (22). Minor side effects include dry mouth, insomnia, and constipation (19).

Orlistat is another commonly used drug in the medical management of obesity. It inhibits intestinal lipase activity, which in turn inhibits absorption of 30% of ingested fat (19). Its side effects include steatorrhoea, increased stool frequency, oily spotting, and derangements in folic acid, vitamin B_{12}, and vitamin D (23–25).

TYPES OF SURGERY

There are two main branches of surgery in bariatric procedures (26–28). Procedures that involve gastric banding result in earlier satiety as a consequence of a decreased gastric volume. This technique was improved with the addition of an adjustable band that enables the surgeon to control the gastric volume based on the patient's response to treatment. Roux-en-Y and "diversion" procedures essentially result in a malabsorption of fat and nutrients. Potential complications of this type of surgery are a continued malabsorptive state and its associated nutritional deficiencies (29). The jejunoileal bypass procedure is no longer performed, because it results in unacceptable malabsorption, deficiency states, fatty liver, and dumping, and carries a relatively high mortality (up to 10%). Both gastric banding and bypass procedures have good success rates (28). However, there is still international variation as to which procedure is favored in various countries (28). Surgery may be carried out laparoscopically (gastric banding or roux loop with gastric stapling) or open (roux loop with gastric stapling). Some surgeons prefer the open technique because of the lower anastomotic failure rate and shorter duration of surgery. Irrespective of the choice of technique, hospital stay seldom exceeds two to five days.

COMPLICATIONS OF OBESITY

Obesity is a systemic disorder with wide ranging effects on multiple organ systems. Of immediate concern to the anesthetist are the effects on the respiratory and cardiovascular systems. Other systems include the endocrine, gastrointestinal, rheumatological, and dermatological systems.

Respiratory

Patients with obesity may be classified into three groups: simple obesity, obesity hypoventilation syndrome (OHS), and OSA (30). Simple obesity refers to obese patients with only minor or no respiratory abnormalities. OHS includes obese patients who have diurnal variation in ventilation and have a $PaCO_2$ greater than 5.9 kPa or 45 mmHg (31). OSA is defined as apnoeic episodes secondary to pharyngeal collapse that occur during sleep and may be obstructive, central, or mixed (32,33).

OSA is the most common of the three and occurs in 2% to 5% of the general population (34). The incidence increases with obesity and increasing age. It occurs in 60% to 90% of obese patients (35,36). Importantly, 95% of cases go unrecognized (37).

Common symptoms of OSA include daytime somnolence, headaches, unrefreshing sleep, nocturnal apnoeic episodes witnessed by a partner, and a history of motor vehicle accidents caused by falling asleep while driving. The patient's partner may recall episodes of snoring and apnoeic episodes during sleep (38,39). The diagnosis is made by formal sleep studies. However, establishing a formal diagnosis can be difficult because it requires an overnight stay in an unfamiliar environment, which may alter the patient's usual sleep pattern, and waiting lists for sleep studies often extend far beyond the intended time for surgery. If it is not possible to assess the patient for OSA, then it should be assumed that the patient suffers from OSA unless it has been proven otherwise. Postoperatively, the patient should be in a monitored environment where ready access to noninvasive ventilation is available (40).

Compliance

The total compliance of the respiratory system is made up of the lung and chest wall compliance with the following relationship:

$$\frac{1}{C_{lung}} + \frac{1}{C_{chest}} = \frac{1}{C_{total}}$$

Lung compliance is decreased in patients with OHS and OSA because of the increase in pulmonary blood volume and the collapse of small airways, thus effectively reducing the functional residual capacity (FRC) (41,42). Under these circumstances, lung compliance can be reduced by almost half in some obese people.

FRC is reduced in obese patients for several reasons. Firstly, there is a cephalad displacement of the diaphragm because of the increased volume of intra-abdominal contents (43). Secondly, the increased abdominal contents cause compression of the inferior vena cava. This leads to an increased venous return and hence an increased thoracic blood volume.

Up to a point, the increased weight of adipose tissue surrounding the thoracic cage decreases chest wall compliance. However, the decrease in chest wall compliance only affects the inspiratory threshold. The inspiratory threshold is the load that the respiratory muscles must overcome in order to initiate flow within the respiratory system. Once this is overcome, the compliance of the chest wall is the same as in non-obese subjects (44).

Attempts to improve compliance during laparoscopic surgery by placing the patient in the reverse Trendelenburg position have not been supported by studies specifically addressing this. In one study, compliance was reduced by 30% in morbidly obese patients on insufflation with 20 mmHg of CO_2. The reverse Trendelenburg position did not alter the compliance. It was hypothesized by the authors that despite placing the patients in the reverse Trendelenburg position, the downward movement of the diaphragm was opposed by the pneumoperitoneum required for laparoscopy (45).

Resistance

Airway, lung, and chest wall resistance are all increased in obese subjects and positively correlate with BMI (46). Resistance is further increased when obese patients are transferred from sitting to the supine position (47). Interestingly, the forced expiratory volume in one second (FEV_1)/forced vital capacity (FVC) are the same in obese and nonobese patients, which suggests that the increase in resistance is related to the reduction in FRC, causing a compression of the small airways (43,48).

End-Tidal CO_2 Monitoring

Correlation between the partial pressure of arterial CO_2 ($PaCO_2$) and end-tidal CO_2 (ET CO_2) is generally reliable under most conditions except at low tidal volumes in the morbidly obese patients where there is an increase in the $PaCO_2$/ET CO_2 gradient. It is postulated that the loss of FRC leads to compression of pulmonary vasculature, which results in an increased ventilation perfusion mismatch. This also occurs in nonobese patients who are ventilated at tidal volumes greater than 800 mL (45).

Work of Breathing

The reduction in respiratory compliance secondary to a decrease in FRC and increase in respiratory resistance and inspiratory threshold is associated with an increase in the work of breathing (49). An increase between 60% and 500% is not unheard of in patients with OHS (49). These factors predispose the morbidly obese patient to a rapid reduction in oxygen saturation during hypoventilation or apnea.

Respiratory Muscle Strength

Respiratory muscle strength is quantified by measuring peak inspiratory and peak expiratory pressures, as well as maximum voluntary ventilation (MVV) (50). Obese patients can have a reduction in respiratory muscle strength up to 30% compared to nonobese patients (41). Factors responsible for this may include overstretching of diaphragm by abdominal contents, preventing optimal Frank–Starling interaction of muscle fibers. Interestingly, there is a case report of fatty infiltration of the diaphragm in an obese patient, which may further explain the impairment in respiratory muscle strength (51).

Spirometry

Compared to mildly obese subjects, patients with OHS often have their total lung capacity reduced by 20%, FRC by 25%, and FEV_1, MVV, and expiratory reserve volume (ERV) all reduced by 40% (50,52–55). Furthermore, changes in respiratory function can be influenced by the distribution of body fat. Fat that is predominantly distributed over the thoracic cage will cause more significant changes in lung function tests compared to a more peripheral fat distribution (56).

General anesthesia causes a reduction in chest wall and diaphragmatic tone (57). In simple obesity, this can be reduced to less than 50% of preinduction values. Furthermore, the incidence of atelectasis and retained secretions increases with reductions in the ERV and FRC. Consequently, these changes can result in a significant reduction in the time required for oxygen saturations (a fall below 90%) (58).

Cardiovascular

Obese patients have an increased risk of ischemic heart disease, hypertension, and atherosclerosis (59). Furthermore, the risk of myocardial infarction and stroke is increased in patients who are moderately overweight, especially amongst patients under the age of 40 (60,61).

Morbidly obese people have an increased total blood volume, cardiac output, oxygen consumption, and blood pressure as a result of the requirements of excess adipose tissue. The increase in cardiac output is typically about 0.01 L/min/kg. The increased blood volume is mainly distributed to excess adipose stores, while cerebral and renal blood flows remain relatively unchanged (62). Initially, there is an increase in left ventricular filling, which results in an increased stroke volume secondary to the Frank–Starling mechanism. The cardiac diameter can be increased between 20% and 55% in morbidly obese subjects (63). However, as body weight increases, further enlargement of the left ventricle can eventually lead to decompensated failure (64). Consequently, these patients are less tolerant to myocardial depression caused by some anesthetic agents, such as propofol (65).

Importantly, changes in position alter cardiovascular and respiratory hemodynamics. Cardiac output, pulmonary artery wedge pressure, and mean pulmonary arterial pressure increase when patients are transferred from the sitting position to supine (66). Some patients may be unable to compensate for these changes and consequently do not tolerate the supine position. This may go unrecognized unless specifically enquired about and examined in the preoperative assessment.

Hepatic

Obesity is associated with macrovesicular fatty liver, which appears as hepatocytes with large empty vacuoles that push the nucleus to the periphery of the cell (67). It is usually reversible with weight loss but can eventually progress to steato-hepatitis and cirrhosis if left untreated. Subjects may be asymptomatic or only have mild right upper quadrant tenderness. Alkaline phosphatase and aminotransferases may be mildly elevated or normal. The risk of hepatic fibrosis is increased when the ratio of aspartate aminotransferase (AST) to alanine aminotransferase (ALT) (AST/ALT) is greater than one (68,69). There are no clear guidelines with regards to the anesthetic management of patients with fatty liver disease. Some authors suggest that further investigation is not warranted, whereas others highlight the increased risk of bariatric surgery and fatty liver disease for postoperative liver dysfunction and its associated morbidity. Further evaluation by computed tomography or ultrasound (US) as well as referral to a gastroenterologist would be the safest option in previously undiagnosed cases.

Obese patients are also susceptible to gastroesophageal reflux, presumably as a consequence of increased intra-abdominal pressure (70). There is an increased risk of osteoarthritis affecting weight-bearing joints. Endocrine dysfunction includes diabetes and polycystic ovarian syndrome (1).

PREOPERATIVE EVALUATION

Emphasis is placed on the fact that bariatric surgery is a last resort after the patient has failed properly conducted dietetic and medical management. In most centers, the patient undergoes an extensive workup prior to bariatric surgery. This often involves the cooperation of a dedicated multidisciplinary team, including a dietician, psychologist, physician, surgeon, and anesthetist. The importance of the psychologist in the team is to assess the likelihood that the patient will cooperate with medical and dietetic advice postoperatively (71). Patients considered to be optimal candidates are highly motivated with evidence of compliance with medical management.

The main reason for preoperative anesthetic evaluation is to allow communication between the patient and the anesthetist. It provides an opportunity for the patient to express any concerns with regards to the anesthetic and the associated procedures, and for the anesthetist to allay some of the fears that the patient may have (72). However, it is interesting to note that there is no conclusive evidence showing that preanesthetic assessment improves outcome (72).

The anesthetist needs to assess the patient's current medical condition and past medical history. A history of angina, ischemic heart disease, congestive cardiac failure, sleep apnea, asthma, and previous anesthetics are important to elicit from the patient (73). The patient should be specifically asked about how many pillows they sleep on at night, because some patients may not be able to tolerate the supine position as discussed above.

Symptoms and signs of OSA are important to elicit, because these patients are more sensitive to the depressant effects of hypnotics and opioids on airway tone and ventilation as well as having lower oxygen reserves because of an associated decrease in FRC. Furthermore, these patients are also associated with an increased incidence of difficult laryngoscopy and mask ventilation. Typical elements in the history include daytime somnolence and headache. Features such as falling asleep during active tasks—for example, driving—are highly significant.

Daytime pulse oximetry showing an SpO_2 less than 96% may be useful in detecting the possibility of OSA. Further investigation with formal respiratory function tests, arterial blood gases, chest X ray, echocardiography, and high-resolution computed tomography of the chest might be considered in these circumstances.

Mouth opening, Mallampatti score, and neck extension and circumference (collar size greater than 17.5 in.) should be assessed and any evidence of temperomandibular disease should be noted. Although there is no one particular characteristic that has a high sensitivity or specificity for predicting a difficult airway, the combined factors help in predicting the possibility of a difficult airway.

Venous access sites should be assessed and documented on the anesthetic sheet. The patient should be counselled on the placement of a central venous catheter if it appears that peripheral access will be difficult. This is particularly important in patients with diabetes where good vascular access for several postoperative days may be required.

Evaluation of the preoperative electrocardiograph may show a low voltage QRS and evidence of left ventricular hypertrophy or strain, prolonged QT interval or prolonged corrected QT interval, and left atrial abnormalities or T-wave flattening in the inferior and lateral leads (74). Right-sided hypertrophy secondary to pulmonary hypertension may be evidenced by right axis deviation or right bundle branch block (75). P pulmonale is usually indicative of pulmonary hypertension and cor pulmonale (76). Varying degrees of atrioventricular (AV) block in combination with left anterior hemiblock have also been reported as complicating morbid obesity.

PERIOPERATIVE MANAGEMENT

Vascular Access

Vascular access is a common problem in obese patients because of increased peripheral distribution of adipose tissue (73). However, bariatric surgery is not an absolute indication for central access if a good peripheral cannula can be sited (77). Good peripheral access is possible in the large majority of cases. A central venous catheter may be placed, and the aid of US guidance has been shown to decrease the number of attempts and complications compared to that occurring during "blind" insertion (78). This should be addressed in the preoperative assessment, and the patient counseled on the options available should peripheral access be a problem. The most accessible sites in the morbidly obese are the internal jugular or subclavian veins.

Invasive blood pressure monitoring is not mandatory if an adequately sized noninvasive cuff is available. However, this may not be possible in some morbidly obese patients. The relative speed of hemodynamic change and the potential for compromise in the reverse Trendelenberg position or following pneumoperitoneum insufflation makes arteria monitoring desirable in all but the simplest cases. Usually, this is a relatively easy process because the area over the radial artery is spared of overlying adipocyte tissue, even in morbidly obese patients (79). In cases of difficulty, US-guided placement represents a feasible option.

Analgesia

Epidural placement for postoperative analgesia was favored in the past. Epidurals were thought to reduce the need for opioids and improve postoperative respiratory function. However, several studies have shown that this is not the case (80). Firstly, placement is usually a difficult process because of lack of the usual bony landmarks. A long needle is often required and because of the excess subcutaneous fat, tactile clues such as the loss of resistance are often lost (81,82). Secondly, epidurals more commonly dislodge in this subgroup of patients because of the increased mobility of the subcutaneous tissue, which results in undesirable movement of the epidural catheter (81). These combined factors result in an increased incidence of failed and dislodged epidurals. There is also an increased risk of complications such as pneumothorax, dural puncture, or spinal cord injury. Furthermore, a well-designed study found that there was no difference in visually assessed pain scores when comparing epidurals to morphine patient-controlled analgesia (PCA) (83).

However, should it be considered desirable by the anesthetist for placement of an epidural, there may be some benefit in placing it under US or fluoroscopic guidance. The total dose of local anesthetic administered should be reduced by 75% to 80% of the dose administered to nonobese patients because the epidural space is reduced in obese patients. This is a function of redistribution of blood from the inferior vena cava to the epidural venous system secondary to the increased intra-abdominal pressure (82,84,85).

Thromboprophylaxis

Obesity in itself is a risk factor for deep venous thrombosis and pulmonary embolism (86,87). Bariatric surgery compounds this by inducing a hypercoagulable state by reducing the level of activated protein C and antithrombin III (88). Consequently, the risk of deep venous thrombosis and pulmonary embolism following gastric bypass surgery is 2.6% and 0.95%, respectively. The recent PROBE study, which evaluated the safety and efficacy of enoxaparin in patients who had undergone bariatric surgery, found that 40 mg every 12 or 24 hours were safe and resulted in a lower incidence of venous thromboembolism compared to the control group (89).

Airway

Obesity is classically associated with difficulties in airway management (82,90). However, there is evidence to suggest that obesity itself is not a reliable predictor of a difficult intubation. Patients with a large neck circumference and a high Mallampatti score were more likely to experience difficulty in intubations (91). It has been recommended that there should be a second anesthetist present or a surgeon skilled in establishing a surgical airway where concern exists about a patient's airway (73). In the author's experience, significant concern is a justification for an awake fiberoptically guided intubation.

Postinduction intubation relies on optimal positioning. With regards to this, some authors have advocated using the ramp technique (92). This involves placing pillows or blankets underneath the patient's upper back and head in order to create a straight line between the sternal angle and the auditory meatus. Importantly, the head, shoulders, and upper body must be significantly higher than the chest in order to obtain the best intubating conditions using this technique (93). The incidence of difficult intubation then approximates the incidence in nonobese patients. Their study demonstrated successful intubation in 99% of morbidly obese patients. Of these, 75% were graded as a Cormack and Lehane Grade I laryngeal view, and none of these required a bougie to intubate them. In the authors' experience, this technique has proved of great value.

A difficult intubation trolley should always be present in the anesthetic room and the anesthetist must be familiar with its contents and their location on the trolley. Other aids to establishing an airway must also be available. These include a full range of Guedel airways, laryngeal masks, endotracheal tubes, stylets, gum elastic bougies, and an emergency percutaneous tracheotomy kit (73). If there is any doubt about establishing an airway, the safest option available remains an awake intubation.

Positioning

The operating table should be assessed for its maximum weight capacity. Average operating tables have a capacity of about 205 kg. In some bariatric cases, specially manufactured "fat tables" with an upper-load capacity of about 450 kg may be required. The patient needs to be adequately secured to the table to prevent the patient from falling off as a result of changes in position. Reverse Trendelenberg tilt should not be a cue for a nautical burial!

Particular attention should be paid to areas that are susceptible to pressure or neural injury. Pressure sores can be prevented with liberal use of gel pads. The more common neural injuries that occur include injuries to brachial plexus, ulnar, and sciatic nerves. Brachial plexus injuries can occur from excessive rotation of the head. Sciatic nerve injuries may be a consequence of ishemic injury from prolonged lateral tilt. Ulnar neuropathies have classically been associated with intraoperative compression or stretching. It is interesting to note that a large retrospective study by the Mayo Clinic and two further prospective studies showed that ulnar neuropathies were not necessarily related to general anesthesia or positioning of the patient (94,95). However, obesity itself is a risk factor for ulnar neuropathy, and adequate padding and positioning of the patient's arm is recommended (96). Fortunately, most neuropathies are transient and usually recover.

Changes in position can result in significant physiological changes in obese patients. Importantly, some obese patients are unable to tolerate the supine position. The physiology behind this has already been discussed above. The possible changes that can occur should also be remembered when patient positioning is altered during surgery. Induction of anesthesia with the table tilted head-up (and the anesthetist standing on a platform) is helpful in severe cases.

Additionally, suitable warming should be used to prevent postoperative hypothermia and shivering, with its attendant increase in oxygen consumption. Forced warm-air overblankets are highly efficient in this setting. Active calf compression should also be employed to minimize the risk of thromboembolism.

Monitoring

Monitoring should include, but is not limited to, an electrocardiogram, pulse oximetry, noninvasive blood pressure monitoring (or invasive monitoring if the patient's body habitus prevents reliable assessment of blood pressure by noninvasive methods), and end-tidal carbon dioxide concentration and temperature. Monitoring of neuromuscular blockade is extremely valuable both intraoperatively and where it is planned to extubate the patient immediately following surgery, as is generally the case. Any blood pressure cuff bladder should encircle 75% to 100% of the upper arm circumference.

Pharmacology

In general, there is limited information regarding anesthetic agents and their effects on the morbidly obese. There is no conclusive evidence showing an advantage of any particular anesthetic technique over another. The important principles in bariatric anesthesia are rapid onset and offset of anesthesia, cardiovascular stability, and minimal respiratory depression. Investigations into pharmacokinetics in morbidly obese patients are also scarce. However, as a rule of thumb, most dosage regimens can be based on the corrected weight [0.4 × excess weight + ideal body weight (IBW)] (97). The IBW is defined as follows:

1. IBW (men) = 49.9 kg + 0.89 kg/cm above 152.4 cm height
2. IBW (women) = 45.4 kg + 0.89 kg/cm above 152.4 cm height (98)

Other sources suggest dosing patients based on lean body mass (99). This is not the same as IBW. In morbidly obese patients, the lean body mass is equal to the IBW plus 20%, because the excess weight is partly due to an increase in lean body mass. Neuromuscular blocking agents can be dosed using this regimen of IBW + 20%. However, for lipophilic drugs, pharmacological studies have not been able to show a consistent relationship between body weight and pharmacokinetics.

Induction Agents

Propofol is a commonly used induction agent for anesthesia. Several small studies have looked at the pharmacokinetics in obese subjects. Importantly, when used as an induction agent as well as for maintenance of anesthesia, it is generally agreed that the induction dose should be based on total body weight rather than lean body mass or corrected body weight (98). Secondly, the volume of distribution (V_d) and clearance (Cl) were positively correlated with weight (100). Therefore, although V_d and Cl were increased in obesity, terminal elimination half-life remained unchanged (100). It also has predictable pharmacokinetics when it is used as an infusion in obese people. While the offset of propofol is not as rapid as desflurane, its pharmacokinetic predictability has been described in the literature (101,102).

In contrast, the pharmacokinetics of thiopentone is altered by morbid obesity. The V_d is increased, which results in an increased terminal elimination half-life (103). Furthermore, obese subjects may need less thiopentone for induction when compared to nonobese subjects (104).

Volatile Agents and Nitrous Oxide

Morbid obesity is associated with an increased metabolism of volatile anesthetic agents. Inorganic fluoride concentrations are higher in obese patients compared to nonobese patients when exposed to the same amount of sevoflurane (105). As mentioned previously, obese patients usually have some degree of fatty infiltration and some may have a degree of liver dysfunction. Under these circumstances, it would seem prudent to avoid volatile agents that have a higher degree of metabolism such as halothane.

Sevoflurane has been compared to isoflurane in bariatric surgery, and the authors concluded that the time to extubation was significantly less for sevoflurane. However, the study was flawed in that it was maldistributed with two-thirds of patients receiving isoflurane and only one-third receiving sevoflurane. Furthermore, the isoflurane group received more than 1 MAC of volatile agent as well as 0.6 MAC N_2O, whereas the sevoflurane group received less than 1 MAC as well as 0.6 MAC N_2O.

Sevoflurane has been compared to desflurane in two studies with respect to emergence from anesthesia in morbidly obese patients. The most recent study found no significant difference between the two agents with respect to cardiovascular stability, time to follow commands and to extubation, and recovery of cognitive abilities between the anesthetic groups during recovery (106).

Conversely, desflurane's low blood gas and lipid solubility, low metabolism, and rapid recovery would appear to make it the logical agent of choice. These characteristics were confirmed by a recent study that demonstrated a significantly shorter time to extubation and higher oxygen saturation when desflurane was compared to sevoflurane (107). The important difference between the two studies was that the second compared the two agents specifically in patients undergoing bariatric surgery. There is still debate over whether desflurane or sevoflurane has superior cardiovascular stability (108,109).

Nitrous oxide was studied in a single-blinded controlled trial in bariatric surgery with regards to bowel distension (110). The surgeon was asked if he or she thought nitrous oxide was being used or not. The results showed that there was no difference compared to chance in the surgeon correctly identifying whether nitrous was being used or not.

In patients with preexisting pulmonary hypertension, consideration should be given before using nitrous oxide because it is associated with pulmonary vasoconstriction (111,112). Furthermore, nitrous oxide is associated with postoperative nausea and vomiting. This would be a distinct disadvantage with regards to the increased risk of wound dehiscence and incisional hernias, as well as the risk of aspiration in a patient who is already at an increased risk for respiratory failure.

Neuromuscular Blockade

Neuromuscular blockers have a low volume of distribution and are thus minimally affected by obesity if dosed appropriately (113,114). Therefore, the dose of nondepolarizing neuromuscular blockers should not be based on absolute body weight, but on the lean body weight plus 20%, as mentioned previously (115). Atracurium and cisatracurium are the drugs of choice in morbid obesity, because they are not reliant on renal or hepatic function or blood flow. Secondly, they are degraded in part by Hoffmann elimination, and hence have a relatively predictable duration of action, provided their dosing is based on IBW rather than actual body weight (116,117). In contrast, vecuronium has a potentially increased duration of action in obese patients because of decreased hepatic clearance (118).

POSTOPERATIVE CARE

Postoperative care should be delivered in a suitable environment. Emergence from anesthesia may be problematic owing to respiratory depression and loss of airway control. Hence the patient should not be extubated until fully awake and able to obey commands. Ideally, this should also be performed in the sitting position. A nasopharyngeal airway may be required in subjects with sleep apnea or a history of airway obstruction. Sufficient numbers of members of staff should be present to help move and position the patient. Equipment should be available for reintubation if necessary. Some patients require extubation directly to a continuous positive pressure system. Subjects should then be transferred to a suitable postoperative care facility with appropriate staffing and skills to manage this group of patients. A high-dependency or intensive care setting may be appropriate, at least for the first hours following surgery.

Emphasis is placed on thromboprophylaxis and analgesia. Low-molecular-weight heparin such as enoxaparin based on lean body weight is appropriate. Elastic support stockings or dynamic compression devices are useful additions, especially where mobility is limited, or anticoagulation is contraindicated.

Analgesia is best managed with a PCA regimen. As mentioned previously, epidurals are often difficult to place in morbidly obese patients and have an increased risk of failure. Satisfactory results have been achieved with morphine PCA using a 20 mg/kg of IBW with a 10-minute lockout and 80% of a calculated four-hour limit (119). Supplemental analgesia using nonsteroidal anti-inflammatory agents (e.g., diclofenac) and paracetamol (acetaminophen) is of value. Additionally, open procedures may also benefit from employment of a rectus sheath block placed by the surgeon immediately prior to wound closure.

Patients presenting for surgery following previous bariatric surgery need to be carefully evaluated because electrolyte and clotting abnormalities sometimes occur secondary to malabsorption.

Vomiting may occur following bariatric surgery (120). Reflux is also a particular problem that is more common in patients who have undergone gastric banding.

The patient needs to be educated on the importance of small-volume meals and adequate time to digest them. Excessive intake or rapid ingestion of meals can lead to vomiting. Short term, this can cause dehydration. Long term, it can lead to protein, iron, and vitamin deficiencies.

Iron deficiency is usually associated with roux-en Y gastric bypass procedures because iron is primarily absorbed in the duodenum and proximal jejunum (29,121). This can be further exacerbated with the use of H_2 antagonists and proton pump inhibitors (122). Patients with a microcytic anemia following bariatric surgery should be further assessed with iron studies, including serum iron, ferritin, total iron-binding capacity, and transferring of iron.

Vitamin B_{12} and folate deficiency is reasonably common in patients who have undergone gastric bypass procedures (121). Vitamin B_{12} is cleaved from food by hydrochloric acid and pepsin and is then bound to intrinsic factor, where it is eventually absorbed in the distal ileum. Deficiencies in B_{12} and folate can cause a megaloblastic anemia, leukopenia, glossitis, and a peripheral neuropathy (123). Regular injections of 1000 mcg of B_{12} and replacement of folate with 1 mg daily can correct these deficiencies (123).

Calcium deficiency and deficiencies in vitamins A, D, E, and K have been noted to occur somewhat insidiously in the years following malabsorptive procedures (124). Hypokalemia has been associated with persistent vomiting after gastric banding (125).

CONCLUSION

Anesthesia for bariatric surgery presents a challenge to the anesthetist and requires careful planning and preparation, as well as a detailed knowledge of how physiology and pharmacological principles are altered by morbid obesity. Despite the major advances in surgical and anesthetic technique, there are still significant areas that require further investigation as to how these patients can best be managed.

REFERENCES

1. http://www.who.int/dietphysicalactivity/publications/facts/obesity/en/.
2. Rosenbaum M, Leibel RL, Hirsch J. Obesity. N Engl J Med 1997; 337(6):396–407.
3. Morley JE. Neuropeptide regulation of appetite and weight. Endocr Rev 1987; 8(3): 256–287.
4. Figlewicz DP, Schwartz MW, Seeley RJ, et al. Endocrine regulation of food intake and body weight. J Lab Clin Med 1996; 127(4):328–332.
5. Boggiano MM, Chandler PC, Oswald KD, et al. PYY3–36 as an anti-obesity drug target. Obes Rev 2005; 6(4):307–322.
6. Morrison CD, Morton GJ, Niswender KD, et al. Leptin inhibits hypothalamic Npy and Agrp gene expression via a mechanism that requires phosphatidylinositol 3-OH-kinase signaling. Am J Physiol Endocrinol Metab 2005; 289(6):E1051–E1057.
7. Kopelman PG. Obesity as a medical problem. Nature 2000; 404(6778):635–643.
8. Wangensteen T, Undlien D, Tonstad S, Retterstol L. Genetic causes of obesity. Tidsskr Nor Laegeforen 2005; 125(22):3090–3093.
9. Leibel RL, Chung WK, Chua SC Jr. The molecular genetics of rodent single gene obesities. J Biol Chem 1997; 272(51):1937–1940.
10. Leiter EH. Carboxypeptidase E and obesity in the mouse. J Endocrinol 1997; 155(2): 211–214.

11. Haslam DW, James WP. Obesity. Lancet 2005; 366(9492):1197–1209.
12. Karmali S, Shaffer E. The battle against the obesity epidemic: is bariatric surgery the perfect weapon? Clin Invest Med 2005; 28:147–156.
13. Banning M. Obesity: pathophysiology and treatment. J R Soc Health 2005; 125(4): 163–167.
14. Halford JC, Harrold JA, Lawton CL, Blundell JE. Serotonin (5-HT) drugs: effects on appetite expression and use for the treatment of obesity. Curr Drug Targets 2005; 6(2):201–213.
15. Connolly HM, Crary JL, McGoon MD, et al. Valvular heart disease associated with fenfluramine-phentermine. N Engl J Med 1997; 337(9):581–588.
16. Tomita T, Zhao Q. Autopsy findings of heart and lungs in a patient with primary pulmonary hypertension associated with use of fenfluramine and phentermine. Chest 2002; 121(2):649–652.
17. Volmar KE, Hutchins GM. Aortic and mitral fenfluramine-phentermine valvulopathy in 64 patients treated with anorectic agents. Arch Pathol Lab Med 2001; 125(12): 1555–1561.
18. Wangsness M. Pharmacological treatment of obesity. Past, present, and future. Minn Med 2000; 83(11):21–26.
19. Klein S. Long-term pharmacotherapy for obesity. Obes Res 2004; 12(suppl):163S–166S.
20. Wadden TA, Berkowitz RI, Womble LG, et al. Randomized trial of lifestyle modification and pharmacotherapy for obesity. N Engl J Med 2005; 353(20):2111–2120.
21. Pereira JL, Lopez-Pardo F, Parejo J, et al. Study of heart valve function on obese patients treated with sibutramine. Med Clin (Barc) 2002; 118(2):57 (spanish).
22. Yanovski SZ, Yanovski JA. Obesity. N Engl J Med 2002; 346(8):591–602 (review).
23. Derosa G, Cicero AF, Murdolo G, et al. Efficacy and safety comparative evaluation of orlistat and sibutramine treatment in hypertensive obese patients. Diabetes Obes Metab 2005; 7(1):47–55.
24. Czerwienska B, Kokot F, Franek E, et al. Effect of orlistat therapy on carbohydrate, lipid, vitamin and hormone plasma levels in obese subjects. Pol Arch Med Wewn 2004; 112(6):1415–1423.
25. Harp JB. Orlistat for the long-term treatment of obesity. Drugs Today (Barc) 1999; 35(2):139–145.
26. Frezza EE, Robinson M. Bariatric and associated operations in private and academic practices. Obes Surg 2004; 14(10):1406–1408.
27. Korenkov M, Sauerland S, Junginger T. Surgery for obesity. Curr Opin Gastroenterol 2005; 21(6):679–683.
28. O'Brien PE, Brown WA, Dixon JB. Obesity, weight loss and bariatric surgery. Med J Aust 2005; 183(6):310–314.
29. Alvarez-Leite JI. Nutrient deficiencies secondary to bariatric surgery. Curr Opin Clin Nutr Metab Care 2004; 7(5):569–575.
30. Koenig SM. Pulmonary complications of obesity. Am J Med Sci 2001; 321(4):249–279.
31. Olson AL, Zwillich C. The obesity hypoventilation syndrome. Am J Med 2005; 118(9): 948–956.
32. Namyslowski G, Scierski W, Mrowka-Kata K, et al. Sleep study in patients with overweight and obesity. J Physiol Pharmacol 2005; 56(suppl 6):59–65.
33. Bradley TD, Logan AG, Kimoff RJ, et al. CANPAP Investigators. Continuous positive airway pressure for central sleep apnea and heart failure. N Engl J Med 2005(Nov 10); 353(19):2025–2033.
34. Young T, Palta M, Dempsey J, et al. The occurrence of sleep-disordered breathing among middle-aged adults. N Engl J Med 1993; 328:1230–1235.
35. Phillips B. Sleep apnea. Underdiagnosed and undertreated. Hosp Pract (Off Ed) 1996; 31:193–194, 197, 201–202.
36. Rajala R, Partinen M, Sane T, et al. Obstructive sleep apnoea syndrome in morbidly obese patients. J Intern Med 1991; 230:125–129.

37. Wake up America: a national sleep alert. Report of the National Commission on Sleep Disorders Research. Washington (DC): U.S. Department of Health and Human Services, 1993.
38. Peppard PE, Young T, Palta M, Skatrud J. Prospective study of the association between sleep-disordered breathing and hypertension. N Engl J Med 2000(May 11); 342(19): 1378–1384.
39. Strollo PJ Jr., Rogers RM. Obstructive sleep apnea. N Engl J Med 1996(Jan 11); 334(2): 99–104.
40. Ebeo CT, Benotti PN, Byrd RP Jr., et al. The effect of bi-level positive airway pressure on postoperative pulmonary function following gastric surgery for obesity. Respir Med 2002; 96(9):672–676.
41. Rochester DF, Enson Y. Current concepts in the pathogenesis of the obesity-hypoventilation syndrome. Am J Med 1974; 57:402–420.
42. Zwillich CW, Sutton FD, Pierson DJ, et al. Decreased hypoxic ventilatory drive in the obesity-hypoventilation syndrome. Am J Med 1975; 59:343–348.
43. Ray CS, Sue DY, Bray G, et al. Effects of obesity on respiratory function. Am Rev Respir Dis 1984; 128:501–506.
44. Suratt PM, Wilhoit S, Hsiao H, et al. Compliance of chest wall in obese subjects. J Appl Physiol 1984; 57:403–407.
45. Sprung J, Whalley DG, Falcone T, et al. The impact of morbid obesity, pneumo-peritoneum, and posture on respiratory system mechanics and oxygenation during laparoscopy. Anesth Analg 2002; 94(5):1345–1350.
46. Sharp JT, Henry JP, Sweany SK, et al. The total work of breathing in normal and obese men. J Clin Invest 1964; 43:728–739.
47. Yap JCH, Watson RA, Gilbey S, et al. Effects of posture on respiratory mechanics in obesity. J Appl Physiol 1995; 79:1199–1205.
48. Kollias J, Boileau RA, Bartlett HL, et al. Pulmonary function and physiological conditioning in lean and obese subjects. Arch Environ Health 1972; 25:146–150.
49. Kress JP, Pohlman AS, Alverdy J, Hall JB. The impact of morbid obesity on oxygen cost of breathing (VO(2RESP)) at rest. Am J Respir Crit Care Med 1999; 160(3):883–886.
50. Weiner P, Waizman J, Weiner M, et al. Influence of excessive weight loss on on after gastroplasty for morbid obesity on respiratory muscle performance. Thorax 1998; 53(1): 39–42.
51. Fadell EJ, Richman AD, Ward WW, et al. Fatty infiltration of respiratory muscles in the Pickwickian syndrome. N Engl J Med 1962; 266:861–863.
52. Pelosi P, Croci M, Ravagnan I, et al. Total respiratory system, lung, and chest wall mechanics in sedated-paralyzed postoperative morbidly obese patients. Chest 1996; 109(1):144–151.
53. Pelosi P, Croci M, Ravagnan I, et al. Respiratory system mechanics in sedated, para-lyzed, morbidly obese patients. J Appl Physiol 1997; 82(3):811–818.
54. Refsum HE, Holter PH, Lovig T, et al. Pulmonary function and energy expenditure after marked weight loss in obese women: observations before and one year after gastric banding. Int J Obes 1990; 14(2):175–183.
55. Biring MS, Lewis MI, Liu JT, Mohsenifar Z. Pulmonary physiologic changes of morbid obesity. Am J Med Sci 1999; 318(5):293–297.
56. Katz I, Stradling J, Slutsky AS, et al. Do patients with obstructive sleep apnea have thick necks? Am Rev Respir Dis 1990; 141(5 Pt 1):1228–1231.
57. Jones JG, Sapsford DJ, Wheatley RG. Postoperative hypoxaemia: mechanisms and time course. Anaesthesia 1990; 45(7):566–573.
58. Jense HG, Dubin SA, Silverstein PI, O'Leary-Escolas U. Effect of obesity on safe duration of apnea in anesthetized humans. Anesth Analg 1991; 72(1):89–93.
59. Whitlock G, Lewington S, Mhurchu CN. Coronary heart disease and body mass index: a systematic review of the evidence from larger prospective cohort studies. Semin Vasc Med 2002; 2(4):369–381.

60. Park HS, Song YM, Cho SI. Obesity has a greater impact on cardiovascular mortality in younger men than in older men among non-smoking Koreans. Int J Epidemiol 2005(Nov 3)(E-pub ahead of print).

61. Fontaine KR, Redden DT, Wang C, et al. Years of life lost due to obesity. JAMA 2003; 289(2):187–193.

62. Morse SA, Bravo PE, Morse MC, Reisin E. The heart in obesity-hypertension. Expert Rev Cardiovasc Ther 2005; 3(4):647–658.

63. Kinner B, Goos H, Ewers P, et al. The relation of anthropometric parameters and echo-cardiography findings in the evaluation of left ventricular form and function in extreme obesity. Z Gesamte Inn Med 1989; 44(5):152–157.

64. Duflou J, Virmani R, Rabin I, et al. Sudden death as a result of heart disease in morbid obesity. Am Heart J 1995; 130(2):306–313.

65. Kirby IJ, Howard EC. Propofol in a morbidly obese patient. Anaesthesia 1987; 42(10): 1125–1126.

66. Paul DR, Hoyt JL, Boutros AR. Cardiovascular and respiratory changes in response to change of posture in the very obese. Anesthesiology 1976; 45(1):73–78.

67. Hamaguchi M, Kojima T, Takeda N, et al. The metabolic syndrome as a predictor of nonalcoholic fatty liver disease. Ann Intern Med 2005; 143(10):722–728. Summary for patients in: Ann Intern Med 2005; 143(10):I70; Ann Intern Med 2005; 143(10):I72.

68. Festi D, Colecchia A, Sacco T, et al. Hepatic steatosis in obese patients: clinical aspects and prognostic significance. Obes Rev 2004; 5(1):27–42.

69. Papadia FS, Marinari GM, Camerini G, et al. Liver damage in severely obese patients: a clinical-biochemical-morphologic study on 1,000 liver biopsies. Obes Surg 2004; 14(7): 952–958.

70. Vaughan RW, Bauer S, Wise L. Volume and pH of gastric juice in obese patients. Anesthesiology 1975; 43(6):686–689.

71. Greenberg I. Psychological aspects of bariatric surgery. Nutr Clin Pract 2003; 18(2): 124–130.

72. Beers RA, Roizen MF. Preoperative evaluation of the patient for bariatric surgery. In: Alvarez AO, ed. Morbid Obesity: Perioperative Management. Part 3. 1st ed. Cambridge, England: Cambridge University Press 2004:9.

73. Oberg B, Poulsen TD. Obesity: an anaesthetic challenge. Acta Anaesthesiol Scand 1996; 40(2):191–200.

74. Fraley MA, Birchem JA, Senkottaiyan N, Alpert MA. Obesity and the electrocardio-gram. Obes Rev 2005; 6(4):275–281.

75. Daniel KR, Courtney DM, Kline JA. Assessment of cardiac stress from massive pulmonary embolism with 12-lead ECG. Chest 2001; 120(2):474–481.

76. Bossone E, Paciocco G, Iarussi D, et al. The prognostic role of the ECG in primary pulmonary hypertension. Chest 2002; 121(2):513–518.

77. Juvin P, Blarel A, Bruno F, Desmonts JM. Is peripheral line placement more difficult in obese than in lean patients? Anesth Analg 2003; 96(4):1218.

78. Gilbert TB, Seneff MG, Becker RB. Facilitation of internal jugular venous cannulation using an audio-guided Doppler ultrasound vascular access device: results from a prospec-tive, dual-center, randomized, crossover clinical study. Crit Care Med 1995; 23:60–65.

79. Brodsky JB. Anesthetic management of the morbidly obese patient. Int Anesthesiol Clin 1986; 24(1):93–103.

80. Schumann R, Shikora S, Weiss JM, et al. A comparison of multimodal perioperative analgesia to epidural pain management after gastric bypass surgery. Anesth Analg 2003; 96(2):469–474.

81. Hood DD, Dewan DM. Anesthetic and obstetric outcome in morbidly obese parturients. Anesthesiology 1993; 79(6):1210–1218.

82. Buckley FP, Robinson NB, Simonowitz DA, Dellinger EP. Anaesthesia in the morbidly obese. A comparison of anaesthetic and analgesic regimens for upper abdominal surgery. Anaesthesia 1983; 38(9):840–851.

83. Charghi R, Backman S, Christou N, et al. Patient controlled i.v. analgesia is an acceptable pain management strategy in morbidly obese patients undergoing gastric bypass surgery. A retrospective comparison with epidural analgesia. Can J Anaesth 2003; 50(7): 672–678.

84. Hodgkinson R, Husain FJ. Obesity, gravity, and spread of epidural anesthesia. Anesth Analg 1981; 60(6):421–424.

85. Taivainen T, Tuominen M, Rosenberg PH. Influence of obesity on the spread of spinal analgesia after injection of plain 0.5% bupivacaine at the L3-4 or L4-5 interspace. Br J Anaesth 1990; 64(5):542–546.

86. Cohen AT, Alikhan R, Arcelus JI, et al. Assessment of venous thromboembolism risk and the benefits of thromboprophylaxis in medical patients. Thromb Haemost 2005; 94(4):750–759.

87. Bauer K. Hypercoagulable states. Hematology 2005; 10(suppl 1):39.

88. Nguyen NT, Owings JT, Gosselin R, et al. Systemic coagulation and fibrinolysis after laparoscopic and open gastric bypass. Arch Surg 2001; 136(8):909–916.

89. Hamad GG, Choban PS. Enoxaparin for thromboprophylaxis in morbidly obese patients undergoing bariatric surgery: findings of the prophylaxis against VTE outcomes in bariatric surgery patients receiving enoxaparin (PROBE) study. Obes Surg 2005; 15(10):1368–1374.

90. Fox GS, Whalley DG, Bevan DR. Anaesthesia for the morbidly obese. Experience with 110 patients. Br J Anaesth 1981; 53(8):811–816.

91. Brodsky JB, Lemmens HJ, Brock-Utne JG, et al. Morbid obesity and tracheal intubation. Anesth Analg 2002; 94(3):732–736.

92. Collins JS, Lemmens HJ, Brodsky JB, et al. Laryngoscopy and morbid obesity: a comparison of the "sniff" and "ramped" positions. Obes Surg 2004; 14(9):1171–1175.

93. Brodsky JB, Lemmens HJ, Brock-Utne JG, et al. Anesthetic considerations for bariatric surgery: proper positioning is important for laryngoscopy. Anesth Analg 2003; 96(6):1841–1842.

94. Warner MA, Warner DO, Harper CM, et al. Ulnar neuropathy in medical patients. Anesthesiology 2000; 92(2):613–615.

95. Warner MA, Warner DO, Matsumoto JY, et al. Ulnar neuropathy in surgical patients. Anesthesiology 1999; 90(1):54–59.

96. Fritzlen T, Kremer M, Biddle C. The AANA Foundation Closed Malpractice Claims Study on nerve injuries during anesthesia care. AANA J 2003; 71(5):347–352.

97. Slepchenko G, Simon N, Goubaux B, et al. Performance of target-controlled sufentanil infusion in obese patients. Anesthesiology 2003; 98(1):65–73.

98. Casati A, Putzu M. Anesthesia in the obese patient: pharmacokinetic considerations. J Clin Anesth 2005; 17(2):134–145.

99. Egan TD, Huizinga B, Gupta SK, et al. Remifentanil pharmacokinetics in obese versus lean patients. Anesthesiology 1998; 89(3):562–573.

100. Servin F, Farinotti R, Haberer JP, Desmonts JM. Propofol infusion for maintenance of anesthesia in morbidly obese patients receiving nitrous oxide. A clinical and pharmacokinetic study. Anesthesiology 1993; 78(4):657–665.

101. Kakinohana M, Tomiyama H, Matsuda S, Okuda Y. Target-controlled propofol infusion for general anesthesia in three obese patients. Masui 2000; 49(7):732–735.

102. Saijo H, Nagata O, Kitamura T, et al. Anesthetic management of a hyper-obese patient by target-controlled infusion (TCI) of propofol and fentanyl. Masui 2001; 50(5):528–531.

103. Jung D, Mayersohn M, Perrier D, et al. Thiopental disposition in lean and obese patients undergoing surgery. Anesthesiology 1982; 56(4):269–274.

104. Dundee JW, Hassard TH, McGowan WA, Henshaw J. The 'induction' dose of thiopentone. A method of study and preliminary illustrative results. Anaesthesia 1982; 37(12): 1176–1184.

105. Martinotti R, Vassallo C, Ramaioli F, et al. Anesthesia with sevoflurane in bariatric surgery. Obes Surg 1999; 9(2):180–182.

106. Arain SR, Barth CD, Shankar H, Ebert TJ. Choice of volatile anesthetic for the morbidly obese patient: sevoflurane or desflurane. J Clin Anesth 2005; 17(6):413–419.

107. Strum EM, Szenohradszki J, Kaufman WA, et al. Emergence and recovery characteristics of desflurane versus sevoflurane in morbidly obese adult surgical patients: a prospective, randomized study. Anesth Analg 2004; 99(6):1848–1853.

108. De Baerdemaeker LE, Struys MM, Jacobs S, et al. Optimization of desflurane administration in morbidly obese patients: a comparison with sevoflurane using an 'inhalation bolus' technique. Br J Anaesth 2003; 91(5):638–650.

109. Casati A, Torri G. Cardiovascular stability during inhalational anaesthesia in morbidly obese patients: which is better, sevoflurane or desflurane? Br J Anaesth 2004; 93(1): 153–154; author reply 154–155.

110. Brodsky JB, Lemmens HJ, Collins JS, et al. Nitrous oxide and laparoscopic bariatric surgery. Obes Surg 2005; 15(4):494–496.

111. Schulte-Sasse U, Hess W, Tarnow J. Pulmonary vascular responses to nitrous oxide in patients with normal and high pulmonary vascular resistance. Anesthesiology 1982; 57(1):9–13.

112. Hilgenberg JC, McCammon RL, Stoelting RK. Pulmonary and systemic vascular responses to nitrous oxide in patients with mitral stenosis and pulmonary hypertension. Anesth Analg 1980; 59(5):323–326.

113. Kisor DF, Schmith VD. Clinical pharmacokinetics of cisatracurium besilate. Clin Pharmacokinet 1999; 36(1):27–40.

114. Roy JJ, Varin F. Physicochemical properties of neuromuscular blocking agents and their impact on the pharmacokinetic-pharmacodynamic relationship. Br J Anaesth 2004; 93(2):241–248.

115. Leykin Y, Pellis T, Lucca M, et al. The pharmacodynamic effects of rocuronium when dosed according to real body weight or ideal body weight in morbidly obese patients. Anesth Analg 2004; 99(4):1086–1089.

116. Varin F, Ducharme J, Theoret Y, et al. Influence of extreme obesity on the body disposition and neuromuscular blocking effect of atracurium. Clin Pharmacol Ther 1990; 48(1):18–25.

117. Leykin Y, Pellis T, Lucca M, et al. The effects of cisatracurium on morbidly obese women. Anesth Analg 2004; 99(4):1090–1094 (table of contents).

118. Weinstein JA, Matteo RS, Ornstein E, et al. Pharmacodynamics of vecuronium and atracurium in the obese surgical patient. Anesth Analg 1988; 67(12):1149–1153.

119. Choi YK, Brolin RE, Wagner BK, et al. Efficacy and safety of patient-controlled analgesia for morbidly obese patients following gastric bypass surgery. Obes Surg 2000; 10(2):154–159.

120. Fujioka K. Follow-up of nutritional and metabolic problems after bariatric surgery. Diabetes Care 2005; 28(2):481–484.

121. Ocon Breton J, Perez Naranjo S, Gimeno Laborda S, et al. Effectiveness and complications of bariatric surgery in the treatment of morbid obesity. Nutr Hosp 2005; 20(6): 409–414.

122. Aymard JP, Aymard B, Netter P, et al. Haematological adverse effects of histamine H_2-receptor antagonists. Med Toxicol Adverse Drug Exp 1988; 3(6):430–448.

123. De Paz R, Hernandez-Navarro F. Management, prevention and control of pernicious anemia. Nutr Hosp 2005; 20(6):433–435.

124. Slater GH, Ren CJ, Siegel N, et al. Serum fat-soluble vitamin deficiency and abnormal calcium metabolism after malabsorptive bariatric surgery. J Gastrointest Surg 2004; 8(1):48–55; discussion 54–55.

125. Reijnen MM, Janssen IM. Cardiac arrhythmias after laparoscopic banding. Obes Surg 2004; 14(1):139–141.

14

Anesthesia for Antireflux Surgery

Johan Raeder

Department of Anesthesia, Ullevaal University Hospital,
Oslo, Norway

INTRODUCTION

Reflux of gastrointestinal contents into the esophagus is a very common phenomenon in the general population. It is seen in all age groups, but most cases presenting for surgery are between the ages of 30 and 60 years (1), males twice as frequent as females. Whereas most episodes of reflux are without symptoms, it has been estimated that 44% of the U.S. population have symptoms of heartburn at least once a month and up to 13%, every day (2). A state of gastroesophageal reflux disease (GORD) is said to exist when reflux causes regular symptoms, e.g., twice a week or more (3). Apart from heartburn, the symptoms may be dysphagia, regurgitation, globus sensation, and nausea. Extraesophageal symptoms may also occur, usually as a result of regurgitation into the pharynx, upper airways, or lungs. These include coughing, hiccups, sore throat, hoarseness, and more severe conditions, such as asthma, recurrent pneumonia, pulmonary fibrosis, or sinusitis (4). The pulmonary complications may evolve to serious conditions, especially in children with genetic disorders of esophageal valve function and reduced upper airways reflexes (5).

PATHOPHYSIOLOGY

During swallowing, a bolus of food or liquor travels through the esophagus due to waves of peristaltic contraction. The lower esophageal sphincter opens in coordination with the peristaltic wave to let the bolus enter the stomach and then closes. GORD may evolve because of inappropriate closure of the sphincter and subsequent reflux of acid stomach juice into the esophagus, but also due to conditions of diminished salivation, improper esophageal peristalsis, or inappropriate transport of the food from the stomach and further down. Usually, the symptoms are more severe when lying flat and after heavy meals.

DIAGNOSIS

The diagnosis is suspected from the clinical symptoms, but some of these are rather unspecific for GORD. Especially important is to rule out other causes of chest pain or airway symptoms, such as coronary disease and primary airway or pulmonary diseases. Relief of symptoms from the use of either antacids or histamine-2 blockers, or proton pump inhibitors is quite specific and sensitive to the diagnosis. In most cases, these treatment modalities will also be sufficient for controlling the disease, together with advice of dietary adjustments and general recommendations of eating and sleeping habits. However, drug treatment will generally not deal with the reflux per se, but only with the resulting symptoms. When the symptoms are poorly controlled or the need for medication is extensive, surgical treatment may be considered. The incidence of surgery has been increasing in most western countries during the last decade, and will typically be in the range of one to two procedures per 10,000 inhabitants per year (6). Before surgery is undertaken, the diagnosis is usually confirmed by more specific measures, such as gastrointestinal endoscopy, radiological filming of contrast passage through the esophagus, contrast reflux from the stomach, or measurements of esophageal pH. Most surgeons also like to have manometric measurements of esophageal peristalsis done preoperatively in order to rule out upper esophageal dysfunction as a major cause of the symptoms (2).

SURGICAL PROCEDURES

The surgical fundoplication procedure is usually without serious risks and complications, and symptom relief is excellent in more than 90% to 95% of the patients (2,7). The dominating surgical technique for relief of symptoms is the Nissen fundoplication. This is nowadays mostly done by laparoscopic approach, due to reduction in postoperative pain and short-term morbidity when compared with an open laparotomy approach. However, the long-term results are equally good with laparotomy (8) and some studies suggest a higher risk of serious complications with the laparoscopic approach (9,10). With fundoplication, the top portion of the stomach is wrapped around the lower esophageal sphincter, forming a plication, which acts as an anatomical valve in preventing regurgitation (Fig. 1). In the last decade, some modification of the Nissen technique has been attempted in order to reduce the incidence of postoperative dysphagia, with a looser and shorter plication (12). Another modification is Toupets method, where only a part of the circumference is plicated (13).

Recent research has looked into more simplified and less invasive endoluminal ways of modifying the lower esophagus (e.g., by radiation or topical drug application) (14). Sometimes the reflux is combined with a hiatal hernia in the diaphragm; in these cases, the hernia is reduced as a first part of the operation before the plication is performed. In some institutions, the fundoplication procedure is more frequently undertaken as an ambulatory procedure, due to the fairly low intensity of pain and other postoperative symptoms (7). However, serious complications may occur, such as pneumothorax, esophageal or stomach perforation, hemorrhage, pneumonia, or severe dysphagia if the plication is made too narrow or tight (2,9,15,16). Other complications may be trapping of swallowed air, hiccups, inability to belch or vomit, early satiety, transient vocal cord paralysis, nausea and diarrhea, or other symptoms of gastrointestinal dysfunction (2,17,18).

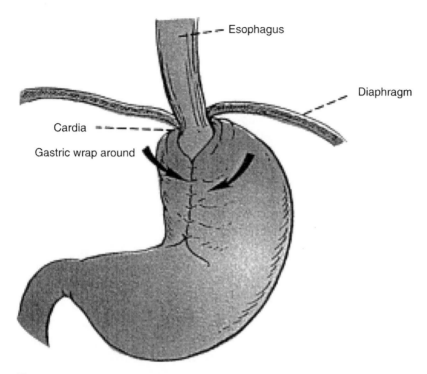

Figure 1 Nissen fundoplication. The gastric fundus is wrapped around the distal esophagus and sutured to itself. *Source*: From Ref. 11.

SPECIAL CONCERNS FOR THE ANESTHESIOLOGIST

Some specific issues with the disease and the cure by laparoscopic surgery are worth mentioning:

Gastric Acid, Ulceration, and Bleeding

Whereas some of these patients have increased gastric fluid acidity and/or reduced mucosal resistance to stomach or intestinal ulceration in general, this may not be the typical case. In most cases, the major problem is a leakage of otherwise normal gastrointestinal fluid, exposing a normal esophageal mucosa to undue amounts of acid, causing symptoms, eventually ulceration, and, in rare cases, bleeding. In most of these patients, the acidity of gastric fluid will be raised preoperatively as a result of medical treatment. Thus, the situation in the individual patient may vary as to whether the use of nonsteroidal anti-inflammatory drugs (NSAIDs), selective cox-2 inhibiting NSAIDs (coxibs), and corticosteroids may be appropriate for perioperative pain prophylaxis and treatment (19). Because these drugs are valuable components of a multimodal pain therapy, their use should be considered. If there is a general hyperacidity or suspicion of reduced mucosal resistance, nonselective NSAIDs should not be used. The coxibs may be an alternative in these cases if symptoms are moderate, as they do not reduce platelet adhesion or promote bleeding, and they are less risky in terms of ulcer formation. If the patient has a normal gastrointestinal acidity and mucosal resistance and is well pretreated with a proton pump inhibitor or other antacid acting drug, there may actually be less risk of gastrointestinal problems with NSAIDs, coxibs, and corticosteroids compared with a general population.

Regurgitation and Aspiration

As these patients have an insufficient valve between the stomach and esophagus, there will be an increased risk of regurgitation upward into the pharynx and eventually into the trachea and lungs, especially when these patients lie flat and have their protective reflexes taken away by sedative acting drugs, opioids, or general anesthesia.

In these patients strict adherence to the fasting routines is mandatory. Whereas the usual two-hour limit for clear fluid and six hours for solid food is valid in most cases (20), some of these patients may have delayed gastric emptying as part of their reflux disease and require prolonged fasting (2). This includes patients with diabetes mellitus, vagotomy, gastrointestinal inflammation, patients on opioid medication, and patients with hypovolemia or pain.

However, even though patients have fasted appropriately, there will be a continuous production of gastric acid that may regurgitate passively. The appropriate approach preoperatively will be to avoid undue sedation in uncontrolled environment, to reduce the amount and acidity of gastric fluid, and to secure the airways properly during induction and maintenance of general anesthesia. For this reason, sedative and opioid premedication are best avoided. However, preoperative proton pump inhibitors, such as esomeprazole, lanzoprazole, pantoprazole, or omeprazole, are useful adjuncts to reduce the volume and acidity of gastric fluid. Use of preoperative oral antacid ingestion is usually not recommended because this can increase the amount of gastric fluid, although the pH value will be improved. In patients with a high risk of regurgitation, preoperative gastric drainage through a nasogastric tube may be considered, but it is usually quite uncomfortable for the patient and does not guarantee against residual gastric content.

As to the anesthetic induction, the risk of passive regurgitation will be reduced by having an elevated head position. This is quite convenient as these patients are usually operated on in a half-sitting position ("beach chair" position) in order to get a better view and access to the upper part of the peritoneal cavity. Also, to ensure proper positioning of the patient in terms of no sharp edges or pressure points, these are good reasons to place the patient in the half-sitting position while awake and keep them there during the induction.

To protect against intra-operative acid aspiration, the airway should be secured by a cuffed endotracheal tube. Although the use of laryngeal masks may be appropriate for other laparoscopic procedures, this is not recommended for reflux patients. This is due to the increased reflux per se, which is further reinforced during the first period of surgery when usually an oro-gastric tube present. Some surgeons will prefer to have a thick oro-gastric tube present throughout the procedure as a template for the plication, whereas others will just like to have the tube for emptying the stomach by the start of the procedure.

Hemodynamics and Pulmonary Function

During pneumoperitoneum there will be an increase in the intraperitoneal pressure with consequences on the circulation and respiratory physics (21). Further, there will be a stretch in the peritoneal wall with the local release of norepinephrine and subsequent pain and stress stimulation (22). As CO_2 is the dominating gas in use for peritoneal insufflation, there will also be absorption of CO_2 into the circulation. This will result in respiratory acidosis if the CO_2 is not removed by increased lung ventilation.

The increased intraperitoneal pressure will press upon arterial and venous vessel walls in the area. This increases the systemic vascular resistance (i.e., afterload). The increase in total resistance may be balanced and usually overcompensated by the vasodilatatory effect of the general anesthetics in use, such as propofol or potent inhalational agents, although this is mainly related to pronounced vasodilatation in other parts of the circulation, leading to shunting. The same anesthetic agents also result in reduced cardiac contractility, unless there is nociceptive or stress-induced sympathetic stimulation. This may result from inadequate anesthesia or analgesia. There is reduced venous return to the heart due to increased pressure transmitted to abdominal veins as well as on the major veins (including the inferior cava) of the posterior abdominal wall. The decrease in venous return may be exaggerated by the semi-sitting position. Summing up, the combined effect of anesthetic induction and establishment of pneumoperitoneum may produce a severe reduction in blood pressure, due to a combination of decreased total peripheral resistance, reduced cardiac contractility, and reduced venous return to the heart. For this reason, it is wise to give these patients a rapid IV fluid load before and during induction of anesthesia, either 0.5 to 1.0 L of a crystalloid, or 200 to 500 mL of a colloid. Frequent measurements of blood pressure are also appropriate and a low threshold for giving vasoconstrictors either ephedrine or phenylephrine, if needed.

The pulmonary compliance will be reduced due to the upward shift of the diaphragm and increased pressure intraperitoneally. To maintain the tidal volume for each breath, the inspiratory peak pressure during controlled ventilation will need to be increased. However, some of the effects on intrathoracic volume and pressure from pneumoperitoneum are counteracted by the semi-sitting position before and after the procedure, but not during anesthesia when compliance is always lowered (21). To maintain normocapnia during CO_2 inflation, the effective minute ventilation [(tidal volume $\div$ deadspace) $\times$ respiratory rate] will need to increase by 25% to 50% after start of pneumoperitoneum, and thereafter remain stable at a plateau (23).

Nausea and Vomiting

This is an issue of special importance in the reflux patients (see Chapter 26). Whereas a few patients may experience nausea preoperatively as part of their disease, all these patients may be at special risk for complications if postoperative nausea and vomiting (PONV) evolve; the worst case being rupture of the plication sutures due to severe retching or vomiting. Choosing an anesthetic technique with decreased risk of PONV as well as using proper prophylaxis is recommended (24,25). PONV may be divided into inherent risk in the patient in question and risks associated with the choice of anesthetic and surgical techniques. Major patient risk factors include female gender, nonsmoking status, and previous susceptibility to nausea or vomiting, either after general anesthesia or during traveling. Risk factors from anesthetic handling are the use of inhalational agents, including nitrous oxide, need of postoperative opioids, and use of high-dose (i.e., ≥ 2.5 mg) neostigmine for neuromuscular block reversal (26). Whereas laparoscopy is associated with less PONV than a similar surgical procedure done by laparotomy (Raeder et al., submitted), there is still an increased risk of PONV with all stimulation and manipulation of the gastrointestinal organs. This may be due to stimulation of the vagal nerve during manipulation and to local and systemic release of serotonin from the numerous serotonergic nerve endings in the mucosa. To reduce the risk of PONV, there may be an argument for not using neuromuscular blockers at all or otherwise avoid the need of reversal by just using a starting dose or a short-acting agent (e.g., mivacurium), ensuring that the train of four (TOF) ratio by the end of the procedure is at least 90% by spontaneous degradation of the relaxant. Another measure is to use total intravenous (IV) techniques instead of inhalational anesthetics, although the extra emetic effect of inhalational agents may be compensated for by adding an extra antiemetic prophylactic agent in addition to what was otherwise planned (24).

Nitrous oxide will expand occasional air pockets inside the gastrointestinal tract and reduce surgical accessibility. This may be an argument for avoiding this agent, in addition to the potential emetic effect of nitrous oxide in high-risk patients (27). A total IV technique will almost always imply using propofol infusion, and this drug is antiemetic per se, providing PONV protection during the first hours after the end of anesthesia (28). Further, any means that reduce the need for postoperative opioids for pain prophylaxis and treatment will also be of benefit in reducing the risk of PONV (see below) (24).

However, even with optimal anesthetic handling in a patient without special risk factors, the risk of PONV will be in the range of 20% to 40%, being substantially higher if individual or anesthetic risk factors are involved. A rough estimation of PONV risk may be done by the modified Apfel score (Table 1). Even though prophylaxis inevitably means that some patients receive drugs that they do not need, there is a strong argument for routine PONV prophylaxis in fundoplication patients because the baseline risk is significant and the consequences of retching and vomiting may be substantial. Droperidol, 5-hydroxytryptamine type 3 (5-HT3) antagonists, and corticosteroids are well-documented antiemetic prophylactics, providing protection for

Table 1 Risk of Postoperative Nausea and Vomiting

Risk factor	Point
Female gender	1
Nonsmoking status	1
Previous susceptibility to nausea or vomiting, either after general anesthesia or during traveling	1
Use of postoperative opioids	1
Inhalational anesthesia	1
Laparotomy	1
Neostigmine ≥ 2.5 mg	1
Add points in each patient to total risk score; 0–7: (risk of PONV)	
0 point: (0–10%)	
1 point: (10–20%)	
2 points: (20–30%)	
3 points: (30–40%)	
4 points: (40–50%)	
5 points: (50–60%)	
6 points: (60–70%)	
7 points: (>70%)	

Abbreviation: PONV, postoperative nausea and vomiting.
Source: From Ref. (24) and Raeder, submitted.

24 hours after a single dose (24). Whereas droperidol and 5-HT3 antagonists are best given by the end of the procedure, the corticosteroids have a slower onset of action and should be given early during the procedure. In a case with medium or high risk of PONV (i.e., more than 30–40%, Table l), giving all the three drugs may be appropriate; the corticosteroids will also protect against pain. Even if just one of these drugs is used, they seem to have a quite similar anti-PONV efficacy, with the possible exception of 5-HT3 agents, which are somewhat better for protection against vomiting and retching than droperidol, which again is slightly better in protecting against nausea (29). Cost issues may also be considered: the 5-HT3 agents are presently in the 10 to 15 Euro range per dose, whereas the other options are in the 1 to 2 Euro range. These differences may change when some of the 5-HT3 agents become generic soon.

Postoperative Pain and Analgesia

The pain after laparoscopic fundoplication is usually moderate, but still there is a need to minimize the pain in order to get an optimal quality for the patient and to get the patient mobilized and discharged as soon as possible (see Chapter 25). As the opioids may provoke PONV (see above), there is a case for achieving maximal pain control with a nonopioid multimodal regimen (30). It has been shown that paracetamol in an optimal dose is a proper basis in this regimen. The starting dose should be 2 g orally or 1 g intravenously, continuing with 1 g four times a day in the adult patient of at least 60 kg weight and less than 60 years of age. Otherwise, dose reduction should be considered. As paracetamol is very rapidly cleared from the stomach, a preoperative oral administration one to two hours ahead of surgery may do, but due to the special concerns with this kind of surgery (see aspiration, above), many will prefer to rather give the first dose as an intra-operative IV infusion. The same argument is valid for NSAID or coxib as well; they may best be given intravenously after induction of anesthesia. It has been shown that the combination of NSAID or coxib with paracetamol has a small additive analgesic effect (31). It has also been shown that adding corticosteroids will have a further analgesic prophylactic effect, in addition to providing protection against PONV and stimulating appetite (Hval K, submitted). Whereas a dose of 3 to 4 mg IV dexamethasone will be appropriate for PONV prophylaxis, the dose should probably be at least 8 mg in an adult to also provide good analgesic protection (32).

Wound infiltration in all port sites should be performed using local anesthesia. Typically, 20 to 40 mL of either bupivacaine (2.5 mg/mL) or ropivacaine (2 mg/mL) is usually recommended, but only documented effective in some studies (33). Although infiltration by the end of the procedure will have a longer postoperative duration per se, there is a controversy claiming that preoperative infiltration is better due to a possible preemptive effect of blocking pain stimulation from surgery in the periphery (34). Some controversy also exists as to the benefits of instilling local anesthesia in the upper peritoneal cavity before closure of all the wounds. Most studies indicate a beneficial effect of installing 40 to 50 mL of diluted local anesthesia after laparoscopic cholecystectomy (35), whereas others do not find a significant analgesic effect (36).

Where postoperative opioids are needed, the choice of agent and dosing strategy may not be very different from any other similar surgical procedure: small, repeated doses of titrated opioid, such as fentanyl 0.5 μg/kg, may be recommended while the patient is in the postoperative care unit (PACU), whereas a rapid conversion to oral drug is appropriate after PACU discharge. Oxycodone may be a better choice than codeine, due to a more predictable absorption and action (37). Further, some 5% to 10% of the Western society population has a genetic failure in converting codeine to active morphine and thus a poor effect of this drug. Oxycodone may be given in 5 to 10 mg tablets for relief of temporary pain or as 10 to 20 mg sustained release formulation if it is expected that the pain will be more long lasting.

CHOICE OF ANESTHETIC TECHNIQUE

For obvious reasons, loco-regional anesthesia is not feasible as the major technique for this type of procedure. However, as discussed above, local anesthesia infiltration is probably useful as a component of multimodal postoperative pain therapy. Intrapleural or intercostal blocks are not as appropriate as they need to be done bilaterally, thus with a high dose need of local anesthetic drug and with inherent risk of pneumothorax. A thoracic epidural technique in the 5th–6th thoracic vertebrae interspace may provide excellent postoperative pain relief and also be an option for intraoperative analgesia with just a "sleep dose" of a suitable anesthetic agent. Still, these patients need to be intubated and extra care should be taken in controlling hypotension, low venous return, and a slowing of the heart rate if an intraoperative thoracic epidural is used. Thus, in most centers a general anesthetic technique is used for fundoplication surgery.

Monitoring

Basic monitoring is appropriate for the routine cases, including continuous electrocardiogram, pulse oximetry, noninvasive blood pressure reading, and basic respiratory monitoring with capnography, oxygen tension, and inhalational agent concentration where a volatile agent is used. Bi-spectral index monitoring (BIS) is the best-documented mode for monitoring anesthetic depth, and is a valuable, although not obligatory, adjunct. BIS is useful both for avoiding awareness if neuromuscular blockers are used (37), and for titration of the anesthetic depth for a rapid emergence (38). Overdosing of the anesthetic drug is less prone to happen with this device active. As the routine patient is young or middle-aged with adequate cardiovascular function, and there is small risk of sudden, major bleeding, an arterial line is not mandatory for this procedure. However, it may be useful for checking blood gas values during pneumoperitoneum and also for controlling rapid changes in blood pressure, which may occur during induction and patient positioning. For the latter reason, two good venous lines should be in use during induction of anesthesia: one for infusion of drugs with an ongoing balanced salt solution running, and the other with a slowly running colloid or crystalloid with the option of rapid rate increase for hemodynamic support. As a typical procedure can take place within two to three hours without major fluid shifts and with rapid recovery, no urinary catheter is needed in the routine case. A central venous line is usually not employed, as the central venous pressure is hard to evaluate in the semi-sitting position and not needed postoperatively. These patients will drink and ambulate within a few hours after a routine case. When neuromuscular blocking agents are used, monitoring of function is recommended, for instance, by the TOF ratio.

As with all anesthetic cases, there may be a need for more extensive monitoring of the patients' respiratory function or hemodynamics in the presence of systemic disease or impairment.

General Anesthetic Agents

Inhalational induction is usually not recommended in patients undergoing esophageal reflux procedures due to the risk of regurgitation. However, in the semi-sitting position, the risk of passive regurgitation is small and a rapid induction–intubation sequence is probably unnecessary. As good venous access is established prior to induction, IV induction techniques are almost universal. Any standard IV induction agent may be used, according to the usual practice of the anesthetist: barbiturate, etomidate, propofol, and in the rare cases of severe hypovolemia, even ketamine together with a benzodiazepine. If a total IV technique is chosen for maintenance, there is a strong case for using propofol throughout, including induction. Compared with inhalational maintenance, propofol maintenance carries a smaller risk of PONV (see above), which is an especially important concern with this procedure (39). Although, propofol is associated with a slightly slower immediate recovery when combined with conventional opioids (39), this is not a major problem. A few minutes delay in eyes opening and extubation do not seem to slow down further recovery end points, such as discharge from the PACU and discharge readiness.

Some studies favor propofol maintenance for these aspects because PONV from inhalational agents may slow down the speed of late recovery (40). Further, most of the studies with propofol reported in recent meta-analyses used fentanyl or sufentanil as the opioid (39). Recent data show a more rapid immediate recovery when propofol is combined with remifentanil (38). As remifentanil allows for a very rapid change in depth of anesthesia, this technique may also allow for intubation without using a neuromuscular blocking agent. A bolus dose of 2 to 3 µg/kg remifentanil given slowly for two to three minutes during or after induction of sleep with propofol will ensure sufficiently profound analgesia and relaxation of the vocal cords to allow for endotracheal intubation.

However, most anesthesiologists will prefer to use a nondepolarizing neuromuscular blocker for intubation. This may also provide the surgeon with better operating conditions during the dissection. A single dose of cisatracurium (0.08 mg/kg) or rocuronuim (0.6 mg/kg) may be sufficient both for intubation and surgery. If the TOF shows at least 90% recovery by the end of the procedure, there is no need of neostigmine reversal. As neostigmine is associated with a dose-related increased risk of PONV, nonreversal may be of benefit. However, if the TOF is less than 90%, a dose of up to 2.5 mg neostigmine with glycopyrrolate should be used.

CONSIDERATIONS IN CHILDREN

Although pediatric anesthesia is beyond the scope of this chapter, laparoscopic fundoplication is presently performed in all the age groups, including neonates. These cases carry most of the same physiological aspects and concerns as the adults, but many of these children will also have other health problems, such as genetic disease, prematurity, and pulmonary problems, which will call for specialized pediatric anesthesia care. Sometimes an open laparotomy is preferred. The pediatric cases will present many additional anesthetic challenges and are definitely cases in need of specialized care from pediatric anesthetists. The reader is referred to specialist pediatric anesthesia texts.

PRACTICAL APPROACH TO ANESTHESIA FOR ANTIREFLUX SURGERY IN THE ADULT

Those patients who take proton pump inhibitors (PPIs) or other drugs for modifying gastric content should take their regular medication, including the evening dose on the day before surgery. A short-acting agent for preoperative night sleep may be added if needed.

As the physiology of gastric emptying may be abnormal, and there is an increased risk of regurgitation during induction, patients are generally maintained nil-by-mouth preoperatively. In severe cases, this includes omission of oral anxiolytics. Alternative management of severe preoperative anxiety may be achieved by establishing venous access in the preoperative holding area and administering a small dose of midazolam (1–2 mg) or low-dose propofol infusion [bolus 20–30 mg, then 2–4 mg/kg/hr or target-controlled infusion (TCI) at 0.5–1.0 μg/mL].

In the operating theater, the patient is positioned in a comfortable "beach chair" position, avoiding any sharp edges and sources of undue pressure on the skin. Then the IV lines are established, starting with a low-dose (see above) infusion of propofol for sedation during the rest of the preparation with mounting of equipment for monitoring and collection of baseline values of vital signs. In the author's center, the patient is allowed to remain in the half-sitting position during induction; this is thought to reduce the risk of passive regurgitation from the stomach to the pharynx.

Induction

The induction is preceded by proper pre-oxygenation (usually deep and normal breathing of 100% oxygen through a mask for three to four minutes). Then the induction is initiated with propofol TCI of 5 μg/mL and remifentanil TCI of 7.5 ng/mL. Without TCI, standard propofol doses should be used: 2 mg/kg followed by 10 mg/kg/min and remifentanil bolus 0.5 μg/kg and 0.3 μg/kg/min. As apnea supervenes, gentle mask ventilation is continued for two minutes; then the trachea can be intubated without the routine use of long-acting neuromuscular blocking agents. Shortly after endotracheal intubation, TCI values are adjusted to 3 μg/mL and 2.5 ng/mL for propofol and remifentanil, respectively. Remifentanil is increased to 7.5 ng/mL again when surgery is about to start. Without TCI, propofol will be reduced to 8 mg/kg/hr after 10 minutes from the start of induction, and then to 6 mg/kg/hr after another 10 minutes, keeping this level for the rest of the procedure. Remifentanil will be reduced to 0.1 μg/kg/min after intubation, and adjusted back to 0.3 μg/kg/min just before start of surgery. In the obese or fragile patient, the author advocates the use of a neuromuscular blocker, for instance, cisatracurium in a single dose of 0.8 mg/kg ideal body weight. A fine-bore gastric tube is in place until the surgeon asks for removal after establishment of pneumoperitoneum. Dexamethasone 8 mg is administered in adult patients for routine pain and PONV prophylaxis.

Maintenance

Further maintenance is effectively managed with propofol and remifentanil; the latter adjusted to the need of the patient as judged by hemodynamic response to ongoing surgery. In the author's center, the propofol dose is fixed unless BIS monitoring is used. A BIS target of 50 (range of 45–55) allows dose titration, although in practical terms, the minimum propofol target is 1.8 μg/mL (or infusion down to 4 mg/kg/hr) even where BIS returns low values, because, at these levels, BIS becomes unreliable and too low levels of propofol may result in sudden awakening. In the author's center, no nitrous oxide or other inhalational agent is used.

Postoperative Care

For postoperative pain prophylaxis, the following drugs are given before the end of anesthesia (in addition to dexamethasone given shortly after induction): paracetamol 1 g IV and ketorolac 30 mg IV, and 20–30 mL of bupivacaine 2.5 mg/mL for wound infiltration. Fentanyl 1 µg/kg is also given because remifentanil has a very rapid decline of its effects. For PONV prophylaxis, the patient will receive ondansetron 4 mg IV and droperidol 1.25 mg IV. Usually, the BIS will be kept in the 50 to 55 range during wound closure, and this will ensure emergence and extubation within few minutes after stopping the remifentanil and propofol infusions. The typical patient will be able to communicate orally and assist themselves in transfer from the operating table to the bed within five minutes from the end of anesthesia.

In the postoperative care unit, the patients receive fentanyl 0.5 µg/kg increments for pain, and eventually ephedrine 5 to 10 mg IV and metoclopramide 10 mg for any nausea or vomiting. The patient may be allowed to drink within one hour if he/she wants to, and to eat "soft" nonheated food after one to two hours. The patients should be kept in the hospital for at least three to four hours, but may then be discharged if they live within one-hour access to an acute surgical service (7). The patients should be thoroughly informed about complications and possible alarm signs before discharge. Day cases should be routinely followed up by a telephone call the day after. Most surgeons like to have the patient back for postsurgical review at two to four weeks after surgery.

REFERENCES

1. Trondsen E, Bakken IJ, Skjeldestad FE. Antireflux surgery in Norway. Tidsskr Nor Laegeforen 2005; 125:1990–1992.
2. Redmond MC. Perianesthesia care of the patient with gastroesophageal reflux disease. J Perianesth Nurs 2003; 18:335–344.
3. Eisen G. The epidemiology of gastroesophageal reflux disease: what we know and what we need to know. Am J Gastroenterol 2001; 96:S16–S18.
4. Kaynard A, Flora K. Gastroesophageal reflux disease. Control of symptoms, prevention of complications. Postgrad Med 2001; 110:42–48,51.
5. Mattioli G, Montobbio G, Pini PA, et al. Anesthesiologic aspects of laparoscopic fundoplication for gastroesophageal reflux in children with chronic respiratory and gastroenterological symptoms. Surg Endosc 2003; 17:559–566.
6. Finlayson SR, Laycock WS, Birkmeyer JD. National trends in utilization and outcomes of antireflux surgery. Surg Endosc 2003; 17:864–867.
7. Trondsen E, Mjaland O, Raeder J, Buanes T. Day-case laparoscopic fundoplication for gastro-oesophageal reflux disease. Br J Surg 2000; 87:1708–1711.
8. Nilsson G, Wenner J, Larsson S, Johnsson F. Randomized clinical trial of laparoscopic versus open fundoplication for gastro-oesophageal reflux. Br J Surg 2004; 91:552–559.
9. Rantanen TK, Salo JA, Sipponen JT. Fatal and life-threatening complications in antireflux surgery: analysis of 5,502 operations. Br J Surg 1999; 86:1573–1577.
10. Sandbu R, Khamis H, Gustavsson S, Haglund U. Long-term results of antireflux surgery indicate the need for a randomized clinical trial. Br J Surg 2002; 89:225–230.
11. Drain CB. Perianesthesia Nursing: A Critical Approach. Philadelphia, PA: Elsevier, 2003:555.

12. Donahue PE, Samelson S, Nyhus LM, Bombeck CT. The floppy Nissen fundoplication. Effective long-term control of pathologic reflux. Arch Surg 1985; 120:663–668.
13. Spivak H, Lelcuk S, Hunter JG. Laparoscopic surgery of the gastroesophageal junction. World J Surg 1999; 23:356–367.
14. Oleynikov D, Oelschlager B, Dibaise J. Endoscopic therapy for gastroesophageal reflux disease: can it replace antireflux surgery? Minerva Chir 2004; 59:427–435.
15. Bittner HB, Meyers WC, Brazer SR, Pappas TN. Laparoscopic Nissen fundoplication: operative results and short-term follow-up. Am J Surg 1994; 167:193–198.
16. Makinen MT, Yli-Hankala A. Respiratory compliance during laparoscopic hiatal and inguinal hernia repair. Can J Anaesth 1998; 45:865–870.
17. Strate T, Langwieler TE, Mann O, et al. Intractable hiccup: an odd complication after laparoscopic fundoplication for gastroesophageal reflux disease. Surg Endosc 2002; 16:1109.
18. Kanski A, Plocharska E, Stanowski E, et al. Transient left vocal cord paralysis during laparoscopic surgery for an oesophageal hiatus hernia. Eur J Anaesth 1999; 16:495–499.
19. White PF. Changing role of COX-2 inhibitors in the perioperative period: is parecoxib really the answer? Anesth Analg 2005; 100:1306–1308.
20. Soreide E, Eriksson LI, Hirlekar G, et al. Pre-operative fasting guidelines: an update. Acta Anaesth Scand 2005; 49:1041–1047.
21. Talamini MA, Mendoza-Sagaon M, Gitzelmann CA, et al. Increased mediastinal pressure and decreased cardiac output during laparoscopic Nissen fundoplication. Surgery 1997; 122:345–352.
22. Myre K, Raeder J, Rostrup M, et al. Catecholamine release during laparoscopic fundoplication with high and low doses of remifentanil. Acta Anaesth Scand 2003; 47:267–273.
23. Joris JL. Anesthetic management of laparoscopy. In: Miller RD, ed. Anesthesia. 4th ed. New York: Churchill Livingstone, 1994:2011–2029.
24. Apfel CC, Korttila K, Abdalla M, et al. A factorial trial of six interventions for the prevention of postoperative nausea and vomiting. N Engl J Med 2004; 350:2441–2451.
25. Apfel CC, Roewer N. Risk assessment of postoperative nausea and vomiting. Int Anesth Clin 2003; 41:13–32.
26. Lovstad RZ, Thagaard KS, Berner NS, Raeder JC. Neostigmine 50 microg kg (–1) with glycopyrrolate increases postoperative nausea in women after laparoscopic gynaecological surgery. Acta Anaesth Scand 2001; 45:495–500.
27. Tramer M, Moore A, McQuay H. Meta-analytic comparison of prophylactic antiemetic efficacy for postoperative nausea and vomiting: propofol anaesthesia vs omitting nitrous oxide vs total i.v. anaesthesia with propofol. Br J Anaesth 1997; 78:256–259.
28. Hammas B, Thorn SE, Wattwil M. Superior prolonged antiemetic prophylaxis with a four-drug multimodal regimen—comparison with propofol or placebo. Acta Anaesth Scand 2002; 46:232–237.
29. Koivuranta M, Laara E, Ranta P, et al. Comparison of ondansetron and droperidol in the prevention of postoperative nausea and vomiting after laparoscopic surgery in women. A randomised, double-blind, placebo-controlled trial. Acta Anaesth Scand 1997; 41:1273–1279.
30. Dahl V, Raeder JC. Non-opioid postoperative analgesia. Acta Anaesth Scand 2000; 44:1191–1203.
31. Breivik EK, Barkvoll P, Skovlund E. Combining diclofenac with acetaminophen or acetaminophen-codeine after oral surgery: a randomized, double-blind single-dose study. Clin Pharmacol Ther 1999; 66:625–635.
32. Bisgaard T, Klarskov B, Kehlet H, Rosenberg J. Preoperative dexamethasone improves surgical outcome after laparoscopic cholecystectomy: a randomized double-blind placebo-controlled trial. Ann Surg 2003; 238:651–660.
33. Moiniche S, Jorgensen H, Wetterslev J, Dahl JB. Local anesthetic infiltration for postoperative pain relief after laparoscopy: a qualitative and quantitative systematic review

of intraperitoneal, port-site infiltration and mesosalpinx block. Anesth Analg 2000; 90: 899–912.

34. Ong CK, Lirk P, Seymour RA, Jenkins BJ. The efficacy of preemptive analgesia for acute postoperative pain management: a meta-analysis. Anesth Analg 2005; 100: 757–773 (table).
35. Cunniffe MG, McAnena OJ, Dar MA, et al. A prospective randomized trial of intraoperative bupivacaine irrigation for management of shoulder-tip pain following laparoscopy. Am J Surg 1998; 176:258–261.
36. Kalso E. Oxycodone. J Pain Symptom Manage 2005; 29:S47–S56.
37. Lennmarken C, Sandin R. Neuromonitoring for awareness during surgery. Lancet 2004; 363:1747–1748.
38. Hoymork SC, Raeder J, Grimsmo B, Steen PA. Bispectral index, serum drug concentrations and emergence associated with individually adjusted target-controlled infusions of remifentanil and propofol for laparoscopic surgery. Br J Anaesth 2003; 91:773–780.
39. Gupta A, Stierer T, Zuckerman R, et al. Comparison of recovery profile after ambulatory anesthesia with propofol, isoflurane, sevoflurane and desflurane: a systematic review. Anesth Analg 2004; 98:632–641 (table).
40. Hofer CK, Zollinger A, Buchi S, et al. Patient well-being after general anaesthesia: a prospective, randomized, controlled multi-centre trial comparing intravenous and inhalation anaesthesia. Br J Anaesth 2003; 91:631–637.

15

Anesthesia for Hepatobiliary Surgery

Chris P. Snowden and David M. Cressey
*Department of Perioperative and Critical Care, Freeman Hospital,
Newcastle upon Tyne, U.K.*

INTRODUCTION

Anesthetic management of patients undergoing hepatobiliary (HPB) procedures is dependent on a complete understanding of the potential benefits, limitations, and perioperative risks of complex surgical procedures, in the context of either preexisting liver disease and/or other coexisting disease states. Surgical criteria for patient selection are important (1). Where malignancy is involved, hepatic resection is established as the only currently available modality of treatment with curative potential. However, because only approximately 10% to 20% of patients presenting with hepatic malignancy are suitable for resection, other types of less invasive HPB surgical techniques are used to achieve reduction of tumor mass and symptomatic control. The following section outlines some surgical aspects for the more frequently encountered HPB operations, but is primarily concerned with hepatic resection. The general features of laparoscopic surgery and liver transplantation anesthesia are beyond the scope of this chapter.

SURGICAL TECHNIQUES

Tumor Ablation Techniques

Radio frequency ablation (2) and cryoablation (3,4) techniques can be performed percutaneously, laparoscopically, or during open laparotomy. The percutaneous approach is usually indicated for palliation, such as pain control, to prolong life (to prevent liver failure caused by tumor growth) or for recurrent tumors. Laparoscopic ablation is selected for smaller, superficially located, or easily accessible tumors with intraoperative ultrasound guidance. Open surgical ablation is indicated for larger or deeply located malignancy and in conjunction with other abdominal organ resections. Tumor ablation probes are inserted into the center of the tumor mass and either cooled (with liquid nitrogen) or heated to temperatures in the region of $100°C$ to $110°C$. This is maintained until the appropriate volume of tissue has been locally destroyed. Potential complications of these techniques include hemorrhage (including hepatic capsular rupture) and biliary leak, and, in more extensive procedures, thrombocytopenia and myoglobinuria have been reported (2).

213

Transjugular Intrahepatic Portosystemic Shunt

This procedure is used to treat complications of portal hypertension usually as a bridge to transplantation (5). Transjugular intrahepatic portosystemic shunt (TIPS) is indicated for acute variceal bleeding or prevention of variceal bleeding when medical therapy or endoscopic therapy (sclerotherapy or ligation) has failed. Ascites that is refractory to medical management, requiring frequent paracentesis, may also be amenable to treatment with TIPS. However, TIPS does not prolong survival without liver transplantation. The main limiting factors when considering TIPS are worsening of liver function and encephalopathy, stent dysfunction or thrombosis, and technical problems during subsequent liver transplantation from misplaced TIPS (5). TIPS placement has a 1% to 2% mortality rate, and because postoperative encephalopathy is a significant risk, high-dependency care is usually required. Post-procedure, TIPS-related encephalopathy occurs in 5% to 35% of patients (secondary to the shunt bypassing blood from the portal vein past what functional liver there is) and is treated either by medical management or by insertion of smaller stents, coils, or balloons into the existing TIPS (6).

Hepatic Resection

Anatomy

Morphologically, the liver is divided into a large right and smaller left lobe by the falciform ligament (Fig. 1). However, a more functional division described in 1957 (7) divides the liver into left and right hemilivers along a line that passes through the gall bladder bed toward the vena cava and through the right axis of the caudate lobe. This follows the line of division of the portal inflow. Further subdivisions of the

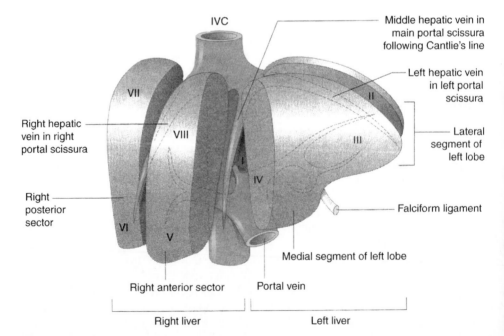

Figure 1 A schematic representation of the surgical hepatic segments as described by Couinand. *Source*: From Ref. 7. *Abbreviation*: IVC, inferior vena cava.

portal inflow divide each hemiliver into two sectors and then each sector into two segments. Divisions in the bile duct and hepatic artery mirror the divisions of the portal inflow forming a series of portal trinities. As each segment of the liver has its own supply from a portal trinity, each can be resected independently.

This segmental picture of the liver clearly demonstrates the relations of the eight segments of the liver often referred to in surgical resections. The left liver comprises segments II and III (also referred to as the left lateral segment) plus IV (which in combination with segment III forms the quadrate lobe). The right liver comprises segments V to VIII. Of note is the caudate lobe which is a distinct anatomical segment, segment I; it receives supply from both left and right liver lobes and drains independently into the vena cava.

The right hepatic vein drains independently into the vena cava, but the middle and left hepatic veins usually join prior to draining into the vena cava. There are often a few small veins draining posteriorly and, occasionally, two or three inferior right hepatic veins of moderate size. If these vessels are not recognized and are torn during hepatic resection, massive blood loss may ensue.

Surgical Incision and Dissection

A laparoscopy is often performed immediately prior to laparotomy to confirm tumor resectability. Unnecessary laparotomy may be avoided in nearly 20% of planned resections where disease was assessed as resectable on preoperative imaging (8). Open resection usually employs bilateral subcostal incisions with extension upward to the sternum (Mercedes-Benz incision) to allow wide surgical access. After the liver has been mobilized, intraoperative ultrasound is used to confirm the expected site of disease and detect any additional lesions (found in 10–50% of cases) (9–11).

The majority of hepatic resections involve either the left or the right hemiliver, but occasionally sectors or segments may be resected. The principal procedures for hepatic resection are outlined in Table 1.

Table 1 Surgical Operations for Hepatic Resection

Operation	Involved segments
Right hemihepatectomy	Segments V–VIII
Extended right hepatectomy	Segments V–VIII plus segment IV
Left hepatectomy	Segments II–IV
Left lateral segmentectomy	Segments II and III
Extended left hepatectomy	Segments II–IV plus V and VIII (among the most challenging of hepatic resections)
Caudate lobe resection	Most commonly removed en bloc as part of a major hepatic resection to achieve tumor clearance, occasionally as an isolated resection
Segmental resection	Each segment can be resected (12)
Central resection	Removal of segments IV, V, and VIII
Resection for hilar cholangiocarcinoma and gall bladder cancer	Tumors of the proximal biliary tree often invade the adjacent hepatic parenchyma or vascular structures within the portahepatis and frequently require partial hepatectomy to achieve negative margins (13,14)
Wedge resections	Have a higher incidence of positive margins and greater blood loss than anatomical resections, and tend to be avoided (15)

Potential Benefits of Hepatic Resection

Hepatic resection can be employed for a number of underlying pathologies. These include benign or malignant primary tumors, secondary metastases, and liver trauma. Patients with untreated but potentially resectable hepatocellular carcinoma have been reported to have a median survival time of less than six months (16), with virtually no five-year survival (17). Surgical treatment prolongs the median survival to 42 months and five-year survival to 32% (18). A 38%, five-year survival can be seen following resection for metastases (19) compared to survival time ranging from 4.5 to 15 months without surgery (16).

Limitations

The aim of resection is to resect clear tumor margins while ensuring adequate remaining residual liver to prevent hepatic insufficiency. Margins of less than 1 cm may be adequate (20), but the relevance of clear resection is reflected in postoperative survival. For patients with tumor-free margins greater than 1 cm, a five-year survival rate of 60% can be expected. Survival rates fall to 30% for patients whose tumor margins are less than 1 cm, and no five-year survivors can be expected when the margins are involved by tumor (21).

Regeneration

The volume of liver that can be safely resected in humans is approximately 80%, assuming good function in the remaining liver, though there are reports of survival after resections of 90% (22). The potential for these massive resections (or extensive ablations) relies on postoperative hepatic regeneration, which has a complex mechanism. Under normal circumstances, the human liver initiates regeneration within three days and has reached its original size by six months (23), although some studies have shown full restoration within three months. Rapid regeneration may allow for complete functional recovery within two to three weeks. In most cases, liver function is restored to almost normal levels within two to three weeks after partial hepatectomy (24).

If there is a predicted risk of liver failure developing after a procedure, then preemptive maneuvers, such as portal embolization of the affected segments some weeks prior to resection, can stimulate regeneration in the proposed liver remnant prior to surgery, thereby enhancing postoperative liver function. An increase of 40% to 60% in the size of the nonembolized liver can be anticipated in noncirrhotic livers (25). Similarly, chemoembolization can be used in potentially unresectable hepatocellular carcinoma to reduce the tumor mass and increase the residual function to an extent that may permit definitive resection.

PREOPERATIVE ASSESSMENT

The majority of HPB surgery is undertaken in otherwise fit patients. Prolonged, preoperative workup for these patients is not required even for extensive resections and, where malignant disease is present, will lead to unacceptable delays in treatment. However, targeted blood tests, including coagulation screen, blood chemistry, and cardiorespiratory investigation, should be performed as indicated by existing guidelines.

Increasingly, more covert forms of liver disease may exist and are relevant to surgical outcome as there is reduced hepatic reserve and an increased susceptibility to hepatic ischemia-reperfusion injury. Steatohepatitis is the third commonest liver disease in the United States and has been estimated to be present in 20% of the U.S. population. The etiology may be secondary to alcohol intake or related primarily to diabetes and/or obesity in the form of nonalcoholic steatohepatitis. The latter is important because it carries a 30% risk of developing cirrhosis within 10 years. The elderly population have reduced liver size and blood flow, decreased drug metabolism (Phase I), and an increased incidence of alcohol-induced cirrhosis. The ultimate diagnosis of covert liver disease depends on histological diagnosis, although a high clinical index of suspicion is often present.

Where preexisting liver disease is present, increased perioperative risk depends on the nature and severity of the disease and the extent of hepatic dysfunction. This requires more specific assessment. Cirrhotics have an increased incidence of surgical intervention for multiple reasons, including variceal bleeding and increased hepatoma formation. Patients with cirrhosis have an insufficient hepatocyte function to meet the increased metabolic demands after partial hepatectomy (26), and have significantly reduced levels of hepatic regeneration after liver resection, making them extremely vulnerable to posthepatectomy liver failure. Regeneration is often defective and may not occur at all in severe disease; conversely, there may simply be a delay in full regeneration. Although chronic liver disease is not an absolute contraindication to resection, the morbidity and mortality increase dramatically with worsening hepatic dysfunction. Childs–Pugh class B or C generally excludes a patient from major resection. However, Childs–Pugh class A patients should be considered for surgery (27), and, in these patients, there is significant incentive toward optimizing preoperative medical care to improve postoperative prognosis. However, in terms of risk prediction for hepatic surgery, none of the preexisting systems relating liver disease severity to perioperative outcome is ideal (Table 2). The original Childs–Turcotte classification was used on patients undergoing portal decompression surgery but has never been validated in other forms of surgery. In contrast, the more recent Childs–Pugh scoring system has demonstrated an association with perioperative risk in patients undergoing esophageal transaction, nonshunt surgery, and abdominal surgery.

Because newer surgical procedures have evolved and the benefits of improved diagnostic facilities, including biochemical parameters, are absent from these predictive scoring systems, the applicability of these systems to newer HPB surgery risk prediction is uncertain. The most up-to-date risk prediction model suggests that renal impairment, bleeding, ascites, American Society of Anesthesiologists (ASA)

Table 2 Components of Liver Disease Severity Assessment as Described by Childs Classifications

Childs–Turcotte (1964)	Childs–Pugh score (1973)
Encephalopathy	Encephalopathy
Jaundice	Jaundice
Albumin	Albumin
Ascites	Ascites
Nutrition	Bleeding (PT time)

Abbreviation: PT, prothrombin time.

grade, histological diagnosis of cirrhosis, and intraoperative hypotension are the most important perioperative factors related to postoperative outcome (28).

Practically, it is perhaps easier to assess the relevance of each preoperative severity marker to an individual's potential risk. Nutritional status and albumin are important factors common to the postoperative recovery of all surgical patients and will not be discussed further.

The specific markers of liver disease severity include the following:

Jaundice

It is important to know if preoperative jaundice is present, because it may be associated with perioperative renal impairment (29,30). The mean incidence of post-operative renal impairment in surgical patients with jaundice is 8% but may be as high as 18%. The mortality for jaundiced patients who go on to develop acute renal failure is estimated at 65%, whereas the overall postoperative mortality rate in surgical patients with jaundice ranges from 0% to 27%. Thus, development of postoperative renal failure is a poor prognostic sign. The etiology of postoperative renal failure in the setting of liver disease is multifactorial and includes central volume depletion, defective renal vascular reactivity, vasoactive mediator imbalance (in which local prostaglandins play a prominent role), and the effect of endotoxin. The proposed deleterious effects of bile acids on renal tubules are thought to be an indirect effect rather than direct toxicity. This makes the renal vasculature intensely susceptible to renotoxic drugs, such as nonsteroidal antiinflammatory drugs (NSAIDs) and contrast media. Whatever the pathophysiological mechanism, the major relevance to anesthesia is the avoidance of hypovolemia. Preoperative measures to prevent the onset of renal impairment have included adequate preoperative hydration, mannitol infusion, bile salts, and lactulose. However, none have demonstrated consistent benefit in adequate clinical trials.

Coagulopathy

Correction of coagulation prior to liver resection is essential where central neuraxial blockade is being considered. Vitamin K, fresh frozen plasma (FFP), or cryoprecipitate may be required preoperatively to correct liver-related coagulopathy. Reduction in platelet counts in these patients is common, but abnormalities in platelet function are often more relevant. Therefore, the preoperative administration of platelets is better guided by laboratory testing (e.g., thromboelastogram) results than by clinical judgment.

Ascites

The development of ascites is a poor prognostic sign in cirrhosis and may adversely influence perioperative respiratory mechanics. Furthermore, ascites, secondary to splanchnic arteriolar vasodilatation, develops at the expense of circulating intra-vascular fluid. In conjunction with medical therapy, including inducing diuresis and paracentesis, there is a real risk of significant intravascular hypovolemia. Attempts should be made to correct this state preoperatively, and it is important to recognize that perioperative fluid limitation does not prevent the development of postoperative ascites.

Encephalopathy

Subclinical hepatic encephalopathy is present in 30% to 70% of cirrhotics and can be detected by subtle psychometric testing. More severe chronic encephalopathy is precipitated by certain drugs, bleeding, sepsis, and surgical stress. Elective hepatic surgery should be deferred until the cause of preoperative encephalopathy is ascertained and effective treatment is provided. Preoperative lactulose may prevent encephalopathy worsening but treatment of the cause (e.g., infection or hemorrhage) is more important. This is particularly relevant wherever postoperative encephalopathy develops de novo, because it is often difficult to distinguish between encephalopathy and drug intoxication. Drug-induced intoxication has a much better prognosis than spontaneous encephalopathy. The use of opioids or benzodiazepines may lead to intoxication, due to increased brain sensitivity, and should be avoided as premedication.

INTRAOPERATIVE CONSIDERATIONS

All but the most minor HPB procedures are performed under general anesthesia with endotracheal intubation and mechanical ventilation. Usual precautionary measures apply for airway protection, while anesthetic maintenance is achieved with newer volatile agents. Nitrous oxide is usually omitted from the inhalational gases, due to its adverse effect on bowel distension. Rapid acting intravenous opiates (e.g., remifentanil, alfentanil) are used for intraoperative analgesia, either in isolation or in combination with neuraxial blockade. On-table extubation is standard in our institution even after extensive resections, and, therefore, measures to enhance recovery (including maintenance of temperature, use of rapidly metabolized anesthetic agents, and adequate reversal of muscle relaxation) are routinely used.

The extent of intraoperative monitoring is dependent on the preoperative state of the patient and the severity of the proposed procedure, including blood loss. Invasive arterial monitoring is used for repeated blood sampling or where rapid changes in hemodynamic status are likely (i.e., during portal vein clamping). Central venous access may be used for both drug access and the control of central venous pressure (CVP) related to blood conservation (see below). Wherever low-CVP techniques are being used, we have found a noninvasive monitor (e.g., esophageal Doppler) to be a useful adjunct to optimize fluid replacement while preventing overt hypovolemia. "Point of contact" blood testing is extremely useful in HPB surgery and allows the rapid recognition of anemia, coagulation deficiencies, metabolic abnormalities, and respiratory dysfunction. The thromboelastogram is particularly relevant and allows targeted correction of coagulation problems. It has also been shown to reduce transfusion requirements during HPB operations.

Surgical procedures and manipulations govern many of the intraoperative anesthetic considerations. However, basic principles can be applied during major hepatic procedures.

Maintaining Hepatic Blood Flow

Hepatosplanchnic blood flow may be altered at three different levels (31).

Systemic

Reduction in hepatosplanchnic blood flow may be demonstrated in globally reduced cardiac output states with redistribution toward vital organs and with more regional changes in vascular resistance of other vascular beds. More importantly for intra-operative anesthetic care, hepatic blood flow may be significantly reduced wherever CVP rises above portal venous critical closing pressure (approximately 3–5 mmHg). Avoidance of an excessive rise in CVP is also important in blood conservation strategies but must be taken in the context of the risks associated with intravascular volume depletion.

Regional

Regional hepatosplanchnic blood flow is altered by hormonal, metabolic, and neurological factors. A major influence on regional hepatic flow during operative procedures is the effect of surgical stress and regional analgesia on the autonomic nerve components of the hepatosplanchnic area. However, some degree of regional auto-regulation of the hepatic blood flow occurs via the hepatic "arterial buffer" response (32,33). Wherever portal flow is reduced, hepatic artery flow is increased to maintain liver blood flow. The mechanism of this response is incompletely understood but is related to hepatic adenosine washout (34). Unfortunately, this blood flow compensatory arrangement is not reciprocal, in that the portal vein does not have any such mechanism to increase hepatic blood flow. Therefore, whenever hepatic arterial pressure falls, there is a reciprocal decrease in liver blood flow. The buffer response is maintained even in severe cirrhosis (35,36). Volatile agents suppress the hepatic artery buffer response to a varying extent, but isoflurane and desflurane are thought to maintain the response better than halothane. Pneumoperitoneum also ablates the buffer response in an experimental setting (37). In most situations, oxygen delivery is surplus to demand, and minor reduction in blood flow is inconsequential. However, in some circumstances (e.g., sepsis and reduced liver reserve, including fatty liver), oxygen dependency may apply and increased demand has to be met by increased oxygen extraction.

Microcirculation

Microcirculatory vascular changes are controlled by multiple hormonal influences, including nitric oxide, endothelins, and carbon monoxide production, which derive predominantly from the hepatic vascular endothelial cells. It has been suggested that a critical balance between vasoconstrictor and vasodilatator substances must exist to maintain a balanced flow at the microcirculatory level. In experimental studies, all volatile agents cause microcirculatory vasoconstriction and, thereby, have the potential to reduce flow. Various agents have been used to promote specific hepatosplanchnic vasodilatation, including dopexamine, prostacyclin, and ET-1 receptor antagonists. However, none of these agents has a proven clinical role in hepatosplanchnic protection. Indeed, action on single mediator pathways is unlikely to cause a beneficial change to microcirculatory flow: it has been suggested that the goal of hepatosplanchnic protection is to attempt for reestablishment of a new vasoactive balance, rather than act upon specific pathways.

Protection of Existing Hepatocellular Function

Glutathione is an important intracellular antioxidant required for hepatocyte function, and cellular stores are often reduced in hepatic disease. N-Acetyl cysteine (NAC) is an exogenous source of glutathione, which may be useful in maintaining existing hepatocellular function as well as protecting against reperfusion injury.

Localized infection in the form of cholangitis may also lead to liver dysfunction, and intraoperative prophylactic antibiotics are important. Excess administration of starch-based colloids may deleteriously reduce Kupffer cell activity, thereby increasing susceptibility to infection (38). Where liver reserve is severely reduced, exogenous provision of coagulation factors (e.g., FFP) may be required.

Reducing Intraoperative Hepatic Injury

In simplest terms, intraoperative hepatic damage may be minimized by resecting the smallest proportion of liver mass required to treat the condition, as discussed previously, while reducing injury to the remaining liver tissue, especially where cirrhosis is an issue. This will enable good postoperative function and the potential for postoperative hepatic regeneration.

Damage to remaining liver tissue is predominantly related to the reduction of tissue injury, secondary to ischemia-reperfusion. Ischemic preconditioning is the process whereby deliberate induction of short-duration ischemia, in anticipation of longer ischemic periods, protects against subsequent hepatic damage (39–42). The mechanism of preconditioning is under much debate, but, intraoperatively, it is practically performed by hepatic artery and portal vein clamping prior to resection (41,43). Some anesthetic agents, including isoflurane, may have pharmacological preconditioning effects (44–46). In contrast, prolonged, sustained liver ischemia will ultimately lead to liver cell death, whereas short periods of ischemia may protect against subsequent liver injury. A normal liver is able to withstand prolonged periods (i.e., up to 60 to 90 minutes) of ischemia. However, even where hepatocyte death does not occur, reperfusion injury is a major cause of subsequent hepatic injury during liver surgery (47). This is caused by multiple interrelated mechanisms, although the release of short-lived oxygen free radicals at reperfusion is the catalyst for a profound inflammatory cytokine response that may impact on distant organs as well as promote local hepatic injury. Free-radical scavengers (e.g., NAC) have been suggested as possible therapeutic options to prevent reperfusion injury, but there is limited clinical evidence to support their use.

Intraoperative Blood Conservation/Management

Significant perioperative blood loss is a potential immediate complication of surgery, and excessive loss is associated with increased perioperative morbidity (48). Where colorectal metastases are involved, it may lead to a shorter disease-free interval (49). Refining anesthetic and surgical techniques to reduce blood loss is, therefore, paramount.

Surgical Techniques

The intraoperative control of blood loss has been facilitated by improved surgical dissection techniques. The Cavitron ultrasonic aspirator is an acoustic vibrator, producing a saline-induced cavitational force to promote liver parenchymal disruption, which is then combined with diathermy. It is very effective in reducing blood loss in hepatic resection (19,50–52). Water jet dissection and ultrasonic cutting have also been used (53,54). The larger vessels are left intact by these techniques and can be individually tied or stapled. Control of residual bleeding of the resected liver surface may be achieved by use of argon beam coagulation (55) or the spray application of fibrin glue (56).

The most important surgical influence on blood conservation has been the isolation of hepatic vascular supply during resection (57). Temporary total inflow occlusion (the Pringle maneuver) isolates inflow at the hepatic pedicle, whereas total vascular exclusion incorporates isolation of suprahepatic subdiaphragmatic and infrahepatic vena cava alongside pedicle clamping. Isolation of liver blood flow may lead to potentially deleterious effects on the normal liver, secondary to prolonged hepatic ischemia; although, occlusion times of up to 60 minutes are considered safe in noncirrhotic livers, postoperative hepatic insufficiency and encephalopathy may occur with shorter durations (58,59). In cirrhotic livers, 30 minutes (and possibly up to 60 minutes) is considered safe in early disease (60,61). Intermittent clamping of 10 to 20 minutes, with 5 minutes declamping may be safer, where more prolonged ischemia is required (62,63). Total vascular exclusion reduces bleeding but carries with it significant pre- and postoperative morbidity (up to 50%) and mortality (up to 10%) (57,59,64). The technique should probably be restricted to cases where tumor is near or involving the retrohepatic vena cava or at the confluence of hepatic veins and vena cava. Approximately, 10% of patients will not tolerate the hemodynamic effects of vena-caval occlusion and may require veno-venous bypass.

Anesthetic Techniques

Reduction of Central Venous Pressure. The reduction of CVP during hepatic resection may dramatically reduce intraoperative blood loss by reducing hepatic venous congestion (65–67). Because restriction of fluid replacement until the resection is completed is a common feature of this technique (68), there is the potential to promote intraoperative hypovolemia and confer susceptibility to reduced renal and hepatosplanchnic blood flow. The concomitant use of vasoconstrictors to maintain any minor reductions in systemic arterial pressure may have a synergistic deleterious effect on gut perfusion in hypovolemia, and may confer susceptibility to postoperative organ failure. However, in most reported series where a low CVP technique has been used, there does not seem to be an increased incidence of acute renal failure or organ failure. Another possible complication of low CVP techniques is air embolus (69). In one series (70), suspected small air emboli were reported in a total of 4 out of 150 patients, with one patient having more marked hemodynamic changes associated with a larger embolus. Diligence in monitoring sudden changes in end-tidal CO_2 and in cauterizing open hepatic vessels is vital, while a combination of epidural anesthesia and intravenous nitroglycerine for vasodilation has been described to achieve a CVP of less than 5 cmH_2O (70).

Control of Coagulopathy. The coagulopathy associated with liver disease can contribute significantly to the potential for perioperative bleeding. The liver is the site of production of all coagulation factors (except von Willebrands factor) and also many coagulation inhibitors, fibrinolytic proteins, and their inhibitors. It is responsible for the breakdown of many of the activated factors of coagulation and fibrinolysis. In addition, platelet abnormalities and thrombocytopenia, secondary to cirrhosis and hypersplenism, are common in liver disease. Hence, it is clear how a complete range of coagulation abnormalities from hypocoagulability and accelerated fibrinolysis, through to diffuse intravascular coagulopathy (DIC) and hypercoagulable states associated with low protein C and S levels can be encountered in liver disease. The complex clotting abnormalities of liver disease are succinctly reviewed by Kang (71). Preoperative assessment of coagulation is a mandatory part of the work-up for major hepatic resection. However, the complex interactions of the numerous aspects of coagulation make interpretation of the simple quantification of each of the factors difficult. Thromboelastography, first used clinically in liver transplant in 1966 (72), provides an on-site method for assessing coagulability of whole blood, including coagulation and fibrinolysis. It provides clinically useful information within 30 minutes of taking a sample, and with the newer multichannel machines, it provides an excellent real-time guide to treating coagulopathy in major hepatic resections and transplantation.

The natural choice for correcting coagulopathy in liver disease is FFP because it contains all the coagulation and inhibitory factors. However, its effects are relatively short lived, and it has the disadvantages of a large volume load and potential cross infection concerns. Cryoprecipitate is a good source of fibrinogen and tends to be administered for documented hypofibrinogenemia. Platelets transfused during major resections will often have only a transient effect, as they are removed rapidly by the spleen and in liver transplantation by the implanted liver. Intraoperatively, platelets are transfused on clinical grounds or when guided by the thromboelastogram. The antifibrinolytic agents, aprotinin and tranexamic acid, have been shown to be effective in reducing transfusion requirement in liver transplantation (73,74) and can be used in hepatic surgery with anticipated high blood loss. Newer agents, such as activated factor VII, have been used to good effect in liver failure with active hemorrhage (75–77). Whenever citrate levels are potentially increased (large citrated blood product transfusions, deficient citrate metabolism due to hepatre dysfunction), it is important to maintain adequate levels of serum calcium to prevent further exacerbation of existing coagulopathy.

Avoidance of Hypothermia. Even mild hypothermia can lead to increased blood loss (78). While platelet numbers remain unchanged, hypothermia impairs platelet function (79). It is worth remembering that because laboratory tests of coagulation are performed at 37°C, these remain normal, unless adjusted to patient temperature (80). Major liver resections are often prolonged, large volumes of fluids are given, and the open abdomen provides an efficient heat sink. Invasive temperature monitoring (esophageal or rectal) and scrupulous attention to active warming of the patient and all infusions must be undertaken pre- and postoperatively.

Autotransfusion. In spite of best efforts to reduce bleeding, transfusion is often necessary during hepatectomy. Autotransfusion, either as preoperative donation or from using cell-saver apparatus, is a safe and effective method for replacing blood loss (81), and it has been used extensively in nonmalignant diseases (82). Because of concern regarding contamination with malignant cells from either method, surgeons were reluctant to use these techniques in patients with tumors. It has been shown that autotransfusion is not responsible for recurrence when a cell-saver apparatus is used in patients with hepatocellular carcinoma (81,82). The practice employed in our hospital is still to wait until the segmental blood supply to the tumor-affected area has been isolated prior to commencing cell-saver collection.

Maintaining Renal Function

Renal dysfunction in patients undergoing hepatic surgery is multifactorial in origin. As discussed previously, the presence of bilirubin salts leading to jaundice may cause renal dysfunction by multiple causes, including changes in vasoconstrictive-vasodilator balance and increasing susceptibility to renotoxic drugs. Prostaglandin inhibitors (e.g., NSAIDs) may reduce renal blood flow and glomerular filtration rate (GFR), and are particularly relevant to patients having hepatic surgery (83) because there may often be a reluctance to prescribe paracetamol as an adjunctive analgesic agent.

In fact, there is no convincing evidence to suggest that therapeutic doses of paraceta-mol are deleterious, even in patients with severe cirrhosis (excepting alcoholics) (84), and are to be preferred over NSAIDs wherever mild analgesia is required following hepatic surgery. Intraoperative measures, including dopamine, mannitol, and loop diuretic therapy, attempting to protect the renal vasculature have been used in HPB surgery, but none have been demonstrated to improve postoperative renal func-tion in prospective clinical trials. In fact some reports have documented a detrimental effect of some therapeutic measures (e.g., dopamine administration).

Use of Nonhepatic Metabolized Drugs

Many anesthetic drugs do not require liver function for adequate metabolism. Because the incidence of covert hepatic disease is increasing, the use of these anes-thetic drugs seems reasonable during hepatic surgery. Atracurium or cisatracurium would seem to be the most obvious first choice nondepolarizing muscle relaxant in patients likely to have disordered liver function, as they are metabolized by esters and excreted through renal system. Remifentanil is a good choice for intraoperative analgesia, because its metabolism is independent of hepatic function and is easily titrated. However, wherever it is used, consideration of postoperative analgesia must be addressed.

Hemodynamic Manipulation

Fluid management is important, and in our institution the use of colloids in prefer-ence to crystalloid is universal. Wherever low CVP practices are used in an attempt to reduce blood loss, there may be requirement for supplementary vasoconstrictors to maintain systemic blood pressure for perfusion of other organs. Vasoconstrictors used including phenylephrine, vasopressin, or noradrenaline may lead to splanch-nic vasoconstriction and secondary hepatic ischemia. Therefore, a complex balance must be maintained between what is considered adequate mean arterial pressure and controlled hypovolemia.

POSTOPERATIVE CARE

Potential immediate postoperative problems specific to patients undergoing major hepatic resection include significant third space fluid shift, ongoing coagulopathy and active bleeding, onset or exacerbation of liver failure with encephalopathy, renal impairment, and biliary leak. Postoperative care in the first 12 to 24 hours should be in a critical care setting with the facility for continuation of invasive hemodynamic monitoring and close observation of renal function. The risks and benefits of any mode of analgesia need to be weighed up for each individual in deciding the best treatment of postoperative pain. Because this group of patients is at risk of renal impairment and coagulation defects, nonsteroidal anti-inflammatory agents should be avoided wherever possible. Hepatically metabolized and renally excreted opiates have the potential disadvantage of accumulation with cerebral depressant effects in a population with a tendency toward encephalopathy. Use of epidural techniques is probably the preferred postoperative analgesic option, given the proposed benefits on postoperative recovery after major surgery and use of large surgical incisions. Each unit or individual must make their own choice on the best option to employ.

In the event of acute liver failure arising after liver resection, attempts should be made to support the patient in hope of buying sufficient time for regeneration of the remaining liver. The main stay of this is ensuring optimal standards of intensive care management, including airway control, adequate hydration, inotropic and renal support as needed, control of coagulopathy and active bleeding, oral gut decontamination, enteral nutrition (low protein diets are no longer considered appropriate in this catabolic state), and consideration of NAC infusion. The use of NAC has been shown to be of benefit when given early and also beyond the first 24 hours in acetaminophen overdose, where it may reduce the incidence of cerebral complications and mortality (85,86). Beneficial effects have also been seen in systemic and cerebral hemodynamics in acute liver failure of other causes, an effect not related to stimulation of liver regeneration or hepato-protection but initially assigned to improvements in systemic oxygen delivery and extraction (87,88). A later study (89) refuted the effects of NAC on oxygen delivery and extraction in hepatic failure, suggesting instead that the microcirculatory effects also seen when NAC is used in sepsis may be more important. Further large-scale trials are probably indicated of this extended use of NAC in non–acetaminophen-induced liver failure.

In addition, a number of specific therapeutic strategies have been investigated. The systems used, other than transplant, can be divided into bioartificial or dialysis methods (including plasmapheresis). Bioartificial systems include extracorporeal liver perfusion (90) and hybrid systems incorporating porcine or human hepatocytes (91). Albumin dialysis incorporated with standard dialysis or hemofiltration, as in the molecular adsorbent recirculation system (MARS) system, has been advocated for removal of water-soluble and albumin bound toxins in acute and acute-on-chronic liver failure. While improvement in biochemical and some clinical features of acute liver failure may be seen with these systems, proof of effect on mortality is still lacking. In a recent systematic review (92) of 528 references on liver support systems, only 2 were randomized controlled trials. Overall, support systems did not appear to have an effect on mortality compared with standard care in cases of acute liver failure.

REFERENCES

1. Van Thiel DH, Wright HI, Fagiuoli S, Caraceni P, Rodriguez-Rilo H. Preoperative evaluation of a patient for hepatic surgery. J Surg Oncol Suppl 1993; 3:49–51.
2. Rossi S, Di Stasi M, Buscarini E, et al. Percutaneous RF interstitial thermal ablation in the treatment of hepatic cancer. AJR Am J Roentgenol 1996; 167:759–768.
3. Ravikumar TS, Kane R, Cady B, Jenkins R, Clouse M, Steele G Jr. A 5-year study of cryosurgery in the treatment of liver tumors. Arch Surg 1991; 126:1520–1523.
4. Adam R, Akpinar E, Johann M, Kunstlinger F, Majno P, Bismuth H. Place of cryosurgery in the treatment of malignant liver tumors. Ann Surg 1997; 225:39–38.
5. Rosado B, Kamath PS. Transjugular intrahepatic portosystemic shunts: an update. Liver Transpl 2003; 9:207–217.
6. Madoff DC, Wallace MJ, Ahrar K, Saxon RR. TIPS-related hepatic encephalopathy: management options with novel endovascular techniques. Radiographics 2004; 24: 21–36.
7. Couinand C. Le fois-etudes anatomiques et chirurgicales. Paris: Masson, 1957.
8. Jarnagin WR, Bodniewicz J, Dougherty E, Conlon K, Blumgart LH, Fong Y. A prospective analysis of staging laparoscopy in patients with primary and secondary hepatobiliary malignancies. J Gastrointest Surg 2000; 4:34–43.

9. Machi J, Isomoto H, Kurohiji T, et al. Accuracy of intraoperative ultrasonography in diagnosing liver metastasis from colorectal cancer: evaluation with postoperative follow-up results. World J Surg 1991; 15:551–556.

10. Makuuchi M, Takayama T, Kosuge T, et al. The value of ultrasonography for hepatic surgery. Hepatogastroenterology 1991; 38:64–70.

11. Parker GA, Lawrence W Jr., Horsley JS III, et al. Intraoperative ultrasound of the liver affects operative decision making. Ann Surg 1989; 209:569–576.

12. Bismuth H, Dennison AR. Segmental liver resection. Adv Surg 1993; 26:189–208.

13. Bismuth H, Nakache R, Diamond T. Management strategies in resection for hilar cholangiocarcinoma. Ann Surg 1992; 215:31–38.

14. Burke EC, Jarnagin WR, Hochwald SN, Pisters PW, Fong Y, Blumgart LH. Hilar cholangiocarcinoma: patterns of spread, the importance of hepatic resection for curative operation, and a presurgical clinical staging system. Ann Surg 1998; 228:385–394.

15. DeMatteo RP, Palese C, Jarnagin WR, Sun RL, Blumgart LH, Fong Y. Anatomic segmental hepatic resection is superior to wedge resection as an oncologic operation for colorectal liver metastases. J Gastrointest Surg 2000; 4:178–184.

16. Savage AP, Malt RA. Survival after hepatic resection for malignant tumours. Br J Surg 1992; 79:1095–1101.

17. Tsao JI, Loftus JP, Nagorney DM, Adson MA, Ilstrup DM. Trends in morbidity and mortality of hepatic resection for malignancy. A matched comparative analysis. Ann Surg 1994; 220:199–205.

18. Zibari GB, Riche A, Zizzi HC, et al. Surgical and nonsurgical management of primary and metastatic liver tumors. Am Surg 1998; 64:211–220.

19. Scheele J, Stang R, Altendorf-Hofmann A, Paul M. Resection of colorectal liver metastases. World J Surg 1995; 19:59–71.

20. Ochiai T, Takayama T, Inoue K, et al. Hepatic resection with and without surgical margins for hepatocellular carcinoma in patients with impaired liver function. Hepatogastroenterology 1999; 46:1885–1889.

21. Cady B, Jenkins RL, Steele GD Jr., et al. Surgical margin in hepatic resection for colorectal metastasis: a critical and improvable determinant of outcome. Ann Surg 1998; 227:566–571.

22. Starzl TE, Putnam CW, Groth CG, Corman JL, Taubman J. Alopecia, ascites, and incomplete regeneration after 85 to 90 per cent liver resection. Am J Surg 1975; 129:587–590.

23. Gove CD, Hughes RD. Liver regeneration in relationship to acute liver failure. Gut 1991; suppl:S92–S96.

24. Nagasue N, Yukaya H, Ogawa Y, Kohno H, Nakamura T. Human liver regeneration after major hepatic resection. A study of normal liver and livers with chronic hepatitis and cirrhosis. Ann Surg 1987; 206:30–39.

25. Kawasaki S, Makuuchi M, Kakazu T, et al. Resection for multiple metastatic liver tumors after portal embolization. Surgery 1994; 115:674–677.

26. Ozawa K. Hepatic function and liver resection. J Gastroenterol Hepatol 1990; 5:296–309.

27. Capussotti L, Polastri R. Operative risks of major hepatic resections. Hepatogastroenterology 1998; 45:184–190.

28. Ziser A, Plevak DJ, Wiesner RH, Rakela J, Offord KP, Brown DL. Morbidity and mortality in cirrhotic patients undergoing anesthesia and surgery. Anesthesiology 1999; 90:42–53.

29. Green J, Better OS. Systemic hypotension and renal failure in obstructive jaundice-mechanistic and therapeutic aspects. J Am Soc Nephrol 1995; 5:1853–1871.

30. Fogarty BJ, Parks RW, Rowlands BJ, Diamond T. Renal dysfunction in obstructive jaundice. Br J Surg 1995; 82:877–884.

31. Pannen BH. New insights into the regulation of hepatic blood flow after ischemia and reperfusion. Anesth Analg 2002; 94:1448–1457.

32. Lautt WW. Mechanism and role of intrinsic regulation of hepatic arterial blood flow: hepatic arterial buffer response. Am J Physiol 1985; 249:G549–G556.

33. Lautt WW. Relationship between hepatic blood flow and overall metabolism: the hepatic arterial buffer response. Fed Proc 1983; 42:1662–1666.
34. Lautt WW, McQuaker JE. Maintenance of hepatic arterial blood flow during hemorrhage is mediated by adenosine. Can J Physiol Pharmacol 1989; 67:1023–1028.
35. Gulberg V, Haag K, Rossle M, Gerbes AL. Hepatic arterial buffer response in patients with advanced cirrhosis. Hepatology 2002; 35:630–634.
36. Richter S, Mucke I, Menger MD, Vollmar B. Impact of intrinsic blood flow regulation in cirrhosis: maintenance of hepatic arterial buffer response. Am J Physiol Gastrointest Liver Physiol 2000; 279:G454–G462.
37. Richter S, Olinger A, Hildebrandt U, Menger MD, Vollmar B. Loss of physiologic hepatic blood flow control ("hepatic arterial buffer response") during CO_2-pneumoperitoneum in the rat. Anesth Analg 2001; 93:872–877.
38. Christidis C, Mal F, Ramos J, et al. Worsening of hepatic dysfunction as a consequence of repeated hydroxyethyl starch infusions. J Hepatol 2001; 35:726–732.
39. Banga NR, Homer-Vanniasinkam S, Graham A, Al Mukhtar A, White SA, Prasad KR. Ischaemic preconditioning in transplantation and major resection of the liver. Br J Surg 2005; 92:528–538.
40. Clavien PA, Selzner M, Rudiger HA, et al. A prospective randomized study in 100 consecutive patients undergoing major liver resection with versus without ischemic preconditioning. Ann Surg 2003; 238:843–850.
41. Koti RS, Seifalian AM, Davidson BR. Protection of the liver by ischemic preconditioning: a review of mechanisms and clinical applications. Dig Surg 2003; 20:383–396.
42. Serafin A, Fernandez-Zabalegui L, Prats N, Wu ZY, Rosello-Catafau J, Peralta C. Ischemic preconditioning: tolerance to hepatic ischemia-reperfusion injury. Histol Histopathol 2004; 19:281–289.
43. Abdalla EK, Noun R, Belghiti J. Hepatic vascular occlusion: which technique? Surg Clin North Am 2004; 84:563–585.
44. Kehl F, Krolikowski JG, Mraovic B, Pagel PS, Warltier DC, Kersten JR. Is isoflurane-induced preconditioning dose related? Anesthesiology 2002; 96:675–680.
45. Hawaleshka A, Jacobsohn E. Ischaemic preconditioning: mechanisms and potential clinical applications. Can J Anaesth 1998; 45:670–682.
46. Cason BA, Gamperl AK, Slocum RE, Hickey RF. Anesthetic-induced preconditioning: previous administration of isoflurane decreases myocardial infarct size in rabbits. Anesthesiology 1997; 87:1182–1190.
47. Serracino-Inglott F, Habib NA, Mathie RT. Hepatic ischemia-reperfusion injury. Am J Surg 2001; 181:160–166.
48. Ekberg H, Tranberg KG, Andersson R, Jeppsson B, Bengmark S. Major liver resection: perioperative course and management. Surgery 1986; 100:1–8.
49. Stephenson KR, Steinberg SM, Hughes KS, Vetto JT, Sugarbaker PH, Chang AE. Perioperative blood transfusions are associated with decreased time to recurrence and decreased survival after resection of colorectal liver metastases. Ann Surg 1988; 208:679–687.
50. Hanna SS, Nam R, Leonhardt C. Liver resection by ultrasonic dissection and intraoperative ultrasonography. HPB Surg 1996; 9:121–128.
51. Fasulo F, Giori A, Fissi S, Bozzetti F, Doci R, Gennari L. Cavitron Ultrasonic Surgical Aspirator (CUSA) in liver resection. Int Surg 1992; 77:64–66.
52. Storck BH, Rutgers EJ, Gortzak E, Zoetmulder FA. The impact of the CUSA ultrasonic dissection device on major liver resections. Neth J Surg 1991; 43:99–101.
53. Baer HU, Stain SC, Guastella T, Maddern GJ, Blumgart LH. Hepatic resection using a water jet dissector. HPB Surg 1993; 6:189–196.
54. Rau HG, Schardey HM, Buttler E, Reuter C, Cohnert TU, Schildberg FW. A comparison of different techniques for liver resection: blunt dissection, ultrasonic aspirator and jet-cutter. Eur J Surg Oncol 1995; 21:183–187.
55. Postema RR, Plaisier PW, ten Kate FJ, Terpstra OT. Haemostasis after partial hepatectomy using argon beam coagulation. Br J Surg 1993; 80:1563–1565.

56. Kohno H, Nagasue N, Chang YC, Taniura H, Yamanoi A, Nakamura T. Comparison of topical hemostatic agents in elective hepatic resection: a clinical prospective randomized trial. World J Surg 1992; 16:966–969.
57. Emond JC, Kelley SD, Heffron TG, Nakagawa T, Roberts JP, Lim RC Jr. Surgical and anesthetic management of patients undergoing major hepatectomy using total vascular exclusion. Liver Transpl Surg 1996; 2:91–98.
58. Bismuth H, Castaing D, Garden OJ. Major hepatic resection under total vascular exclusion. Ann Surg 1989; 210:13–19.
59. Delva E, Camus Y, Nordlinger B, et al. Vascular occlusions for liver resections. Operative management and tolerance to hepatic ischemia: 142 cases. Ann Surg 1989; 209:211–218.
60. Nagasue N, Yukaya H, Ogawa Y, Hirose S, Okita M. Segmental and subsegmental resections of the cirrhotic liver under hepatic inflow and outflow occlusion. Br J Surg 1985; 72:565–568.
61. Nagasue N, Uchida M, Kubota H, Hayashi T, Kohno H, Nakamura T. Cirrhotic livers can tolerate 30 minutes ischaemia at normal environmental temperature. Eur J Surg 1995; 161:181–186.
62. Man K, Fan ST, Ng IO, et al. Tolerance of the liver to intermittent Pringle maneuver in hepatectomy for liver tumors. Arch Surg 1999; 134:533–539.
63. Cunningham JD, Fong Y, Shriver C, Melendez J, Marx WL, Blumgart LH. One hundred consecutive hepatic resections. Blood loss, transfusion, and operative technique. Arch Surg 1994; 129:1050–1056.
64. Habib N, Zografos G, Dalla SG, Greco L, Bean A. Liver resection with total vascular exclusion for malignant tumours. Br J Surg 1994; 81:1181–1184.
65. Jones RM, Moulton CE, Hardy KJ. Central venous pressure and its effect on blood loss during liver resection. Br J Surg 1998; 85:1058–1060.
66. Matsumata T, Itasaka H, Shirabe K, Shimada M, Yanaga K, Sugimachi K. Strategies for reducing blood transfusions in hepatic resection. HPB Surg 1994; 8:1–6.
67. Chen H, Merchant NB, Didolkar MS. Hepatic resection using intermittent vascular inflow occlusion and low central venous pressure anesthesia improves morbidity and mortality. J Gastrointest Surg 2000; 4:162–167.
68. Melendez JA, Arslan V, Fischer ME, et al. Perioperative outcomes of major hepatic resections under low central venous pressure anesthesia: blood loss, blood transfusion, and the risk of postoperative renal dysfunction. J Am Coll Surg 1998; 187:620–625.
69. Hatano Y, Murakawa M, Segawa H, Nishida Y, Mori K. Venous air embolism during hepatic resection. Anesthesiology 1990; 73:1282–1285.
70. Rees M, Plant G, Wells J, Bygrave S. One hundred and fifty hepatic resections: evolution of technique towards bloodless surgery. Br J Surg 1996; 83:1526–1529.
71. Kang Y. Coagulopathies in hepatic disease. Liver Transpl 2000; 6:S72–S75.
72. Von Kaulla KN, Kaye H, von Kaulla E, Marchioro TL, Starzl TE. Changes in blood coagulation. Arch Surg 1966; 92:71–79.
73. Findlay JY, Rettke SR, Ereth MH, Plevak DJ, Krom RA, Kufner RP. Aprotinin reduces red blood cell transfusion in orthotopic liver transplantation: a prospective, randomized, double-blind study. Liver Transpl 2001; 7:802–807.
74. Boylan JF, Klinck JR, Sandler AN, et al. Tranexamic acid reduces blood loss, transfusion requirements, and coagulation factor use in primary orthotopic liver transplantation. Anesthesiology 1996; 85:1043–1048.
75. Chuansumrit A, Chantarojanasiri T, Isarangkura P, Teeraratkul S, Hongeng S, Hathirat P. Recombinant activated factor VII in children with acute bleeding resulting from liver failure and disseminated intravascular coagulation. Blood Coagul Fibrinol 2000; 11(suppl 1):S101–S105.
76. White B, McHale J, Ravi N, et al. Successful use of recombinant FVIIa (Novoseven) in the management of intractable post-surgical intra-abdominal haemorrhage. Br J Haematol 1999; 107:677–678.

77. Bernstein DE, Jeffers L, Erhardtsen E, et al. Recombinant factor VIIa corrects prothrombin time in cirrhotic patients: a preliminary study. Gastroenterology 1997; 113:1930–1937.
78. Schmied H, Kurz A, Sessler DI, Kozek S, Reiter A. Mild hypothermia increases blood loss and transfusion requirements during total hip arthroplasty. Lancet 1996; 347: 289–292.
79. Valeri CR, Feingold H, Cassidy G, Ragno G, Khuri S, Altschule MD. Hypothermia-induced reversible platelet dysfunction. Ann Surg 1987; 205:175–181.
80. Bunker JP, Goldstein R. Coagulation during hypothermia in man. Proc Soc Exp Biol Med 1958; 97:199–202.
81. Fujimoto J, Okamoto E, Yamanaka N, et al. Efficacy of autotransfusion in hepatectomy for hepatocellular carcinoma. Arch Surg 1993; 128:1065–1069.
82. Zulim RA, Rocco M, Goodnight JE Jr., Smith GJ, Krag DN, Schneider PD. Intraoperative autotransfusion in hepatic resection for malignancy. Is it safe? Arch Surg 1993; 128:206–211.
83. Perazella MA. COX-2 selective inhibitors: analysis of the renal effects. Exp Opin Drug Saf 2002; 1:53–64.
84. Lauterburg BH. Analgesics and glutathione. Am J Ther 2002; 9:225–233.
85. Keays R, Harrison PM, Wendon JA, et al. Intravenous acetylcysteine in paracetamol induced fulminant hepatic failure: a prospective controlled trial. BMJ 1991; 303: 1026–1029.
86. Makin AJ, Wendon J, Williams R. A 7-year experience of severe acetaminophen-induced hepatotoxicity [1987–1993]. Gastroenterology 1995; 109:1907–1916.
87. Harrison PM, Wendon JA, Gimson AE, Alexander GJ, Williams R. Improvement by acetylcysteine of hemodynamics and oxygen transport in fulminant hepatic failure. N Engl J Med 1991; 324:1852–1857.
88. Wendon JA, Harrison PM, Keays R, Williams R. Cerebral blood flow and metabolism in fulminant liver failure. Hepatology 1994; 19:1407–1413.
89. Walsh TS, Hopton P, Philips BJ, Mackenzie SJ, Lee A. The effect of N-acetylcysteine on oxygen transport and uptake in patients with fulminant hepatic failure. Hepatology 1998; 27:1332–1340.
90. Horslen SP, Hammel JM, Fristoe LW, et al. Extracorporeal liver perfusion using human and pig livers for acute liver failure. Transplantation 2000; 70:1472–1478.
91. Busse B, Smith MD, Gerlach JC. Treatment of acute liver failure: hybrid liver support. A critical overview. Langenbecks Arch Surg 1999; 384:588–599.
92. Kjaergard LL, Liu J, Als-Nielsen B, Gluud C. Artificial and bioartificial support systems for acute and acute-on-chronic liver failure: a systematic review. JAMA 2003; 289: 217–222.

16
Anesthesia for Pancreatic Surgery

Iain Jones and Andrew Berrill
*Department of Anesthesia, St. James's University Hospital,
Leeds, U.K.*

ANATOMY

The pancreas is a tapered organ from 12 to 15 cm in length. It lies in the upper abdomen, posteriorly to the stomach and duodenum. The gland is divided into four parts. These are the head, neck, body, and tail. The pancreas is widest at the head, which lies within the curve of the duodenum. The body of the pancreas tapers upward to terminate at the tail, located in relationship to the spleen. The uncinate process projects to the left from its lowest portion. The pancreas derives its blood supply from the superior pancreaticoduodenal artery (arising from the gastroduodenal artery) and from the inferior pancreaticoduodenal artery (arising from the inferior mesenteric artery). There is also a contribution from the splenic artery. Venous drainage passes to the portal venous system.

FUNCTIONS

Two predominant tissue types constitute the pancreas. These are exocrine tissue, which is involved in the production and secretion of digestive enzymes, and endocrine tissue (islets of Langerhans), responsible for the secretion of hormones into the circulation.

Patients presenting for pancreatic surgery represent a major challenge to the anesthetist, both because of the anatomical complexity of the surgery and because of potential derangement of pancreatic function. There are several indications for surgery, including exocrine tumors (often adenocarcinoma), endocrine tumors, acute pancreatitis, and pancreatic drainage.

GENERAL CONSIDERATIONS

All patients presenting for pancreatic surgery require large-bore intravenous access and intubation and controlled ventilation. Consideration should be given to the use of invasive monitoring. Appropriate arrangements should be made for postoperative pain relief, and consideration should be given to the requirement for postoperative high-dependency care.

EXOCRINE TUMORS

Pancreatic cancer is the fourth most common type of cancer death in the United States and the sixth in the United Kingdom. The peak incidence is in the 65-to-75-year age group. Many patients present with advanced disease, which results in low resection rates. Late presentation is responsible in part for the median survival of less than six months, and five-year survival rate of 0.4% to 5%. Between 2.6% and 9% of patients undergo pancreatic resection with a median survival of 11 to 20 months, and a five-year survival rate of 7% to 25%.

Pancreatic ductal adenocarcinoma is the most common epithelial exocrine pancreatic tumor, and accounts for more than 85% of all malignant pancreatic tumors. About 80% to 90% of tumors are located within the head of the gland. The most common sites for metastases are liver and peritoneum. The most common extraperitoneal site for metastases is the lung.

Diagnosis and Investigation

In most patients, the diagnosis is fairly straightforward (painless obstructive jaundice and weight loss, with back pain). Other associated conditions, such as late onset diabetes mellitus or an unexplained attack of acute pancreatitis, may point to an underlying cancer. Clinical features, such as persistent back pain, marked and rapid weight loss, abdominal mass, ascites, and supraclavicular lymph nodes, are often indicative of an unresectable tumor (1).

Initial investigation involves abdominal ultrasound, which may detect the primary pancreatic tumor, extrahepatic bile duct dilatation, or liver metastases. Endo-luminal ultrasonography and magnetic resonance cholangiopancreatography are now replacing endoscopic retrograde cholangiopancreatography (ERCP). Both techniques are used to visualize ampullary tumors directly. Biopsy is easier with ERCP. Other pancreatic tumors are detectable by ERCP only if they impinge on the pancreatic duct, so small early cancers or those in the uncinate process can be missed. Contrast-enhanced computed tomography (CT) remains the investigation of choice for clinical staging; it accurately predicts resectability in 80% to 90% of patients, although it is less accurate at predicting the resectability of small pancreatic tumors. Factors contraindicating resection include liver, peritoneal or other metastases, distant lymph node metastasis, and major venous encasement. Enlargement of lymph nodes alone is a poor indicator of metastatic disease. Factors that do not necessarily contraindicate resection include local invasion (if the duodenum, stomach, colon, or lymph nodes lie within the operative field); venous impingement or minimal invasion of the superior mesenteric vein, splenic vein, or hepatic vein trifurcation; gastroduodenal artery encasement; or age of the patient. Magnetic resonance imaging (MRI) has similar diagnostic and staging accuracy to CT, but may be superior in the detection of liver metastasis.

Laparoscopy, including laparoscopic ultrasonography, can detect occult metastatic lesions in the liver and peritoneal cavity not detected by other imaging modalities in 10% to 35% of patients, but the place of laparoscopy remains controversial.

ANESTHESIA FOR PANCREATIC CARCINOMA

Pancreatic resection can now be performed with considerable safety and a low rate of pancreatic complications. Patients presenting for resection of pancreatic carcinomas often suffer multiple comorbidities and have reduced physiological reserve to deal with a significant surgical insult. Patients may have poor nutritional status as a consequence of an insidious disease course.

Detailed preoperative evaluation is mandatory, with particular attention to cardiorespiratory status. Patients with jaundice are prone to fatigue, and accurate assessment of exercise tolerance may be difficult. Coagulation may be deranged, therefore, preoperative coagulation screening is recommended (1).

Access to the operative site is usually via a bilateral subcostal incision. Maintenance of anesthesia with either volatile agents or total intravenous anesthesia is appropriate. The authors maintain anesthesia using a volatile agent in conjunction with a continuous epidural infusion.

FLUID THERAPY AND INOTROPES

Fluid therapy is aimed at correction of preoperative fluid losses from fasting and bowel preparation, perioperative fluid losses from bleeding, insensible and "third-space" tissue losses. Additionally, fluids are administered for "standard" maintenance requirements. Markers of adequate fluid resuscitation include central venous pressure (CVP) and response to a fluid challenge and urine output. Pulmonary artery wedge pressure provides similar information regarding fluid status as the CVP; however, insertion of a pulmonary artery catheter is known to be associated with significant complications, and routine use is not recommended unless there is a specific clinical indication (2).

Perioperative hypotension is common as a result of the combined effects of preoperative fluid depletion and general and epidural anesthesia. The judicious use of vasopressors, such as ephedrine and phenylephrine, is often required. The routine use of inotropes, such as dopamine and dopexamine, has been advocated by some to improve outcome by increasing hepatosplanchnic blood flow and optimizing global oxygen delivery. Thus the blind use of "prophylactic" dopamine is inadvisable on present evidence (3), though "guided" goal-directed therapy is likely to have a major place (Chapter 8).

ROLE OF SOMATOSTATIN ANALOGUES IN PANCREATIC SURGERY

The value of somatostatin analogues in the prevention and treatment of pancreatic fistulae and other complications following pancreatoduodenectomy is not established. Of six randomized placebo-controlled trials from Europe, five showed a benefit in reducing overall complications. However, three studies from the United States did not show benefit from the use of somatostatin analogues. Differences in study design may account for the different outcomes, although the current balance of evidence tends to favor the use of octreotide for this indication. Octreotide is first administered intraoperatively, and is continued postoperatively (1).

POSTOPERATIVE ANALGESIA

Thoracic epidural analgesia (TEA) with an epidural sited in the mid-thoracic region provides excellent pain relief (Chapter 25). Alternatively, a patient-controlled analgesia (PCA) system with opioids may be used. With TEA, a combination of local anesthetic and opioid provides the best analgesia on movement and less hypotension than with local anesthetic alone, and halves the duration of ileus compared with epidural opioid alone or PCA. Our combination of choice is 0.15% bupivacaine with fentanyl $2\,\mu g/mL$ at a variable rate of 8 to $15\,mL/hr$. A continuous infusion is associated with sensory block regression, particularly with local anesthetic alone. Patient-controlled epidural analgesia, usually with a background infusion, allows patient self-titration and sparing of local anesthetic consumption (4).

In patients with well-preserved renal function, a balanced postoperative pain regimen may also include a nonsteroidal anti-inflammatory drug (e.g., diclofenac as "rescue" analgesia), and regular paracetamol (acetaminophen).

POSTOPERATIVE CARE

Postoperatively, patients are initially managed in a high-dependency facility capable of performing invasive monitoring and regular observations. Step-down to ward-based care may occur after several days and depends on clinical status and recovery on an individual basis.

COMPLICATIONS

Intra-abdominal Abscess

Intra-abdominal abscess following pancreatic resection occurs in 1% to 12% of patients. The usual cause is an anastomotic leak, and is often heralded by a right subhepatic or left subdiaphragmatic collection. Contrast-enhanced CT is indicated when an intra-abdominal leak is suspected. The preferred management of intra-abdominal collections is CT-guided percutaneous drainage.

Hemorrhage

Postoperative hemorrhage occurs in 2% to 15% of patients after pancreatic resection. Bleeding within the first 24 hours is usually due to insufficient intraoperative hemostasis or bleeding from an anastomosis. Free intraperitoneal hemorrhage requires immediate reoperation, but the management of anastomotic bleeding is initially conservative. Stress ulceration is rare and can usually be managed medically or endoscopically. Secondary hemorrhage (1–3 weeks after surgery) often has a more sinister underlying cause. It is commonly related to an anastomotic leak, secondary erosion of the retroperitoneal vasculature, or a pseudoaneurysm with a mortality rate of 15% to 58%. Treatment options include angiography and embolization if a bleeding point can be identified. However bleeding from a pancreaticojejunostomy is particularly problematic, and a complete pancreatectomy or refashioning of the anastomosis may be necessary.

Fistula After Pancreaticoduodenectomy

The reported incidence of pancreatic fistula ranges from 2% to 24%. The mortality risk from a major pancreatic fistula may be as high as 28%, principally due to retroperitoneal sepsis or hemorrhage.

Delayed Gastric Emptying

The incidence of delayed gastric emptying ranges from 14% to 70% after pancreatic resection, although the definition has not been standardized. The incidence may be reduced by using intravenous erythromycin. Delayed gastric emptying almost always resolves with conservative treatment; however, surgical correction is occasionally required. Some studies have suggested that a pylorus-preserving operation increases the risk of delayed gastric emptying, but two large randomized studies comparing pylorus preservation with the standard operation did not show any significant differences. Many series have shown that delayed gastric emptying is related to the presence of intra-abdominal complications, particularly pancreatic leak, and also to extended surgery.

SURVIVAL AFTER RESECTION

Current perioperative mortality in high-volume centers varies from 1% to 4%. Intraoperative blood loss, preoperative serum bilirubin level, diameter of the main pancreatic duct, and occurrence of complications are independent prognostic factors. Many postoperative complications can be effectively managed by medical treatment or radiological and/or endoscopic intervention. Complications requiring reoperation are associated with a mortality rate of between 23% and 67% (5,6).

Patients who undergo resection for nonmetastatic disease have a five-year survival of 7% to 25%, with a median survival of 11 to 20 months. Patients with irresectable locally advanced, nonmetastatic disease have a median survival of 6 to 11 months, and those with metastatic disease have a median survival of two to six months. The majority of patients develop disease recurrence within two years after resection. Liver metastases frequently develop early, suggesting the presence of micrometastases at the time of surgery, whereas local recurrences tend to appear later (1,5,6).

PALLIATION OF ADVANCED PANCREATIC CANCER

Many patients with pancreatic cancer present with advanced disease not amenable to resection. The major symptom requiring intervention is obstructive jaundice. A number of studies have compared operative bypass procedures with biliary stenting, and have shown that complications such as cholangitis and bile leak are more common with bypass procedures, whereas recurrent jaundice is a feature of stenting because of stent occlusion or migration. No significant difference has been found in median survival or procedure-related deaths between operative bypass and biliary stenting. Self-expanding metal stents have greatly reduced the risk of obstruction and acute cholangitis. Nevertheless, surgical bypass may be advantageous for the patient with locally advanced disease because it may maximize complication-free time to be spent at home without hospital readmission for recurrent jaundice.

SPECIALIST CENTERS AND THE "VOLUME-OUTCOME" RELATIONSHIP

The development of high-volume specialist centers is thought to be a major reason for the reduction in perioperative mortality over the past decade. The evidence base supporting surgery in specialist units has grown substantially and now clearly shows a reduced mortality. There is less postoperative morbidity, reduced postoperative length of hospital stay, an increased resection rate, and improved long-term survival (1).

ENDOCRINE TUMORS

Neuroendocrine tumors of the pancreas are uncommon, with an estimated incidence of between 6 and 10 per million population per year. The pancreatic Islets of Langerhans cells are part of the amine precursor uptake and decarboxylation (APUD) system. Thus islet-cell tumors are known collectively as APUDomas. Pancreatic islets may produce hormones that are not normally present in the pancreas, such as gastrin, adrenocorticotropin (ACTH), vasoactive intestinal polypeptide, and growth hormone–releasing hormone. Neuroendocrine cells are also found in the proximal portion of the duodenum and the antrum of the stomach, where they produce gastrin and somatostatin.

Although many pancreatic islet-cell tumors are multihormonal, one peptide generally predominates and is responsible for the clinical syndrome. Approximately 10% to 20% of islet-cell tumors arise in association with multiple endocrine neoplasia type 1 (MEN-1).

MEN-1 is inherited as an autosomal dominant trait and is characterized by tumors of multiple endocrine organs, including pancreas, pituitary, and parathyroid. In patients with MEN-1, islet-cell tumors are always multifocal, occurring in the pancreas, duodenum, or both. Gastrinoma is the most common functional tumor in these patients. The presence of MEN-1 should be excluded by testing for other components of the syndrome, which include primary hypoparathyroidism, other endocrine pancreatic tumors, pituitary tumors, lipomas, and carcinoid tumors of the gut. Careful history taking, including family history, examination for lipomas, and measurement of serum calcium, prolactin, pancreatic polypeptide, and gastrin, is indicated (7,8).

Insulinomas

Insulinomas are the most common pancreatic islet tumor, with an incidence of approximately three to six per million populations per year. The mean age of patients with insulinoma is 45, but it can occur at any age, and younger in MEN-1 patients. They are generally small solitary benign tumors located within the pancreas. Fewer than 10% are malignant. Malignant tumors are relatively indolent, and cure is possible in a large number of cases. Even in nonresectable disease, debulking may provide effective palliation, and debulking alone has been shown to improve survival. Liver resection in patients with metastatic disease can also improve survival. Hepatic resection and transplantation have been described in metastatic disease. Patients with insulinoma have symptoms caused by hypoglycemia. Presenting symptoms include seizures, difficulty awakening, visual disturbances, confusion, lethargy, and weakness. Hypoglycemia also causes catecholamine release leading to sweating, anxiety, and palpitations. Symptoms tend to occur early in the morning after an overnight fast or during exercise.

Medical Treatment

Diazoxide controls hypoglycemia effectively in around 60% of patients. It may cause prolonged hypotension during anesthesia and should be discontinued at least one week before surgery. However, it may not block secretion from abnormal (i.e., non-B) cells, and can also suppress glucagon secretion, thus exacerbating symptoms. Other dose-dependant side effects include sodium retention, hypotension, cardiac disturbance, and weight gain. Numerous other drugs have been used to assist in insulinoma management with limited success, including calcium channel blockers, beta-blockers, and phenytoin. Octreotide, a somatostatin analogue, has unpredictable effectiveness in suppressing insulin release from insulinomas, probably because only 50% of insulinomas express somatostatin receptors.

Surgical Treatment

The operation required may vary from distal pancreatectomy to enucleation. If the tumor transgresses the major pancreatic duct, pancreaticoduodenectomy may be required. The spleen is preserved whenever possible, but splenectomy may be unavoidable. Planning for this should include vaccination against meningococcus and hemophilus influenzae. Prophylactic therapies include antibiotics and possibly somatostatin.

Close monitoring of glucose intake and blood glucose is started the evening before surgery and continued throughout the perioperative period. During this period of starvation and at operation when the tumor is handled, glucose 50% solution should be available. Intravenous glucose and potassium should be infused, and blood glucose, electrolytes, and fluid input and output monitored at least hourly to avoid hypoglycemia, fluid overload, and hyponatremia. On excision of the tumor, a progressive increase in blood glucose has been described within minutes. Maintenance of normoglycemia is more important than the observation of rebound hyperglycemia (7–9).

There has been some interest in the choice of anesthetic agents, and their effects on blood glucose. Methoxyflurane has been used historically because of its tendency to increase blood glucose. More recently, sevoflurane has been recommended because it appears to suppress the spontaneous release of insulin. Isoflurane also has a favorable metabolic profile if liver blood flow or function is disturbed. Intravenous anesthesia with propofol and epidural anesthesia are reported not to interfere with blood glucose control (7). Postoperative complications, which may alter blood glucose homeostasis, include diabetes mellitus (as a result of pancreatic insufficiency), acute pancreatitis, and intra-abdominal abscesses. Pancreatic fistula is a serious complication because it can lead to electrolyte imbalance and the need for further surgery. Over 90% of patients have "successful" surgery with complete correction of hypoglycemia. Furthermore, because as much pancreas as possible is preserved, there is a low prevalence of diabetes mellitus postoperatively (~2%). Complications of the excision are primarily those associated with uncontrolled pancreatic drainage, which include abscess, fistula, pseudocyst, and wound infection.

Surgery may also be indicated in patients with islet-cell tumors and life threatening symptoms, such as gastrointestinal hemorrhage, bile, or intestinal obstruction. In these instances, the tumor may be resected or bypassed to relieve symptoms (7–9).

Gastrinoma

In the initial description of the Zollinger–Ellison syndrome in 1955, Zollinger and Ellison included a triad of clinical findings: peptic ulceration of the jejunum, gastric acid hypersecretion, and an islet-cell tumor of the pancreas. Around one to three persons per million develop gastrinoma each year. Approximately 20% of those with gastrinoma have MEN-1. Sporadic Zollinger–Ellison syndrome occurs most commonly in the fifth decade of life. Most patients complain of epigastric pain and indigestion. Perforated peptic ulcer occurs in approximately 10%; conversely, 10% of patients never have any signs or symptoms of peptic ulcer disease. Diarrhea and steatorrhea leading to weight loss often occur as a result of excessive acid production, which inactivates pancreatic enzymes. Presentation with esophagitis occurs less commonly. Gastrinomas are malignant and may be extrapancreatic. Eighty percent arise within the "gastrinoma triangle," which includes both the head of the pancreas and the duodenum. Liver metastases are a survival-limiting feature: patients without liver metastases rarely die from the tumor; those with liver metastases have a 10-year survival of 30%.

Preparation for surgery requires dose titration of proton pump inhibitors, such as omeprazole or lansoprazole, to achieve normal basal acid secretion. Anemia can occur from bleeding gastric ulceration. A full coagulation screen and liver function tests are required because alterations in fat absorption may influence vitamin K–dependant clotting factor production. Liver function may be further disturbed by intrahepatic disease. Intravenous ranitidine is useful both immediately before and after surgery to prevent gastric acid hypersecretion. The goal of surgery is complete resection of gastrinoma; cure may be achieved in patients with both localized and metastatic disease. An upper abdominal incision is made, and adequate exposure of the entire abdomen is indicated because extrapancreatic primary gastrinomas have been identified within the ovary, mesentery, liver, and stomach. Overall surgery produces disease-free survival in approximately 60% of patients. Fifty percent of patients will experience a recurrence, with a long-term cure rate of 30%.

Glucagonoma

Glucagonoma is a malignant tumor that usually presents in the fifth or sixth decade of life. Patients have a characteristic raised red itchy rash called necrolytic migratory erythema. The rash is typically seen on the lower extremities. It is initially erythematous and scaly, but can progress to sloughing bullous lesions. Patients also have hypoaminoacidemia, weight loss, type 2 diabetes mellitus, severe muscle wasting, and a high probability of deep venous thrombosis and pulmonary embolism. Ketoacidosis is rare because insulin release is increased. The cachexia is often so severe that patients require nutritional support, and may require total parenteral nutrition to correct protein and trace element deficiencies for several weeks before surgery, otherwise infection and poor wound healing may occur. Anemia is also common, possibly as a result of bone marrow suppression.

Glucagonomas are usually located within the pancreas and are often metastatic and unresectable at the time of diagnosis; the majority of patients have liver metastases at presentation. Treatment is by debulking. Somatostatin analogues give rapid relief at first, but increasing doses may be required later.

Vasoactive Intestinal Peptide Tumor

The vasoactive intestinal peptide tumor (VIPOMA) syndrome is also called the pancreatic cholera syndrome, the Verner–Morrison syndrome, or the watery diarrhea, hypokalemia, and achlorhydria syndrome. VIPOMAs produce severe secretory diarrhea that causes hypokalemia, hypochlorhydria, hypovolemia, and dehydration.

Patients with this condition can produce 5 to 10 L of stool per day. The diarrhea will persist even when oral intake is restricted. These patients can also complain of abdominal cramping, weakness, and flushing. The weakness is caused by hypokalemia and dehydration. They may also have hypercalcemia. Most VIPOMAs arise within the pancreas but extrapancreatic tumors have been described. The dehydration and fluid abnormalities are severe, and it is necessary to correct these before surgery. Octreotide dramatically reduces the secretory diarrhea, making presurgical correction relatively straightforward. A response normally occurs in 24 to 48 hours. If octreotide fails, other treatment options include steroids, such as methylprednisolone, indomethacin (prostaglandin inhibitor), or metoclopramide. Preoperatively, they require treatment with an H_2-receptor antagonist to prevent rebound gastric acid hypersecretion. The coexistence of VIPOMA and gastrinoma in MEN-1 should be excluded by preoperative investigations and tumor localization. Vasoactive intestinal peptide (VIP) relaxes smooth muscle and dilates splanchnic and peripheral vascular beds; it can induce hypotension from this mechanism, as well as fluid losses from circulating blood volume. Death has resulted from delayed diagnosis rather than from the tumor itself. Resuscitation in a critical care environment is often required. Fluid resuscitation should be guided by central venous monitoring. Electrolyte disturbances (such as potassium and magnesium deficiency) and acidosis require correction. As 60% of VIPOMAs are malignant, albeit slow growing, and often copresent with liver metastasis, surgical resection is indicated (Table 1).

Somatostatinoma

Somatostatinomas are very rare tumors of pancreatic islet δ cells. The tumors are often large at presentation, with signs of biliary obstruction. When jaundice is present, stenting may be required before surgery to reduce coagulopathy and postoperative renal failure.

Nonfunctioning Islet-Cell Tumors

Nonfunctioning islet-cell tumors of pancreatic polypeptide-producing tumors do not have a clinical syndrome related to excessive hormone secretion. They are usually malignant and large at the time of diagnosis, and produce symptoms secondary to their mass effects, such as extrahepatic bile duct obstruction, intestinal bleeding secondary to invasion of a major vessel within the gut, or intestinal obstruction.

Table 1 The Features of Vasoactive Intestinal Peptide Tumors and Their Main Causes

Features	Cause
Diarrhea	VIP stimulated
Hypokalemia	Passive K^+ loss, active secretion by colon, secondary to hyperaldosteronism
Hypochlorhydria	Inhibition of gastric mucosal function
Metabolic acidosis	Excess bicarbonate loss
Flushing	VIP vasodilatation
Hyperglycemia	VIP glycogenolysis (structurally similar to glucagon)
Hypercalcemia (tetany)	Hyperparathyroidism, acidosis
Hypomagnesemia (tetany)	Loss in stool

Abbreviation: VIP, vasoactive intestinal peptide.
Source: From Ref. 7.

Patients may also have hepatic metastasis. Diabetes may occur due to suppression of insulin release, and these tumors can present in conjunction with phaeochromocytoma and von Recklinghausen's disease in the MEN-2 syndrome.

Rare islet-cell tumors can produce a variety of unusual hormones, including growth hormone releasing factor, ACTH, parathyroid hormone-related peptide, neurotensin, and serotonin. Carcinoid tumors can also be localized to the pancreas. ACTH-producing islet-cell tumors may be controlled by drugs, such as ketoconazole and aminoglutethimide. However, medical control of hypercortisolism is usually inadequate, and these patients often require bilateral adrenalectomy if complete resection of the ACTH-releasing tumor is impossible. Serotonin-producing islet-cell tumors require octreotide as a premedication at the time of surgical resection to prevent the occurrence of carcinoid crisis (Chapter 18) (7,8,10).

Medical Management

Evidence relating to managing the complex problems associated with endocrine tumors is limited mainly to retrospective reviews and case reports. Whenever possible, patients should be treated in specialist centers, with local experience in endocrine surgery.

Medical therapy can be used to control the signs and symptoms of excessive hormonal secretion. In this respect, somatostatin analogues (such as octreotide), which inhibit hormone release, have revolutionized anesthetic management. Octreotide is given parenterally as 100 μg every eight hours or 100 μg/hr during surgery. In an emergency, 50 μg/hr as an intravenous bolus before surgical manipulation can be given where no preoperative prophylaxis has been used (7).

Anesthesia

The most common procedures for pancreatic endocrine tumors are pancreatoduodenectomy, distal pancreatectomy, and enucleation, and may include resection of metastasis. Surgical assessment should have defined the type of endocrine dysfunction and the site of tumor, and predicted the surgical intervention and the need for prophylactic immunization before splenectomy. Preparation for anesthesia involves correction of fluid and electrolyte abnormalities and hypovolemia. Blood loss during surgery depends on metastatic involvement of hepatic and portal vessels, preexisting coagulation abnormalities, the presence of portal hypotension, and oozing from raw surface areas. Average blood loss is often around 2 L. Adequate provision for monitoring, cross-matched blood, and suitable postoperative care should be available (7,8).

Multidisciplinary care from surgeons, endocrinologists, anesthetists, radiologists, and pathologists necessitates an agreed management plan in a tertiary referral center because of the rare and varied nature of the disorders. Surgery is the only approach, which can achieve a definitive cure. The role of the anesthetist in preoperative preparation, maintenance of perioperative hemostasis, and postoperative high-dependency or intensive care is important in securing a favorable outcome (7).

SURGERY FOR ACUTE PANCREATITIS

Acute pancreatitis represents a spectrum of disease, ranging from a mild self-limiting course, requiring only brief hospitalization, to a rapidly progressive fulminant disease, resulting in multiorgan dysfunction syndrome, with or without accompanying sepsis. Only a minority of patients with pancreatitis have disease severe enough to require admission to an intensive care unit (ICU). These patients have mortality rates in the range of 30% to 50% and a mean hospital stay of more than one month, attesting to the severity of severe pancreatitis. An accepted definition of severe acute pancreatitis (SAP) is that it is associated with complications that are either local (e.g., peripancreatic fluid collection, necrosis, abscess, and pseudocyst) or systemic (e.g., organ dysfunction).

There are several incontrovertible indications for operative intervention in patients with SAP: suspected or confirmed intra-abdominal catastrophe, including intestinal infarction or perforation, severe hemorrhage, or abdominal compartment syndrome. In acute pancreatitis, the extensive inflammatory process in the retroperitoneum leads to the development of peripancreatic fluid collections and pancreatic necrosis. Routine operative or percutaneous drainage of the former is not necessary because it may infect otherwise sterile tissues. Necrosis develops in approximately 10% to 20% of patients with acute pancreatitis and in a significantly greater proportion of those with severe clinical disease. The presence of tissue necrosis further exacerbates or impairs the resolution of the systemic inflammatory response. Necrotic tissue may also become seeded with enteric organisms, resulting in infected pancreatic necrosis. Necrosis in the context of severe disease mandates repeated assessment of the need for operative debridement of the pancreas and peripancreatic tissues. Later in the disease, the necrotic pancreas demarcates from viable tissue, leading to an easier and safer debridement with a greater likelihood of sparing pancreatic tissue. Over time, the area of necrosis undergoes liquefaction, resulting in a pancreatic abscess that might be more amenable to percutaneous rather than operative drainage. Thus the optimal intervention depends on the clinical course and the precise timing of the proposed intervention.

SAP represents an example of a sterile inflammatory process leading to organ dysfunction. The clinical picture is often one of systemic inflammatory response syndrome (SIRS), and can be indistinguishable from severe sepsis. The potential for development of infected pancreatic necrosis and/or extrapancreatic sites of infection further complicates management of these patients. Several case series describe the course of patients with SAP and sterile pancreatic necrosis treated without debridement. Patients without evidence of pancreatic infection can be managed without operation, with low mortality and morbidity rates, even in the presence of organ dysfunction. Clinical deterioration is not necessarily an indication for operative debridement. The significant risk of iatrogenic bowel injury, hemorrhage, and risk of infecting sterile pancreatic necrosis should be considered before proceeding with operative debridement of sterile necrosis.

Several large case series suggest that the diagnosis of infected pancreatic necrosis warrants consideration of a single or series of interventions designed to achieve pancreatic debridement and/or drainage. Percutaneous drainage may be the only intervention necessary, if the necrosis has demarcated and liquefied. Several case series suggest that necrotomy should be delayed to facilitate this, suggesting a reduction in the relative risk of death of 37% to 69% associated with "late" necrotomy (two to three weeks after presentation). There are as yet no randomized trials to confirm these observations.

Access to the peritoneum via laparotomy represents the conventional operative approach. There are recent reports of selected relatively stable patients undergoing laparoscopic debridement in conjunction with percutaneous drainage. Percutaneous drainage with or without percutaneous debridement might also offer advantages by minimizing the morbidity of laparotomy or temporizing, until the retroperitoneal process has sufficiently demarcated such that operative management is simpler.

Ultrasound or CT-guided fine needle aspirate (FNA) with Gram stain and culture of pancreatic or peripancreatic tissue is used to discriminate between sterile and infected necrosis in patients, with radiological evidence of pancreatic necrosis and clinical features consistent with infection. Debridement or drainage is not recommended in patients with sterile necrosis. For patients with infected pancreatic radiologically or FNA-confirmed necrosis, debridement is recommended. Clinical criteria and judgment determine the timing of intervention (11).

SAP patients suffer the SIRS and may progress to multiorgan dysfunction. The majority come to the operating theater from a critical care unit.

The Role of the Anesthetist

The role of the anesthetist is to continue supportive strategies instituted in critical care to limit SIRS and organ damage.

Fluid Resuscitation

There is no evidence to support one type of fluid over another. Fluid challenges in patients with suspected hypovolemia may be given at a rate of 500 to 1000 mL of crystalloid or 300 to 500 mL of colloid over 30 minutes and repeated based on response (increase in blood pressure and urine output) and tolerance (evidence of intravascular volume overload). Large volumes of fluid may be required. Fluid challenge requires close monitoring to evaluate the response and avoid overload, resulting in tissue and pulmonary edema. The degree of intravascular fluid deficit in patients with SIRS varies with venodilatation and ongoing capillary leak.

Vasopressors

When an appropriate fluid challenge fails to restore adequate blood pressure and organ perfusion, therapy with vasopressor agents should be considered. Norepinephrine and dopamine have both been recommended as the first choice vasopressor to correct hypotension in septic shock. There is no high-quality evidence to recommend one catecholamine over another. Animal and human studies suggest some advantages of norepinephrine and dopamine over epinephrine (potential tachycardia and a possible disadvantageous effect on splanchnic circulation) and phenylephrine (decrease in stroke volume). Norepinephrine is more potent than dopamine and may be more effective at reversing hypotension in patients with septic shock. Dopamine may be particularly useful in patients with compromised systolic function, but may cause more tachycardia and be more arrhythmogenic.

Vasopressin use may be considered in patients with refractory shock, despite adequate fluid resuscitation and high-dose conventional vasopressors.

Blood Product Administration

The optimum hemoglobin for patients with severe sepsis has not been specifically investigated; however, the transfusion requirements in critical care trial suggest that hemoglobin of 7.0 to 9.0 g/dL is adequate for most critically ill patients. A transfusion threshold of 7.0 g/dL was not associated with increased mortality. Red blood cell transfusion in critically ill patients increases oxygen delivery but does not usually increase oxygen consumption. In theater, blood should be cross-matched, available, and transfused depending on ongoing losses.

Fresh frozen plasma is recommended for coagulopathy when there is a documented deficiency of coagulation factors and the presence of active bleeding, or prior to surgical or invasive procedures.

Platelet counts of more than $50,000/mm^3$ are typically required for surgery or invasive procedures.

Mechanical Ventilation

High tidal volumes and inflation pressures should be avoided in acute lung injury/acute respiratory distress syndrome (ALI/ARDS), and probably in other patients at risk of developing these conditions. An initial tidal volume of 6 mL/kg of lean weight, in conjunction with end-inspiratory plateau pressures <30 cmH$_2$O, are commonly accepted. Hypercapnia can be tolerated in patients with ALI/ARDS if required to minimize plateau pressures and tidal volumes.

A minimum amount of positive end expiratory pressure should be set to prevent lung collapse at end expiration. Similar strategies should be employed in the operating theater as in the ICU.

Glucose Control

Significant improvements in survival have been shown in postoperative surgical patients when continuous insulin infusion is used to maintain blood glucose between 4.4 and 6.1 mmol/L. Logically, tight glycemic control should be maintained intra- as well as postoperatively.

Correction of Acidosis

Patients with SAP often have a severe metabolic acidosis. Bicarbonate therapy for the purpose of improving hemodynamics or reducing vasopressor requirements is not recommended for hypoperfusion-induced lactic acidemia when the pH is more than 7.15 (12); this is because there is a risk of sodium accumulation and paradoxical intracellular acidosis, together with an unfavorable left shift of the oxygen–hemoglobin dissociation curve.

SURGERY FOR CHRONIC PANCREATIC CONDITIONS

Pancreatic pseudocysts may develop after acute or chronic pancreatitis, or after abdominal trauma. Patients may present with an abdominal mass, abdominal pain, or loss of appetite. Pleural effusion is a common coexisting finding. Rarely, patients may present with jaundice or sepsis due to an infected pseudocyst. Drainage procedures may be indicated to alleviate symptoms. Conventionally, this is achieved at open operation by anastomosis of the wall of the cyst to a neighboring viscus (stomach, duodenum, and jejunum). Interest is growing in the use of laparoscopic techniques for drainage procedures of the pancreas.

CONCLUSIONS

Surgery remains the treatment of choice for many pancreatic conditions, including most malignancies. This is high-risk, with relatively high associated morbidity and mortality. Anesthesia for pancreatic surgery presents real challenges to the anesthetist, and mandates a combined approach with the surgeon and intensivist to ensure best outcomes. Important features remain meticulous attention to detail, including volume status and metabolic and thermal requirements. Suitable provision needs to be made for the potential management of massive blood loss. Given these provisos, good short-to-mid-term outcomes are possible, and these allow better long-term outcomes within the limits imposed by the biology of the underlying disease.

REFERENCES

1. Alexis N, Halloran M, Raraty P, et al. Current standards of surgery for pancreatic cancer. Br J Surg 2004; 91:1419–1427.
2. Al-Khafajia A, Webb AR. Fluid resuscitation. Br J Anaesth CEPD 2004; 4:127–131.
3. Mackenzie SJ. Should perioperative management target oxygen delivery? Br J Anaesth 2003; 91:615–619.
4. Macleod G, Cumming C. Thoracic epidural anaesthesia and analgesia. Br J Anaesth CEPD 2004; 4:16–19.
5. Gouma DJ, van Geenen RC, van Gulik TM, et al. Rates of complications and death after pancreaticoduodenectomy: risk factors and the impact of hospital volume. Ann Surg 2000; 232(6):786–795.
6. Bottager TC, Junonger T. Factors influencing morbidity and mortality after pancreatico-duodenectomy, critical analysis of 221 resections. World J Surg 1999; 23:164–172.
7. Holdcroft A. Hormones and the gut. Br J Anaesth 2000; 85:56–68.
8. Norton JA, Le H. Insulinoma and other tumours. In: Morris PJ, Wood WC, eds. Oxford Textbook of Surgery. Vol. 2. 2d ed. Oxford, United Kingdom: Oxford University Press, 2001:1809–1819.
9. Bliss R, Carter P, Lennard W. Insulinoma: a review of current management. Surg Oncol 1997; 6:49–59.
10. Phan G, Yeo C, Hruban R, et al. Surgical experience with pancreatic and peripancreatic neuroendocrine tumours, review of 125 patients. J Gastrointest Surg 1998; 2:473–482.
11. Avery N, Randall C, Beale R. Management of the critically ill patient with severe acute pancreatitis. Crit Care Med 2004; 32:2524–2536.
12. Dellinger R, Carlet J, Masur H. Surviving sepsis campaign guidelines for management of severe sepsis and septic shock. Intensive Care Med 2004; 30:536–555.

17

Anesthesia for Laparoscopic Surgery

John C. Berridge
Department of Anesthetics, The General Infirmary at Leeds, Leeds, U.K.

INTRODUCTION

Laparoscopy is now a common minimally invasive technique in an increasing number of operations. This chapter will briefly outline the benefits of laparoscopic surgery to the patient, the pathophysiological effects of abdominal insufflation, the anesthetic management of laparoscopy, in general, and general surgical procedures, in particular. Postoperative pain management will be briefly outlined.

BENEFITS OF LAPAROSCOPIC SURGERY

Laparoscopic surgery has a number of benefits to the patient and some to the delivery of health care. It is associated with a shorter length of hospital stay, less postoperative pain, fewer pulmonary complications, and earlier return to normal activity. This is in part achieved by a reduced inflammatory response compared to open surgery, and a much reduced "trauma of access." The range of operations now performed laparoscopically is increasing both in type and in numbers of surgeons performing such operations. The common procedures in general surgery are listed in Table 1.

PHYSIOLOGICAL EFFECTS OF LAPAROSCOPIC SURGERY
Hemodynamic Effects of Abdominal Insufflation and Position

To perform laparoscopic surgery it is necessary to create a pneumoperitoneum by insufflating a gas, almost always carbon dioxide, into the abdominal cavity. The abdomen is filled with gas until the intra-abdominal pressure (IAP) is sufficient to allow space to perform the surgery. This is usually between 12 and 15 mmHg. Different levels of IAP have varying effects. The effect of the pneumoperitoneum on the cardiovascular system also depends on the position required for surgery and the extent to which artificial ventilation needs to be increased to achieve normocapnia. There are also a

Table 1 Common Laparoscopic Procedures

Cholecystectomy
Hernia repair
Appendicectomy
Hemicolectomy
Adrenalectomy
Bariatric surgery

number of patient-related factors that determine the size of any adverse cardiovascular events. These include morbid obesity, age, and cardiorespiratory comorbidity.

During laparoscopic cholecystectomy, the usual pressure achieved is 12 to 15 mmHg. The patient is also often positioned with a head-up tilt of up to 20°. This increased IAP and Trendelenburg position lead to a reduction in venous return with a fall in cardiac output and cardiac filling pressures (1). Blood pressure, however, is maintained or increases, because carbon dioxide in the peritoneum leads to an increase in sympathetic tone and elevated systemic vascular resistance (2). There is further evidence of reduced cardiac filling from echocardiographic studies that have shown a reduced left ventricular end-diastolic volume during laparoscopic cholecystectomy (3). One study comparing low-pressure insufflation with high-pressure insufflation showed interesting results (4). Where low-pressure insufflation of 7 mmHg was used there was, on average, a 10% increase in stroke volume with a 28% increase in cardiac output. At 15 mmHg, there was a fall in stroke volume of 26% and cardiac output of 28%. Both groups showed a rise in heart rate and mean arterial pressure. It is hypothesized that at low IAP there is little reduction in venous return but that the sympathetic stimulation from the intraperitoneal carbon dioxide leads to an increase in heart rate and stroke volume. As well as low pressure insufflation techniques, other procedures that prevent the adverse hemodynamic changes are lifting the abdominal wall (5) and using pneumatic venous compression devices to increase venous return (6). The hemodynamics changes are summarized in Table 2.

Regional Blood Flow

As well as global effects on hemodynamics, elevated IAP and carbon dioxide load have effects on blood flow to individual organs. The most obvious effect is on the intra-abdominal organs, with consistent findings of decreased portal vein, hepatic artery, and mesenteric artery flow (7). These effects can lead to subclinical hepatic dysfunction after cholecystectomy and colectomy (8).

Renal function is even more sensitive to the rise in IAP with consistent reductions in urine output, renal blood flow, and creatinine clearance (9,10). The primary cause of impaired renal function is the effect of raised IAP on reducing renal vein

Table 2 Hemodynamic Changes at Differing Intra-abdominal Pressures During Laparoscopic Cholecystectomy

Intra-abdominal pressure	Heart rate	Stroke volume	Cardiac output	Central venous pressure	Mean arterial pressure	Systemic vascular resistance
7	↑	↑	↑	Unknown	↑	↑
15	↑↑	↓↓	↓	↓	↑	↑

flow (11). There is further evidence of renal hypoperfusion, such as decreased urinary oxygen tension (12) and renal parenchymal hypoxia (13). Prolonged periods of high IAP may lead to impairment of both hepatic and renal function.

Laparoscopic surgery is sometimes performed in pregnancy. Animal studies suggest that a carbon dioxide pneumoperitoneum leads to a profound reduction in uterine blood flow with maternal and fetal acidosis (14). However, if the arterial partial pressure of carbon dioxide is kept within the normal range, this does not appear to occur (15).

It has yet to be determined whether elevating the cardiac output or using techniques that either prevent or reverse the adverse hemodynamics effects of elevated IAP can attenuate these potentially harmful effects.

Respiratory Effects

Laparoscopic surgery affects respiration in two main ways. First, there is the effect of the carbon dioxide load and the consequent need for an increase in alveolar ventilation to maintain normocapnia. Then, there are the changes in lung mechanics from the raised IAP and the patient position.

Carbon Dioxide Load

Carbon dioxide absorption is a consistent finding in laparoscopic surgery (16). The volume of carbon dioxide used varies according to the procedure, and is greatest in extraperitoneal procedures, such as nephrectomy and hernia repair (17,18). Absorption of carbon dioxide necessitates increased alveolar ventilation to maintain normocapnia. The extent of this is variable but is approximately 30% in cholecystectomy and 55% in hernia repair (19). Where there is extensive subcutaneous emphysema, the extra CO_2 load, and hence alveolar ventilation required to maintain "normocapnia," can be up to 400%. This translates to a minute volume of 30 L (20). Interestingly, a significant proportion of the carbon dioxide load is excreted after surgery when the patients are not mechanically ventilated. This is most pronounced in subjects who develop intraoperative subcutaneous emphysema (20). The effect of carbon dioxide absorption on ventilation implies that some patients with compromised respiratory function may be at risk for postoperative respiratory failure or require a period of ventilation until the carbon dioxide load is excreted.

Lung Mechanics

General anesthesia with mechanical ventilation is associated with characteristic changes in lung volumes, leading to impaired gas exchange (21). The main changes relate to reduced ventilation of the well-perfused basal areas, leading to an increase in intrapulmonary shunt. The relative increased ventilation of the upper regions leads to an increase in dead space. The combination of these effects is a reduction in functional residual capacity and total compliance of about 20%.

This results in a fall in arterial oxygen tension unless the inspired oxygen is increased. Laparoscopy with a pneumoperitoneum considerably worsens these effects (22,23). The changes with anesthesia and laparoscopy can be partly offset by applying positive end-expiratory pressure (PEEP) (24,25). Of course, the adverse hemodynamics effects of PEEP may compound the adverse hemodynamics effects of raised IAP.

Paradoxically, although the raised IAP with laparoscopy worsens intraoperative gas exchange, there is consistent evidence of better postoperative function.

The changes after surgery are much less, with vital capacity falling by about 21% in the first 24 hours after laparoscopic cholecystectomy, as compared with 50% following open surgery (26).

This improvement in lung mechanics is reflected in a lower incidence of postoperative lung infiltrates and atelectasis (26,27). This suggests that the postoperative advantages of the laparoscopic approach outweigh the disadvantages intraoperatively in patients with compromised pulmonary function.

Endocrine Changes

Laparoscopic surgery, although associated with less of an inflammatory response than open surgery, shows no difference in the hormonal stress response (28–30). There is a considerable stress response with inflation of the abdomen. Plasma catecholamines, cortisol, and antidiuretic hormone rise on inflation of the abdomen (31,32). Renin is released due to the changes in renal perfusion (33).

The extent to which circulating concentrations of these hormones rise in laparoscopy is related to the severity of the physiological insult. One study shows a relationship between the rise of stress hormones and the rise in mean arterial blood pressure (34), suggesting that it is the stressful nature of the carbon dioxide pneumoperitoneum that is responsible for this acute stress response. Against this is the fact that vasopressin levels were similar in patients who had a wall-lift procedure compared to pneumoperitoneum, when there were similar changes in mean arterial pressure (33). However, it has been argued that vasopressin release may be due to changes in cardiac filling and not be a sensitive indicator of painful stress.

Markers of tissue trauma differ greatly between open and laparoscopic procedures. C-reactive protein levels, erythrocyte sedimentation rate, and leucocytosis are lower after laparoscopic surgery compared to open, as is interleukin-6 (28). The lower levels of interleukin-6 are probably fundamental to this reduction in inflammatory response. It is conceivable that the reduced response is responsible for the shorter period of convalescence required after laparoscopic surgery.

ANESTHESIA FOR LAPAROSCOPIC SURGERY

The peculiarities of laparoscopic surgery require some, if minimal, adaptation of anesthesia for open surgery. There is a debate about the suitability of laryngeal mask anesthesia for laparoscopy. When the procedure is short and diagnostic, and there is no risk factor for regurgitation, there is considerable evidence that laryngeal mask anesthesia is safe. However, if there is going to be intra-abdominal surgery, most anesthetists would opt for endotracheal intubation and muscle relaxation. Indeed, the respiratory effects of the carbon dioxide insufflation and the need for hyperventilation during the surgery are further indications for endotracheal intubation.

The anesthetic technique utilized is a matter for the individual. However, because the patient is expected to mobilize earlier, the use of long-acting sedatives or techniques that carry a risk of severe postoperative nausea and vomiting (PONV) should be avoided. Some people advocate total intravenous anesthesia as a means to reduce the incidence of PONV (35). A well-conducted balanced anesthetic avoiding nitrous oxide, however, produces acceptably low levels of PONV (36).

Because laparoscopic surgery is extremely painful during carbon dioxide insufflation and because this occurs near the very end of surgery, there is a need for profound analgesia throughout the procedure. To allow rapid recovery from anesthesia, it is therefore desirable that the method of intraoperative analgesia not have an appreciable hangover effect. The only opioid that allows such flexibility is remifentanil. Due to its unique pharmacokinetic profile, it is possible to infuse remifentanil throughout the procedure, yet have no delay in offset after cessation of the infusion (37). The drawback of providing postoperative analgesia after stopping remifentanil can be overcome by using various local anesthetic techniques, nonopioid analgesics, and morphine at least 15 minutes before stopping the infusion; although a recent paper suggests that giving morphine 45 minutes prior to the end of the infusion leads to better analgesia after laparoscopic cholecystectomy (38).

Similar considerations apply to the choice of muscle relaxant. Muscle relaxation assists in the development of the pneumoperitoneum and retrieval of the products of surgery. However, as wound closure is relatively swift, there may be insufficient time to allow the effects of the relaxant to wear off during wound closure. Relaxants that reverse easily or are eliminated rapidly are an attractive option.

An alternative strategy is to use muscle relaxants only at the start of surgery, and to use a combination of remifentanil and volatile anesthesia without neuromuscular block to provide sufficient relaxation at the end of surgery. It is important that there be no residual neuromuscular blockade prior to the cessation of anesthesia because this is a cause of severe postoperative distress in patients. To that end, monitoring of neuromuscular block is desirable.

The use of a volatile agent should be controlled by end-tidal monitoring, and the use of remifentanil will reduce the necessary end-tidal concentration by about 50% (39). The choice of the volatile agent lies between isoflurane, sevoflurane, and desflurane. For any procedure that lasts for over an hour, there are distinct advantages to desflurane. Its low blood-gas solubility prevents any appreciable accumulation, allowing more rapid recovery. This is especially the case in patients undergoing bariatric surgery (Chapter 13).

Nitrous oxide is best avoided in laparoscopic surgery because it distends the hollow viscera (40) and can delay the resolution of gaseous air embolism (41), which may be clinically relevant in some forms of surgery (42).

POSTOPERATIVE PAIN

Although laparoscopic surgery allows rapid recovery and early return to work, there is still a considerable amount of pain soon after surgery (43). This pain is much less as soon as two hours after surgery. The pain intensity after laparoscopic cholecystectomy may be similar to that after open surgery, immediately following the day of surgery but declines rapidly thereafter.

An interesting specific problem is that of shoulder tip pain after pneumoperitoneum. Many patients find this more troublesome than pain from the trochar sites. It is likely that shoulder tip pain is due to subdiaphragmatic irritation from gas or blood. Strategies to reduce this specific pain have included instillation of bupivacaine into the peritoneum (44) and interpleural injection of bupivacaine (45). Rigorous surgical washout at the end of the procedure is also effective at limiting the pain of peritoneal irritation.

Nonsteroidal anti-inflammatory drugs are widely used in patients who do not have a contraindication. These are safe and effective for most patients. When used in combination with a regular paracetamol (acetaminophen), there is a considerable reduction in the requirement for opioid analgesia (46). Due to the rapid recovery after laparoscopic surgery, there is little place for the routine use of epidural analgesia. However, in patients with severe respiratory disease, an argument can be made for epidural analgesia to allow better early postoperative respiratory function.

CONCLUSIONS

An increasing range of procedures is now safely carried out using laparoscopic or laparoscopically assisted techniques, many as day-case or short-stay procedures. Good anesthesia for laparoscopic surgery requires an understanding of the pathophysiology of the pneumoperitoneum, as well as some modification of standard anesthetic practice to allow safe and rapid recovery. Rapid early mobilization and hospital discharge are possible, particularly where special attention is paid to minimizing the surgical stress response.

REFERENCES

1. Joris JL, Noirot DP, Legrand MJ, et al. Hemodynamic changes during laparoscopic cholecystectomy. Anesth Analg 1993; 76:1067–1071.
2. Reid CW, Martineau RJ, Hull KA, Miller DR. Hemodynamic consequences of abdominal insufflation with CO_2 during laparoscopic cholecystectomy. Can J Anaesth 1992; 39:A132.
3. Cunningham AJ, Turner J, Rosenbaum R, et al. Transoesophageal echocardiographic assessment of haemodynamic function during laparoscopic cholecystectomy. Br J Anaesth 1993; 70:621–625.
4. Dexter SP, Vucevic M, Gibson J, et al. Hemodynamic consequences of high- and low-pressure capnoperitoneum during laparoscopic cholecystectomy. Surg Enosc 1999; 13: 376–381.
5. Uemura N, Nomura M, Inoue S, et al. Changes in hemodynamics and autonomic nervous activity in patients undergoing laparoscopic cholecystectomy: differences between the pneumoperitoneum and abdominal wall lifting method. Endoscopy 2002; 34:643–650.
6. Alishahi S, Francis N, Crofts S, et al. Central and peripheral adverse hemodynamic changes during laparoscopic surgery and their reversal with a novel intermittent sequential pneumatic compression device. Ann Surg 2001; 233:176–182.
7. Junghans T, Bohm B, Grundel K, et al. Does pneumoperitoneum with different gases, bodypositions and intraperitoneal pressures influence renal and hepatic flow? Surgery 1997; 121:206–211.
8. Kotake Y, Takeda J, Matsumoto M, et al. Subclinical hepatic dysfunction in laparoscopic cholecystectomy and colectomy. Br J Anesth 2001; 87:774–777.
9. Koivusalo AM, Kellokumpu I, Ristkari S, et al. Splanchnic and renal deterioration during and after laparoscopic cholecystectomy: a comparison of the carbon dioxide pneumoperitoneum and the abdominal wall lift method. Anesth Analg 1997; 85:886–891.
10. Lindberg F, Bergqvist D, Bjorck M, et al. Renal hemodynamics during carbon dioxide pneumoperitoneum: an experimental study in pigs. Surg Endosc 2003; 17:480–484.
11. McDougall EM, Monk TG, Wolf JS, et al. The effect of prolonged pneumoperitoneum on renal function in an animal model. J Am Coll Surg 1996; 182:317–328.
12. Leonhardt KO, Landes RR. Oxygen tension of the urine and renal structures. Preliminary report of clinical findings. N Engl J Med 1963; 269:115–121.
13. Laisalmi M, Koivusalo AM, Valta P, et al. Clonidine provided opiod-sparing effect, stable hemodynamics and renal integrity during laparoscopic cholecystectomy. Surg Endosc 2001; 15:1331–1335.

14. Curet M, Vogt DA, Schob O, et al. Effects of CO_2 pneumoperitoneum in pregnant ewes. J Surg Res 1996; 63:339–344.
15. Cruz AM, Southerland LC, Duke T, et al. Intraabdominal carbon dioxide insufflation in the pregnant ewe. Uterine blood flow, intraamniotic pressure and cardiopulmonary effects. Anesthesiology 1996; 85:1395–1402.
16. Kazama T, Ikeda L, Kato T, et al. Carbon dioxide output in laparoscopic cholecystectomy. Br J Anaesth 1996; 760:530–535.
17. Streich B, Decaillot F, Perney C, et al. Increased carbon dioxide absorption during retroperitoneal laparoscopy. Br J Anaesth 2003; 91:793–796.
18. Kazama T, Ikeda K, Sanjo Y. Comparative carbon dioxide output through injured and noninjured peritoneum during laparoscic procedures. J Clin Monit Comput 1998; 14:171–176.
19. Debois P, Sabbe MB, Wouters P, et al. Carbon dioxide adsorption during laparoscopic cholecystectomy and inguinal hernia repair. Eur J Anaesthesiol 1996; 13:191–197.
20. Sumpf E, Crozier TA, Ahrens D, et al. Carbon dioxide absorption during extraperitoneal and transperitoneal endoscopic hernioplasty. Anesth Analg 2000; 91:589–595.
21. Hedenstierna G. Gas exchange during anaesthesia. Br J Anaesth 1990; 64:507–514.
22. Drummond GB, Martin LV. Pressure volume relationships in the lung during laparoscopy. Br J Anaesth 1978; 50:261–266.
23. Pelosi P, Foti G, Cereda M, et al. Effects of carbon dioxide insufflation for laparoscopic cholecystectomy on the respiratory system. Anaesthesia 1996; 51:744–749.
24. Tokics L, Hedenstierna G, Strandberg A, et al. Lung collapse and gas exchange during general anesthesia; effects of spontaneous breathing, muscle paralysis ans positive endexpiratory pressure. Anesthesiology 1987; 66:157–167.
25. Loeckinger A, Kleinsasser A, Hermann C, et al. Inert gas exchange during pneumoperitoneum at incremental values of positive end-expiratory pressure. Anesth Analg 2000; 90:466–471.
26. Schauer PR, Lana J, Ghiatas AA, et al. Pulmonary function after laparoscopic cholecystectomy. Surgery 1993; 114:389–397.
27. Johnson D, Litwin D, Osachoff J, et al. Postoperative respiratory function after laparoscopic cholecystectomy. Surg Laparosc Endosc 1992; 2:221–226.
28. Zengin K, Taskin M, Sakoglu N, et al. Systemic inflammatory response after laparoscopic and open application of adjustable banding for morbidly obese patients. Obes Surg 2002; 12:276–279.
29. Dionigi R, Domimioni L, Benevento A, et al. Effects of surgical trauma of laparoscopic vs open cholecystectomy. Hepatogastroenterology 1994; 41:471–476.
30. Mealy K, Gallagher H, Barry M, et al. Physiological and metabolic responses to open and laparoscopic cholecystectomy. Br J Surg 1992; 79:1061–1064.
31. Donald RA, Perry EG, Wittert GA, et al. The plasma ACTH, AVP, CRH and catecholamineresponses to conventional and open cholecystectomy. Clin Endocrinol Oxf 1993; 38:609–615.
32. Marana E, Scambia G, Maussier ML, et al. Neuroendocrine stress response in patients undergoing benign ovarian cyst surgery by laparoscopy, mini laparotomy and laparotomy. J Am Assoc Gynecol Laparosc 2003; 10:159–165.
33. Koivusalo AM, Kellokumpu I, Scheinin M, et al. Randomised comparison of the neuroendocrine response to laparoscopic cholecystectomy using either conventional or abdominal wall lift techniques. Br J Surg 1996; 83:1532–1536.
34. Walter A, Aitkenhead AR. Role of vasopressin in the haemodynamic response to laparoscopic cholecystectomy. Br J Anaesth 1997; 78:128–133.
35. Apfel CC, Korttila K, Abdalla M, et al. An international multicenter protocol; to assess the single and combined benefits of antiemetic strategies in a controlled clinical trial of a 2 x 2 x 2 x 2 x 2 factorial design (IMPACT). Cntrol Clin Trial 2003; 24:736–751.
36. Divatia JV, Vaidya JS, Badwe RA, Hawalder RW. Omission of nitrous oxide during anaesthesia reduces the incidence of post operative nausea and vomiting. A metaanalysis. Anesthesiology 1996; 85:1066–1062.

37. Egan TD, Lemmens HJ, Fiset P, et al. The pharmacokinetics of the new short-acting opioid remifentanil (GI87084B) in healthy adult male volunteers. Anesthesiology 1993; 79:881–892.
38. Munoz HR, Guerrero ME, Brandes, V, Cortinez LI. Effect of timing of morphine administration during remifentanil-bases anaesthesia on early recovery from anaesthesia and post-operative pain. Br J Anaesth 2002; 88:814–818.
39. Lang E, Kapila A, Shlugman D, et al. Reduction of isoflurane minmum alveolar anaesthetic concentration by remifentanil. Anesthesiology 1996; 85:721–728.
40. Eger EI, Saidman LJ. Hazards of nitrous oxide in bowel obstruction and pneumothorax. Anaesthesiology 1965; 26:61–66.
41. Steffey EP, Johnson BH, Eger EI. Nitrous oxide intensifies the pulmonary arterial pressure response tovenous injection of carbon dioxide in the dog. Anesthesiology 1980; 52:52–55.
42. Greville AC, Clements EAF, Erwin DC, et al. Pulmonary air embolism during laparoscopic laser cholecystectomy. Anaesthesia 1991; 46:113–114.
43. Ure BM, Troidl L, Spangenberger W, et al. Pain after laparoscopic cholecystectomy. Intensity and localisation of pain and predictors in preoperative symptoms and intraoperative events. Surg Endosc 1994; 8:90–96.
44. Narchi P, Benhamou D, Fernandez H. Intraperitoneal local anaesthetic for shoulder pain after day case laparoscopy. Lancet 1991; 38:1569–1570.
45. Schulte-Steinberg H, Weninger E, Jokisch D, et al. Intraperitoneal versus interpleural morphine or bupivacaine for pain after laparoscopic cholecystectomy. Anesthesiology 1995; 82:634–640.
46. Hahn TW, Mogensen T, Lund C, et al. Analgesic effect of i.v. paracetamol: possible ceiling effect of paracetamol in post-operative pain. Acta Anaesthesiol Scand 2003; 47:138–145.

18
Anesthesia for the Carcinoid Syndrome

Lennart Christiansson
Department of Anesthesiology, University Hospital, Uppsala, Sweden

INTRODUCTION

How anesthetic management of patients with carcinoid tumors has evolved over recent decades is well summarized in several good reviews (1–3). The early concept of a relatively benign gastrointestinal (GI) tumor producing a single hormone (serotonin) has changed into a complex picture, in which we know that numerous mediators are involved and surgery is becoming increasingly extensive. The perioperative course, on the other hand, has become considerably less dramatic since somatostatin analogues were introduced to the therapeutic arsenal. One study (4) summarizes the perianesthetic risks and outcomes of 119 patients that underwent surgery in 1983 to 1996 at a tertiary center. It was shown that the intraoperative use of octreotide (Food and Drug Administration approval in 1988) reduced the incidence of complications during surgery. The two main risk factors for complications were found to be carcinoid heart disease and high preoperative urinary serotonin metabolite 5-Hydroxyindolacetic acid (5-HIAA) output. It should be noted, however, that the overall incidence of perioperative complications or death was low (12%).

TUMOR BIOLOGY, DIAGNOSIS, AND TREATMENT

Tumor Biology

The first description of carcinoid tumors dates back to more than 100 years, and the carcinoid syndrome as an entity can be found in the literature of the last 50 years. The incidence is in the region of 20 per 1 million people (3) in the western world, and the carcinoids are normally slow-growing, potentially malignant tumors with distinctive biological features and clinical characteristics. Excellent background information on most aspects of carcinoid tumors is found in recent reviews (5–9). The tumors are derived from neuroendocrine cells. Common to these cells is their affinity to silver salts (i.e., enterochromaffin) and the property of producing amines and polypeptides. Chromogranin A (CgA) is a general tumor marker that can be detected in most patients with a carcinoid tumor. Foregut carcinoids (intrathoracic, gastric, and proximal duodenum) are more common in patients with familial multiple neoplasia type 1 (10) where deletions are found on chromosome 11, whereas

o Tryptophan
   ➢ *Tryptophan hydroxylase*
⇩ 5-Hydroxytryptophan (5-HTP)
   ➢ *L-aromatic amino acid decarboxylase*
⇩ 5-Hydroxytryptamine (Serotonin)
   ➢ *Monoamine oxidase (MAO)*
⇩ 5-Hydroxyindole acetaldehyde
   ➢ *Aldehyde dehydrogenase*
⇩ 5-Hydroxyindole acetic acid (5-HIAA)

Figure 1 The metabolic pathway for serotonin.

changes in chromosome 18 are seen in midgut tumors (small intestine, appendix, and proximal colon) (7,9,11). Other genetic conditions associated with neuroendocrine tumors are von Hippel–Lindau syndrome and von Recklinghausen disease (neurofibromatosis type 1).

Tumors of foregut and midgut embryonic origins produce serotonin, neurokinin, and substance P. In addition to these mediators, midgut carcinoids produce kallikrein/bradykinin and prostaglandins. Foregut tumors are less commonly causing the carcinoid syndrome but the list of secretory products found in these tumors includes histamine, glucagon, gastrin, and several releasing peptides.

Serotonin [5-Hydroxytryptamine (5-HT)] has a complex role as transmitter in the central nervous system and regulator of smooth muscle tone in the cardiovascular and GI systems. It is also very important for platelet function. The metabolic pathway for serotonin is described in Figure 1.

Serotonin is metabolized by monoamine oxidase (MAO) in the liver, and any amount that survives this "first pass effect" in the liver will normally be rapidly removed by the endothelium of lung capillaries. The serotonin receptor subtypes 1, 2, and 4 are coupled via G proteins, whereas the $5-HT_3$ receptor is a ligand-gated ion channel. The activation of $5-HT_1$ receptors induces nitric oxide and causes vasodilatation, but the classical response to serotonin is vasoconstriction via the $5-HT_{2A}$ receptor. Figure 2 gives an overview of how serotonin is handled by the carcinoid tumor cell. The fact that its release is mediated by cell surface β-adrenoceptors is important for the understanding of how stress can induce a carcinoid crisis. This effect is counter regulated by stimulation of somatostatin receptors (SSTR) on the cell membrane.

The clinical tumor presentation is either by localization (bowel obstruction, pain, bleeding, etc.) or by hormone secretion. The vast majority (more than 75%) of carcinoid tumors are found in the GI tract (3), and metastases are more frequently occurring if the primary tumor is more than 2 cm in diameter. A carcinoid syndrome might manifest foregut and midgut carcinoid tumors, but the overall incidence is less than 10%. Rare intrathoracic tumors might secrete adrenocorticotropic hormone (ACTH), which can cause a Cushing syndrome.

Diagnosis

In patients with the carcinoid syndrome, the levels of urinary 5-HIAA per 24 hours are usually increased, particularly so in midgut carcinoids. In other cases, measurements of serotonin levels in urine or platelets can be helpful. Plasma CgA has a higher

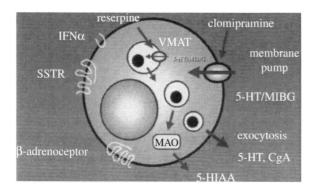

Figure 2 The midgut carcinoid tumor cells express on its surface adrenoceptors, which mediate the release of 5-HT, and SSTR, which inhibit the release of secretory products and receptors for IFN. Serotonin, or its precursor 5-HTP, can be taken up by the tumor cell via a membrane pump (inhibited by clomipramine) and incorporated into secretory granules via VMAT (inhibited by reserpine). Cytosolic 5-HT can be degraded within the tumor cell by MAO to 5-HIAA. Serotonin stored within granules is released by exocytosis together with CgA. The tumor cell can also handle catecholamines or analogs (MIBG). *Abbreviations*: 5-HT, 5-Hydroxytryptamine; SSTR, somatostatin receptors; IFN, interferon; VMAT, vesicular monoamine transporters; MAO, monoamine oxidase; 5-HIAA, 5-Hydroxyindolacetic acid; CgA, chromogranin A; MIBG, meta-iodobenzylguanidine. *Source*: From Ref. 12.

sensitivity than 5-HIAA, but the specificity is lower. For tumor localization, specialized techniques are now in use where standard imaging is insufficient (8,9). These sophisticated methods are somatostatin-receptor scintigraphy, iodinated meta-iodobenzylguanidine (^{131}I-MIBG) scanning, and the highly sensitive positron emission tomography using an ^{11}C-labeled 5-Hydroxytryptophan (5-HTP) serotonin precursor.

The presence of symptoms and the site of origin affect outcome (13). The size of the primary tumor and the presence of distant (liver) metastases are important for prognosis but have not been shown to be independent predictors of survival (14). Histochemical prognostic indicators are the expression of certain cellular proteins (e.g., Ki-67) (11,15) and the concentrations of secreted markers (plasma Chromogranin A and urinary 5-HIAA), and clinical predictors are the carcinoid syndrome and carcinoid heart disease.

Medical Treatment

Since the introduction of somatostatin analogues, serotonin inhibitors or receptor antagonists are not routinely used any more. In countries where the 5-HT$_{2A}$ receptor blocker ketanserin is available, the drug has been used with reported success in patients with mainly serotonin-related hypertension. Ketanserin also has high affinity for α-adrenergic and histamine H$_1$ receptors. Blocking of α$_1$-receptors is more likely to be the explanation of its property to lower blood pressure than the 5-HT$_{2A}$ antagonism. 5-HT$_3$ receptor antagonists (e.g., ondansetron) are the routinely administered antiemetics and, for carcinoid patients, theoretically, the drug of choice for prevention or treatment of nausea.

Cyproheptadine is a histamine H$_1$ receptor antagonist that also has combined effect on the serotonin system with vascular response (5-HT$_{2A}$) and central depressant properties. A combination of histamine H$_1$ and H$_2$ blockers is occasionally prescribed for patients with a foregut carcinoid secreting both histamine and gastrin. Sometimes, a histamine H_2 blocker (e.g., ranitidine) is prescribed even in the absence of hyperacidity, because it has been shown that both H_1 and H_2 receptors are involved in histamine vasodilatation.

In more recent years, interferon (IFN) α has been shown to reduce tumor growth in patients, with a specific protein kinase activity, responding to treatment (7,8). Chemotherapy is normally avoided but can be tried in foregut carcinoids with aggressive tumor growth. Conventional irradiation has a very limited effect, but the use of radiolabeled MIBG or octreotide to concentrate irradiation to tumors or metastases is currently tested in clinical series (5,8).

Somatostatin

Somatostatin was first identified in 1968 and its chemical structure was defined in 1982. Like somatostatin, octreotide (16,17) suppresses release of pituitary [growth hormone (GH), thyroid stimulating hormone (TSH)] and various pancreatic hormones (e.g., glucagon, insulin, cholecystokinin, and pancreatic polypeptide). It reduces gastric acid secretion, splanchnic blood flow, GI motility, and pancreatic exocrine function. Octreotide must be used with caution in patients at risk of developing cholecystitis, cholestatic hepatitis, or pancreatitis. In diabetics, dose adjustments of oral medication or insulin may be necessary.

Circulating octreotide is 65% protein bound, and the plasma levels peak within minutes after intravenous (IV) injection and about 30 minutes following subcutaneous (SC) administration. The elimination half-life of IV octreotide is approximately 75 minutes, compared with two to three minutes for somatostatin. Upon SC administration of octreotide, the plasma disappearance $t_{\frac{1}{2}}$ is more than or equal to 90 minutes. The use of octreotide for the treatment of neuroendocrine GI tumors was first reported in 1985, preceded, however, by reports of successful use of somatostatin in 1978.

The clinically available analogues (octreotide and lanreotide) have tumor antiproliferative and antiangiogenetic effects via pathways such as mitogen-activated protein kinases, tyrosine phosphatases, and ion fluxes. The release of tumor markers and mediators is decreased and systemic effects are blocked on a receptor level. Five subtypes of SSTR (6) have been characterized. Octreotide binds primarily to subtypes 2, 3, and 5, but the binding to the former appears to be essential for its clinical efficacy. With doses of 300 to 3000 µg/day, the carcinoid syndrome can be kept under control in most patients. This treatment has also reduced the incidence of carcinoid crisis. Long-acting formulations of analogues are now available for injection with a two to four week interval, and have been shown to control symptoms, as well as SC octreotide once steady-state concentrations are achieved (18). In terms of symptom control, quality of life, and reduction in tumor cell markers, both analogues are equally efficacious, but most patients prefer lanreotide because of the simplified mode of administration (8,19).

When tumor interventions are performed, it is advocated that octreotide prophylaxis is given with incremental boluses as necessary during the procedure, should signs of carcinoid crisis develop. In larger doses, octreotide can have significant effects on blood pressure and heart rate. The physiologic importance of somatostatin in the neurohumoral control of cardiac impulse formation and conduction is well known (20). Activation of the G-protein–coupled SSTR results in changes in calcium and potassium conductance (17). Octreotide can increase the risk of bradycardia via an interaction with β-blockers and calcium channel blockers (21). Symptomatic bradycardia due to atrioventricular-block Mobitz type II or complete heart block has been reported (20).

Surgery

Symptomatic patients often have malignant tumors. Surgery is thus often not curative, but resections or debulking procedures are still indicated for control of symptoms. With the same aim, to gain quality of life, surgery can be justified for metastatic disease (22–24). Liver transplantation is considered an alternative if the tumor is limited to the liver and not accessible to surgery or responding to other treatments (25,26). The same strategy is applicable to the management of primary carcinoid tumors of the liver (27).

In selected patients with peritoneal carcinomatosis, maximal cytoreductive surgery in combination with intraperitoneal chemotherapy has shown good palliative results (28). Arterial embolization (29), chemoembolization, cryotherapy, and radiofrequency ablation are optional techniques (12), used either alone or in combination with surgery.

THE CARCINOID SYNDROME

The classical syndrome includes flushing, diarrhea, abdominal pain, right-sided valvular heart disease, teleangiectasia, bronchial constriction, pellagra-like skin changes, and increased levels of 5-HIAA in urine (7,30). The syndrome occurs in malignant midgut carcinoids with liver metastases or other tumors that bypass the portal circulation, such as ovarian, bronchial, or retroperitoneal carcinoids. Flushing is caused by the vasodilatory tachykinins (neurokinin, neuropeptide K, or substance P), bradykinin, or histamine. The role of bradykinin with respect to flushing has been questioned (31), but methodology and problems with artifactual cascade activation or inhibition make data difficult to compare. Diarrhea is more common in serotonin-secreting tumors. Serotonin and tachykinins are probably responsible for the fibrotic complications unique to this syndrome. It affects the endocardium of the right heart, retroperitoneal connective tissue, and mesenteric vasculature.

Carcinoid Heart Disease

This entity was first recognized in 1952, when a young man with pulmonic stenosis, tricuspid regurgitation, asthma, and cyanosis was found to have metastatic carcinoid disease (32). The endocardial plaques are composed of smooth muscle cells, myofibroblasts, and an overlying endothelial cell layer. Cardiac involvement is seen in 30% to 60% of patients with metastatic disease, and there is an apparent correlation with 5-HIAA levels, or perhaps with the duration of exposure to elevated serotonin levels (33,34). The patients with the most severe right heart disease also had higher plasma levels of the tachykinins neuropeptide K and substance P (35).

Both diagnosis and follow-up of carcinoid heart disease are best made by echocardiography (32,34,36–38). The most common finding is tricuspid (60% or more) valve involvement (often regurgitation combined with stenosis) followed by pulmonary stenosis (20% or more) or insufficiency (38). Valve replacement surgery is a feasible option but associated with substantial mortality and major morbidity (21). The left side of the heart was not often affected, and if so, it was mainly in patients with bronchial carcinoids (serotonin) or in those with an atrial defect (32). In other patients, the assumed causative mediators are either metabolized (serotonin) or inactivated (kinins and growth factors) (7,9) in the pulmonary circulation. Conflicting data exist on the extent to which modern treatment with octreotide, α-interferons, and active surgery has reduced the incidence of clinically significant carcinoid heart disease (33,52).

Carcinoid Crisis

This life-threatening situation with flushing, oedema, severe hypotension, and tachycardia might occur when larger quantities of mediators are released into the systemic circulation. This can be triggered by all kinds of manipulations of a carcinoid tumor or its metastases. Kallikrein is an enzyme found in carcinoid tumors. It stimulates plasma kininogen to liberate bradykinin, which is thought to cause the symptoms of the crisis together with prostaglandins, histamine, and various tachykinins (in particular, substance P). Reports (39,40) from the mid-1980s beautifully illustrate the refractoriness of carcinoid hypotension and the comparison of conventional treatment with the novel octreotide. Since the introduction of pretreatment with somatostatin analogues (41–43), carcinoid crisis is far less commonly seen, but during surgery and other tumor interventions (44) one always has to be prepared to give additional boluses of octreotide.

ANESTHETIC AND PERIOPERATIVE ASPECTS

Preoperative Assessment and Optimization

Examination should aim to uncover any signs of carcinoid syndrome with a liberal use of echocardiography to detect carcinoid heart disease (2). Antibiotic prophylaxis is recommended if valvular involvement is present. A symptomatic cardiac dysfunction will of course have impact on patient selection and intraoperative management. Fluid and electrolyte abnormalities are occasionally encountered in cases of diarrhea. Another problem is histamine-induced asthma. Because β-receptors are found on carcinoid tumor cells, adrenergic stimulation can possibly cause mediator release and elicit or worsen a carcinoid crisis. β-agonists are therefore normally avoided when treating mild bronchoconstriction or hemodynamic disturbances.

Historically, a number of drugs have been used to block the production, release, or action of mediators of carcinoid cells. When there is known or suspected histamine release (foregut tumors), a combination of H_1 and H_2 blockers can be effective. Treatment with serotonin-receptor antagonists and steroids has been difficult to be proven effective. Ketanserin (approved in some European countries) counteracts both histamine and serotonin, and has been tried with some success in preventing and treating $5\text{-}HT_2$ receptor–induced constriction of bronchi and vasculature. Hence, this option can still be useful in cases with octreotide-refractory asthma and hypertension. Intraoperatively, the more common and severe reaction is flushing and bradykinin-induced hypotension. The trigger for the kinin production is kallikrein formed in the tumor. Aprotinin is a known serine protease inhibitor (kallikrein) and has thus been tried to treat or prevent hypotension. The high incidence of anaphylactoid reactions to aprotinin makes its use controversial.

The cornerstone of medical treatment of carcinoid tumors is the use of somatostatin analogues. This treatment is equally important in the perioperative phase, as described in a recent consensus report (45). Patients already on long-acting treatment and with the condition well controlled are given a bolus of 250 to 500 µg SC two hours before elective surgery. In emergency surgery, patients not pretreated with analogues; 50 to 100 (–1000!)µg octreotide can be given IV prior to induction.

Intraoperative Management

Premedication

All usual preoperative medication should be continued (2). A benzodiazepine can be used for anxiolysis, and is often combined with the sedative effect of an antihistamine. All drugs known to release histamine are best avoided. Ondansetron is the preferred antiemetic because of its serotonin antagonistic effect (3).

Monitoring

In addition to standard monitoring, intra-arterial pressure recording should be started prior to induction and continued into the early postoperative period. A central venous line is not mandatory but can be very helpful when patients with the carcinoid syndrome are undergoing major resections or treated for liver metastases. IV administration of vasoactive drugs is thereby made safer, and central venous pressure monitoring can to some extent help differentiating between hypovolemia and mediator-induced hypotension (2). For patients with symptomatic cardiac dysfunction, further monitoring with ST-segment analysis, a pulmonary artery catheter, or transesophageal echocardiography is advocated. Placement of a urinary catheter and a temperature probe is routine care and so is the use of a warming blanket.

Induction

Most routine techniques can be used, but drugs known to have the capacity to set free histamine are best avoided. A combination of propofol and fentanyl is considered safe, and for muscle relaxation, vecuronium and cis-atracurium have theoretical advantages. Depolarizing relaxants will increase intra-abdominal pressure, which can confer a squeezing effect on the tumor or its metastases. For rapid sequence induction, one should therefore consider using rocuronium instead of suxamethonium. Glycopyrrolate would be the first choice if an anticholinergic agent is indicated.

Maintenance

The commonest technique is to use balanced anesthesia with an inhalational agent, an opioid, and a nondepolarizing muscle relaxant (2). Replacing the volatile anesthetic with a propofol infusion appears to be equally safe. Modern short-acting opioids, especially remifentanil (46), have successfully been tried instead of the standard drug fentanyl. Remifentanil can be part of total IV anesthesia with propofol, combined with an inhalational agent, or used to top up the effect of a thoracic epidural analgesia. The fact that recovery might be delayed in patients with high serotonin levels speaks in favor of using short-acting agents for maintenance. Nitrous oxide is considered safe but its use in the combinations mentioned above would be superfluous.

Regional anesthesia (46–48) can be used in these patients in the same way as in most patients having GI surgery. The catheter should be inserted at a thoracic level that provides congruent analgesia. Routine testing is recommended. The circulatory consequences should be minimized to avoid confounding the hemodynamic situation during tumor manipulations. It might be safer to use relatively more opioid than local anesthetic for the neuraxial block. If it becomes necessary to treat hypotension, an α_1-agonist (phenylephrine, methoxamine, or metaraminol) should be used, in order not to risk triggering the release of mediators by stimulation of β-receptors. In accordance with the experience from thoracic procedures and upper GI surgery in general, good analgesia at emergence will facilitate fast-track extubation and possibly improve outcome.

Carcinoid Crisis

Hypotension is the commonest problem encountered during carcinoid surgery (40,47). Because treatment differs, it is important to distinguish the carcinoid crises from anaphylactic shock or hypotension caused by histamine release. If carcinoid crisis develops during surgery, incremental IV boluses of 50 to 200 μg octreotide are given with a few minutes intervals. According to the recent consensus report (45), IV boluses of as much as 500 to 1000 μg can be given, depending on the severity

Table 1 Carcinoid Syndrome: Key Facts

Most secreting *carcinoid tumors* are of foregut or midgut embryonic origin, and they produce serotonin, neurokinin, and substance P. Midgut carcinoids also produce kallikrein/ bradykinin and prostaglandins. The list of secretory products found in foregut tumors includes histamine, glucagon, gastrin, and several releasing peptides.

The classical *carcinoid syndrome* includes flushing, diarrhea, abdominal pain, right-sided valvular heart disease, and bronchial constriction. The syndrome occurs in malignant midgut carcinoids with liver metastases or other tumors that bypass the portal circulation. Surgery is thus not always curative, but resections or debulking procedures are still indicated for control of symptoms.

Clinical *prognostic predictors* are the carcinoid syndrome, carcinoid heart disease, and high concentrations of secreted markers (plasma CgA and urinary 5-HIAA).

Serotonin and tachykinins are probably responsible for the *fibrotic complications* unique to this syndrome. It affects the endocardium of the right heart, retroperitoneal connective tissue, and mesenteric vasculature. Carcinoid heart disease is seen in 30% to 60% of patients with metastatic tumors. The most common findings are tricuspid regurgitation and pulmonic valve stenosis.

Carcinoid crisis is a life-threatening situation with flushing, edema, severe hypotension, and tachycardia that might occur when larger quantities of mediators are released into the systemic circulation. This can be triggered by all kinds of manipulations of a carcinoid tumor or its metastases. Kallikrein stimulates plasma kininogen to liberate bradykinin, which is thought to cause the symptoms of the crisis together with prostaglandins, histamine, and various tachykinins.

Since the introduction of *somatostatin analogues*, carcinoid symptoms are normally well controlled, and antihistamines or serotonin inhibitors are not routinely used any more. In more recent years, IFN α has also been shown to reduce tumor growth in a subset of patients. Like somatostatin, octreotide suppresses release of pituitary (GH and TSH) and various pancreatic hormones. It reduces gastric acid secretion, splanchnic blood flow, GI motility, and pancreatic exocrine function.

The *perioperative* use of *octreotide* has reduced the incidence and severity of complications during surgery. The fact that more patients now are manageable has led to more extensive surgery, either curative or palliative debulking for alleviation of symptoms.

Abbreviations: CgA, chromogranin A; 5-HIAA, 5-Hydroxy indolacetic acid; IFN, interferon; GH, growth hormone; TSH, thyroid stimulating hormone; GI, gastrointestinal.

and refractoriness of the hypotension. Controlled studies regarding dosing are scarce, but in case reports (49,50), older recommendations are questioned and possible intraoperative tachyphylaxis reported. If not started when commencing surgery, the boluses are followed up by an IV infusion of octreotide, 100 to 200 µg/hr, for the duration of the remaining operation. Initial management also includes fluid therapy and α_1-agonistic vasopressors.

Table 2 Practical Approaches to the Patient with Carcinoid Syndrome

Pretreatment
If the patient has not been treated for at least two weeks with a somatostatin analogue or if
    they are still symptomatic, octreotide 500 µg is administered subcutaneously
    preoperatively, two hours before surgery. In urgent cases, 100 µg octreotide is given IV
    prior to induction. An octreotide infusion is started at a rate of 100 µg/hr
Premedication
Most patients receive a combination of a benzodiazepine tranquilizer (diazepam) and a
    5-hydroxytryptamine$_3$ antiemetic (ondansetron). If sedation is not a concern, an
    antihistamine (cyproheptadine) can be added
Monitoring
Routine monitoring and invasive recording of arterial pressure and central venous pressure is
    advocated. If the patient has a symptomatic cardiac dysfunction or coronary disease, ST-
    segment monitoring and transesophageal echocardiography may be added or a pulmonary
    arterial catheter inserted
Epidural analgesia
The catheter is inserted 3–5 cm at a thoracic level that provides congruent analgesia. This will
    be T8–10 for most mesenterial tumors, with the higher level preferred if surgery also
    includes liver resection. After routine testing, a bolus of opioid (e.g., fentanyl 1 µg/kg) is
    given and an infusion (e.g., 0.15% bupivacaine +2 µg/mL fentanyl) started for
    continuation into the postoperative phase
Inductions
Glycopyrrolate is the preferred anticholinergic. Propofol, fentanyl, and vecuronium are all
    suitable drugs for induction and intubation
Maintenance
For hypnosis, either an inhalational agent or a propofol infusion is used. Analgesia is
    provided with the combination of a thoracic epidural block and a remifentanil infusion. If
    no epidural is used, an opioid with somewhat longer lasting effect (fentanyl) is more
    appropriate
Carcinoid crisis
Hypotension
    Octreotide 50–200 µg IV boluses plus increased infusion rate
    Phenylephrine 50–200 µg IV boluses plus infusion 0.1–2 µg/kg/min
    Arginin–vasopressin, antihistamine, steroid, and calcium chloride, if unresponsive
Bronchospasm
    Octreotide 50–200 µg IV boluses.
    Antihistamine, nebulized ipratropium, and steroid, if unresponsive
Hypertension
    Octreotide 50–200 µg IV boluses.
    Labetalol, esmolol, and GTN-infusion, if unresponsive
Postoperative aspects
All symptomatic patients are observed in a high dependency or intensive care unit and the
    octreotide infusion is continued at 50–100 µg/hr. Normothermia and active pain
    management is important for avoiding stress and allowing early extubation

Abbreviations: IV, intravenous; GTN, glyceryl trinitrate.

One additional vasopressor that works via a different mechanism should be available. Arginin–vasopressin (AVP) is probably available in many departments but angiotensin II is a very powerful alternative vasoconstrictor. An antihistamine and a corticosteroid should also be kept ready for IV use. Calcium chloride can be tried if ionized calcium is low, or in an attempt to improve cardiovascular responsiveness when inhalational anesthesia was used in a patient on calcium blockers.

Mediator-induced bronchospasm is in first line treated with octreotide, antihistamine, nebulized ipratropium bromide, and possibly steroids (3). β-agonists are second line, because they may precipitate mediator release and thereby worsen the spasm.

Hypertension is a less frequently occurring intraoperative event (47) and the first-line intervention is to give octreotide boluses IV. If no response is noted, a short-acting β-blocker (esmolol or labetalol) is given and if necessary a vasodilator (glyceryl trinitrate infusion) started. Where available, the serotonin- and α_1-receptor antagonist ketanserin (51) can be tried.

Hyperglycemia can be seen in patients with high serotonin levels (1) due to its adrenaline-like metabolic effect or the release of glucagon from the tumor. This situation can occur even in the absence of obvious adrenergic stress. The response to insulin treatment is usually normal.

Postoperative Care and Analgesia

Postoperative requirements depend on whether any carcinoid tumor or metastases remain unresected, or whether the surgical intervention was unrelated to the patient's carcinoid disease. All patients showing signs of mediator release into the systemic circulation during surgery should be observed in a high dependency or intensive care unit, postoperatively. Intraoperative fluid shifts may still warrant monitoring and correction. Patients who have required supplemental dosing of octreotide during surgery should have their infusion of octreotide, 50 to 100 μg/hr, continued for the next 24 hours or until the preoperative treatment schedule can be resumed. Good pain relief is vital to prevent sympathetic stress and is probably best achieved with a patient-controlled opioid analgesia system or a continuous regional block. For neuraxial blocks, a mixture of fentanyl with low-concentration bupivacaine can provide safe analgesia.

Key facts and summary of carcinoid can be seen in Tables 1 and 2.

REFERENCES

1. Mason RA, Steane PA. Carcinoid syndrome: its relevance to the anaesthetist. Anaesthesia 1976; 31:228–242.
2. Vaughan DJ, Brunner MD. Anesthesia for patients with carcinoid syndrome. Int Anesthesiol Clin 1997; 35(4):129–142 (review).
3. Graham GW, Unger BP, Coursin DB. Perioperative management of selected endocrine disorders. Int Anesthesiol Clin 2000; 38(4):31–67 (review).
4. Kinney MA, Warner ME, Nagorney DM, et al. Perianaesthetic risks and outcomes of abdominal surgery for metastatic carcinoid tumours. Br J Anaesth 2001; 87(3):447–452.
5. Caplin ME, Buscombe JR, Hilson AJ, et al. Carcinoid tumour. Lancet 1998; 352: 799–805.
6. Kulke MH, Mayer RJ. Carcinoid tumors. N Engl J Med 1999; 340(11):858–868 (review).
7. Öberg K. Carcinoid tumors, carcinoid syndrome, and related disorders. In: Larsen PR, Kronenberg HM, Melmed S, Polonsky KS, eds. Williams Textbook of Endocrinology. 10th ed. Saunders, 2002.

8. Öberg K. Diagnosis and treatment of carcinoid tumors. Expert Rev Anticancer Ther 2003; 3(6):863–877 (review).
9. Modlin IM, Kidd M, Latich I, et al. Current status of gastrointestinal carcinoids. Gastro-enterology 2005; 128(6):1717–1751.
10. Doherty GM. Multiple endocrine neoplasia type 1. J Surg Oncol 2005; 89:143–150.
11. Öberg K. Carcinoid tumors: molecular genetics, tumor biology, and update of diagnosis and treatment. Curr Opin Oncol 2002; 14(1):38–45 (review).
12. Ahlman H, Nilsson O, Olausson M. Interventional treatment of the carcinoid syndrome. Neuroendocrinology 2004; 80(suppl 1):67–73 (review).
13. Onatis MW, Kirshbom PM, Hayward TZ, et al. Gastrointestinal carcinoids: characteriza-tion by site of origin and hormone production. Ann Surg 2000; 232(4):549–556.
14. Van Gompel JJ, Sippel RS, Warner TF, Chen H. Gastrointestinal carcinoid tumors: fac-tors that predict outcome. World J Surg 2004; 28(4):387–392.
15. Rorstad O. Prognostic indicators for carcinoid neuroendocrine tumors of the gastrointest-inal tract. J Surg Oncol 2005; 89(3):151–160 (review).
16. Katz MD, Erstad BL. Octreotide, a new somatostatin analogue. Clin Pharm 1989; 8(4):255–273 (review).
17. Lamberts SWJ, van der Lely AJ, de Herder WW, Hofland LJ. Octreotide. NEJM 1996; 334(4):246–254.
18. Rubin J, Ajani J, Schirmer W, et al. Octreotide acetate long-acting formulation versus open-label subcutaneous octreotide acetate in malignant carcinoid syndrome. J Clin Oncol 1999; 17:600–606.
19. O'Toole D, Ducreux M, Bommelaer G, et al. Treatment of carcinoid syndrome: a pro-spective crossover evaluation of lanreotide versus octreotide in terms of efficacy, patient acceptability, and tolerance. Cancer 2000; 88(4):770–776.
20. Dilger JA, Rho EH, Que FG, Sprung J. Octreotide-induced bradycardia and heart block during surgical resection of a carcinoid tumor. Anesth Analg 2004; 98(2):318–320.
21. Di Luzio S, Rigolin VH. Carcinoid heart disease. Curr Treat Options Cardiovasc Med 2000; 2(5):399–406.
22. Hellman P, Lundstrom T, Ohrvall U, et al. Effect of surgery on the outcome of midgut carcinoid disease with lymph node and liver metastases. World J Surg 2002; 26(8):991–997.
23. Sarmiento JM, Que FG. Hepatic surgery for metastases from neuroendocrine tumors. Surg Oncol Clin N Am 2003; 12(1):231–242 (review).
24. Åkerstrom G, Hellman P, Hessman O, Osmak L. Management of midgut carcinoids. J Surg Oncol 2005; 89(3):161–169 (review).
25. Claure RE, Drover DD, Haddow GR, et al. Orthotopic liver transplantation for carcinoid tumour metastatic to the liver: anesthetic management. Can J Anaesth 2000; 47(4):334–337.
26. Olausson M, Friman S, Cahlin C, et al. Indications and results of liver transplantation in patients with neuroendocrine tumors. World J Surg 2002; 26:998–1004.
27. Fenwick SW, Wyatt JI, Toogood GJ, Lodge JP. Hepatic resection and transplantation for primary carcinoid tumors of the liver. Ann Surg 2004; 239(2):210–219.
28. Elias D, Sideris L, Liberale G, et al. Surgical treatment of peritoneal carcinomat-osis from well-differentiated digestive endocrine carcinomas. Surgery 2005; 137(4):411–416.
29. Schell SR, Camp ER, Caridi JG, Hawkins IF Jr. Hepatic artery embolization for control of symptoms, octreotide requirements, and tumor progression in metastatic carcinoid tumors. J Gastrointest Surg 2002; 6(5):664–670.
30. Van der Horst-Schrivers ANA, Machteld Wymenga AN, Links TP, et al. Complications of midgut carcinoid tumors and carcinoid syndrome. Neuroendocrinology 2004; 80(Suppl 1):28–32.
31. Gustafsen J, Boesby S, Nielsen F, Giese J. Bradykinin in carcinoid syndrome. Gut 1987; 28(11):1417–1419.

264   **Christiansson**

32. Anderson AS, Krauss D, Lang R. Cardiovascular complications of malignant carcinoid disease. Am Heart J 1997; 134(4):693–702 (review).
33. Moller JE, Connolly HM, Rubin J, et al. Factors associated with progression of carcinoid heart disease. N Engl J Med 2003; 348(11):1005–1015.
34. Denney WD, Kemp WE, Anthony LB, Oates JA, Byrd III BF. Echocardiographic and biochemical evaluation of the development and progression of carcinoid heart disease. J Am Coll Cardiol 1998; 32:1017–1022.
35. Lundin L, Norheim I, Landelius J, et al. Carcinoid heart disease: relationship of circulating vasoactive substances to ultrasound-detectable cardiac abnormalities. Circulation 1988; 77(2):264–269.
36. Lundin L. Carcinoid heart disease: a clinical, biochemical and morphological study. Comprehensive summaries of uppsala dissertations from the faculty of medicine. Acta Univ Upsal 1989; 206:52.
37. Botero M, Fuchs R, Paulus DA, Lind DS. Carcinoid heart disease: a case report and literature review. J Clin Anesth 2002; 14(1):57–63 (review).
38. Westberg G, Wangberg B, Ahlman H, et al. Prediction of prognosis by echocardiography in patients with midgut carcinoid syndrome. Br J Surg 2001; 88(6):865–872.
39. Kvols LK, Martin JK, Marsh HM, Moertel CG. Rapid reversal of carcinoid crisis with a somatostatin analogue. N Engl J Med 1985; 313(19):1229–1230.
40. Marsh HM, Martin JK Jr., Kvols LK, et al. Carcinoid crisis during anesthesia: successful treatment with a somatostatin analogue. Anesthesiology 1987; 66(1):89–91.
41. Roy RC, Carter RF, Wright PD. Somatostatin, anaesthesia, and the carcinoid syndrome. Peri-operative administration of a somatostatin analogue to suppress carcinoid tumour activity. Anaesthesia 1987; 42(6):627–632.
42. Parris WC, Oates JA, Kambam J, et al. Pre-treatment with somatostatin in the anaesthetic management of a patient with carcinoid syndrome. Can J Anaesth 1988; 35(4):413–416.
43. Gray J, Jahr JS, Schneider P. Carcinoid syndrome and the anesthetic use of octreotide: a review. Am J Anesthesiol 1999; 26(8):377–380.
44. Kharrat HA, Taubin H. Carcinoid crisis induced by external manipulation of liver metastasis. J Clin Gastroenterol 2003; 36(1):87–88.
45. Öberg K, Kvols L, Caplin M, et al. Consensus report on the use of somatostatin analogs for the management of neuroendocrine tumors of the gastroenteropancreatic system. Ann Oncol 2004; 15:966–973.
46. Farling PA, Duairaju AK. Remifentanil and anaesthesia for carcinoid syndrome. Br J Anaesth 2004; 92(6):893–895.
47. Veall GR, Peacock JE, Bax ND, Reilly CS. Review of the anaesthetic management of 21 patients undergoing laparotomy for carcinoid syndrome. Br J Anaesth 1994; 72(3):335–341 (review).
48. Orbach-Zinger S, Lombroso R, Eidelman LA. Uneventful spinal anesthesia for a patient with carcinoid syndrome managed with long-acting octreotide. Can J Anaesth 2002; 49(7):678–681.
49. Zimmer C, Kienbaum P, Wiesernes R, Peters J. Somatostatin does not prevent serotonin release and flushing during chemoembolisation of carcinoid liver metastases. Anesthesiology 2003; 98:1007–1011.
50. Cortinez LI. Refractory hypotension during carcinoid resection surgery. Anaesthesia 2000; 55(5):489–518.
51. Hughes EW, Hodkinson BP. Carcinoid syndrome: the combined use of ketanserin and octreotide in the management of an acute crisis during anaesthesia. Anaesth Intensive Care 1989; 17(3):367–370.
52. Quaedvlieg PF, Lamers CB, Taal BG. Carcinoid heart disease: an update. Scand J Gastroenterol Suppl 2002; 236:66–71 (review).

19

Anesthesia for Pheochromocytoma Resection

Lennart Christiansson
Department of Anesthesiology, University Hospital, Uppsala, Sweden

INTRODUCTION

Less than 0.1% of all cases of hypertension are caused by pheochromocytomas. Nevertheless, these tumors are clearly important to the anesthetist because a significant number of hospital deaths in patients with pheochromocytoma occur during the induction of anesthesia for resection or during operative procedures for other causes (1). In a recent case report (2), an undiagnosed pheochromocytoma was considered to be "the anesthesiologist's nightmare." The author of an editorial (3) asks the rhetorical question whether pheochromocytoma are specialist cases that all must be prepared to treat. The management of this tumor is analogous to that of malignant hyperthermia, a disease now well understood and manageable with modern protocols. Comparably, the perioperative fatality rate for pheochromocytomas has dropped considerably over the last decades. The increasing use of very sensitive tests for metabolites of circulating catecholamines in combination with genetic screening will bring down the number of unsuspected cases admitted for surgery. Furthermore, improvements in the localization of tumors have accompanied surgical advances. How anesthetic management of patients with pheochromocytomas has advanced over the last four decades is described in several reviews (4–17).

Ever since the introduction of pretreatment with phentolamine in the early 1950s and the α-antagonist phenoxybenzamine (18) in the late 1960s, intraoperative handling has been refined. The perioperative mortality rate for elective resection of pheochromocytomas has been reduced from about 25% to 0–3% today, but for undiagnosed or ill-prepared patients, mortality can still be as high as 50% (1,9). The plethora of vasoactive drugs in use makes it obvious that we still have not reached consensus. Most experts agree that we intraoperatively have to protect the patient against a hypertensive crisis. The evidence base, however, for how long (if at all) to treat prior to surgery and which drugs to use is still sadly lacking.

Controlled studies dealing with pheochromocytoma issues are rare. However, several retrospective studies (15,19–22) analyze the perianesthetic risks and outcomes for patients who underwent pheochromocytoma surgery in the time between 1964 and 2001 at tertiary centers in Europe and the United States. Very few perioperative deaths were reported, a fact particularly noteworthy as no pretreatment with α-adrenergic blockers was used in the first study of 102 patients (19) and in 29 of 63 patients in the second study (20). It is claimed that zero mortality can be achieved even without pretreatment. Consistent finding in these studies was that control of blood volume and active use of vasodilating drugs, short-acting β-blockers and vasopressors, had the greatest impact on outcome, whereas the type of anesthetic was of secondary importance. Preoperative systolic blood pressure, increased levels of urinary metanephrines, and prolonged anesthesia (large tumor size) were found to be independent risk factors. Despite pretreatment, a considerable number of patients experienced intraoperative hemodynamic lability. The improved outcome (fewer deaths and major morbidity) was in these studies attributed not only to the perioperative handling and monitoring of the circulation, but also to improved technology for tumor localization and surgical techniques, allowing less tumor manipulation. In a long-term follow-up of 121 patients who underwent surgery between 1950 and 1997, mortality was linked to age at primary surgery, cardiovascular disease, and unrelated malignancies. The only pheochromocytoma-related risk factor for death was the preoperative level of urinary-secreted methoxycatecholamines (23).

TUMOR BIOLOGY, DIAGNOSIS, AND TREATMENT

Tumor Biology and Genetics

The word "pheochromocytoma" is derived from the Greek words for dusky (phaios), color (chroma), and cell tumor (cytoma). This term was introduced by Pick in 1912, but the first description probably dates back to Frankel in 1886 (15). Excellent background information on most aspects of pheochromocytomas is found in recent reviews (24–28). Pheochromocytomas occur in both sexes, and the highest incidence is at 30 to 50 years of age. The incidence is about 1 to 2 per million per year, but the true incidence may in the future prove to be considerably higher when all "incidentalomas" are accounted for. Approximately 10% of the tumors are familial, either inherited as an autosomal-dominant trait or as part of a neoplastic endocrine syndrome (Table 1). Recent research developments have challenged the traditional "10% rule" (i.e., 10% malignant; 10% bilateral; 10% extra-adrenal, and of those 10% extra-abdominal; 10% not hypertensive; and 10% hereditary). The risk of malignancy substantially exceeds the 10% in patients with extra-adrenal disease and in carriers of the germ-line succinyl dehydrogenase (SDH) subunit B mutations (28).

The adrenal cortex and the medulla have separate embryologic origins. The medullary portion stems from the chromaffin ectodermal cells of the neural crest. Although usually found in the adrenal medulla, these vascular tumors can occur anywhere along the sympathetic adrenal axis, such as in the right atrium, the spleen, the broad ligament of the ovary, or the ganglia of Zuckerkandl at the bifurcation of the aorta. Pheochromocytomas and abdominal paragangliomas are catecholamine-producing tumors of the sympathetic nervous system (SNS), whereas head and neck paragangliomas (chemodectomas, glomus-, and carotid-body tumors) are nonsecreting tumors of parasympathetic origin (28).

The diagnosis of benign versus malignant cannot be determined by histologic appearance. It is instead dependent on whether metastases are present or not. Other prognostic factors are local invasiveness, tumor size, and DNA ploidy pattern (7). Malignancy is recognized in about 10% of pheochromocytomas, and in 15% to

Table 1 Hereditary Syndromes Associated with Pheochromocytomas

MEN type II A (RET-gene, chromosome 10) (Sipple syndrome)	Parathyroid adenoma or hyperplasia/ hyperparathyroidism
	Medullary carcinoma of thyroid pheochromocytoma; incidence 30–50% (often bilateral but very rarely malignant or extra-adrenal)
MEN type II B (RET-gene, chromosome 10)	Medullary carcinoma of thyroid (familial type)
	Mucosal neuromata
	Pheochromocytoma; incidence 30–50%
	Intestinal ganglioneuromas
	Marfanoid habitus
Von Hippel-Lindau syndrome (chromosome 3) (=retinal cerebellar hemangioblastomatosis)	Hemangioblastoma of the central nervous system
	Retinal angiomatosis
	Pheochromocytoma ($\leq$50% bilateral); incidence 15–25%
	Renal carcinoma
	Pancreatic and renal cysts
Von Recklinghausen (neurofibromatosis type 1-gene, chromosome 17)	Multiple neurofibromas
	Café-au-lait spots
	Pheochromocytoma (solitary); incidence 1–5%
Mutations of SDH (SDHB chromosome 1 or SDHD chromosome 11)	Familial paraganglioma syndrome (carotid body tumor)
	Pheochromocytoma; incidence $\leq$20%

Abbreviations: MEN, multiple endocrine neoplasia; SDH, succinyl dehydrogenase.

35% of abdominal paragangliomas. Metastases are most frequently found in the spine, lungs, liver, kidneys, or the central nervous system (CNS).

In patients with pheochromocytoma, blood pressure does not correlate directly with circulating catecholamines because sympathetic reflexes are intact. The activity of the SNS may even be enhanced because excessive amounts of norepinephrine are stored in its nerve terminals. This easier access of norepinephrine, released from the postganglionic neuron, can result in marked symptoms with relatively small increments in circulating catecholamines (16). As a consequence, any condition that leads to a stimulation of the SNS (e.g., anxiety or pain) results in excessive release of transmitter and an exaggerated physiologic response, which can be just as problematic as the unpredictable release of vasoactive hormones from the tumor itself. The eliciting situations in the operating room (e.g., invasive procedures, intubation, and incision) must be approached with caution, preparation, and vigilance (3).

Virtually all epinephrine-secreting tumors are adrenal in origin. This is because the converting enzyme, phenylethanolamine-*N*-methyltransferase (Fig. 1), is glucocorticoid dependent and found only in the adrenal gland and groups of adrenergic neurons in the CNS. Dopamine-secreting pheochromocytomas are very rare and should, if present, always raise suspicion of malignancy. In addition to catecholamines, pheochromocytomas produce a variety of hormones, such as enkephalins, neuropeptide Y, vasoactive intestinal peptide, gastrin, somatostatin, and adrenocorticotrophic hormone.

Secretion of norepinephrine normally causes hypertension, but when symptoms are those of hypermetabolism, epinephrine cosecretion should be suspected (4).

o L-TYROSINE
> *Tyrosine hydroxylase*
⇩ L-DOPA
> *L-aromatic amino acid decarboxylase*
⇩ DOPAMINE
> *Dopamine β-hydroxylase*
⇩ NOREPINEPHRINE (Noradrenaline)
> *Phenylethanolamine-N-methyltransferase*
⇩ EPINEPHRINE (Adrenaline)

Figure 1 The pathway of catecholamine synthesis.

The clinical features of the rare dopamine-secreting tumors are also of a nonspecific "inflammatory" or "hypermetabolic" nature, and the patients are not hypertensive (29). In pheochromocytoma, patients fasting blood glucose concentration is increased, and the tolerance curve is abnormal. High catecholamine concentrations lead to glycogenolysis, lipolysis, and inhibition of insulin release (α_1-agonism). In cases involving epinephrine, this effect is partly opposed by the β_2-agonistic promotion of insulin release (6).

Clinical Presentation

The classical triad of pheochromocytoma presentation is paroxysmal sweating, hypertension, and headache. Hypertension is sustained in 50% and paroxysmal in 30%, and blood pressure is normal in 20% of patients. In rare cases when mainly epinephrine or dopamine is secreted, orthostatic hypertension may be the presenting symptom (30). Further symptoms include weight loss, hyperglycemia, tachycardia or tachyarrhythmias, tremor, pallor, and flushing, depending on which catecholamine is secreted. Other clues to the diagnosis are hypertension, which is episodic (spells) or difficult to treat, glucose intolerance, nausea, palpitations, and problems with blood pressure in connection with induction of anesthesia, labor, abdominal examination, surgery, or other forms of stress. A pressor response to particular drugs can also suggest the presence of this tumor. These drugs include histamine, glucagon, droperidol, metoclopramide, tyramine (in food or wine), cytotoxic drugs, saralasin, tricyclic antidepressants and phenothiazines, cocaine, alcohol, ephedrine, ketamine, pancuronium, halothane, morphine, atracurium, and suxamethonium (1).

Mortality in pheochromocytoma is usually caused by a malignant hypertensive crisis with cerebrovascular accidents or dissecting aortic aneurysm, myocardial infarction, arrhythmias, heart failure, acute renal failure, or irreversible shock leading to multiple organ dysfunctions.

Diagnosis

Provocation or suppression tests are not often used in modern practice. In the common clinical setting, combined measurement of 24-hour urinary metanephrines and catecholamines may be the best screening, due to low likelihood of false-positive results. In patients at high risk of having pheochromocytoma, measurements of fractionated plasma metanephrines may be preferable, as its sensitivity approaches

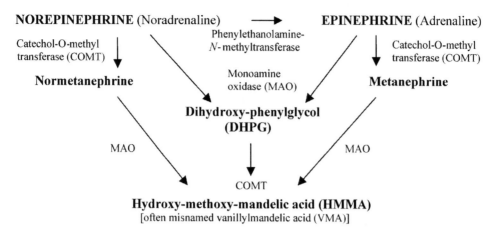

Figure 2 Catecholamine metabolism (simplified). *Abbreviations*: COMT, catechol-O-methyl transferase; MAO, monoamine oxidase.

100% (26). The introduction of high-pressure liquid chromatography to diagnostic methods has largely removed the problem of drug and dietary interference with results (15).

It is important to first appreciate that under normal conditions, catecholamines released by nerve cells are mainly subject to neuronal reuptake (24). Only minor amounts are metabolized or escape into circulation. The first step of metabolism (Fig. 2) is deamination, but in the adrenal medulla, where catechol-O-methyl transferase (COMT) is present, methylation results in the formation of metanephrines. Other intermediate metabolites undergo conjugation to glucuronides and sulfates that are excreted in the urine. Dopamine metabolism normally constitutes just a minor pathway (Fig. 3). A negative feedback mechanism regulates catecholamine synthesis via tyrosine hydroxylase in normal adrenal medullas, but not in pheochromocytomas where the enzyme activity also is much higher.

Variable secretion of catecholamines by tumors and the contribution of leakage to metabolism explain the much stronger relationship of tumor mass to levels of metabolites than the catecholamines themselves. In contrast to sympathetic nerves, pheochromocytoma cells contain both monoamine oxidase (MAO) and high concentrations of membrane-bound COMT. The latter explains the abundance of methylated free metanephrine in plasma from these patients. This considerable production of metanephrines provides a much more sensitive diagnostic signal than other

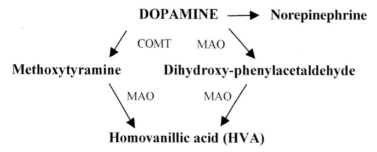

Figure 3 Dopamine metabolism (simplified). *Abbreviations*: COMT, catechol-O-methyl transferase; MAO, monoamine oxidase.

pheochromocytoma-derived catecholamine metabolites. The continuous intratumoral production of metanephrines makes possible the detection of pheochromocytomas in patients with normal plasma or urinary levels of catecholamines.

After the diagnosis of pheochromocytoma is confirmed by biochemical testing, imaging techniques are employed for tumor localization. These techniques include magnetic resonance imaging (MRI), computed tomography (CT), iodinated meta-iodobenzylguanidine scanning (^{131}I-MIBG), or ^{111}In-DTPA-octreotide somatostatin-receptor scintigraphy. Increased knowledge of the expression of specific catecholamine transport and storage systems by pheochromocytoma cells provides the basis for the scintigraphic imaging techniques, and has led more recently to the development of several positron emission tomography ligands.

Pheochromocytomas are typically large tumors (2–5 cm in diameter) and may contain areas of hemorrhage or necrosis. Tumors in hereditary syndromes tend to be smaller and bilateral. About 98% of the tumors are intra-abdominal and 90% originate within the adrenal gland (29). CT has good sensitivity, 93% to 100%, for detecting adrenal pheochromocytomas, but sensitivity decreases for extra-adrenal tumors. MRI is superior to CT for detecting extra-adrenal tumors and is also used as method of choice in pregnant patients (13). MIBG scans are often negative for the very rare dopamine-secreting tumors, and so are routine biochemical tests. Dopamine has to be specifically measured in these cases.

Medical Treatment

Somatostatin receptors are expressed on pheochromocytoma tumor cells. Octreotide has antisecretory potential (Chapter 18) in various endocrine tumors and has been tested for its inhibiting capacity in pheochromocytoma. The results have been ambiguous, however. Patients who show positive testing for somatostatin receptors and positive scintigraphy may benefit from somatostatin-targeted chemotherapy.

Medical treatment is used mainly in the preparation for surgery. Chemotherapy (cyclophosphamide, vincristine, and dacarbazine) has been tried for inoperable tumors. Irradiation with radiolabeled MIBG was used for malignant tumors with or without metastases. Even with good initial regression of tumors, no long-lasting effects could be shown so far for either approach (16).

Metyrosine (α-methylparatyrosine) inhibits tyrosine hydroxylase and may decrease catecholamine synthesis by up to 80%. It is very effective but used mainly in malignant or inoperable cases because of the many side effects (sedative fatigue, anxiety, depression, extrapyramidal signs, and tremor).

Surgery

The treatment of choice for adrenal tumor in general is surgical resection, once the tumor has reached a certain size (>3–5 cm) and becomes symptomatic, or if imaging, genetic testing, or history is suspicious for malignancy (31). For secreting pheochromocytomas, less invasive techniques, such as arterial embolization, chemoembolization, cryotherapy, and radiofrequency ablation, are normally not considered safe to use, because the circulatory effects can be difficult to control.

Traditionally open surgery was performed, but since the first report of laparoscopic adrenalectomy for pheochromocytoma in 1992, practices have changed. Several studies have shown that the two techniques are comparable with regard to intraoperative hemodynamic changes, but the postoperative recovery is faster for the laparoscopic approach (32–34). In many centers, laparoscopic adrenalectomy is the preferred technique for pheochromocytomas and all other benign tumors of up to a size of 6 to 8 cm (35–37). However, hand-assisted laparoscopy has been used to remove pheochromocytomas as large as 15 cm. Adrenocortical-sparing surgery may be performed using laparoscopy in patients with hereditary forms of pheochromocytoma (38).

The laparoscopic technique has also been used with success in patients who presented with malignant hypertension and acute heart failure. A release of noradrenaline was elicited by pneumoperitoneum, but hypertension could be controlled safely even in this type of patients (39). However there are also reports on how pneumoperitoneum can cause massive noradrenaline release leading to acute heart failure, despite treatment with α_1-, β-, and calcium channel blockers (40).

Catecholamine-Induced Cardiomyopathy

The sustained norepinephrine release will lead to hypertrophic cardiomyopathy in 20% to 30% of the patients, the condition being at least partially reversible by the use of adrenergic blockade and tumor removal. Patients may present with symptoms ranging from palpitations and nonspecific electrocardiogram (ECG) changes to severe dysrhythmias and congestive heart failure. The myocardial dysfunction may be secondary to activation (or down regulation) of adrenoreceptors, coronary vasospasm, or relative ischemia due to hypertrophy and increased myocardial oxygen demands (8). Even young patients are at risk of developing myocardial ischemia or sustaining a myocardial infarction (41). Microscopy shows interstitial edema, hemorrhage, and inflammatory infiltrates. The criteria for myocarditis are normally not met. The myocytes show contraction-band necrosis, and later fibrosis and calcification may follow (6). Intracellular calcium overload appears to be the main abnormality involved (42).

Both hypertrophic and dilated cardiomyopathies have been reported as complications of pheochromocytoma. The latter might worsen in the perioperative period in which case congestive heart failure ensues. With tailored vasoactive support, cardiac failure may resolve within a week and the cardiomyopathy will, to some extent, reverse over a few months (13,43). In most cases, left ventricular hypertrophy due to norepinephrine-induced hypertension is associated with this condition. The many exceptions to this rule have led to speculations whether congestive cardiomyopathy and nonhypertrophic malignant hypertension are linked to tumors mainly secreting adrenaline rather than noradrenaline (44).

Pheochromocytoma in Pregnancy

This condition is associated with considerable morbidity and mortality. In a retrospective study, maternal mortality was 17% and fetal loss 26%. With antepartum diagnosis, the former was reduced to 0% and fetal loss to 15% (45). The tumor should be excised during the first trimester, or fetal maturity is awaited so that cesarean section can be performed followed by adrenalectomy (46).

Aside from the classical presentation, pregnant women with pheochromocytomas complain more frequently of headaches, palpitation, sweating, and dyspnea. The condition may be confused with preeclampsia. Pheochromocytomas should be suspected in any pregnant patient who develops hypertension before 20 weeks of gestation, without concomitant proteinuria, and whose hypertension is unusual or labile. After biochemical confirmation of diagnosis, ultrasonography and MRI can be safely employed for tumor localization in pregnancy. Most α-adrenergic blockers cross the placenta, but have been shown to be safe. β-blockers can also be used for pretreatment as required. Sodium nitroprusside is associated with decreased placental perfusion, acidosis, and cyanide accumulation in the fetus (14). Nitroglycerin and magnesium are considered ideal agents for intraoperative blood pressure control in the pregnant with pheochromocytoma (46).

Pediatric Aspects

Pheochromocytoma is a rare tumor in children accounting for 10% of the annual incidence of approximately 2 per million in the general population. Children are more likely to have tumors that are bilateral, multiple, and/or extra-adrenal, but the incidence of malignancy appears to be lower. The associated hypertension is more commonly sustained than in adults (47). Neuroblastomas are rare malignant tumors, predominantly occurring in childhood. They can secrete catecholamines, and, even if the likelihood of a severe hypertensive reaction to tumors manipulation is much less, the preparedness should be the same as for pheochromocytoma. In a very interesting case report, a five-year-old boy with pheochromocytoma is described (48). On admission, there was a six months history of paroxysmal symptoms, sustained hypertension (186/126 mmHg), tachycardia, retinopathy, and left ventricular hypertrophy. During surgery, the hemodynamic changes were accompanied by a spectacular rise in body temperature to 40°C. The author discusses the mechanisms by which pyrexia can be an early sign of a developing "pheochromocytoma multisystem crisis." The hyperpyrexia is thought to be induced by the release of interleukin-6 and tumor necrosis factor in combination with hypermetabolism and impaired heat loss during catecholamine secretion (cutaneous vasoconstriction).

Phenoxybenzamine is used for preoperative blood pressure control, but the criteria for normalization or end points for the treatment are less well defined in children (47). In a retrospective study of 16 consecutive pediatric patients with pheochromocytomas, α-antagonists were used for pretreatment with good results, either alone or in combination with β-blockers or calcium channels blockers (49). There are reports of successful perioperative use of clonidine in children. From a theoretical standpoint, the properties of α2-agonists should be ideal in the management of pheochromocytoma (47). Referring to the suppression test, it is questionable whether clonidine will have the anticipated effect (inhibition of norepinephrine release) or not in pheochromocytoma patients. There are surprisingly few reports of their use in adults. The drugs best documented for intraoperative blood pressure control in children are sodium nitroprusside and magnesium sulfate (47). Esmolol has reportedly been effective in treating both hypertension and tachyarrhythmias. Even for children, invasive arterial and central venous monitoring is considered mandatory. If possible, the arterial line should be inserted under local anesthesia and sedation prior to induction. There are also reports on the use of pulmonary artery catheters and peroperative echocardiography. Laparoscopic adrenalectomy has been described in children, and the hypertensive response to the creation of pneumoperitoneum was the same as for adults, and it was managed with nicardipine, esmolol, or magnesium (47,50).

ANESTHETIC AND PERIOPERATIVE ASPECTS

Examination should aim to uncover any signs of pheochromocytoma sequelae. Liberal use of echocardiography may detect cardiomyopathy. Asymptomatic cardiac dysfunction impacts on both selection and duration of pretreatment and intraoperative management. If catecholamine secretion remains uncontrolled, a life-threatening crisis may develop (51). The pressor effect will cause end-organ damage, such as hypertensive encephalopathy and cardiomyopathy. Since the introduction of aggressive antihypertensive treatment, this crisis is far less commonly seen, but during surgery and other tumor interventions, one always has to be prepared to give additional acute treatment (6). The events of greatest concern are anesthesia induction, insufflation of pneuomoperitoneum, tumor manipulation, and loss of endogenous catecholamine stimulation in combination with residual α_1-adrenergic blockade after tumor removal.

Tumor manipulation is the main risk factor during adrenalectomy because large amounts of catecholamines are released into the circulation, with plasma concentration in some patients exceeding normal values by a factor of more than 1000. Although specific anesthetic drugs have been recommended, the most important factors still are optimal preoperative preparation, gentle induction of anesthesia, and good communication between the surgeon and anesthesiologist. Virtually all anesthetic drugs and techniques (including isoflurane, sevoflurane, sufentanil, remifentanil, fentanyl, and regional anesthesia) have been used with satisfactorily results (1). Theoretically, desflurane might cause sympathetic stimulation and crisis, though this has not been reported.

Preoperative Optimization

α-Adrenergic Blockade

The α-adrenergic blocker phenoxybenzamine became the standard drug for pretreatment soon after the publication of the first series of patients in 1967 (18). However, the drug has two characteristics that make it less than ideal.

First, it is a nonselective α-blocker, so it prevents both the presynaptic α_2-mediated inhibition of catecholamine release and the postsynaptic α_1-mediated vasoconstriction. The increased release of norepinephrine at adrenergic terminals may become a problem in patients with marginal coronary perfusion. Thus, most patients treated with phenoxybenzamine need simultaneous β-adrenergic blockade. The same logic is applied if the tumor is secreting clinically relevant amounts of adrenaline. In patients with severe cardiomyopathy, however, β-blockade has been shown to precipitate cardiac failure (6).

Secondly, phenoxybenzamine is a noncompetitive inhibitor that binds covalently to the α-receptor. This causes more frequent and more resistant postoperative hypotension of longer duration than other alternative therapies. The plasma half-life of phenoxybenzamine is 24 hours, and the drug should therefore be withheld for at least 12 hours before surgery. Common side effects of nonselective α-blockade include postural hypotension, reflex tachycardia, headache, somnolence, constipation, dry mouth, stuffy nose, and nausea (13).

No controlled, randomized, prospective clinical studies have investigated the value of pretreatment with adrenergic receptor–blocking drugs. It is often forgotten that the use of phenoxybenzamine in the original publication (18) was for three days only, prior to surgery. These drugs probably reduce the incidence of hypertensive crisis, the wide blood pressure fluctuations during manipulation of the tumor, and the myocardial dysfunction that occur perioperatively. The reduction in perioperative mortality (from ~50% to the current 0–6%) is often used as an indirect proof of its efficacy. α-adrenergic receptor blockade restores plasma volume by counteracting the vasoconstrictive effects of high levels of catecholamines. The efficacy of therapy should be judged by the reduction in symptoms and stabilization of blood pressure. For patients who exhibit ST-T changes on ECG, long-term (one to six months) preoperative α-adrenergic receptor blockade has produced ECG normalization and clinical resolution of catecholamine-induced cardiomyopathy (52). The optimal duration of preoperative therapy with phenoxybenzamine has not been studied. Criteria for the treatment have been recommended (1). Accordingly, one should aim at a blood pressure of not higher than 165/90 mmHg and with orthostatic hypotension present. The ECG should be free of ST-T changes that are not permanent and of frequent premature ventricular contractions or symptomatic arrhythmia.

There is still dogmatic insistence on the use of phenoxybenzamine for at least two weeks preoperatively, although many experts find a shorter treatment period adequate. The length of treatment can be tailored to the patient's condition (3). A few days of treatment to allow regulation of adrenergic receptors is sufficient for some, whereas prolonged treatment may be necessary to facilitate remodeling in case of severe hypertrophy of the heart or cardiac dysfunction. Some authors concluded that advances in anesthetic and monitoring techniques and the availability of fast-acting drugs capable of correcting sudden changes in cardiovascular variables have eliminated the need for the use of phenoxybenzamine or other drugs to produce profound and long-lasting α-blockade (20,21). In one study (53), patients who were treated with phenoxybenzamine for more than 10 days did not have better perioperative stability than patients who had treatment for less than a week. Neither did the degree of postural hypotension after pretreatment predict operative stability. Alternative drugs should be considered for pretreatment of patients with congestive heart failure, in whom α-adrenergic blockade leads to tachycardia and β-adrenergic blockade diminishes cardiac performance (13). In a report of two complicated cases, it is pointed out how important it is that the anesthesiologist carefully monitors the end points of the patients pretreatment and alerts the team of potential factors that may impact the intraoperative course (54).

When comparing two series of patients, doxazosin was found to be as effective as phenoxybenzamine in controlling arterial pressure and heart rate both before and after surgery. Doxazosin, a selective and competitive blocker, also had fewer undesirable side effects (55). No significant differences were found in the operative and postoperative blood pressure control and plasma volume when three groups of patients with phenoxybenzamine, prazosin, or doxazosin pretreatment were compared (56). In another study, doxazosin used either alone or in combination with a β-blocker produced excellent hemodynamic control with only minor and transient adverse reactions (57). If patients were not hypertensive before surgery, no blockade of any form was instituted (58). Recently, intravenous (IV) use of the selective α_1-receptor blocker urapidil ($t\frac{1}{2}$ is three hours) for pretreatment was described. The drug replaced prazosin and bisoprolol for three days before surgery, and was maintained throughout anesthesia. Hypertensive peaks were handled with boluses of nicardipine and esmolol as required. It was concluded that it was safe to use urapidil for perioperative control of blood pressure (59).

Calcium Channel Blockade

Several calcium channel blockers have been tried in the preoperative preparation of pheochromocytoma. More than 20 years ago, a case was reported where nifedipine was used for pretreatment of a patient with hypertrophic cardiomyopathy (60).

In another case, diltiazem was used preoperatively in a patient with hypertensive crisis due to hepatic metastases from a pheochromocytoma. Intraoperatively, great fluctuations in blood pressure were noted (61). In a study of 113 patients, calcium channel blockers were used as the primary mode of antihypertensive therapy with good result. Selective α-antagonists were added only if the hypertension was not adequately controlled. A β-blocker was used, where a cardiac dysrhythmia was noted.

One of the most effective calcium channel blockers appears to be nicardipine. In several series of patients, pretreatment with nicardipine was successful with little need for additional drugs to control hypertension and without the risk of prolonged hypotension after tumor removal (33,62,63). However, the putative mechanism—prevention of increased free plasma catecholamine levels—could not be demonstrated (63). Calcium channel blockers also proved safe in laparoscopic adrenalectomy when comparing with groups treated with α-blocker and/or β-blocker (32). In a retrospectively studied series of more than 100 patients, the use of nicardipine (pre- and peroperative) was associated with low mortality and morbidity even when not all hemodynamic changes were prevented (64).

β-Adrenergic Blockade

β-adrenergic receptor blockade has been suggested for patients who have persistent arrhythmias or tachycardia (often epinephrine or dopamine secretion), because these conditions can be precipitated or aggravated by nonselective α-adrenergic receptor blockade. Similarly, nonselective β-blockade, when given before α-blockade in cases of norepinephrine-secreting tumors, can give rise to an unopposed vasoconstrictor effect. This can increase the risk of dangerous hypertension. The same phenomenon can occur when labetalol is used (65).

The short-acting β-blocker esmolol has been successfully used in combination with sodium nitroprusside to control circulation during surgery for pheochromocytoma (66). Onset is rapid and its effect largely reversed within 30 minutes. Recently, the use of landiolol, an even shorter-acting and more highly β_1-selective adrenergic blocker, was reported for treating intraoperative tachyarrhythmias (67).

Metyrosine (See Medical Treatment)

Tumors secreting adrenaline, and, in particular, dopamine, are very rare. In non-hypertensive patients with adrenaline or dopamine-secreting pheochromocytomas, no preoperative α-antagonists are given (68) because they can worsen the situation (unopposed β-adrenergic activity). If pretreatment is necessary for arrhythmias or other symptoms that do not respond to β-blockers, metyrosine can be tried, because it blocks the conversion of tyrosine to the dopamine precursor dihydroxyphenylalanine.

Magnesium

Although magnesium sulphate has been used for preoperative preparation, its main application is intraoperatively. This drug is described further in the section on intraoperative management.

Intraoperative Management

Premedication

All usual preoperative medication should be continued, but phenoxybenzamine (if used) is normally stopped the day before surgery. Avoiding stress is very important in these patients, and a benzodiazepine is a good choice for anxiolysis. All drugs known to release histamine are best avoided, as are droperidol and metoclopramide.

Monitoring

Intra-arterial pressure recording should be started, and a large-bore venous catheter inserted, prior to induction of anesthesia, and continued into the postoperative period. A central venous line is mandatory for safe administration of IV vasoactive drugs. Central venous pressure monitoring can be helpful for guiding volume replacement during surgery. For patients with catecholamine-induced cardiomyopathy or any other symptomatic cardiac dysfunction monitoring may include cardiac output monitoring or transesophageal echocardiography. Measurements of cardiac output, filling pressures, and vascular resistance can give valuable information, when myocardial compliance and vascular capacity are altered and circulating blood volume difficult to estimate. Arterial blood gases and glucose concentration need to be checked regularly. Monitoring of ventilation, urine output, and body temperature are all part of routine setup.

Induction

Most routine techniques can be used, but drugs known to have the capacity to set free histamine are best avoided. Halothane sensitizes the myocardium to the effects of catecholamines and may thus have proarrhythmogenic properties. A combination of propofol and a short-acting opioid is considered safe, and lidocaine is often added. For muscle relaxation, vecuronium and cisatracurium have theoretical advantages. Depolarizing relaxants increase intra-abdominal pressure, which might trigger catecholamine release from the tumor. For rapid sequence induction, one should, therefore, consider either using rocuronium or suxamethonium with precurarization. Ketamine should be avoided. Glycopyrrolate would be the first choice of anticholinergic agent because atropine can elicit tachycardia.

Maintenance

The most common technique to use is balanced anesthesia with an inhalational agent, an opioid, and a nondepolarizing muscle relaxant. Isoflurane, sevoflurane, nitrous oxide, fentanyl, sufentanil, alfentanil, remifentanil, and propofol are all considered being safe. Isoflurane in combination with nitrous oxide has been used together with an infusion of sufentanil 0.5 µg/kg/hr (69). Another author concluded that alfentanil is a good choice of drug, having a rapid onset of action, good vasodilating properties, and a short elimination halftime (6). The dosage was 25 mg/hr for the first 15 minutes as a bolus and was followed up by a continuous infusion of 4 mg/hr. Replacing the volatile anesthetic with a propofol infusion appears to be equally safe. Modern short-acting opioids (particularly remifentanil) have successfully been tried as alternatives to the standard drug fentanyl. Remifentanil can be combined with propofol, with an inhalational agent or to top-up a thoracic epidural analgesia that for hemodynamic reasons is not fully activated.

Nowadays many adrenalectomies are performed with laparoscopic technique, and epidural blocks are often not necessary. For open resections, regional anesthesia can be used in the same way as in most patients having major abdominal surgery. Preoperative placement of epidural catheters can cause dramatic increases in sympathetic activity. Good local anesthesia and proper sedation must therefore be provided.

The epidural catheter should be inserted at a thoracic level that provides congruent analgesia. Routine testing is recommended. The circulatory consequences should be minimized to avoid confusion with hemodynamic changes that occur during tumor manipulations. It might be safer to use relatively more opioid than local anesthetic for the neuraxial block. If it becomes necessary to treat hypotension, an α_1-agonist with direct action (noradrenaline, phenylephrine, and methoxamine) should be used. If circulation is stable toward the end of the operation, the depth of the epidural block can be increased with a local anesthetic. In accordance with experience from thoracic procedures and upper gastrointestinal surgery, in general, good analgesia at emergence facilitates fast-track extubation and may possibly improve outcome.

Hypertensive Crisis

Pheochromocytoma crisis ranges from severe hypertension, circulatory failure, pulmonary edema, acute myocardial infarction, and encephalopathy to multiple organ dysfunctions. The reported mortality is very high (70). The anesthetist has to be fully prepared to intervene and to have an armory of vasoactive drugs readily available. Because of ease of use, many prefer to give sodium nitroprusside or nitroglycerin to curtail hypertensive episodes. Phentolamine is not an ideal agent because it has too long onset time and duration of action (1). Calcium channel blockers are thought to inhibit the release of catecholamine from tumor cells by blocking calcium entry, and may possibly prevent catecholamine-induced vasospasm (7). Nicardipine is a good vasodilator when given as an infusion at a rate of 1 to 3 μg/kg/min. If insufficient response is noted, a short-acting β-blocker (esmolol; $t_{\frac{1}{2}} \sim 9$ minutes) is given, and, if necessary, a vasodilator is started as well. For patients in cardiac failure or with ventricular arrhythmias, lidocaine is possibly a better alternative. Two recent additions to the therapeutic options, magnesium and adenosine, will be described in greater detail below.

Magnesium

Magnesium is a common enzyme cofactor and as such involved in gating of calcium channels, ion fluxes, neuromuscular activity, control of vasomotor tone, and cardiac excitability. 1 g of magnesium sulfate is equivalent to 4 mmol, 8 mEq, or 98 mg of elemental magnesium. Normal concentrations are assumed to be approximately 0.7 to 1 mmol/L, and the therapeutic range is in the region of 2 to 4 mmol/L. Magnesium interacts with storage and release of catecholamines from the adrenal medulla and peripheral adrenergic nerve endings (71).

The use of magnesium in eclampsia is well documented, but its use has also been extensively studied in cardiology (reperfusion and arrhythmias). In pheochromocytoma, magnesium is used (since 1985) as an antiarrhythmic vasodilator, and because of its antiadrenergic effect, that is either direct or indirect, via calcium antagonism on the level of binding sites within channel pores. This helps preserving adenosine triphosphate (ATP) and glycogen stores in general and limits lactate production in the myocardium. It is important to note that its use is associated with increased sedation and muscular weakness that can prolong postoperative ventilation (8).

Magnesium has also been used successfully in patients presenting with pheochromocytoma crisis with either hypertensive encephalopathy or catecholamine-induced cardiomyopathy. The doses given was 40 to 60 mg/kg for loading plus an infusion of 2 g/hr with further boluses of 20 mg/kg as required. The total perioperative dose ranged from 8 to 18 g (70). Another author combined epidural analgesia with magnesium sulfate for the perioperative treatment of a pheochromocytoma patient with severe coronary artery disease. This was the first reported use of magnesium for this kind of surgery in the United States (72). In a case report of a patient who stopped phenoxybenzamine because of side effects, preoperative preparation of less than one day was described using a combination of labetalol and magnesium sulfate. It was also used for hemodynamic control during surgery with good stability reported (73).

Adenosine and Adenosine Triphosphate

Adenosine has a global role as a paracrine homeostatic regulator, and its physiological responses are depending on receptor subtype ($A_1/A_{2A-B}/A_3$), metabolic state of the tissue, tonus of the SNS, and whether the administration is endogenous or exogenous and if the person studied is awake or anesthetized. In ischemic tissue, adenosine decreases oxygen demand (A_1) and increases its oxygen supply (A_{2A}) via vasodilation. In the cardiovascular system, adenosine is not only a potent vasodilator, but also has antiarrhythmic and negative chronotropic effects. Adenosine is either hydrolyzed from ATP/adenosine diphosphate/adenosine monophosphate or converted from adenosylhomocysteine (74). In the pulmonary circulation, adenosine can produce both vasoconstriction and relaxation depending on basal tone of the blood vessels (75). Dipyridamole is an adenosine uptake inhibitor, and some of its effects can be explained by changes in adenosine concentration. Adenosine receptor agonists attenuate the stimulatory effects of catecholamines on the heart and inhibit norepinephrine release from nerve terminals (76,77).

During anesthesia, adenosine causes dose-dependent hypotension, due to inadequate sympathetic reflex response. In an interesting study of healthy awake volunteers, adenosine caused systemic vasodilation, paralleled by a reflex increase in cardiac output at infusion rates of up to 80 μg/kg/min (78). Mean blood pressure was unaffected, but the pulse pressure increased. Adenosine infusion has been successfully used for controlled hypotension in cerebral aneurysm surgery (79,80). No tachyphylaxis or rebound hypertension was noted, as compared to sodium nitroprusside. The plasma half-life of adenosine is less than 10 seconds. Its use in pheochromocytoma surgery was first described in 1988 (81). An infusion of 50 to 500 μg/kg/min during inhalational anesthesia could control rapid elevation of blood pressure in all 10 patients. In the absence of arrhythmias, no β-blockers or other additional drugs were required. The same approach has also been used during resection of a norepinephrine-secreting neuroblastoma in a child (82). The combined use of ATP and sevoflurane anesthesia for pheochromocytoma resection was reported in 1989 (83). Recently a very interesting review was published on the use of ATP in conjunction with magnesium chloride in intensive care (84). Potentially beneficial effects, noted in several (mainly experimental) studies, were presented for the ischemia-reperfusion and sepsis-organ failure complex. The authors also speculated that ATP–$MgCl_2$ might be suitable for the control of acute pulmonary hypertension and blood pressure during aortic crossclamping.

Hypotension

It is important to distinguish the postligation fall in blood pressure from hypovolemia, anaphylactic shock, or hypotension caused by histamine release. Initial management includes fluid therapy and α_1-agonistic vasopressors. For treatment of hypotension or any other symptom of withdrawal, it is logical to use the same catecholamine after ligation as was endogenously secreted by the tumor. This can occasionally be epinephrine or dopamine, but normally either norepinephrine or phenylephrine hydrochloride is used to treat hypotension. One must be prepared that the initially required dose can be much higher than what is normally used. This is not often the case, but it sometimes happens when the patient is deeply blocked with phenoxybenzamine. One further vasopressor that works via a different mechanism should be available (e.g., arginine-vasopressin). An antihistamine and a corticosteroid should also be kept ready for IV use. Calcium chloride may be needed to improve cardiovascular responsiveness, if calcium channel blockers or magnesium were used, and, in particular, if it was in combination with inhalational anesthesia.

Arrhythmia

The most commonly occurring pheochromocytoma-associated rhythm disturbances intraoperatively are tachycardias and tachyarrhythmias. The main treatment objective is to reduce catecholamine stress, and β-blockers are thus the first-line drugs in tachycardia and supraventricular tachyarrhythmias. In unresponsive cases, trying amiodarone can be justified. If the arrhythmia is of ventricular origin, or if the patient has cardiac dysfunction or congestive failure, lidocaine has traditionally been preferred. However, experience is growing with the use of magnesium, and this drug may well prove to be an even safer option.

Blood Glucose Control

Hyperglycemia is common owing to the metabolic effects of catecholamines. This situation can occur even in the absence of obvious adrenergic stress. The response to insulin treatment is usually less than normal because of increased glucose production and peripheral insulin resistance.

A drop in blood glucose levels in the postligation period is thought to result from insulin production being freed from the inhibitory effects of catecholamine excess. This effect is intensified by a concurrent use of a nonselective β-blocker, such as propranolol (6). Infusion of glucose-containing solutions will be necessary at this stage of the operation, with continuation into the postoperative phase.

Postoperative Care and Analgesia

Pheochromocytoma patients should be observed in a high dependency or intensive care unit postoperatively. Intraoperative fluid shifts may still warrant advanced monitoring and continued correction. With good pain relief provided and normothermia maintained, most patients are expected to be extubated in the operating room or as a fast-track procedure. Analgesia is probably best achieved with a patient-controlled opioid system or a continuous regional block. For neuraxial blocks, a mixture of fentanyl with low concentration of bupivacaine or ropivacaine can provide safe analgesia.

Most important in the management of the circulation is the correct interpretation of hemodynamic changes, so that fluid requirement can be balanced against vasomotor tone. The aim is to maintain normal circulating blood volume, but if the patient still requires a vasopressor infusion, this can normally be tapered off over a few hours. In the exceptional case, regeneration and/or re-regulation of α-receptors may take one to two days. Some patients leave the operating theater with no adrenocortical function and require replacement therapy from the outset (6). In many treatment protocols, a dexamethasone test is advocated as part of preoperative investigations. It is also important to continue the monitoring for hypoglycemia.

As with all such specialist procedures, best results for pheochromocytoma surgery are obtained by concentrating cases into specialist centers. With attention to detail, anesthesia for pheochromocytoma can be safely performed as a routine with low morbidity and mortality.

REFERENCES

1. Roizen MF, Fleisher LA. Anesthetic implications of concurrent diseases. In: Miller RD, ed. Anesthesia. 6th ed. Philadelphia, Pennsylvania: Churchill Livingstone, 2004.
2. Myklejord DJ. Undiagnosed pheochromocytoma: the anesthesiologist nightmare. Clin Med Res 2004; 2(1):59–62.
3. Bogdonoff DL. Pheochromocytoma: specialist cases that all must be prepared to treat? J Cardiothorac Vasc Anesth 2002; 16(3):267–269 (editorial).
4. Schull LG, Bailey JC. Anesthesia for patients having pheochromocytoma. Anesth Analg 1960; 39:400–408.
5. Bingham W, Elliott J, Lyons SM. Management of anaesthesia for phaeochromocytoma. Anaesthesia 1972; 27(1):49–60.
6. Hull CJ. Phaeochromocytoma. Diagnosis, preoperative preparation and anaesthetic management. Br J Anaesth 1986; 58(12):1453–1468 (review).
7. Werbel SS, Ober KP. Pheochromocytoma. Update on diagnosis, localization and management. Med Clin North Am 1995; 79(1):131–153.
8. O'Riordan JA. Pheochromocytomas and anesthesia. Int Anesthesiol Clin 1997; 35(4): 99–127 (review).
9. Singh G, Kam P. An overview of anaesthetic issues in phaeochromocytoma. Ann Acad Med Singapore 1998; 27:843–848 (review).
10. Walther MM, Keiser HR, Linehan WM. Pheochromocytoma: evaluation, diagnosis, and treatment. World J Urol 1999; 17(1):35–39 (review).
11. Prys-Roberts C. Pheochromocytoma-recent progress in its management. Br J Anaesth 2000; 85:44–57.
12. Pacak K, Linehan WM, Eisenhofer G, et al. Recent advances in genetics, diagnosis, localization and treatment of pheochromocytoma. Ann Intern Med 2001; 134:315–329.
13. Kinney MAO, Narr BJ, Warner MA. Perioperative management of pheochromocytoma. J Cardiothorac Vasc Anesth 2002; 16(3):359–369 (review).
14. Jalbout M, Siddik-Sayyid S, Baraka A. Perianesthetic management of patients undergoing resection of pheochromocytoma. Middle East J Anesthesiol 2003; 17(3):329–346 (review).
15. Williams DT, Dann S, Wheeler MH. Phaeochromocytoma—views on current management. Eur J Surg Oncol 2003; 29(6):483–490. Erratum in: Eur J Surg Oncol 2003; 29(10):933.
16. Bravo EL, Tagle R. Pheochromocytoma: state-of-the-art and future prospects. Endocr Rev 2003; 24(4):539–553.
17. Connery LE, Coursin DB. Assessment and therapy of selected endocrine disorders. Anesthesiol Clin North Am 2004; 22(1):93–123 (review).
18. Ross EJ, Prichard BNC, Kaufman L, et al. Preoperative and operative management of patients with phaeochromocytoma. BMJ 1967; 1:191–198.
19. Desmonts JM, le Houelleur J, Remond P, Duvaldestin P. Anaesthetic management of patients with phaeochromocytoma. A review of 102 cases. Br J Anaesth 1977; 49(10): 991–998.

20. Boutros AR, Bravo EL, Zanettin G, Straffon RA. Perioperative management of 63 patients with pheochromocytoma. Cleve Clin J Med 1990; 57:613–617.
21. Kinney MA, Warner ME, vanHeerden JA, et al. Perianesthetic risks and outcomes of pheochromocytoma and paraganglioma resection. Anesth Analg 2000; 91(5):1118–1123.
22. Plouin PF, Duclos JM, Soppelsa F, et al. Factors associated with perioperative morbidity and mortality in patients with pheochromocytoma: analysis of 165 operations at a single center. J Clin Endocrinol Metab 2001; 86(4):1480–1486.
23. Khorram-Manesh A, Ahlman H, Nilsson O, et al. Long-term outcome of a large series of patients surgically treated for pheochromocytoma. J Int Med 2005; 258:55–66.
24. Schulz C, Eisenhofer G, Lehnert H. Principles of catecholamine biosynthesis, metabolism and release. In: Lehnert H, ed. Pheochromocytoma: Pathophysiology and Clinical Management. Frontiers of Hormone Research. Vol. 31. 1st ed. Basel, Switzerland: S. Karger, 2004:1–25.
25. Gertner ME, Kebebew E. Multiple endocrine neoplasia type 2. Curr Treat Options Oncol 2004; 5(4):315–325 (review).
26. Peczkowska M, Januszewicz A. Multiple endocrine neoplasia type 2. Fam Cancer 2005; 4:25–36 (review).
27. Bertherat J, Gimenez-Roqueplo A-P. New insights in the genetics of adrenocortical tumors, pheochromocytomas and paragangliomas. Horm Metab Res 2005; 37:384–390.
28. Elder EE, Elder G, Larsson C. Pheochromocytoma and functional paraganglioma syndrome: no longer the 10% tumor. J Surg Oncol 2005; 89:193–201.
29. Dubois LA, Gray DK. Dopamine-secreting pheochromocytomas: In search of a syndrome. World J Surg 2005; 29(7):909–913.
30. Dluhy RG, Lawrence JE, Williams GH. Endocrine hypertension. In: Larsen PR, Kronenberg HM, Melmed S, Polonsky KS, eds. Williams Textbook of Endocrinology. 10th ed. Saunders, 2002 (ISBN 0721691846).
31. Shen WT, Sturgeon C, Duh Q-Y. From incidentaloma to adrenocortical carcinoma: the surgical management of adrenal tumors. J Surg Oncol 2005; 89:186–192.
32. Sprung J, O'Hara JF Jr., Gill IS, et al. Anesthetic aspects of laparoscopic and open adrenalectomy for pheochromocytoma. Urology 2000; 55(3):339–343.
33. Inabnet WB, Pitre J, Bernard D, Chapuis Y. Comparison of the hemodynamic parameters of open and laparoscopic adrenalectomy for pheochromocytoma. World J Surg 2000; 24(5):574–578.
34. Jaroszewski DE, Tessier DJ, Schlinkert RT, et al. Laparoscopic adrenalectomy for pheochromocytoma. Mayo Clin Proc 2003; 78(12):1501–1504.
35. Möbius E, Nies C, Rothmund M. Surgical treatment of pheochromocytomas: laparoscopic or conventional? Surg Endosc 1999; 13(1):35–39.
36. Cheah WK, Clark OH, Horn JK, et al. Laparoscopic adrenalectomy for pheochromocytoma. World J Surg 2002; 26(8):1048–1051.
37. Kazaryan AM, Kuznetsov NS, Shulutko AM, et al. Evaluation of endoscopic and traditional open approaches to pheochromocytoma. Surg Endosc 2004; 18(6):937–941 (review).
38. Waltner MM. New therapeutic and surgical approaches for sporadic and hereditary pheochromocytoma. Am NY Acad Sci 2002; 970:41–53 (review).
39. Col V, de Canniere L, Messaoudi L, et al. Heart failure induced by pheochromocytoma: laparoscopic treatment and intraoperative changes of several new cardiovascular hormones. Horm Res 1999; 51(1):50–52.
40. Tauzin-Fin P, Sesay M, Gosse P, Ballanger P. Effects of perioperative alpha1 block on haemodynamic control during laparoscopic surgery for phaeochromocytoma. Br J Anaesth 2004; 92(4):512–517.
41. Biccard BM, Gopalan PD. Phaeochromocytoma and acute myocardial infarction. Anaesth Intensive Care 2002; 30(1):74–76.
42. Frustaci A, Loperfido F, Gentiloni N, et al. Catecholamine-induced cardiomyopathy in multiple endocrine neoplasia. Chest 1991; 99:382–385.
43. Quezado Z, Keiser H, Parker M. Reversible myocardial depression after massive catecholamine release from a pheochromocytoma. Crit Care Med 1992; 20:549–551.

44. Shapiro L, Singh S, Trethowan N. Normotensive cardiomyopathy and malignant hypertension in phaeochromocytoma. Postgrad Med J 1982; 58:110–111.

45. Dugas G, Fuller J, Singh S, Watson J. Pheochromocytoma and pregnancy: a case report and review of anesthetic management. Can J Anaesth 2004; 51(2):134–138.

46. Hamilton A, Sirrs S, Schmidt N, Onrot J. Anaesthesia for phaeochromocytoma in pregnancy. Can J Anaesth 1997; 44(6):654–657.

47. Hack HA. The perioperative management of children with phaeochromocytoma. Paediatr Anaesth 2000; 10(5):463–476 (review).

48. Matsota P, Avgerinopoulou-Vlahou A, Velegrakis D. Anaesthesia for phaeochromocytoma removal in a 5-year-old boy. Paediatr Anaesth 2002; 12(2):176–180.

49. Ciftci AO, Tanyel FC, Senocak ME, Buyukpamukcu N. Pheochromocytoma in children. J Pediatr Surg 2001; 36(3):447–452.

50. Minami T, Adachi T, Fukuda K. An effective use of magnesium sulfate for intraoperative management of laparoscopic adrenalectomy for pheochromocytoma in a pediatric patient. Anesth Analg 2002; 95(5):1243–1244.

51. Kizer JR, Koniaris LS, Edelman JD, St. John Sutton MG. Pheochromocytoma crisis, cardiomyopathy, and hemodynamic collapse. Chest 2000; 118:1221–1223.

52. Roizen MF, et al. The effect of alpha-adrenergic blockade on cardiac performance and tissue oxygen delivery during excision of pheochromocytoma. Surgery 1983; 94(6): 941–945.

53. Russell W, Metcalfe I, Tonkin A, Frewin D. The preoperative management of phaeochromocytoma. Anaesth Intensive Care 1998; 26:196–200.

54. Shupak RC. Difficult anesthetic management during pheochromocytoma surgery. J Clin Anesth 1999; 11(3):247–250.

55. Prys-Roberts C, Farndon JR. Efficacy and safety of doxazosin for perioperative management of patients with pheochromocytoma. World J Surg 2002; 26(8):1037–1042.

56. Kocak S, Aydintug S, Canakci N. Alpha blockade in preoperative preparation of patients with pheochromocytomas. Int Surg 2002; 87(3):191–194.

57. Miura Y, Yoshinaga K. Doxazosin: a newly developed, selective alpha 1-inhibitor in the management of patients with pheochromocytoma. Am Heart J 1988; 116(6 Pt 2):1785–1789.

58. Ulchaker J, Goldfarb D, Bravo E, Novick A. Successful outcomes in pheochromocytoma surgery in the modern era. J Urol 1999; 161:764–767.

59. Tauzin-Fin P, Hilbert G, Krol-Houdek M, et al. Mydriasis and acute pulmonary oedema complicating laparoscopic removal of phaechromocytoma. Anaesth Intensive Care 1999; 27(6):646–649.

60. Serfas D, Shoback D, Lorell B. Phaeochromocytoma and hypertrophic cardiomyopathy: apparent suppression of symptoms and noradrenaline secretion by calcium-channel blockade. Lancet 1987; 2:711–713.

61. Munro J, Hurlbert B, Hill G. Calcium channel blockade and uncontrolled blood pressure during phaeochromocytoma surgery. Can J Anaesth 1995; 42:228–230.

62. Colson P, Ryckwaert F, Ribstein J, et al. Haemodynamic heterogeneity and treatment with the calcium channel blocker nicardipine during phaeochromocytoma surgery. Acta Anaesthesiol Scand 1998; 42(9):1114–1119.

63. Proye C, Thevenin D, Cecat P, et al. Exclusive use of calcium channel blockers in preoperative and intraoperative control of pheochromocytomas: hemodynamics and free catecholamine assays in ten consecutive patients. Surgery 1989; 106(6):1149–1154.

64. Lebuffe G, Dosseh ED, Tek G, et al. The effect of calcium channel blockers on outcome following the surgical treatment of phaeochromocytomas and paragangliomas. Anaesthesia 2005; 60(5):439–444.

65. Chung PC, Li AH, Lin CC, Yang MW. Elevated vascular resistance after labetalol during resection of a pheochromocytoma. Can J Anaesth 2002; 49(2):148–150.

66. Nicholas E, Deutschman C, Allo M, Rock P. Use of esmolol in the intraoperative management of pheochromocytoma. Anesth Analg 1988; 67:1114–1117.

67. Ogata J, Yokoyama T, Okamoto T, Minami K. Managing a tachyarrhythmia in a patient with pheochromocytoma with landiolol, a novel ultrashort-acting β-adrenergic blocker. Anaesth Analg 2003; 97:291–304 (letter to the editor).
68. Kantorovich V, Pacak K. A new concept of unapposed β-adrenergic overstimulation in a patient with phaeochromocytoma. Ann Internal Med 2005; 142(12):1026–1028 (letter to the editor).
69. Joris JL, Hamoir EE, Hartstein GM, et al. Hemodynamic changes and catecholamine release during laparoscopic adrenalectomy for pheochromocytoma. Anesth Analg 1999; 88(1):16–21.
70. James MF, Cronje L. Pheochromocytoma crisis: the use of magnesium sulfate. Anesth Analg 2004; 99(3):680–686.
71. Fawcett WJ, Haxby EJ, Male DA. Magnesium: physiology and pharmacology. Br J Anaesth 1999; 83:302–320 (review).
72. Pivalizza EG. Magnesium sulfate and epidural anesthesia in pheochromocytoma and severe coronary artery disease. Anesth Analg 1995; 81(2):414–416.
73. Poopalalingam R, Chin EY. Rapid preparation of a patient with pheochromocytoma with labetolol and magnesium sulfate. Can J Anaesth 2001; 48(9):876–880.
74. Poulsen S-A, Quinn RJ. Adenosine receptors: new opportunities for future drugs. Bioorg Med Chem 1998; 6:619–641 (review).
75. Tabrizchi R, Bedi S. Pharmacology of adenosine receptors in the vasculature. Pharmacol Ther 2001; 91:133–147 (review).
76. Shyrock JC, Belardinelli L. Adenosine and adenosine receptors in the cardiovascular system: biochemistry, physiology and pharmacology. Am J Cardiol 1997; 79(12A):2–10.
77. Pelleg A, Katchanov G, Xu J. Autonomic neural control of cardiac function: modulation by adenosine and adenosine 5′-triphosphate. Am J Cardiol 1997; 79(12A):11–14.
78. Edlund A, Sollevi A, Linde B. Haemodynamic and metabolic effects of infused adenosine in man. Clin Sc 1990; 79:131–138.
79. Sollevi A, Lagerkranser M, Irestedt L, et al. Controlled hypotension with adenosine in cerebral aneurysm surgery. Anesthesiology 1984; 61:400–405.
80. Öwall A, Gordon E, Lagerkranser M, et al. Clinical experience with adenosine for controlled hypotension during cerebral aneurysm surgery. Anesth Analg 1987; 66:229–234.
81. Gröndal S, Bindslev L, Sollevi A, Hamberger B. Adenosine: a new antihypertensive agent during pheochromocytoma removal. World J Surg 1988; 12:581–585.
82. Selldén H, Kogner P, Sollevi A. Adenosine for per-operative blood pressure control in an infant with neuroblastoma. Acta Anaesthesiol Scand 1995; 39:705–708.
83. Doi M, Ikeda K. Sevoflurane anesthesia with adenosine triphosphate for resection of pheochromocytoma. Anesthesiology 1989; 70:360–363.
84. Nalos M, Asfar P, Ichai C, et al. Adenosine triphosphate-magnesium chloride: relevance for intensive care. Intensive Care Med 2003; 29:10–18 (review).

20

Anesthesia for Colorectal Surgery

Stuart D. Murdoch
Department of Anesthesia, St. James's University Hospital, Leeds, U.K.

INTRODUCTION

Colorectal surgery is associated with both a significant mortality and morbidity (1). Patients usually present suffering from inflammatory bowel disease (IBD) (Crohn's or ulcerative colitis), diverticulitis, or neoplasia. The nature of surgery is often similar (i.e., resection of the affected area of bowel), and patients' demographic characteristics can differ significantly. Colorectal conditions can present as emergencies, perforation of the bowel, or obstruction, or for elective surgery. As well as resection of the colon or rectum, surgery in this area includes formation and closure of stomas, formation of pouches to mimic colorectal function, and treatment of incontinence and rectal bleeding. This chapter will deal mainly with resection of the large bowel, although the principles described for perioperative management can be applied for other surgery on the bowel (Chapter 21).

PATHOLOGY

Colorectal cancer is one of the leading causes of death from cancer; it has an incidence, which rises with age, reported at 20 per 100,000 in the under-65 age group, rising to 337 per 100,000 in the over-65 group (2). Diverticular disease is a disease of the Western world, being largely unrecognized in Africa. Its incidence increases with age, affecting 30% of 60-year-olds and up to 65% of individuals at the age of 85. The diverticulum represents a defect in the colonic mucosa, typically affecting the sigmoid colon. Diverticula can become inflamed and infected, leading to a spectrum of conditions from simple contained abscess to generalized peritonitis. Inflammation and infection of diverticula do not always necessitate surgery and can often be managed by nonoperative measures. With the increase in age of the general population, the number of patients presenting with diverticular disease or colorectal cancer will increase significantly, often with other significant comorbidity.

IBD affects a younger age group, with a peak incidence between 10 and 40 years of age for both ulcerative colitis and Crohn's. The reported incidence of ulcerative colitis is 10 to 20 per 100,000/yr, and Crohn's disease is reported at 5 to 10 per 100,000/yr. It is believed that up to 240,000 people suffer from IBD in the

United Kingdom (3). The mainstay of management is medical treatment, usually aminosalicylates and steroids. Other immune-modifying agents (such as cyclosporin, azathioprine, and infliximab) are used in severe disease. These treatments can have significant implications in the postoperative period, especially for wound healing. Despite advances in medical treatment, many patients still require surgery.

This chapter will focus on those patients undergoing elective surgery. This area has attracted significant attention recently, with numerous well-conducted clinical trials examining practice, such that class I evidence is now available to inform clinical decision-making (4). Most evidence relates to perioperative care rather than anesthetic management. The majority of this work has been aimed at rapid mobilization of the patient, the return to oral diet, and earlier hospital discharge. Such techniques have earned the name "fast-track" surgery, although the term is not exclusive to colorectal surgery. The significant aspects of elective surgery in these conditions are usually aimed at resecting diseased bowel, returning the bowel to continuity following the formation of a stoma or the creation of a pouch.

PREASSESSMENT

General Considerations

Neoplasia of the colon and rectum and diverticular disease are diseases of old age. Therefore, this population suffers significant comorbidity such as ischemic heart disease, respiratory disease, and diabetes (Chapters 7 and 21). Any method of analyzing perioperative risk [American Society of Anesthesiology (ASA) classification, physiological and operative severity score for the enumeration of mortality and morbidity (POSSUM) (5), Goldman, etc.] will therefore identify a high-expected incidence of both morbidity and mortality.

Patients with IBD are younger and with less coexisting disease. They might have recently taken or are on long-term steroids or other immunosuppressive drug treatment, which can cause many long-term problems. Although drug dosing is aimed to minimize this, the occurrence of complications is often an indication for surgery. Immunosuppressive agents are also associated with poor wound healing postoperatively. Patients with IBD may also have had multiple previous surgeries. Recently, the National Institute of Clinical Excellence (6) has reviewed the use of investigations prior to elective surgery; however, the evidence base to support their recommendations is relatively poor, and there is little evidence to show how the results of perioperative tests should change anesthetic management in the vast majority of patients (7).

All patients who are having major surgery, including all undergoing bowel resection, should have a medical history taken and a clinical examination carried out. Blood should be taken for a full blood count and base-line urea and electrolytes. Apart from those patients who fall into the ASA 1 and under 60 years of age, all patients should have an electrocardiogram performed. The American Society of Cardiologists has produced extensive guidelines for the preoperative investigation and intervention in patients presenting for noncardiac surgery but with cardiac disease. However, when compared with European countries, this represents a significantly greater number of investigations.

Cardiovascular Investigations

Cardiopulmonary exercise testing may be able to identify those high-risk patients who are most at risk of developing complications. In a study of 548 patients with cardiovascular disease or aged over 60 undergoing intra-abdominal surgery, all patients underwent exercise testing using a standard protocol for six minutes or until significant ST depression. The authors used an anaerobic threshold of 11 mL/min/kg to categorize patients into one of three groups. This figure was chosen as indicative of moderate cardiac failure (8). The overall mortality was 3.9% (21 patients). Of the 11 deaths due to cardiopulmonary causes, 9 were in patients who had an anaerobic threshold of less than 11 mL/min/kg or who had significant myocardial ischemia on testing. Even in the group of deaths not related to cardiopulmonary disease, all but one patient had an anaerobic threshold of less than 11 mL/min/kg and/or significant myocardial ischemia. This study directed patients postoperatively to the intensive care unit, high dependency unit (i.e., level 3 or level 1–2 critical care facility), or the ward, based on the results of exercise testing; there was no mortality due to cardiovascular reasons in the patients sent to the ward immediately postoperatively. This seems a way in which the inexorable demand for critical care beds can be met, by selecting out patients who are at risk based on validated criteria, rather than on the nature of the surgery and relatively poorly defined underlying pathology.

RISK PREDICTION

Recently, three large multicenter trials have collected data on a total of 16,606 patients presenting with disease of the colon and rectum. The largest of these was a study conducted on behalf of the Association of Coloproctology of Great Britain and Ireland, which analyzed data on 8077 patients with a new diagnosis of colorectal cancer over a 12-months period (9). The factors associated with 30-day mortality were advanced age, high ASA classification, advanced Duke's stage, urgency of the operation, and inability to resect the cancer. Overall mortality was 7.5%, 5.6% for elective cases, and 14% for emergencies. The authors produced a model in which risk was adjusted for the above factors to predict operative mortality.

The second large study (10) examined data collected from 15 U.K. hospitals in the period 1993–2001, the data was for all patients undergoing colorectal surgery. Of the 6883 patients studied, 35.9% had malignant disease and 68.2% of all patients had elective surgery. Mortality in all patients undergoing elective surgery was 2.8%, in those undergoing emergency surgery it was 12.0%. The aim of this study was to produce a dedicated risk-adjustment score for colorectal surgery (colorectal POSSUM). The factors found to influence the outcome included the physiological variables: advanced age, the presence of cardiac failure, systolic blood pressure, pulse rate, urea, and hemoglobin. The significant operative factors were Duke's staging, operative urgency, peritoneal soiling, and operative severity. This model overcame some of the known shortcomings of P-POSSUM, particularly the under prediction of mortality in the high-risk group and the over prediction in the low-risk patient (11).

The third large study looked solely at patients presenting with large bowel obstruction secondary to colorectal cancer. Data was available for 1046 patients, of which 989 patients had surgery, over a 12-month period. The mortality in this group was 15.7%; again, the factors associated with adverse outcome were advanced age, urgency of surgery, and ASA classification.

PREOPERATIVE CARE

Supplemental nutrition is ineffective in reducing complications in most patients prior to surgery (12,13). There is, therefore, no benefit in delaying surgery in the hope of improving the patient's condition. However, there may be a small number of patients with nutrient deficiency, who will benefit from supplementation prior to surgery.

Mechanical Bowel Preparation

Traditionally all patients undergoing bowel resection have had mechanical bowel preparation (14) prior to surgery as a means of reducing the incidence of infection, as the bowel is normally colonized with bacteria and contains fecal material. Bowel preparation will result in the removal of fecal material and stool, but will not result in a sterile bowel. As a consequence of bowel preparation, the patient may experience pain and discomfort as well as dehydration, electrolyte imbalance, and the possibility of bowel perforation. This practice is not well supported by the available evidence; indeed, two large randomized studies have been performed, examining the incidence of postoperative complications in patients with and without bowel preparation and have failed to find a significant difference in postoperative infectious or anastomotic complications (15,16). Despite this evidence, mechanical bowel preparation is still widely used in the surgery of the colon (17). In a survey in five European countries, the heads of surgery from 200 centers belonging to the Enhanced Recovery After Surgery group responded to questions related to their practice in colorectal surgery, and the vast majority of centers still used mechanical bowel preparation for a left hemicolectomy. However, it may be that some surgeons have changed practice, in that patients for right-sided operations are no longer receiving bowel preparation prior to surgery. It is also important to point out that the two randomized studies were only reported in 2003 and 2005. Although previous small-scale studies have reported similar results, it is unlikely that overnight change of long held beliefs will change.

Antibiotics

Antibiotics are used prophylactically in all operations to prevent wound infection. This practice is supported by many studies and has been subject to a systematic review (18). A total of 147 studies were identified, the studies varied significantly in their design and the antibiotic regimens tested. The authors concluded that antibiotics chosen should be effective against aerobic and anaerobic bacteria, and should be given so that their concentration is sufficient when bacterial contamination occurs and that multiple-dose regimens may be no more efficient than single dose. A surgical unit should have a protocol for all patients to optimize compliance with these recommendations.

Preoperative Fasting

Just as it is traditional for all patients about to undergo bowel surgery to have mechanical bowel preparation, it is equally traditional for all patients to be starved from the midnight before their operation. This is to ensure an empty stomach and reduce the risk of aspiration. However, this period of starvation is associated with alterations in carbohydrate metabolism and insulin sensitivity (19). There is limited evidence that giving the patient a carbohydrate drink on the night prior to surgery and the day of surgery, at least two hours prior to the start of surgery, alters this response.

In a group of patients given a carbohydrate drink prior to surgery, the evening before and two to three hours prior to the start of anesthesia, the reduction in insulin sensitivity seen in all patients postsurgery was statistically less compared to that in the placebo group. The degree of postoperative insulin resistance has been shown to be an independent predictor of length of stay (20). Insulin resistance is also an indicator of the severity of stress of surgery. In a recent study of 65 patients given a carbohydrate drink prior to surgery, there was a significantly greater loss of muscle mass in the placebo group compared to the treatment group. However, there was no difference in plasma insulin or glucose or in the incidence of complications. While length of stay was ten days in the control group [inter-quartile range (IQR = 6)] and eight days in the treatment group (IQR = 4), it was not statistically significant. Further studies need to be performed before this practice can unequivocally be said to benefit the patient in terms of significant end points. The value of reduced insulin resistance and improved glucose control may be similar to that seen in critical care patients, where improved glycemic control has been shown in a large randomized trial to result in a significant reduction in mortality (21).

Preoptimization

In recent years, several studies have examined the benefits of targeting hemodynamic variables (oxygen delivery, cardiac output, and stoke volume) (22,23) prior to surgery (Chapter 8). Patients may be transferred to a dedicated area prior to surgery, invasive monitoring initiated, and the patient treated with fluids or inotropes until an end point is reached or the attempt abandoned when the patient is not capable of reaching the protocol end point. This compares with the conventional approach of administering fluids according to "a recipe" to all patients with the aim of simply maintaining a blood pressure or a central venous pressure. It has been established that the presence of a normal blood pressure does not preclude hypovolemia and impaired blood flow (24).

A meta-analysis (25) has demonstrated that in patients where mortality in the control group is greater than 20%, hemodynamic optimization is of benefit in reducing mortality and morbidity. In patients where mortality is less than this, a clear benefit has not been demonstrated, although there was a trend toward a reduced mortality. As the mortality for any procedure decreases, it becomes increasingly more difficult to be able to demonstrate a benefit in mortality from any single procedure. As the expected mortality from elective colorectal surgery is nearer 5% for all patients, it may be difficult to demonstrate a significant survival advantage when preoptimization is used routinely. However, in selected patients, the use of goal-directed therapy to maximize oxygen delivery and tissue perfusion is likely to be of survival benefit. Despite this, it is unclear that how many units are identifying high-risk patients and optimizing them in clinical practice, because the resource implications of doing it in terms of manpower and high dependency beds are not inconsiderable [even though it has been argued that optimization, by reducing morbidity, ultimately uses less resource than nonoptimization (26)]. Some units do, however, seem to be using optimization to a given end point during surgery itself, which overcomes many of the problems of admitting the patient to high dependency prior to surgery.

ANESTHESIA

Prior to the commencement of anesthesia, specific consent should be obtained for anesthesia. This will depend on the anesthetist having first decided what, if any, invasive procedures will be needed. This will vary depending mostly on the patients underlying comorbidity: there are no overwhelming reasons why all patients will need invasive monitoring because blood loss can often be small, and hemodynamic disturbance in a fit patient relatively minor. In a patient with significant comorbidity, it may be advantageous to have a more detailed knowledge of the hemodynamic variables obtainable by invasive monitoring. This will enable the anesthetist to tailor the technique to the individual patient. It is also important that the patient is aware of the planned postoperative analgesic technique and the advantages and potential harm of the technique.

Induction and Maintenance

There is no evidence for an "optimal" anesthetic technique. The method employed should be that which ensures the safety of the patient and which the anesthetist is familiar with. It should avoid hemodynamic compromise and long-lasting effects. Any of the modern induction agents and methods of maintenance of anesthesia can potentially achieve these goals.

Temperature Maintenance

During anesthesia, body temperature should be maintained at near normal values. There is a tendency for body temperature to fall during anesthesia (poikilothermia), due to vasodilation and a distribution of blood away from the core, lack of thermoregulatory control, and loss of heat to the environment. Hypothermia is associated with an increase in wound infection (27), delayed removal of sutures, and prolonged hospital stay. To prevent hypothermia, fluids should be warmed, and two forced air-warming devices used, one for the upper body and one below the incision (28).

PERIOPERATIVE CARE

Analgesia

It is usual for a midline incision to be performed for lower intestinal surgery, although a Pfannenstiel incision is occasionally appropriate for some open procedures. Laparoscopically assisted procedures, likewise, commonly employ a low abdominal transverse incision for removal of the specimen (Chapter 17).

Where the common midline incision is employed, it crosses several dermatomes and is associated with significant pain. Pain is not only unpleasant, and needs to be relieved for humanitarian reasons, but can also contribute to potential morbidity and mortality. The effects of pain can affect every organ system and include impaired respiratory function, because deep breathing will exacerbate the pain; the patient therefore avoids this and fails to expand their lung bases. This effect is believed to lead to the retention of respiratory tract secretions and an increase in the incidence of pneumonia and respiratory failure. Hemodynamic changes can occur because the pain results in an enhanced stress response, tachycardia, and hypertension.

There are two main approaches to the control of severe pain following major surgery: the use of regional anesthetic techniques, usually in the form of a thoracic epidural, or the use of opiates (Chapter 25). There is much debate over the benefits of one technique over the other. A few studies have demonstrated a survival benefit, whereas others have shown no difference. A systematic review of epidural analgesia and anesthesia in a wide range of surgery did demonstrate a benefit (29). Two recent large randomized controlled trials have attempted to address this and have been unable to demonstrate any significant difference in mortality or major complications (30,31), although both studies also failed to demonstrate significant problems with the use of epidural analgesia. The study by Rigg et al. (30) in high-risk surgical patients, demonstrates an improvement in analgesia, as judged by visual analogue scores, and a significant reduction in postoperative respiratory failure. The Veterans administration study also showed an improvement in analgesia and a reduction in complications in the group of patients having repair of aortic aneurysm, but not general abdominal surgery. In this study, local anesthetic agents were not infused epidurally in the postoperative period, analgesia being achieved by 3 to 6 mg morphine given epidurally every 12 to 24 hours.

While there is insufficient evidence to recommend epidural analgesia for a reduction in mortality, the benefit in analgesia and the subjective difference in patients postoperatively make epidural analgesia desirable. Patients may seem more awake, quicker to mobilize, and less compromised by the nausea and vomiting associated with opiates. It is essential that the patient is nursed in an area where the staff are familiar with epidurals and their complications, and have the time and expertise to look after the patient. This may be a ward area and not necessarily a high dependency area. Even if epidural analgesia is recommended, some patients decline consent for the procedure. This may be due to previous experience of "failed" and inadequate epidurals or a simple reluctance to let "anyone near their back with a needle." This group of patients and others, where epidural analgesia is not possible, are best managed with an opiate regime.

A combination of local anesthetic and opiate is the optimal combination of drugs (32) for epidural administration, though no study has demonstrated the advantage of one mixture over another. The epidural should be sited in the dermatome, corresponding to the middle of the expected surgical incision.

Recently, there has been an interest in performing large bowel surgery laparoscopically. This results in a much smaller incision, usually in a single dermatome and possibly below the umbilicus. A recent large multicenter trial, however, demonstrated little benefit in the laparoscopic group (33). Although 30% of the group intended to have laparoscopic surgery were converted to open surgery, the incidence of conversion decreased with time, presumably as surgical experience increased. There were increased complications and length of stay in the group which had laparoscopic surgery converted to open surgery. Overall length of stay was two days longer in the open group than in the laparoscopic group.

Fluids

The aim of fluid management perioperatively is to maintain hydration, electrolyte homeostasis, hemodynamic stability, and organ perfusion and function. Urinary losses as well as third-space loss, fluid sequestration into the gut, and loss from high-output stoma sites all need to be considered in terms of fluid and electrolyte therapy. Loss of potassium, chloride, magnesium, and phosphate, together with malabsorption may all be issues in the perioperative and postoperative periods.

Wet vs. Dry Approaches

Fluid management in the peri- and postoperative period has stimulated considerable controversy. One body of opinion favors a stroke volume optimization approach, which may result in the administration of considerable volumes of fluid (34,35). The use of epidural analgesia and its concomitant vasodilatation may also necessitate the use of fluids to maintain blood pressure.

An alternative approach favors the early commencement of oral fluids post-operatively, and supplementary fluids only to ensure fluid balance (36,37). This strategy in part depends on the use of vasopressors to maintain blood pressure (38), an option unlikely to be available in the vast majority of general surgical wards. The study by Nisaanevich examined the use of two different fluids regimens on outcome following intra-abdominal surgery. The first group received an initial bolus of 10 mL/kg and then 12 mL/kg/hr. The second group received 4 mL/kg/hr. The post-operative fluid management was determined by the surgical staff unaware of the patient's fluid management intraoperatively. The group of patients receiving least fluid passed flatus more quickly than the liberal fluid group, and perhaps, more importantly, had statistically fewer complications and a statistically significant shorter length of hospital stay median of eight days versus nine days $p < 0.01$. The paper by Brandstrup also examined two groups of patients, where one group had limited fluids intraoperatively, and then fluids to maintain body weight. Oral fluids were encouraged. The second group of patients had more fluid given intraoperatively, according to a protocol based on body weight and fluid loss, and postoperatively received further fluid. Postoperatively, hypotension was treated by both the fluid boluses and the use of inotropic agents. Although there were protocol violations, which have cast some doubt over the validity of the results, the study demonstrated fewer complications in the restricted fluid group, including cardiopulmonary and wound-healing complications.

However, other studies have shown a benefit to some groups of patients when given a liberal fluid regimen, compared to more restricted fluid use. In patients undergoing laparoscopic cholecystectomy (39), it has been demonstrated that liberal fluid administration of 40 mL/kg intraoperatively as opposed to 15 mL/kg was associated with improved pulmonary function, exercise capacity, and a shorter length of hospital stay.

There is therefore conflicting evidence as to how to manage the fluids of patients undergoing colorectal surgery. How do we resolve this? It is likely that we are considering different patient populations. The study by Branstrup had only 4 deaths in a total of 172 studied patients, and the study by Nisanevich had 0 deaths in 152 patients; in contrast to the study by Wilson, which had 11 deaths in 138 patients. It is only in the group of patients, where a mortality rate of greater than 20% has been demonstrated in the control group, that a difference in mortality has been demonstrated. It is very difficult to reliably compare the epidemiological data of one group of patients with another in a different center in a different country. It may also reflect a difference in the degree of monitoring of patients. Areas where inotropes can be routinely used to manage hypotension imply a greater level of supervision. This may allow periods of hypotension to be more quickly treated and prevent tissue hypoperfusion and associated complications. Close observation of patients and early treatment of abnormalities of physiology in a high dependency area have been shown to reduce cardiorespiratory complications, and have a trend toward shorter length of hospital stay (40).

The fluid regimen employed cannot be viewed as a single aspect of patient care, and one regimen cannot be used for all patient groups. It may be that the transfusion of liberal amounts of fluids prevents some complications on the ward at the expense of a group of patients receiving more fluid than needed. This latter group of patients may benefit from being kept relatively dry. It is also important to appreciate that whatever fluid protocol is employed, hypovolemia must be treated with restoration of the circulating volume.

Oxygen

Oxygen has traditionally been given to patients to prevent postoperative hypoxemia and myocardial ischemia (41). Supplemental oxygen is usually given at a rate of $2\,L/min$ for 72 hours or the patient receives opiates. This greatly reduces the incidence of both the hypoxemia and the subsequent ischemia.

High concentrations of oxygen have been associated with a decreased incidence of wound infection and postoperative nausea and vomiting. In a study (42) of 500 patients undergoing colorectal resection, half received 30% oxygen intraoperatively and two hours afterwards, and half received 80%. Otherwise treatment was identical in the two groups. Oxygen saturations in both groups were the same; the arterial and tissue partial pressure of oxygen was higher in the group receiving the higher quantity of oxygen. In the control group, 28 patients (11.2%; 95% confidence interval 7.3–15.1) developed a culture-positive wound infection with pus, compared to only 13 patients given 80% oxygen (5.2%; 95% confidence interval 2.4–8.0%). This was a statistically highly significant result $p < 0.01$, but did not result in any decrease in length of hospital stay. There was no difference in the incidence of atelectasis in the two groups. Supplemental oxygen has also been shown to decrease the incidence of postoperative nausea and vomiting (43). It therefore seems appropriate to use a high level of oxygen intraoperatively and in the recovery phase.

Nasogastric Tubes

The use of a tube inserted into the stomach prophylactically to drain gastric contents following major surgery has long been routine, and is standard practice in the majority of centers (44). Nasogastric tube usage has also been used, in the belief that it will hasten the return of gut function, reduce the risk of pulmonary complications by reducing the risk of aspiration, and reduce the incidence of anastomotic leakage. This is despite a meta-analysis in 1995, which demonstrated little difference in patients, treated with or without a nasogastric tube; although an increase in vomiting and distension were reported in those patients not receiving a tube. Since this report, more randomized studies have been performed, and a further systematic review conducted in 2005 (45). This review examined data on over 4000 patients. The data indicated, in those patients who did not receive a nasogastric tube, there was an earlier return of bowel function ($p < 0.001$) and a trend toward decreased pulmonary complications ($p = 0.07$), but an increase in wound infection ($p = 0.08$). Of the 28 studies examined (3 studies examined the incidence of anastomotic leak in patients having colonic surgery), no difference was demonstrated between the two groups. Nineteen studies reported on pulmonary complication. In those without a nasogastric tube, there was a tendency for a reduced incidence of complications [risk reduction 1.35 (95% confidence interval 0.98–1.86) $p = 0.07$]. In those patients having colonic surgery, there was no difference $p = 0.73$. Therefore, there seems little advantage in the routine use of nasogastric tubes in all patients; they may have a place in a small number of patients with vomiting and discomfort, and, indeed, there may be several advantages to not employing them.

Feeding

Following surgery, there is inevitably a period of gut dysmotility that prevents normal oral intake (46). Dysmotility has been managed by using a nasogastric tube, intravenous fluids, and start oral intake, once bowel sounds are heard and flatus has been passed. This can serve to deny an already malnourished patient calorific intake during a period when they are overcoming the stress of surgery. The fear is that early feeding will contribute to anastomotic leak and ileus. It has long been known that patients can tolerate feeding after 24 hours with few side effects (47). In a study of 105 patients comparing patient choice of when to start an oral diet versus a protocol-driven policy where normal diet was not started until day 5, patients resumed a normal diet on average in the third day of operation (48). There was no significant difference in the rate or nature of complications in the two groups, but there was also no difference in time to hospital discharge.

A meta-analysis of early enteral feeding (any type of enteral feed within 24 hours of surgery) versus nil by mouth has identified 11 studies with 837 patients. In six of these studies, feeding was directly into the small bowel. The analysis looked at the incidence of complications as well as hospital stay and mortality. There was no difference in the rate of anastomotic dehiscence, wound infection, or pneumonia. There was an increase in the incidence of vomiting in the group receiving early feeding relative risk 1.27 (95% confidence interval 1.01–1.61), with a decrease in the number of infections relative risk 0.72 (95% confidence interval 0.54–0.98). There was a reduction in the hospital length of stay in those patients fed early by 0.84 days (95% confidence interval 0.36–1.31 days $p = 0.001$). There was no statistically significant difference in mortality. There was a trend to reduced mortality in the group fed early, relative risk 0.48 (95% confidence interval 0.18–1.29); it was unlikely that the numbers involved in the studies would be sufficiently powered to detect such a difference.

In conclusion, the standard approach to feeding has few advantages and several disadvantages. Early feeding is safe, may improve tissue healing, and may reduce septic episodes and length of hospital; larger studies are needed to look at its effect on mortality.

ENHANCED RECOVERY OR FAST-TRACK SURGERY

In recent years, several groups (49,50) have utilized developments in all aspects of anesthetic and surgical care to minimize discomfort to patients, to reduce complications suffered, and minimize hospital stay. The discharge criteria for patients remain the same, but are achieved sooner (51). These studies seem to show a general improvement in patient condition compared to conventional surgery, with not only a shorter hospital stay but also a lower mortality when compared to the general mortality for colorectal resection from the Association of Coloprocotology audit. This reduction in mortality may, however, reflect patient selection, for the control groups also have a low mortality. As yet, most of the studies performed have had relatively small numbers of patients enrolled.

One concern is that care is being shifted from the hospital to the community, and this has been demonstrated in other patient groups (52). There are also concerns about complications occurring in the community, and it has been suggested that 10% to 20% of patients may need to be readmitted for a period of time, although not necessarily overnight. It is also difficult to determine how many patients are suitable for early discharge following surgery from the total population of patients undergoing colorectal surgery, especially in areas where patient's needs cannot be readily met in the community. The shifting of care from one sector to another is potentially politically difficult. Despite these reservations, the recommendations from the groups advocating fast-track surgery are hard to dispute (53). It may be possible to dispute individual aspects of the recommendations; they are effectively evidence-based medicine in practice. However, it is important that large-scale evaluation of the concept and practice is undertaken to examine not only its economic impact but also how it works outside a clinical trial, how many patients are suitable, how often does care deviate from the ideal, and what impact will this have on the patient in terms of complications, length of stay, and mortality. Despite this, many of the recommendations should be adapted anyway as best practice.

REFERENCES

1. Alves A, Panis Y, Mathieu MP, et al. Association Française de Chirurgie. Postoperative mortality and morbidity in French patients undergoing colorectal surgery. Arch Surg 2005; 14:278–283.
2. Mulcahy HE, Farthing MJ, O'Donoghue DP. Screening for asymptomatic colorectal cancer. BMJ 1997; 314(7076):285–291.
3. Carter MJ, Lobo AJ, Travis SPL. IBD Section of the British Society of Gastroenterology. Guidelines for the management of inflammatory bowel disease in adults. Gut 2004; 53(suppl V):v1–v16.
4. Kehlet H, Wilmore DW. Multimodal strategies to improve surgical outcome. Am J Surg 2002; 183:630–641.
5. Copeland CP, Jones D, Walters M. POSSUM: a scoring system for surgical audit. Br J Surg 1991; 78(3):755–760.
6. NCCAC. Preoperative Tests, the Use of Routine Preoperative Tests for Elective Surgery—Evidence, Methods and Guidance. London: NICE, 2003.
7. Carlisle J. Guidelines for routine preoperative testing. BJA 2004; 93(4):495–497.
8. Older PO, Smith RER, Courtney PG, et al. Preoperative evaluation of cardiac failure and ischemia in elderly patients by cardiopulmonary exercise testing. Chest 1993; 104:701–704.
9. Tekkis P, Poloniecki JD, Thompson MR, et al. Operative mortality in colorectal cancer: prospective national study. BMJ 2003; 327:1196–1201.
10. Tekkis PP, Prytherch DR, Kocher HM, et al. Development of a dedicated risk-adjustment scoring sytem for colorectal surgery (colorectal POSSUM). Br J Surg 2004; 91:1174–1182.
11. Tekkis PP, Kessaris N, Kocher HM, et al. Evaluation of POSSUM and P-POSSUM scoring systems in patients undergoing colorectal surgery. Br J Surg 2003; 90(3):340–345.
12. Hytlander A, Bosaeus I, Svedlund J, et al. Supportive nutrition on recovery of metabolism, nutritional state, health-related quality of life, and exercise capacity after major surgery: a randomized study. Clin Gastroenterol Hepatol 2005; 3(5):466–474.
13. Veteran's Affairs Total Paretenteral Nutrition Study Group. Perioperative total parenteral nutrition in surgical patients. N Engl J Med 1991; 325:525–532.
14. Platell C, Hall J. What is the role of mechanical bowel preparation in patients undergoing colorectal surgery? Dis Colon Rectum 1998; 41:875–883.
15. Ram E, Sherman Y, Weil R, et al. Is mechanical bowel preparation mandatory for elective colon surgery? A prospective randomised study. Arch Surg 2005; 140:285–288.
16. Zmora O, Mahajna A, Bar-Zakai B, et al. Colon and rectal surgery without mechanical bowel preparation: a randomized prospective trial. Ann Surg 2003; 237(3):363–367.
17. Lassen K, Hannermann P, Ljungqvist O, et al. Patterns in current perioperative practice survey of colorectal surgeons in five northern European countries. BMJ 2005; 330: 1420–1421.

18. Song F, Glenny AM. Antimicrobial prophylaxis in colorectal surgery: a systematic review of randomized controlled trials. Br J Surg 1998; 85:1232–1241.
19. Nygren J, Soop M, Thorell A, et al. Preoperative oral carbohydrates and postoperative insulin resistance. Clin Nutr 1999; 18(2):117–120.
20. Thorell A, Nygren J, Ljungqvist O. Insulin resitance: a marker of surgical stress. Curr Opinion Clin Nutr Metab Care 1999; 2:69–78.
21. Van den Berghe G, Wouters PJ, Bouillon R, et al. Outcome benefit of intensive insulin therapy in the critically ill: insulin dose versus glycemic control. Crit Care Med 2003; 31(2):359–366.
22. Wilson J, Woods I, Fawcett J, et al. Reducing the risk of major elective surgery: randomised controlled trial of preoperative optimisation of oxygen delivery. BMJ 1999; 318(7191):1099–1103.
23. Boyd O, Grounds RM, Bennett ED. A randomized clinical trial of the effect of deliberate perioperative increase of oxygen delivery on mortality in high-risk surgical patients. JAMA 1993; 270:2699–2707.
24. Hamilton-Davies C, Mythen MG, Salmon JB, et al. Comparison of commonly used clinical indicators of hypovolaemia with gastrointestinal tonometry. Intensive Care Med 1997; 23:276–281.
25. Kern JW, Shoemaker WC. Meta-analysis of hemodynamic optimisation in high-risk patients. Crit Care Med 2002; 30(8):1686–1692.
26. Fenwick E, Wilson J, Sculpher M, et al. Pre-operative optimisation employing dopexamine or adrenaline for patients undergoing major elective surgery: a cost-effectiveness analysis. Intensive Care Med 2002; 28(5):599–608.
27. Kurz A, Sessler DI, Lenhardt R. Perioperative normothermia to reduce the incidence of surgical-wound infection and shorten hospitalization. N Engl J Med 1996; 334:1209–1215.
28. Kurz A, Kurz M, Poeschl G, et al Forced air warming maintains intraoperative normothermia better than circulating-water mattresses. Anesth Analg 1993; 77:89–95.
29. Rodgers A, Walker N, Schug S, et al. Reduction of post-operative mortality and morbidity with epidural or spinal anaesthesia: results from overview of randomised trials. BMJ 2000; 321:1493–1497.
30. Rigg JRA, Jamrozik K, Myles PS, et al. MASTER Anaesthesia Trial Study Group. Epidural anaesthesia and analgesia and the outcome of major surgery: a randomised trial. Lancet 2002; 359:1276–1282.
31. Park WY, Thompson J, Lee KK. Effect of epidural anaesthesia and analgesia on perioperative outcome. A randomised controlled Veterans Administration study. Ann Surg 2001; 234:560–571.
32. Kaneko M, Saito Y, Kirhara Y, et al. Synergistic antinocioceptive interaction after epidural coadministration of morphine and lidocaine in rats. Anesthesiology 1994; 80:137–150.
33. Guillou PJ, Quirke P, Thorpe H, et al. Short-term endpoints of conventional versus laparoscopic assisted surgery in patients with colorectal cancer (MRC CLASICC trial): multicentre, randomised controlled trial. Lancet 2005; 365:1718–1726.
34. Grocott MPW, Mythen MG, Gan TJ. Perioperative fluid management and clinical outcomes in adults. Anesth Analg 2005; 100:1093–1106.
35. Wilson J, Woods I, Fawcett J, et al. Reducing the risk of major elective surgery: randomised controlled trial of perioperative optimisation of oxygen delivery. BMJ 1999; 318(7191):1099–1103.
36. Nisanevich V, Felsenstein I, Almogy G, et al. Effect of intraoperative fluid management on outcome after intra-abdominal surgery. Anesthesiology 2005; 103:25–32.
37. Branstrup B, Tonnessen H, Bejer-Holgersen R, et al. Effects of intravenous fluid restriction on postoperative complications: comparison of two perioperative fluid regimens: a randomized assessor-blinded multicenter trial. Ann Surg 2003; 238(5):641–648.

38. Holte K, Foss NB, Svensen C, et al. Epidural anesthesia, hypotension, and changes in intravascular volume. Anesthesiology 2004; 100(2):281–286.
39. Holte K, Klrskov B, Christensen DS, et al. Liberal versus restrictive fluid administration to improve recovery after laparoscopic cholecystectomy. A randomised, double-blind study. Ann Surg 2004; 240:892–899.
40. Jones HJS, Coggins R, Lafuente J, et al. Value of a surgical high-dependency unit. BJS 1999; 86:1578–1582.
41. Reeder MK, Muir AD, Foex P, et al. Postoperative myocardial ischaemia: temporal association with nocturnal hypoxaemia. Br J Anaesth 1991; 67(5):626–631.
42. Greif R, Akça O, Horn EP, et al. Supplemental perioperative oxygen to reduce the incidence of surgical-wound infection. N Engl J Med 2000; 342:161–167.
43. Greif R, Laciny S, Rapf B, et al. Supplemental oxygen reduces the incidence of postoperative nausea and vomiting. Anesthesiology 1999; 91:1246–1252.
44. Sakamandis AK, Ballas KD, Kabaroudis AG. Role of nasogastric intubation in major operations: a prospective study. Med Sci Res 1999; 27:789–791.
45. Nelson R, Tse B, Edwards S. Systematic review of prophylactic nasogastric decompression after abdominal operations. Br J Surg 2005; 92:673–680.
46. Catchpole BN. Smooth muscle and the surgeon. Aust N Z J Surg 1989; 59:199–208.
47. Moss G. Maintenance of gastrointestinal function after bowel surgery and immediate enteral full nutrition. Vol. II. Clinical experience, with objective demonstration of intestinal absorption and motility. J Parenter Enteral Nutr 1981; 5:215–220.
48. Hans-Guerts IJM, Jeekel J, Tilanus HW, Brouwer KJ. Randomized clinical trial of patient-controlled versus fixed regimen feeding after elective abdominal surgery. Br J Surg 2001; 88:1578–1582.
49. Kehlet H, Wilmore DW. Multimodal strategies to improve surgical outcome. Am J Surg 2002; 183:630–641.
50. Anderson ADG, McNaught CE, MacFie J, et al. Randomised clinical trial of multimodal optimisation and standard peroperative surgical care. Br J Surg 2003; 90:1497–1504.
51. Kehlet H, Wilmore DW. Fast-track surgery. Br J Surg 2005; 92:3–4.
52. Bohmer RM, Newell JM, Torchina DF. The effect of decreasing length of stay on discharge destination and readmission after coronary artery bypass operation. Surgery 2002; 132:10–15.
53. Fearon KCH, Ljungqvist O, Von Meyenfeldt M, et al. Enhanced recovery after surgery: a consensus review of clinical care for patients undergoing colonic resection. Clin Nutr 2005; 24:466–477.

21

Anesthesia for Colorectal Surgery in the Elderly

Dave Murray
Cleveland School of Anesthesia, The James Cook University Hospital, Middlesbrough, U.K.

INTRODUCTION

In Western countries, approximately 25% of surgical patients are over 65 years of age (1). Not only is the proportion of elderly patients per head of population increasing, but the number of elderly patients undergoing surgery is also increasing independently of this rise (2). Data for Great Britain and Ireland show that over 70% of patients undergoing surgery for colorectal cancer are older than 65 years (3). In addition, the incidence of bowel cancer is also increasing (4). Hence, the elderly population represents a considerable consumer of health-care resources.

AGING PROCESS

Aging is associated with loss of function in all organ systems, which may be clinically invisible until there has been almost complete loss of reserve. This results in the elderly suffering the highest incidence of postoperative cardiovascular, respiratory, and cerebral complications of all surgical populations (5). Even so-called "fit" elderly patients have very definite limits to their tolerance of anesthesia, surgery, and the associated stress response. This has led some clinicians to grade even healthy patients over 80 as minimum of American Society of Anesthesiology (ASA) grade 3.

Neurological System

Blindness, largely due to cataract and glaucoma, affects nearly 30% of the elderly. Deafness is more common—severe in about 35%—and may be completely denied by the patient. These may severely restrict the ability to obtain consent, provide an accurate history, and comprehend details of anesthetic technique, such as epidural insertion. It may also contribute to impairment of the cognitive function of the patient. Cognitive impairment itself increases with aging, and dementia may affect up to 20% of patients over the age of 80.

299

Autonomic integrity is compromised with advancing age, and reflexes such as the baroreceptor response are attenuated. The effects of general anesthesia may unmask presymptomatic failure. Postural effects are accentuated, and may be profound, leading to a poor response to acute hypovolemia. Other autonomic systems affected include temperature regulation and gut motility.

Cardiovascular System

Atrial fibrillation is common in the elderly due to the decline in atrial pacemaker cells to approximately 10% of the adolescent level. Myocytes are reduced in both number and contractility. Cardiac output is increased by increasing stroke volume, via the starling mechanism, rather than by increases in heart rate or contractility. The elderly are more dependent on preload as the ventricle becomes less compliant. Increases in intrathoracic pressure, for instance, due to high pressures during ventilation, may reduce cardiac output precipitously. Isolated systolic hypertension is common as large and medium arterial vessels become stiffer and increase peripheral resistance. There is concentric left-ventricular hypertrophy to compensate for this. The increase in basal sympathetic outflow leads to downregulation of β-adrenergic receptors. This causes a fall in sympathetic responsiveness and the unpredictable action of indirectly acting agonists, such as ephedrine. However response to α-adrenergic agonists remains relatively unaffected (1).

Respiratory System

The loss of elastic tissue supporting the airways leads to an increase in the collapsibility of alveoli and terminal airways at higher pulmonary volumes than in younger patients. This results in the closing capacity encroaching into tidal ventilation when supine by the age of 65. An increase in venous admixture and shunting leads to an increase in the alveolar to arterial oxygen gradient that increases with advancing age. The detrimental effects of the supine position on oxygenation can be attenuated by sitting the patient up.

There is a progressive increase in the number of episodes of airway collapse and arterial oxyhemoglobin desaturation during sleep with advancing age. Snoring (partial upper airway obstruction) is almost universal. Silent aspiration may occur due to the fall in sensitivity of the cough reflexes and increased esophageal reflux with aging. The negative intrathoracic pressure necessary to overcome the high resistance of the collapsed upper airway further aggravates these problems.

Renal System

There is a reduction in the ability of the kidney to both excrete and conserve water and electrolytes. Reduced mobility, incontinence, and prostate disease also produce complex behavioral effects with regard to the need to pass urine. Self-imposed fluid restriction is quite common in an attempt to limit the impact of these conditions. This has implication in both the pre- and postoperative environment. Clear fluid balance charting is essential, and the use of a urinary catheter may allow for a more accurate fluid balance to be kept. Fluid retention in the postoperative period may be estimated by daily weighing the patient.

Locomotor and Connective Tissue

Arthritis is almost universal in the elderly. This will limit their ability to exercise and may make accurate assessment of exercise tolerance difficult. Hence a reduction in exercise tolerance due to cardiorespiratory disease may go undetected. Joint mobility should be assessed because restriction of movement may lead to difficulty in positioning the patient for surgery. Excessive manipulation may lead to severe pain postoperatively. Spinal landmarks should be assessed because performing regional blockade may be challenging due to difficulty in patient positioning, calcification of spinous ligaments, and vertebral collapse due to osteoporosis. The elderly often have thin fragile veins, and ease of securing adequate venous access should be assessed preoperatively.

Drug Metabolism

Virtually all aspects of drug handling are potentially affected by the physiology of aging (6). Reduced protein binding leads to an increase in free drug concentration in the plasma. There is an increase in the volume of distribution of lipophilic drugs because of the increase in body lipid content in the elderly. Organ-based elimination is also increased. This results in virtually all narcotic drugs, intravenous agents, and benzodiazepines exhibiting an age-related increase in their $t_{1/2}$ β elimination half-life. This may result in a prolonged duration of action and recovery. For instance, premedication with benzodiazepines may lead to prolonged sedation in the postoperative period. The dosing interval of fentanyl, if used for perioperative analgesia, will be increased.

PREOPERATIVE ASSESSMENT OF ELDERLY PATIENT

The primary aim of assessment is to identify the effects of both the aging and the disease process in individual organ systems. Initial assessment should be by thorough history taking and examination, with the intention of detecting potentially serious conditions or an acute deterioration, particularly cardiac and respiratory disorders. Opportunities to optimize the patient's condition for the planned surgery or to modify the operative plan to reduce the potential perioperative and postoperative complications should also be considered in preoperative assessment. There may be time constraints, if the proposed surgery is for cancer resection, and planned investigations should therefore be targeted to provide maximal clinical information where the results are likely to affect patient management, without causing an undue delay (7). Those factors that are modifiable, such as weight loss and smoking cessation, should also be considered in evaluation.

Assessment of Specific Organ Systems

Neurological Assessment

Advanced age and a history of delirium or confusion following previous surgery convey a higher risk of early postoperative cognitive dysfunction (POCD) (8,9), although the incidence of POCD after one to two years is low (10). This may indicate the avoidance of a general anesthetic if feasible. Adequacy of vision and hearing should be assessed in order that anaesthetic technique may be explained appropriately. Cerebrovascular disease, especially of the vertebral and carotid arteries, should be assessed, particularly if flexion or extension of the neck is likely. This is particularly relevant if the prone position is intended during surgery, and alternatives should be considered if the patient has evidence of vertebrobasilar insufficiency. The ability of the patient to look up toward you from a chair without going dizzy is as good a test as any.

Assessment of autonomic dysfunction is difficult. There is a dearth of tests available that can identify presymptomatic failure. The results of previous tilt testing may help but is unlikely to be available routinely in the preoperative period.

Cardiac Assessment

The incidence of ischemic heart disease and valve disease increases with age and is associated with increased morbidity and mortality. This compounds the effects of aging on the cardiovascular system. The electrocardiogram (ECG) is a useful investigation that is easy to perform and noninvasive. Many of the elderly display a significant abnormality. Echocardiography is another highly useful modality in assessing the function of the myocardium and heart valves.

While severity of disease may be usefully gauged by exercise tolerance, concomitant diseases in the elderly, such as severe arthritis or blindness, may prevent normal daily activities, such as shopping or climbing stairs. In situations where the patient is unable to exercise, an inotrope-induced stress test, such as a dobutamine stress echo, is a suitable alternative. More complex investigations, such as dipyridamole thallium scanning, transesophageal echo, or Holter monitoring, probably do not have a role in colorectal surgery, and are more appropriate for patients undergoing surgery where there is a high cardiovascular risk, such as large-vessel vascular surgery.

Cardiac Drugs. Many elderly patients will be taking drugs for treatment of hypertension, ischemic heart disease, and heart failure. It is important that these drugs are given on the day of surgery and not omitted due to the patient being "nil-by-mouth." All drugs should be continued in the perioperative period; withdrawal may actually be harmful; for instance, the sudden withdrawal of β-blocker drugs. The exception to this is with angiotensin-converting enzyme (ACE) inhibitors, which can safely be discontinued on the day of surgery. Continuation of ACE inhibitors may lead to difficulty in maintaining blood pressure during the perioperative period (11). The evidence for commencement of β-blocker drugs prior to colorectal surgery is controversial (12–14). In addition, there are significant logistical difficulties in commencing these drugs in an elderly population in an outpatient setting. Anticoagulants are often used in atrial fibrillation and valvular heart disease. These will need to be stopped to ensure that clotting function is normal prior to surgery, particularly if an epidural or spinal technique is used. Antiplatelet agents, such as clopidogrel, should also be stopped prior to epidural insertion. Recommencement of anticoagulants, such as warfarin, after surgery should balance risk of postoperative bleeding against further thrombosis. It should be remembered that warfarin therapy for cardiac disease is based on a long-term risk reduction.

Respiratory Assessment

Chest disease is common in the elderly, and pulmonary complications are more common in the elderly in the postoperative period compared to younger patients. A history of smoking, active chest disease, recent chest infection, or hospital admissions with pulmonary symptoms suggests the need for further investigation. Of the more "routine" investigations, arterial blood gases and chest X ray provide useful information. Formal pulmonary function testing for peak flow rate, forced expiratory volume in one second (FEV_1), and forced vital capacity allow an estimation of physiological reserve to be made by comparison with expected age-adjusted values. The presence of reversibility following bronchodilators suggests that there is potential for improvement. Preoperative physiotherapy and incentive spirometry may also be useful in reducing postoperative pulmonary complications (15,16).

A history of snoring and observed pauses in breathing suggests that the patient may be prone to postoperative sleep apnea, particularly if opioid-based analgesia is instituted. The patient may benefit from continuous pulse oximetry to detect nighttime desaturation.

In extreme cases, there may be a requirement for postoperative ventilatory support. However in the absence of reliable predictors of the need for postoperative ventilation, this needs to be a clinical decision. In these cases, there may be a need to alter the surgical plan to perform less invasive surgery to reduce the metabolic demand and maintain effective pulmonary function.

Functional Capacity

While many of the above investigations of cardiac and respiratory function are useful, they only provide snapshots of a clinical continuum. The concept of assessing functional reserve is a more useful tool for assessing these systems and the ability of the patient to cope with the oxygen demand of the perioperative period.

The impact of cardiorespiratory disease on postoperative recovery is not just limited to cardiorespiratory complications, but may also lead to gastrointestinal (GI), renal, and central nervous system complications. Major surgery generates a strong systemic inflammatory response that is associated with a rise in oxygen requirements from an average of $110 \, mL/min/m^2$ at rest to an average of $170 \, mL/min/m^2$ in the postoperative period (17). Inability to meet this rise in postoperative requirements creates an oxygen debt, the magnitude and duration of which correlates with the incidence of organ failure and death.

The elderly patient who has limited cardiorespiratory reserve may be unable to increase their cardiac output and oxygen delivery to meet this oxygen debt in the postoperative period. This functional limitation is likely to be evident in the preoperative period, and is frequently assessed as the number of metabolic equivalents (METs) that the patient can achieve (18,19). One MET represents a resting oxygen consumption of $3.5 \, mL/kg/min$. An ability to perform exercise at greater than 4 METs is associated with a low risk of complications. An inability to climb two flights of stairs has a good positive predictive value for the development of complications (20). METs may be objectively measured by tests such as ECG exercise testing, or questionnaires such as the Duke Activity Status may similarly be utilized (21). However, the difficulty still remains in assessing functional capacity in those patients whose daily activities are limited by arthritis, blindness, or previous cerebrovascular disease.

Preoperative Blood Tests

Estimation of hemoglobin and platelet concentration should be carried out in all patients. Tests of clotting function are unlikely to be abnormal without significant liver disease or anticoagulant therapy. Hemoglobin levels are often low due to GI losses from the tumor site, and patients may not have sufficient hematinic stores to restore their hemoglobin levels themselves in the postoperative period. Serum urea and electrolyte values should also be obtained. Abnormal values are relatively common. Diuretic use may lead to low serum potassium values. However, normal urea and creatinine values do not necessarily mean that renal function is normal. Reduced dietary intake and muscle mass means that the respective values of urea and creatinine are lower in the elderly. In addition, renal function needs to deteriorate markedly before urea and creatinine levels are elevated beyond normal values.

Predictive Value of Preoperative Investigations

The increased perioperative morbidity in the elderly necessitates some assessment of risk in order that the most appropriate course of action may be undertaken. However, this is not easily carried out. Specific preoperative tests are of limited value in predicting risk, although they can guide perioperative management by defining pathophysiology more fully. Cardiopulmonary exercise testing may be used to objectively measure an individual patient's ability to mount a cardiovascular and respiratory response to an increase in oxygen demand. Patients with a low anaerobic threshold have a correspondingly higher mortality rate, and may benefit from preoperative optimization and admission to the intensive care unit (17,22).

There has been a variety of scoring systems developed in order that the clinician might predict which patients are at risk of postoperative complications (23), but they generally have poor positive predictive values and are more useful at determining those patients not at risk of complications. However, the ASA classification remains a very good predictor of outcome in the elderly. The decision as to whether to proceed with surgery is based on a consideration of the risks of surgery, the risks of delay to allow for further investigation or improvement, and the risks of not proceeding. This is particularly relevant for emergency colorectal surgery. In elderly patients with severe cardiorespiratory disease, the life expectancy due to their disease may be shorter than that due to the planned surgery. For instance, in chronic obstructive pulmonary disease, less than 50% of patients with an FEV_1 less than 30% of predicted will survive five years (24). It may be more appropriate to consider a less invasive technique or a palliative procedure if this is felt likely to reduce postoperative risk. A transverse rather than a longitudinal abdominal incision may be used. Obstructive symptoms may be relieved by a loop ileostomy or colostomy without the need to undergo a full laparotomy. Surgery can be avoided altogether by stenting the bowel lumen at the tumor site. Models, such as that developed by the Association of Coloproctology of Great Britain and Ireland, may be helpful in estimating operative mortality (3). Ultimately a final assessment must be made by the anesthetist and surgeon guided by preoperative evaluation, and based on clinical experience.

PERIOPERATIVE CARE

Choice of Anesthetic Technique

There are few anesthetic techniques that are used in younger adults, which cannot be used to anesthetize the elderly patient. However, these are likely to require an alteration in technique to take account of age-related changes of normal physiology and the effects of any active disease process.

The nature of surgery usually dictates that a general anesthetic technique is required, although colorectal resection is feasible under a regional technique. Rectal surgery, such as that for rectal prolapse, is more amenable to a regional technique, and may be appropriate in the elderly. However, care is required to ensure that hemodynamic instability does not occur and receives prompt treatment. Surgery, such as examination under anesthesia and per-anal resection of polyp, may precede more invasive surgery depending on the operative and histological findings. This provides the anesthetist with the opportunity to assess the patient's response to anesthesia prior to more invasive surgery. Duration of surgery may vary; minor procedures may take less than 30 minutes, colonic resection is frequently performed within two hours, while an abdominoperineal resection may take over four hours.

Premedication

The duration of action of benzodiazepines is prolonged. However, clinically the effects are less pronounced with temazepam then diazepam (25). Concern that the use of premedication may lead to the development of POCD appears unfounded (26).

Intravenous Anesthetic Agents

Care should be taken when inducing anesthesia. Induction agents in the elderly should be administered more slowly than in the younger patient, because prolongation of arm-brain circulation time increases the time taken for the patient to lose consciousness. Reduced protein binding coupled with a contracted blood volume leads to a higher free drug concentration. This, coupled with the reduction in dose requirement (27) means that inadvertent overdose may easily occur, leading to marked cardiorespiratory side effects (28,29). The choice of induction agent is less important than the way in which it is administered. Etomidate may have advantages due to its improved cardiovascular stability, particularly in patients in whom there is considerable cardiac compromise. However, concern has been raised over adrenal suppression following administration of a single dose (30). The incidence of side effects is similar with propofol and thiopentone, if administered with care (31). The use of short-acting opioids such as fentanyl or alfentanil reduces the dose of induction agent required, and attenuates the stress response to laryngoscopy.

Inhalational Anesthetic Agents

The minimum alveolar concentration of all inhalational anesthetic agents is reduced by 20% to 40% from young adult values (32–34). Again the choice of agent is largely theoretical, with few clear clinical advantages to any one agent. Desflurane may allow earlier extubation, particularly after prolonged surgery; however, the earlier recovery characteristics compared to other agents are short lived (35,36). Of the newer agents, sevoflurane has been more extensively studied in the elderly. The use of sevoflurane, being relatively nonirritant, for both induction and maintenance of anesthesia appears to be an attractive option and may avoid the cardiovascular side effects seen with intravenous induction agents. However, the more easily lost airway in the edentulous elderly patient can cause problems. Gaseous induction is likely to be slower in the elderly due to ventilation-perfusion mismatch and shunt, and is exacerbated by the elderly supine patient having their closing capacity within tidal breathing. An air or oxygen mixture is frequently used as a carrier gas rather than nitrous oxide.

Neuromuscular Blockade

Ageing is associated with a reduction in muscle mass, which may be expected to lower the dose requirement of neuromuscular blocking drugs. However, the potency of neuromuscular blocking drugs is similar in all adult populations, due to the development of extrajunctional cholinergic receptors in the elderly (37,38). Vecuronium and rocuronium demonstrate a slower onset and longer duration of action than in younger patients compared to atracurium and cisatracurium (39–41). Atracurium is probably the preferred drug because its duration of action is little different to that seen in younger patients. Hoffman degradation and spontaneous ester hydrolysis compensate for the reduction in hepatic clearance (42). Further doses of neuromuscular blocker beyond the intubating dose are frequently unnecessary, because general anesthesia itself may provide sufficient muscle relaxation, due to the reduction in muscle mass in the elderly, particularly if an epidural is used during surgery. Reversal of neuromuscular blockade with anticholinesterase drugs tends to be similar to that in younger adults, with less increase in heart rate from the accompanying anticholinergic drugs (43). Neuromuscular monitoring is recommended, particularly when using steroid-based drugs.

Airway Management

An endotracheal tube will obviously be required for major colorectal resection. Care needs to be taken when securing endotracheal tubes, because adhesive tape may damage the frail skin found in the elderly. Airway management may be difficult due to arthritic changes that reduce neck mobility. The use of smaller endotracheal tubes reduces the incidence of sore throat in the postoperative period. Normal levels of oxygenation and normocapnia should be maintained. Ventilation pressures should be kept as low as possible. The addition of positive end-expiratory pressure may be useful to maintain normal oxygenation.

Minor colorectal surgery may be carried out using a laryngeal mask airway. However, intubation and controlled ventilation may be the preferred choice. The elderly are more susceptible to the respiratory depressant effects of general anesthesia and may fail to maintain normocarbia and adequate oxygenation. This can be prevented by controlled ventilation. The obtunded protective airway reflexes, reduction in gastric emptying, and reduced gastroesophageal sphincter tone all make reflux of gastric contents and subsequent aspiration more likely in the elderly. This is compounded by the use of Lloyd-Davies patient positioning to perform even minor colorectal surgery. However, a balance needs to be struck between protection against risk of pulmonary aspiration, and avoidance of the stress response and laryngeal trauma that may be inherent in the process of intubation.

Monitoring

Standard patient monitoring should be instituted upon entering the anesthetic room. Invasive monitoring should be guided by the patient's clinical status and planned surgery. The beat-to-beat real time information obtained from invasive monitoring of arterial blood pressure may be beneficial in these high-risk patients. Atrial fibrillation, common in the elderly, may render automated noninvasive blood pressure monitoring inaccurate and prone to delay due to the beat-to-beat variation in pulse pressure. Arterial access also allows near-patient testing of hemoglobin concentration and acid–base status. Central venous pressure monitoring may most easily be achieved via the internal jugular vein, whereas the use of a long-line sited in the antecubital fossa is an alternative, less invasive approach.

Fluid Management

Large bore intravenous access will be required unless for minor surgery. Securing intravenous cannulae may be difficult, due to skin fragility. Care needs to be taken if fluids are administered under pressure, because fragile vessel walls may rupture, leading to extravasation of fluids. These patients require careful attention to fluid management. The National Enquiry into Perioperative Deaths (44) has highlighted the need for careful fluid management. Hypovolemia is a major contributor to hypotension during the perioperative and postoperative period. The elderly are less able to compensate for hypovolemia, due to the effects of aging on cardiovascular and renal systems. The use of purgative bowel preparation prior to surgery may exacerbate fluid depletion. This can be minimized by administering a liter of intravenous crystalloid fluids the night before surgery. A urinary catheter should be used throughout the perioperative period, although the presence of adequate urine output may only indicate an adequate, rather than an optimum, fluid balance. Central venous pressure monitoring may be beneficial in the elderly, but may not be a reliable guide to fluid status. A worsening base deficit from arterial blood gas analysis may imply that organ perfusion is compromised, due to hypovolemia. Patient positioning may have an impact on adequacy of fluid replacement. The increase in venous return, seen when the patient is placed in the head-down position, may falsely elevate central venous and arterial blood pressures, resulting in reduced fluid replacement unless these postural changes are taken into consideration. The use of esophageal Doppler as a less invasive way of monitoring cardiac output to direct fluid replacement has received attention and, appears to offer benefits over conventional invasive monitoring (45,46).

There is currently a debate as to whether intravenous fluids should be administered in a liberal or restricted fashion. The use of Doppler to guide fluid therapy results in increased volumes of fluid being administered, with quicker recovery of bowel function and shorter postoperative stay (46). However, in nontargeted fluid administration, liberal fluid regimes have been associated with more complications and longer postoperative stay, compared to restrictive regimes (47,48). Fluid is similarly restricted within accelerated recovery programs that allow early discharge from hospital. Many of these trials include elderly patients undergoing colorectal surgery; however, it is difficult to draw firm conclusions, especially when one considers the differing anesthetic regimes used (particularly in accelerated recovery programs). Given the effects of aging on cardiovascular and renal physiology, the elderly are less tolerant of both hypovolemia and hypervolemia. The margin for error is smaller, and hence the ability to target fluid replacement by use of techniques, such as Doppler monitoring, may be particularly beneficial.

Blood Loss

Blood loss may vary with the type of surgery. A straightforward hemicolectomy may result in as little as 300 mL, whereas a difficult abdominoperineal resection may result in 3000 mL, due to difficulty in pelvic dissection (particularly if there has been previous pelvic surgery or radiotherapy). Blood loss is often insidious with little measured blood loss in suction containers. Swabs should be weighed throughout surgery to obtain accurate estimates of blood loss. Blood replacement is better instituted using transfusion triggers based on near-patient testing of hemoglobin or hematocrit. While a hemoglobin concentration of 7 to 8 g/dL may be well tolerated in the younger population, this may be less acceptable in the elderly, due to the presence of cardiac disease and reduced cardiac reserve. It may be more appropriate to aim for a target of 10 g/dL in the elderly, particularly if there is an evidence of cardiac ischemia at lower hemoglobin levels (49). Target hemoglobin levels should also take into account anticipated ongoing blood loss in the postoperative period.

Temperature Management

Maintenance of body temperature is essential during the perioperative period, and should start when the patient enters the theater environment. Hypothermia is more common in the elderly (50), and they are less able to conserve body temperature, due to the effects of aging. While they have reduced muscle bulk that reduces the oxygen demand created by shivering, this may still impose a requirement that exceeds respiratory and cardiac reserve, although the effects may not be as great as once thought (51). The elderly may also lack the metabolic and muscular reserve to restore their body temperature back to normal levels. Failing to maintain normal body temperature may result in increased cardiac morbidity, length of hospital stay, wound infection rates, and blood loss (52). Core temperature monitoring is easily achieved with nasopharyngeal temperature probes. Patients will frequently be hypothermic by the time they enter theater from the anesthetic room, particularly if anesthetic time is prolonged from establishing an epidural and inserting invasive monitoring. Further evaporative heat losses occur from the exposed surgical site, and it may be difficult to restore normothermia unless all available measures are used. Passive measures, such as reflective drapes and warmed intravenous fluids, can only help to prevent heat loss. The use of epidural anesthesia during the perioperative period means that heat loss from the lower extremities is increased, due to sympathetically mediated vasodilatation. To restore a hypothermic patient to normothermia, forced warm air systems and warming mattresses are more useful, particularly if placed on the lower extremities. However, patient positioning, particularly the Lloyd-Davis position, means that it can be difficult to utilize all these methods. In this case, the author's preference is to use reflective drapes on the legs and head, and a forced air blower on the torso. The core temperature should be within normal limits before the patient leaves the recovery area.

Patient Positioning

This may present a challenge due to the reduction in joint mobility, arthritic changes, and previous prosthetic joint replacement. While this is unlikely to present difficulties in the supine position, surgery often takes place in the Lloyd-Davies, left lateral, or prone jack-knife positions (Chapter 23). Care should be taken to ensure that pressure areas are well padded to avoid nerve injury and pressure sores. The latter may be debilitating and entail a hospital stay longer than that for the original surgery.

Perioperative and Postoperative Analgesia

Oral analgesia may be sufficient for less invasive procedures. Single-shot caudal injections are useful in surgery such as repair of rectal prolapse. Patients undergoing colorectal resection will require significant levels of perioperative and postoperative analgesia. Perioperatively, options include morphine, remifentanil infusion, or epidural analgesia (Chapter 25). Inadequate postoperative analgesia may increase the risk of adverse outcomes (5), in addition to being inhumane. This is most easily achieved with patient-controlled analgesia (PCA) using morphine (53), or patient-controlled epidural analgesia (PCEA). However, the presence of confusion and cognitive dysfunction may make assessment of pain and treatment with PCA/PCEA techniques problematic. Nonsteroidal anti-inflammatory drugs are useful adjuncts. However, the benefits need to be balanced against the risk of renal complications caused by using these drugs in patients with preexisting age-related renal dysfunction, impaired fluid handling, and the potential for postoperative hypovolemia. The benefits of newer cyclooxygenase-2 inhibitors with regard to renal function may be offset by concerns over increased cardiac morbidity, and these drugs remain controversial (54,55).

The choice of analgesic technique should weigh up all risks and benefits including patient preference. The evidence supporting that epidural analgesia is associated with improved outcomes is not very clear (56). Reduced respiratory complications and thrombotic complications have been demonstrated; however, long-term improvement in outcome has not (57). This may be in part due to the high levels of care that patients receive, regardless of analgesic regime. Epidural analgesia may offer better quality postoperative analgesia than other regimens (56); however, there is little evidence from trials carried out exclusively in the elderly (5). Epidural analgesia may be associated with a significant failure rate unless intensive and active follow-up is implemented (58). PCA is an acceptable form of analgesia in the elderly, and is associated with good quality pain relief (59).

A variety of agents may be used to provide epidural analgesia. The use of low-dose local anesthetic combined with low-dose opioid is commonly used. Epinephrine may be added to improve the quality of block (60). The use of higher-strength solutions of local anesthetic agent such as 0.5% bupivacaine is more likely to be associated with a greater drop in blood pressure, depending on the degree of sympathetic blockade produced. This may be offset by the reduction in end-tidal volatile anesthetic agent needed, because a stronger solution in effect provides epidural anesthesia rather than epidural analgesia, as would be expected with more dilute solutions. However, significant fall in blood pressure may be associated with a reduction in colonic blood flow, which may have implications for subsequent anastomotic healing and ischemic reperfusion injury of the gut (61). Placing the epidural catheter at a level appropriate to the surgical incision can minimize the extent of the block and reduce such cardiovascular changes. For colorectal surgery, the catheter is most appropriately placed at lower thoracic spaces (T8–T11). The author's preference is to use 0.1% levobupivacaine with 2 µg/mL fentanyl. Once the epidural catheter has been inserted, 10 mL of solution is injected as a test dose. A further 5 to 10 mL is given prior to the start of surgery to establish a sufficient block. The local anesthetic solution is then infused at a rate of 5 to 8 mL/hr. The cardiovascular effects of this regimen are usually minimal. In the postoperative period, a patient-controlled bolus of 5 to 8 mL, with a 20-minute lockout period, is added.

The epidural should ideally be inserted in the awake patient. This allows the catheter to be sited at the appropriate level for surgery, while minimizing the risk of spinal cord damage (62). In addition, the patient is able to cooperate for allowing optimum body positioning during insertion. This is important when one considers the limited mobility in the elderly may make insertion more problematic than in younger more mobile patients.

POSTOPERATIVE CARE

The elderly should receive postoperative care in an environment that is appropriate to the degree of comorbidity and type of surgery. These patients are more likely to require high dependency and even intensive care postoperatively. Continuation of invasive monitoring allows closer attention to be paid to oxygenation, fluid balance, acid–base status, and analgesia, and may allow the recognition of postoperative complications to occur sooner. Chest physiotherapy and incentive spirometry may also be appropriate. Early mobilization should be encouraged. The patient should receive continuous humidified oxygen, particularly while epidural or PCA opiates are being used. Epidural analgesia is usually continued for three to five days, supplemented by simple oral analgesics, such as paracetamol.

CONCLUSIONS

The elderly patient preparing for colorectal surgery presents a significant challenge. This group of patients is extremely heterogenous. On one hand, the elderly have been successfully included in accelerated recovery programs (63). On the other, the elderly undergoing intra-abdominal surgery are considered to be in one of the highest-risk groups for cardiac complications (18). This group of patients are most appropriately managed by considering the range of pathophysiological processes at work and tailoring the anesthetic and the surgery accordingly.

REFERENCES

1. Priebe HJ. The aged cardiovascular risk patient. Br J Anaesth 2000; 85:763–778.
2. Klopfenstein CE, Herrmann FR, Michel JP, Clergue F, Forster A. The influence of an aging surgical population on the anesthesia workload: a ten-year survey. Anesth Analg 1998; 86:1165–1170.
3. Tekkis PP, Poloniecki JD, Thompson MR, Stamatakis JD. Operative mortality in colorectal cancer: prospective national study. BMJ 2003; 327:1196–1201.
4. Boyle P, Langman JS. ABC of colorectal cancer: Epidemiology. BMJ 2000; 321:805–808.
5. Jin F, Chung F. Minimizing perioperative events in the elderly. Br J Anaesth 2005; 87:608–624.
6. Jones AG, Hunter JM. Anaesthesia in the elderly. Special considerations. Drugs Aging 1996; 9:319–331.
7. Hollenberg SM. Preoperative cardiac risk assessment. Chest 1999; 115:51S–57S.
8. Dodds C, Allison J. Postoperative cognitive deficit in the elderly surgical patient. Br J Anaesth 1998; 81:449–462.
9. Moller JT, Cluitmans P, Rasmussen LS, et al. Long-term postoperative cognitive dysfunction in the elderly ISPOCD1 study. ISPOCD investigators. International Study of Post-Operative Cognitive Dysfunction. Lancet 1998; 351:857–861.
10. Abildstrom H, Rasmussen LS, Rentowl P, et al. Cognitive dysfunction 1–2 years after non-cardiac surgery in the elderly. ISPOCD group. International Study of Post-Operative Cognitive Dysfunction. Acta Anaesth Scand 2000; 44:1246–1251.
11. Colson P, Ryckwaert F, Coriat P. Renin angiotensin system antagonists and anesthesia. Anesth Analg 1999; 89:1143–1155.
12. Devereaux PJ, Beattie WS, Choi PT, et al. How strong is the evidence for the use of perioperative beta blockers in non-cardiac surgery? Systematic review and meta-analysis of randomised controlled trials. BMJ 2005; 331:313–321.

13. Howell SJ, Sear JW, Foex P. Peri-operative beta-blockade: a useful treatment that should be greeted with cautious enthusiasm. Br J Anaesth 2001; 86:161–164.
14. Warltier DC. Beta-adrenergic-blocking drugs: incredibly useful, incredibly underutilized. Anesthesiol 1998; 88:2–5.
15. Doyle RL. Assessing and modifying the risk of postoperative pulmonary complications. Chest 1999; 115:77S–81S.
16. Warner DO. Preventing postoperative pulmonary complications: the role of the anesthesiologist. Anesthesiol 2000; 92:1467–1472.
17. Older P, Smith R, Courtney P, Hone R. Preoperative evaluation of cardiac failure and ischemia in elderly patients by cardiopulmonary exercise testing. Chest 1993; 104:701–704.
18. Eagle KA, Berger PB, Calkins H, et al. ACC/AHA guideline update for perioperative cardiovascular evaluation for noncardiac surgery—executive summary a report of the American College of Cardiology/American Heart Association Task Force on Practice Guidelines (Committee to Update the 1996 Guidelines on Perioperative Cardiovascular Evaluation for Noncardiac Surgery). Circulation 2002; 105:1257–1267.
19. Chassot PG, Delabays A, Spahn DR. Preoperative evaluation of patients with, or at risk of, coronary artery disease undergoing non-cardiac surgery. Br J Anaesth 2002; 89:747–759.
20. Girish M, Trayner EJ, Dammann O, Pinto-Plata V, Celli B. Symptom-limited stair climbing as a predictor of postoperative cardiopulmonary complications after high-risk surgery. Chest 2001; 120:1147–1151.
21. Hlatky MA, Boineau RE, Higginbotham MB, et al. A brief self-administered questionnaire to determine functional capacity (the Duke Activity Status Index). Am J Cardiol 1989; 64:651–654.
22. Older P, Hall A, Hader R. Cardiopulmonary exercise testing as a screening test for perioperative management of major surgery in the elderly. Chest 1999; 116:355–362.
23. Ridley S. Cardiac scoring systems—what is their value? Anaesthesia 2003; 58:985–991.
24. Brewis RAL, Corrin B, Geddes DM, Gibson GJ, eds. Respiratory Medicine. 2d ed. London: WB Saunders, 1995:1029.
25. Clark G, Erwin D, Yate P, Burt D, Major E. Temazepam as premedication in elderly patients. Anaesthesia 1982; 37:421–425.
26. Rasmussen LS, Steentoft A, Rasmussen H, Kristensen PA, Moller JT. Benzodiazepines and postoperative cognitive dysfunction in the elderly. ISPOCD Group. International Study of Postoperative Cognitive Dysfunction. Br J Anaesth 1999; 83:585–589.
27. Homer TD, Stanski DR. The effect of increasing age on thiopental disposition and anesthetic requirement. Anesthesiol 1985; 62:714–724.
28. Christensen JH, Andreasen F, Jansen JA. Pharmacokinetics and pharmacodynamics of thiopentone, a comparison between young and elderly patients. Anaesthesia 1982; 37:398–404.
29. Dundee JW, Robinson FP, McCollum JS, Patterson CC. Sensitivity to propofol in the elderly. Anaesthesia 1986; 41:482–485.
30. Morris C, McAllister C. Etomidate for emergency anaesthesia; mad, bad and dangerous to know? Anaesthesia 2005; 60:737–740.
31. Steib A, Freys G, Beller JP, Curzola U, Otteni JC. Propofol in elderly high risk patients. A comparison of haemodynamic effects with thiopentone during induction of anaesthesia. Anaesthesia 1988; 43(suppl 4).
32. Nakajima R, Nakajima Y, Ikeda K. Minimum alveolar concentration of sevoflurane in elderly patients. Br J Anaesth 1993; 70:273–275.
33. Strum DP, Eger EI, Unadkat JD, Johnson BH, Carpenter RL. Age affects the pharmacokinetics of inhaled anesthetics in humans. Anesth Analg 1991; 73:310–318.
34. Walpole R, Logan M. Effect of sevoflurane concentration on inhalation induction of anaesthesia in the elderly. Br J Anaesth 1999; 82:20–24.

35. Conzen P, Peter K. Inhalation anaesthesia at the extremes of age: geriatric anaesthesia. Anaesthesia 1995; 50(suppl 33).
36. Juvin P, Servin F, Giraud O, Desmonts JM. Emergence of elderly patients from prolonged desflurane, isoflurane, or propofol anesthesia. Anesth Analg 1997; 85:647–651.
37. Bell PF, Mirakhur RK, Clarke RS. Dose-response studies of atracurium, vecuronium and pancuronium in the elderly. Anaesthesia 1989; 44:925–927.
38. Bevan DR, Fiset P, Balendran P, Law-Min JC, Ratcliffe A, Donati F. Pharmacodynamic behaviour of rocuronium in the elderly. C J Anaesth 1993; 40:127–132.
39. Matteo RS, Ornstein E, Schwartz AE, Ostapkovich N, Stone JG. Pharmacokinetics and pharmacodynamics of rocuronium (Org 9426) in elderly surgical patients. Anesth Analg 1993; 77:1193–1197.
40. Slavov V, Khalil M, Merle JC, Agostini MM, Ruggier R, Duvaldestin P. Comparison of duration of neuromuscular blocking effect of atracurium and vecuronium in young and elderly patients. Br J Anaesth 1995; 74:709–711.
41. Sorooshian SS, Stafford MA, Eastwood NB, Boyd AH, Hull CJ, Wright PM. Pharmacokinetics and pharmacodynamics of cisatracurium in young and elderly adult patients. Anesthesiol 1996; 84:1083–1091.
42. Kitts JB, Fisher DM, Canfell PC, et al. Pharmacokinetics and pharmacodynamics of atracurium in the elderly. Anesthesiol 1990; 72:272–275.
43. Mirakhur RK. Antagonism of neuromuscular block in the elderly. A comparison of atropine and glycopyrronium in a mixture with neostigmine. Anaesthesia 1985; 40:254–258.
44. Extremes of Age. The 1999 Report of the National Confidential Enquiry into Perioperative Deaths, London, 1999.
45. Conway DH, Mayall R, Abdul-Latif MS, Gilligan S, Tackaberry C. Randomised controlled trial investigating the influence of intravenous fluid titration using oesophageal Doppler monitoring during bowel surgery. Anaesthesia 2002; 57:845–849.
46. Gan TJ, Soppitt A, Maroof M, et al. Goal-directed intraoperative fluid administration reduces length of hospital stay after major surgery. Anesthesiol 2002; 97:820–826.
47. Brandstrup B. Effects of intravenous fluid restriction on postoperative complications: comparison of two perioperative fluid regimens: a randomized assessor-blinded multicenter trial. Ann Surg 2003; 238:641–648.
48. Nisanevich V, Felsenstein I, Almogy G, Weissman C, Einav S, Matot I. Effect of intraoperative fluid management on outcome after intraabdominal surgery. Anesthesiol 2005; 103:25–32.
49. Walsh TS, McClelland DB, Lee RJ, et al. Prevalence of ischaemic heart disease at admission to intensive care and its influence on red cell transfusion thresholds: multicentre Scottish Study. Br J Anaesth 2005; 94:445–452.
50. Vaughan MS, Vaughan RW, Cork RC. Postoperative hypothermia in adults: relationship of age, anesthesia, and shivering to rewarming. Anesth Analg 1981; 60:746–751.
51. Frank SM, Fleisher LA, Olson KF, et al. Multivariate determinants of early postoperative oxygen consumption in elderly patients. Effects of shivering, body temperature, and gender. Anesthesiol 1995; 83:241–249.
52. Harper MH, McNichols T, Gowrie-Mohan S. Maintaining perioperative normothermia. BMJ 2003; 326:722–723.
53. Gagliese L, Jackson M, Ritvo P, Wowk A, Katz J. Age is not an impediment to effective use of patient-controlled analgesia by surgical patients. Anesthesiol 2000; 93:601–610.
54. Juni P, Reichenbach S, Egger M. COX 2 inhibitors, traditional NSAIDs, and the heart. BMJ 2005; 330:1342–1343.
55. Jones R. Efficacy and safety of COX 2 inhibitors. BMJ 2002; 325:607–608.
56. Ballantyne JC. Does epidural analgesia improve surgical outcome? Br J Anaesthesia 2004; 92:4–6.
57. Kehlet H, Holte K. Effect of postoperative analgesia on surgical outcome. Br J Anaesth 2001; 87:62–72.

58. Rigg JR, Jamrozik K, Myles PS, et al. Epidural anaesthesia and analgesia and outcome of major surgery: a randomised trial. Lancet 2002; 359:1276–1282.
59. Mann C, Pouzeratte Y, Boccara G, et al. Comparison of intravenous or epidural patient-controlled analgesia in the elderly after major abdominal surgery. Anesthesiol 2000; 92:433–441.
60. Niemi G, Breivik H. Epinephrine markedly improves thoracic epidural analgesia produced by a small-dose infusion of ropivacaine, fentanyl, and epinephrine after major thoracic or abdominal surgery: a randomized, double-blinded crossover study with and without epinephrine. Anesth Analg 2002; 94:1598–1605.
61. Gould TH, Grace K, Thorne G, Thomas M. Effect of thoracic epidural anaesthesia on colonic blood flow. Br J Anaesth 2002; 89:446–451.
62. Fischer HB. Regional anaesthesia—before or after general anaesthesia? Anaesthesia 1998; 53:727–729.
63. Basse L, Thorbol JE, Lossl K, Kehlet H. Colonic surgery with accelerated rehabilitation or conventional care. Dis Col Rectum 2004; 47:271–277.

22

Rapid Recovery After Major Abdominal Surgery

Susan M. Nimmo

Department of Anesthesia, Critical Care and Pain Medicine, Western General Hospital, Edinburgh, U.K.

INTRODUCTION

Current anesthetic and surgical practice allows us to modify and control many of the factors that continue to lead to physiological compromise, morbidity, and death following major surgery. Multimodal programs that address these factors have been reported for a variety of operations, and can lead to a more rapid recovery from surgery (and in some instances, earlier hospital discharge) (1). Rapid recovery is generally considered in the context of time to discharge from hospital, with length of stay used as a surrogate marker of fitness following surgery. The speed of recovery is not however the only consideration. Quality of recovery is also relevant and, particularly in the elderly and patients with significant comorbidities, improving the quality of recovery may not result in a dramatic reduction in hospital stay. Time to discharge is influenced by a multitude of other factors, including availability of carers and an appropriate care package, and the patient's own desire to return home. What we are attempting to achieve with a rapid recovery program is perioperative care, which limits as far as possible an individual patient's physiological compromise (due to surgery and anesthesia) and optimizes their recovery, allowing them to return to their normal level of function as quickly as possible. For many patients, this combination will make earlier discharge from hospital possible.

The causes of delayed discharge following major colorectal surgery include ongoing pain, nausea, continued ileus, and fatigue. A holistic consideration of the factors, which contribute to these and institution of perioperative care packages involving both surgical and anesthetic practice, which attempt to limit these factors as far as possible, have succeeded in reducing length of hospital stay from the traditional 7 to 14 days to as short a time as two to three days in some studies. It is important to note that earlier return home is associated with earlier achievement of normal activities and reported well-being, so that differences between groups of patients in rapid recovery programs versus those receiving more traditional care continue to be demonstrable up to around six weeks following major surgery. It is the purpose of this chapter to specifically address the contribution of anesthesia.

Table 1 Issues Related to Anesthesia, Which Need to Be Considered in a Rapid Recovery
Program for Colorectal Resection

Preoperative issues	Patient information
	Preoperative assessment
	Premedication
	Fasting times and fluids
	Nutrition and carbohydrate loading
Anesthetic factors	Epidural block and remifentanil
	Analgesia
	Stress response to surgery
	Fluids balance
	Vasoactive agents
	Monitoring
	Temperature maintenance
	Antiemetics
Postoperative management	Fluid balance
	Analgesia
	Nutrition
	Postoperative ileus
	Anastomotic leak
	Mobilization

However, implementing a rapid recovery program is a team effort involving the
patient, surgeon, anesthetist, nursing and other staff caring for the patient during
the perioperative period. Similarly, although many of the issues related to the anesthetic contribution are discussed individually below, it is unlikely that any one factor
alone will influence enhanced patient recovery. It is the institution of the entire
package of care, which is important. Many of the individual components have been
subjected to experimental studies, and the results show significant evidence of
benefit. However, this type of research is difficult to achieve for a multimodal care
package. In this context, beneficial end points, such as patient satisfaction and
quality of life and length of hospital stay combined with a lack of demonstrable complications as a result of application of the package, need to be available. Effective
data collection and audit should be a mandatory part of a rapid recovery program
(2). A number of anesthetic related issues are relevant to rapid recovery (Table 1).

PREOPERATIVE ISSUES

Patient Information

Provision of adequate information to the patient and an understanding of the
concepts and process involved are fundamental to the success of rapid recovery programs. Many patients, particularly the elderly, take a relatively passive role when
admitted to hospital for surgery, and expect to be in hospital for some time and
certainly for longer than three days following major surgery. If patients are to be
successfully discharged from hospital within a week of surgery, then arrangements
have to be in place early for this to be possible. Similarly, patients have to know
what to expect and what is expected of them in terms of mobilization, pain relief,
and nutrition. Good patient information preoperatively is provided both in the
preadmission clinic and following admission to the ward. This should be undertaken

by an individual who is fully conversant with the rapid recovery program and is able to give patients clear information and answer concerns. Similarly, it is essential that all staff caring for these patients provide a consistent approach, and are motivated to assist them with nutrition and mobilization while ensuring that other aspects of their perioperative care, in particular analgesia, are optimal. Patients require specific information regarding the proposed anesthetic, and informed consent for the administration of epidural analgesia and anesthesia needs to be obtained (3).

Preoperative Assessment

It is the purpose of preoperative assessment to address patient factors, which may be improved prior to embarking on major surgery. Medical treatment of significant conditions, such as ischemic heart disease, chronic obstructive pulmonary disease, and diabetes mellitus, should be optimal for the individual patient. Generally, a patient's usual medications should be continued with the obvious exception of anticoagulants. Diabetic therapies will need to be modified. It remains uncertain whether it is preferable to discontinue angiotensin-converting enzyme inhibitors preoperatively, but if significant hypotension is a concern, it may be preferable to do so. If regional anesthesia is contemplated, as is likely, then antiplatelet agents, such as clopidogrel, should be stopped a minimum of 10 days preoperatively. Low-dose aspirin therapy is not considered a risk factor on its own for epidural hematoma formation. Protocols must be in place for the safe timing of deep venous thrombosis (DVT) prophylaxis in a patient who is to receive an epidural block (4).

Considerable research effort is being directed at the introduction of perioperative drug treatments to improve outcome from major surgery. Studies have shown that perioperative beta-blockade can improve outcome, following major vascular surgery in patients with ischemic heart disease (5). Similarly the introduction of a statin may be beneficial. However, these results have not as yet been extended to a more general surgical population, and the place of such perioperative therapy for colorectal surgery is not yet known.

Premedication

The use of an anxiolytic or sedative premedication in these patients depends on the perceived balance between excessive preoperative anxiety and increased postoperative sedation, secondary to the continued action of these agents. Generally, because the aim is to mobilize patient early following surgery, any unnecessary sedation should be avoided. The need for sedative premedication is often removed or at least reduced by provision of good preoperative information.

Fasting Times and Fluids

It has been increasingly demonstrated in studies that optimal volume replacement is mandatory in improving outcome from major surgery, including colorectal surgery. Patients admitted for colorectal surgery will often receive preoperative bowel preparation (usually a potent laxative), which can cause significant fluid losses, particularly in an elderly patient who may also be on diuretic therapy for example. If this is combined with prolonged preoperative fasting, then the patient may be unable to compensate, and will arrive in the anesthetic room significantly volume depleted, with the potential for cardiovascular instability and impaired perfusion intra- and postoperatively.

The requirement for bowel preparation prior to colorectal resection is currently a subject of debate, and in many centers has been reduced or abandoned altogether (6). In addition, it is unnecessary for patients to be fasted for clear fluids beyond two hours preoperatively. Patients should be actively encouraged to take fluids up until this time. By applying these strategies, the majority of colorectal patients would arrive in theater without preoperative fluid depletion.

Nutrition and Carbohydrate Loading

One aspect of the stress response to surgery is a relative resistance to the effects of the anabolic hormone insulin. This is mediated by catabolic hormones, such as steroids and glucagon. Clinical work looking at carbohydrate loading within two to three hours of surgery has shown a reduction in insulin resistance (7). This may lead to a reduction in postoperative muscle catabolism, contributing to improved wound healing, improved respiratory function, and enhanced mobility postoperatively. Carbohydrate-rich drinks preoperatively have the further advantage of encouraging oral fluid intake preoperatively. In diabetic patients, we replace carbohydrate loading with an equivalent volume of clear fluid taken orally just before commencing fluid fasting.

Significant malnutrition preoperatively leads to an increase in postoperative complications and mortality. This may be seen in elderly patients with malignant disease. If this is recognized early enough prior to surgery, enhanced preoperative nutrition should improve it.

ANESTHETIC FACTORS

There are a number of interrelated aims of anesthetic management for enhanced recovery after colorectal surgery:

- Limit or minimize the stress response to surgery
- Optimize analgesia to allow patient mobilization from the day of surgery without being limited by pain
- Minimize the use of systemic opioids, which have the dual effect of:
  1. slowing recovery of gastrointestinal function following surgery and limiting the patients ability to recommence enteral nutrition as a result of this and
  2. increasing the incidence of nausea and vomiting
- Maintain physiologic parameters as close to normal as possible, including temperature and fluid homeostasis
- Avoid sedative premedication
- A suggested anesthetic protocol is outlined in Table 2.

Epidural Blockade and Remifentanil

The stress response to surgery is a neuroendocrine response to tissue damage, inflammation, and pain. It is initiated both by sympathetic afferents from the site of injury and by chemical mediators, released as a result of tissue damage and inflammation (8). As some of the neurotransmitters responsible for pain transmission are proinflammatory, and because inflammatory mediators sensitize and recruit nociceptors, pain is a major driver of the stress response to surgery. This effect is not limited to the

Table 2 Suggested Anesthetic Protocol for Rapid Recovery After Colorectal Resection

Epidural	T10–T11 for anterior resection and left hemicolectomy
	T9–T10 for right hemicolectomy
	Morphine bolus 2–6 mg, dependent on the patient
	Up to 15 mL of either 0.125% or 0.25% bupivacaine in increments, dependent on the patient
	Commence infusion, 0.1% bupivacaine with 2 µg/mL fentanyl (6–16 mL/hr)
Induction	Remifentanil 1 µg/kg
	Propofol target-controlled infusion or bolus
	Vecuronium
Maintenance	Oxygen/air mix
	Propofol infusion or sevoflurane
	Remifentanil 0.1 µg/kg/min, varied as necessary
	Vecuronium boluses if indicated
	If necessary, additional boluses of either epidural infusion solution or remifentanil, as indicated
Antiemetic	Ondansetron 4 mg and cyclizine 50 mg
Hypotension	Ephedrine/metaraminol/noradrenaline to maintain adequate BP in normovolemic patient

Note: Routine monitoring (arterial and central venous pressure monitoring only if clinically indicated). Warming blanket and blood warmer. *Abbreviation*: BP, blood pressure.

immediate period of surgery, because the stress response will continue to be activated by significant postoperative pain. Hypothermia is also a significant trigger of the surgical stress response.

The stress response, with activation of the sympathetic nervous system and the hypothalamic pituitary adrenal axis, in particular, evolved to enable an organism to survive recoverable injury by promoting factors, such as mobilization of nutrients for healing, activation of coagulation for hemostasis, a sympathetically mediated support of the circulation allowing flight from ongoing injury, and maintenance of an effective circulation in the face of blood and fluid loss. The descending inhibitory pain pathways and endogenous opioid system have evolved for similar reasons. In the much more controlled environment of major surgery, it is postulated that many of these responses are unnecessary, and may be precursors of postoperative organ dysfunction. Patients with significant ischemic heart disease may not tolerate the hypertension and tachycardia associated with sympathetic nervous system activity, and perioperative myocardial ischemia and infarction may result. A procoagulant state is unnecessary if bleeding is controlled surgically, but it is a contributory factor for thromboembolic complications. Similarly, if patients are fed both preoperatively and postoperatively, then there is no requirement for them to mobilize body protein for repair. Muscle catabolism and poor nutrition contribute to wound infections and dehiscence, and muscle weakness contributes to poor mobility. Respiratory muscle weakness, specifically, will reduce a patient's ability to cough and clear secretions, potentially contributing to postoperative atelectasis, chest infection, and respiratory failure. The stress response and protein catabolism also have an immunosuppressive effect resulting in an increased likelihood of postoperative infection.

It can be seen from the above discussion that far from being of benefit to a surgical patient, the stress response is a contributory factor to a variety of potential postoperative complications, which are likely to be more severe in an elderly population and/or those with significant comorbidity (9). One of the aims of anesthesia is to reduce the stress response to surgery, and stress response reduction must also be continued into the postoperative period.

A number of interventions have been shown to reduce the sympathetic and endocrine responses to major surgery. These include the use of high-dose opioids, beta-blockade, and regional anesthesia. High-dose opioid infusions have been shown to reduce the stress response to cardiac surgery. With the advent of remifentanil (a potent opioid with a very short half-life, due to rapid metabolism by blood and tissue esterases), it has become possible to administer high-dose opioid analgesia without having to commit a patient to a period of postoperative ventilation.

Neuraxial blockade has been shown to effectively block the stress response to major lower limb and pelvic surgery (10). Neuraxial blockade is less effective at blocking the stress response following major abdominal surgery. There are a number of possible reasons for this, including:

- failure to achieve complete neural blockade
- epidural analgesia not inhibiting inflammatory mediators of the stress response

The meta-analysis by Rodgers et al. (11) suggested a beneficial outcome in terms of reduced mortality, if neuraxial blockade was used for lower limb and pelvic surgery. The situation is less clear for abdominal surgery. Rigg et al. (12) in the Master trial failed to demonstrate a reduction in mortality following major abdominal surgery and esophagogastrectomy in high-risk patients utilizing epidural anesthesia and analgesia. However, they did confirm good effective dynamic analgesia and a reduction in respiratory complications. Combining high-dose opioids in the form of remifentanil and neuraxial epidural blockade could provide an effective additive effect.

Central to rapid recovery from colorectal surgery is the provision of effective analgesia (13). This is optimally achieved with a low thoracic epidural. A combination of local anesthetic and opioid appears to provide an optimal combination of effective dynamic analgesia, allowing patients to mobilize comfortably while limiting side effects (14). The epidural serves a number of additional beneficial functions:

- By limiting systemic opioid use, ileus and postoperative nausea and vomiting are reduced, both of which facilitate return to normal oral intake of diet and fluids (which is often a rate limiting step in postoperative recovery)
- Studies looking at the combined effect of epidural analgesia and feeding early postoperatively demonstrate an optimal effect when these are combined. Provision of nutrition in the face of ongoing activity by catabolic hormones, and obtunding the stress response without providing nutrition, have both been shown to be less effective (15)
- Epidural analgesia reduces postoperative respiratory complications (16)
- Epidural analgesia reduces the incidence of DVT and pulmonary embolism
- Epidural analgesia limits myocardial ischemia following major surgery (17)

In the light of all the above perceived benefits, it is disappointing that epidural analgesia has not been shown to have an unequivocal benefit on morbidity and mortality following major surgery. However, provision of good analgesia, while very important, may be insufficient on its own to change outcome. It remains to be seen whether epidural analgesia as part of a multimodal package of care, facilitating early nutrition and mobilization, can contribute to a reduction in postoperative morbidity and mortality. Similarly, the benefits to be gained from epidural analgesia must be balanced against the well-documented risks (18).

It is also important to consider management strategies for patients in whom effective epidural analgesia cannot be achieved. There are a number of absolute contraindications to epidural analgesia, including:

- patient refusal
- patients who are anticoagulated, either therapeutically or due to their illness
- patients who are at high risk of epidural abscess formation as a result of local or systemic infection
- patients with significant musculoskeletal or neurological disease

In addition, studies and audits have shown that it may only be possible to achieve and maintain effective epidural analgesia in 60% to 70% of the patients for whom it is intended (19). One of the causes of failure of epidural analgesia is the catheter falling out prematurely. If we are to actively mobilize these patients, the catheter must be secure. Either tunnelling or epidural fixation devices are appropriate. In patients for whom epidural analgesia cannot be achieved or is contraindicated, it is important to consider how we can facilitate early recovery of gut function and mobilization without the benefits of this.

The critical issues here are provision of good dynamic analgesia, while limiting the use of opioids, which will inevitably delay recovery of gut function.

Multimodal analgesia, using a combination of opioid, paracetamol, and nonsteroidal anti-inflammatory agents (NSAIDs) (provided these are not contraindicated), will be necessary. This can usefully be combined with local anesthesia to the wound. Local anesthetic wound infiltration can be undertaken at the time of surgery, and continued into the postoperative period via wound catheters placed during wound closure. The administration of local anesthetic, either by infusion or by regular bolus doses, has been shown both to enhance analgesia and to provide some opioid-sparing effect. It is noteworthy that some studies looking at multimodal rehabilitation programs have demonstrated the practicality and efficacy of applying these protocols in the absence of epidural analgesia (20). The efficacy of a nonepidural technique will, to an extent, depend on the amount of surgical trauma, and is likely to be more successful for smaller wounds. It will also depend on how effectively multimodal analgesia can be delivered. For example, NSAIDs are often contraindicated in patients presenting for colorectal resection due to age and other co-morbidities. If a patient cannot be given NSAIDs, it is likely to result in increased opioid use, which may be counterproductive in terms of recovery of gastrointestinal function, as discussed earlier.

Perioperative beta-blockade reduces components of the stress response and may be part of the explanation for improved outcome of patients able to commence perioperative beta-blockers prior to high-risk vascular surgery, as shown by Poldermans et al. (5). However, because hypotension (see below) is one of the major limiting factors in mobilizing patients following colorectal resection, with ongoing epidural analgesia, it is unlikely that the addition of perioperative beta-blockers in this group would be practical. Perhaps it should be considered and studied in patients for whom epidural blockade is contraindicated.

Fluid Balance

A number of studies have shown that excessive salt and water loading perioperatively in a variety of different surgical procedures, including, colorectal resection, slows recovery, and, in the latter case specifically, slows return of gastrointestinal function secondary to edema of the bowel wall (21). It is known from animal studies that hypoalbuminemia, and salt and water overload with edema cause a delay in gastric emptying, which improves with salt and water restriction and a high protein intake. Lobo et al. (22) assessed gastric emptying, time to passage of flatus and stool, and length of hospital stay in a small prospective randomized controlled trial of 20 patients undergoing elective colonic resections. One group was randomized to a standard postoperative fluid regime receiving 1 L of 0.9% saline and 2 L of 5% glucose daily, in contrast to the group on restricted postoperative fluids, who received 0.5 L of 0.9% saline and 1.5 L of 5% glucose daily. They showed a weight gain of 3 kg in the "unrestricted" fluid group, with lower hemoglobins and serum albumin, as compared to the group on restricted fluids. This was associated with slower gastric emptying, slower return of gastrointestinal function, and longer hospital stay in this study. The premise is that excess fluid infusion in the face of a reduced ability to excrete sodium and water in the immediate postoperative period results in bowel edema and delays recovery of bowel function. The patients in this study were relatively young (ages ranging from 52 to 67) and those with significant comorbidity likely to affect fluid balance, such as preexisting cardiac failure or renal impairment, were excluded.

In contrast, studies investigating optimization of cardiovascular status preoperatively, using invasive monitoring to guide fluid loading and vasoactive drug therapy (so-called "preoptimization"), have shown an improvement in outcome in patients where this was undertaken successfully (23). The most significant intervention appeared to be volume loading. More recent studies assessing the effect of intraoperative volume loading guided by esophageal doppler monitoring have also suggested that volume loading is beneficial, resulting in shorter hospital stay (24).

These results and those of an increasing number of similar studies are probably not mutually exclusive. The common theme of these studies is to identify the intravenous fluids appropriate to the individual patient. Fit and otherwise healthy younger patients, provided they have not undergone prolonged preoperative fluid fasting or aggressive bowel preparation with associated fluid loss, should be appropriately hydrated preoperatively, and should only require to receive maintenance fluids (which, as Lobo et al. (22) have shown, are less than traditional perioperative fluid regimens have provided). Conversely, for patients who have reason to be volume deplete preoperatively [for example, following bowel preparation, excessive fluid fasting, fluid losses related to their pathology (e.g., obstruction or diarrhea), or in those patients who have related comorbidities e.g., cardiac failure and renal impairment], there may be a greater requirement for intravenous fluids. For many of these patients, the combination of general anesthesia and epidural sympathetic blockade further complicates assessment of fluid balance and requirement for fluids, particularly because vasodilation will exaggerate the hypotensive effect of even mild hypovolemia.

Similarly, epidural-induced vasodilation may produce unacceptable levels of hypotension, even with optimal fluid loading. In this context, it is more appropriate to provide counterbalancing vasoconstriction rather than continue to give more intravenous fluids. This approach is supported by provisional evidence, suggesting that splanchnic blood flow and by inference flow to the anastomosis are best maintained by maintenance of mean arterial pressure (25). In fit patients, intraoperative fluid requirements can be guided by measurement of intraoperative losses, including an estimate of insensible loss, cardiovascular parameters, pulse and blood pressure, and urine output. Provided volume status is considered adequate, residual hypotension can be treated with bolus doses of ephedrine or metaraminol if this is considered necessary.

In less fit patients, there is a need for increased cardiovascular monitoring, and the placement of arterial and central venous lines is dictated by the preoperative condition of the patient, as for any other anesthetic and operation. It should be remembered, however, that for purely logistic reasons, postoperative mobilization may be more restricted where invasive monitoring is in place. It is increasingly apparent that for patients undergoing major surgery, an intraoperative monitor of flow would be of benefit. The current gold standard for monitoring cardiac output is pulmonary artery catheterization; however, in this type of program, it would be not only impractical but also counterproductive to undertake pulmonary artery catheterization. A number of less invasive alternatives are being developed and may be useful for intraoperative monitoring. One such alternative is the esophageal doppler, which measures blood velocity in the descending aorta and provides an esti-mate of flow from this measurement combined with an estimate of the cross-sectional area of the aorta (26). There are a number of sources for error in these measurements, and absolute values should be interpreted with care. Despite this, studies of the use of the esophageal doppler intraoperatively to guide fluid therapy have suggested an improvement in cardiovascular parameters, associated with improved recovery and shorter length of hospital stay (27). Alternative monitors of cardiac output, such as lithium dilution, have not been so widely assessed in this context but might be useful.

For patients with cardiovascular compromise, who may be acutely sensitive to changes in volume status, particularly in the context of a sympathetic block secondary to epidural analgesia, optimizing volume loading guided by appropriate monitoring (as discussed) is the first step to treatment. Often, however, this will not restore an adequate blood pressure, and we have utilized low-dose infusions of noradrenaline in this situation titrated to maintain mean arterial pressure at not less than 15% of the patients normal. Some units use peripheral infusions of phenyleph-rine titrated to effect. Signs of end-organ function, such as urine output and base excess, should be monitored carefully to ensure that vasoconstriction is not detrimen-tal to organ perfusion. Central venous oxygen saturations have been shown to be predictive of outcome in high-risk critical care patients, and may be of benefit during major surgery (28). Measurement can be continuous using a fibreoptic catheter; how-ever, spot measurements can be made using a standard central venous line. The utility of central venous oxygen saturation, in terms of improving outcome following major surgery, has not been established.

Intraoperative blood loss should be replaced as appropriate to the patient. The optimal hemoglobin level for such patients remains the subject of debate. However, for elderly patients with a high incidence of cardiorespiratory comorbidity, it is likely that they will be intolerant of hemoglobin levels maintained below 9 g/dL (29). Currently in the United Kingdom, red cell concentrate is leukocyte deplete, so that the issue of immunocompromise following transfusion is of less concern and should not influence transfusion practice.

Temperature Maintenance

Temperature should be routinely measured intraoperatively. All patients should be actively warmed intraoperatively, and intravenous fluids should be warmed to maintain normothermia.

Antiemetics

Because postoperative nausea and vomiting is both distressing to the patient and precludes early enteral fluid intake, antiemetic therapy should be given routinely intraoperatively.

POSTOPERATIVE ISSUES

Fluid Balance

Maintenance of postoperative fluid balance is also very important, particularly in avoiding excess volume replacement to counteract hypotension, due to the effects of the epidural-induced vasodilation. For patients already receiving an infusion of vasoactive agent from theater, this can be continued to maintain an optimal blood pressure postoperatively in conjunction with appropriate fluids and patient monitoring. One of the difficult issues at this stage is postural hypotension, which limits the ability of patients with epidural analgesia to be mobilized. Once again, it is preferable to avoid fluid overload in managing this issue. In our unit, a 30 mg dose of oral ephedrine is a very effective agent in these circumstances. The dose is given 30 minutes prior to mobilization and usually prevents an acute fall in blood pressure when the patient assumes an upright position. Oral ephedrine has been used successfully for some time in quadriplegic patients with postural hypotension to facilitate mobilization (Dr. Ian Grant, personal communication). It is also critical that elderly patients being mobilized for the first time postoperatively, with an epidural in place, are acclimatized gradually; we have a protocol for sequential mobilization from lying to standing to transfer to a chair over 30 minutes.

One of the fundamental elements for rapid recovery is reinstitution of oral fluids and diet. Patients are allowed to recommence oral clear fluids immediately on waking, provided there are no contraindications from surgery. The avoidance of systemic opioids as a result of using epidural analgesia and prophylactic antiemetic therapy minimizes the incidence of postoperative nausea and vomiting to facilitate this strategy. If patients can tolerate adequate volumes of oral fluids, then the intravenous fluid infusion can be discontinued, which further limits the potential for fluid overloading these patients.

Analgesia

Epidural analgesia should be continued effectively for 48 to 72 hours in these patients. The contribution of an acute pain team in optimizing analgesia while limiting the side effects of epidural analgesia is absolutely critical. Provision of good step-down analgesia is then very important, and can be difficult for those patients who have achieved a pain-free postoperative course up to this point. Again multimodal analgesia should be prescribed and can be given orally. For bowel function, it is optimal to avoid as far as possible the constipating effects of opioids. Tramadol has been shown to have less constipating effect than other opioids and may be useful in this situation (30); however, if this agent does not provide adequate analgesia to allow the patient to continue mobilizing actively, more potent opioids should be used sparingly.

Nutrition

Early postoperative nutrition has the dual effect of reducing the metabolic consequences of fasting and enhancing bowel function. Early postoperative oral nutrition has been shown to reduce gut permeability and hence reduce gut translocation of bacteria and endotoxins. Coordinated peristalsis and secretion of gut hormones are encouraged by enteral nutrition, which will therefore have a beneficial effect in reducing ileus and improving gut function further (31).

Early work suggests that specific nutrients may be beneficial in improving immune function, and some groups advocate the use of probiotics to favorably influence the composition of gut flora (32). The beneficial effects of such strategies require further study for confirmation.

Postoperative protein catabolism can be reduced by the combination of obtunding the stress response to surgery and providing nutrition to the patient. Limiting fasting times both pre- and postoperatively is one of the cornerstones of rapid-recovery programs.

Postoperative Ileus

Ileus following colonic surgery has a multifactorial etiology (33). An increased understanding of this allows us to manipulate perioperative care to limit ileus as far as possible. This has produced concerns that enhanced bowel activity could compromise a colorectal anastomosis. Multiple studies in the literature refute this and confirm the safety of early enteral nutrition, demonstrating that this does not put the anastomosis at risk. This is in contrast to waiting until gut function has returned (as demonstrated by passage of flatus and stool), which has been the traditional signal for recommencing oral nutrition (Chapter 6). Because this usually takes four days or more, this practice increases the negative metabolic effects of major surgery.

Early feeding alone, as with other individual interventions, is unlikely to make a substantial difference to recovery. However, it is beneficial in combination with strategies to reduce nausea, ileus, and the catabolic response to surgery. Carli et al. (34) have shown, for example, that patients receiving significant systemic opioids were unable to recommence an adequate oral intake in the early postoperative period, and showed a larger loss of body weight and exercise capacity in comparison to patients receiving epidural analgesia in whom systemic opioids were avoided. In patients following major abdominal surgery, Barratt et al. (15) have demonstrated that reduction of the catabolic effects of the stress response with epidural analgesia was necessary for patients to benefit from parenteral nutrition, as shown by reduced negative nitrogen balance.

Anastomotic Leak

Anastomotic leak occurs in between 1.8% and 5% of colorectal resections. It is a dreaded complication, due to the morbidity and mortality associated with it. In a study of risk factors for anastomotic leak, Makela et al. (35) identified that preoperative malnutrition (defined as >5 kg weight loss in the months prior to surgery), low albumin, cardiovascular comorbidity, and excess alcohol consumption were all associated with an increased risk of anastomotic leak. A low rectal anastomosis, prolonged surgery, the requirement for major perioperative blood transfusion, and gross peritoneal soiling were also risk factors. This group has found no association with bowel preparation and no longer use this routinely. They did not, however, comment on oral nutrition or anesthetic factors.

Mobilization

Provided that patients are cardiovascularly stable and comfortable, mobilization can begin on the day of surgery. This is facilitated by the use of short-acting anesthetic agents, which limits the hangover effect of general anesthesia.

Postural hypotension is a limiting factor in mobilization, and strategies to limit this have been discussed earlier.

Early mobilization may help maintain muscle strength postoperatively (36).

RESULTS OF THE APPLICATION OF MULTIMODAL CARE PATHWAYS FOR RAPID RECOVERY FOLLOWING MAJOR SURGERY

The individual components that should be considered in commencing a rapid recovery program for colorectal resection of particular relevance to anesthetic management have been outlined. It is obvious from this discussion that there is much overlap between these issues: the optimum effect of one component being achieved only if another is effective, resulting in a multimodal and multidisciplinary approach. There is increasing evidence in the literature that such multimodal programs are both effective and safe. The initial description of a rapid recovery program for colorectal surgery came from Basse et al. in Denmark (37). They described their program and enrolled 60 consecutive patients scheduled for bowel resection into it. Focusing on effective thoracic epidural analgesia, early enteral feeding, and enforced early mobilization, they aimed at a 48-hour postoperative hospital stay. This was achieved in over 50% of the study group; the majority of the rest were discharged from hospital within five days of surgery. Subsequent studies by this group and others to assess outcome markers, such as pulmonary function, indices of weight loss, and exercise capacity, have revealed significant differences between cohorts of patients managed with a multimodal pathway (such as that described) in contrast to a group receiving a more traditional postoperative care package. The multimodal care group shows evidence of significantly less deterioration in organ function, body mass, and exercise capacity (38). Follow-up studies have shown that this difference is sustained for up to six weeks postoperatively, and manifests as earlier return to normal levels of function at home and improved scoring in quality of life questionnaires (39).

Trials that look at physiological end points, such as exercise testing and walking times are much more convincing than measurements of length of stay. While the issues discussed earlier are relevant, it is likely that the surgical approach (allowing limitation of tissue trauma either by utilizing laparoscopic techniques or by limiting the size of surgical incisions) will have a much more profound effect than variations in anesthetic technique, emphasizing yet again the need for a concerted team approach (40,41).

It is perhaps disappointing that the majority of studies looking at both the benefits of epidural analgesia and of rapid recovery programs do not show an impressive reduction in overall morbidity and mortality. This may be a feature of the numbers of patients studied, and at least one rapid recovery program is currently undertaking extensive audit of patients enrolled in multiple centers in Europe, with the intention of both demonstrating effectiveness of such a program on a wide scale and documenting any associated complications. However, what the studies do show is a significantly better quality of recovery, which lasts beyond the duration of hospital care and into the first six weeks of convalescence. Also, of critical importance is the fact that despite the increasing application of these perioperative care programs, there has been no increase in serious complication rates.

An additional and very important advantage of this type of recovery program is that it fosters and enhances good teamwork between all those clinicians and nurses responsible for the patient, and provides a platform for the anesthetist to be more involved throughout the patient's perioperative care and decision making.

REFERENCES

1. Kehlet H, Wilmore DW. Multimodal strategies to improve surgical outcomes. Am J Surg 2002; 183:630–641.
2. Fearon KCH, Ljungqvist O, Von Meyenfeldt M, et al. Enhanced recovery after surgery: a consensus review of clinical care for patients undergoing colonic resection. Clin Nutr 2005; 24:466–477.
3. Epidurals for Pain Relief After Surgery. The Royal College of Anaesthetists, The Association of Anaesthetists of Great Britain and Ireland, March 2004.
4. Checketts MR, Wildsmith JAW. Regional block and DVT prophylaxis. Cont Educ Anaesth Crit Care Pain 2004; 4:48–51.
5. Poldermans D, Boersma E, Bax JJ, et al. The effect of bisoprolol on perioperative mortality and myocardial infarction in high-risk patients undergoing vascular surgery. N Engl J Med 1999; 34:1789–1794.
6. Wille-Jorgensen P, Guenaga KF, Castro AA, Matos D. Clinical value of preoperative mechanical bowel cleansing in elective colorectal surgery: a systematic review. Dis Colon Rectum 2003; 46:1013–1020.
7. Nygren J, Soop M, Thorell A, et al. Preoperative oral carbohydrates and postoperative insulin resistance. Clin Nutr 1999; 18:117–120.
8. Desborough JP. The stress response to trauma and surgery. Br J Anaesth 2000; 85: 109–117.
9. Wilmore D. From Cuthbertson to fast track surgery: 70 years of progress in reducing stress in surgical patients. Ann Surg 2002; 236:643–648.
10. Holte K, Kehlet H. Epidural anaesthesia and analgesia-effects on surgical stress responses and implications for postoperative nutrition. Clin Nutr 2002; 21:199–206.
11. Rodgers A, Walker N, Schug S, et al. Reduction of postoperative mortality and morbidity with epidural or spinal anaesthesia: results from overview of randomised trials. Br Med J 2000; 321:1493–1533.
12. Rigg JRA, Jamrozik K, Myles PS, et al. Epidural anesthesia and analgesia and outcome of major surgery: a randomised trial. Lancet 2002; 359:1276–1282.
13. Nimmo SM. Benefit and outcome after epidural analgesia. Cont Educ Anaesth Crit Care Pain 2004; 4:44–47.
14. Crews J, Hord A, Denson D, et al. A comparison of the analgesic efficacy of 0.25% levobupivacaine combined with 0.005% morphine, 0.25% levobupivacaine alone, or 0.005% morphine alone for the management of postoperative pain in patients undergoing major abdominal surgery. Anesth Analg 1999;89:1504–1512.
15. Barratt SM, Smith RC, Kee AJ, et al. Multimodal analgesia and intravenous nutrition preserves total body protein following major upper gastrointestinal surgery. Region Anesth Pain Med 2002; 27:15–22.
16. Ballantyne JC, Carr DB, deFerranti S, et al. The comparative effects of postoperative analgesic therapies on pulmonary outcome: cumulative meta-analyses of randomised, controlled trials. Anesth Analg 1998; 86:598–612.
17. Beattie WS, Badner NH, Choi P. Epidural analgesia reduces postoperative myocardial infarction: a meta-analysis. Anesth Analg 2001; 93:853–858.
18. Wheatley RG, Schug SA, Watson D. Safety and efficacy of postoperative epidural analgesia. Br J Anaesth 2001; 87:47–61.

19. McLeod G, Davies H, Munnoch N, et al. Postoperative pain relief using thoracic epidural analgesia: outstanding success and disappointing failures. Anaesthesia 2001; 56:75–81.
20. Delaney CP, Fazio VW, Senagore AJ, et al. "Fast track" postoperative management protocol for patients with high co-morbidity undergoing complex abdominal and pelvic colorectal surgery. Br J Surg 2001; 88:1533–1538.
21. Brandstrup B, Tonneson H, Beier-Holgersen R, et al. Effects of intravenous fluid restriction on postoperative complications: a comparison of two perioperative fluid regimens. Ann Surg 2003; 238:215–219.
22. Lobo DN, Bostock KA, Neal KR, et al. Effect of salt and water balance on recovery of gastrointestinal function after elective colonic resection: a randomised controlled trial. Lancet 2002; 359:1812–1818.
23. Wilson J, Woods I, Fawcett J, et al. Reducing the risk of major elective surgery: randomised controlled trial of preoperative optimisation of oxygen delivery. Br Med J 1999; 318:1099–1103.
24. Wakeling HG, McFall MR, Jenkins CS, et al. Intraoperative oesophageal Doppler guided fluid management shortens postoperative hospital stay after major bowel surgery. Br J Anaesth 2005; 95:634–642.
25. Gould TH, Grace K, Thorne G, Thomas M. Effect of thoracic epidural anaesthesia on colonic blood flow. Br J Anaesth 2002; 89:446–451.
26. Wigfull J, Cohen AT. Critical assessment of haemodynamic data. Cont Educ Anaesth Crit Care Pain 2005; 5(3):84–88.
27. Gan TJ, Soppitt A, Maroof M, et al. Goal-directed intraoperative fluid administration reduces length of hospital stay after major surgery. Anesthesiology 2002; 97:820–826.
28. Rivers E, Ander DS, Powell D. Central venous oxygen saturation monitoring in the critically ill patient. Curr Opin Crit Care 2001; 7:204–211.
29. McLellan SA, McLelland DB, Walsh TS. Anaemia and red blood cell transfusion in the critically ill. Blood Rev 2003; 17:195–208.
30. Wilder-Smith CH, Bettiga A. The analgesic tramadol has minimal effect on gastrointestinal motor function. Br J Clin Pharmacol 1997; 43:71–75.
31. Lewis SJ, Egger M, Sylvester PA, Topic ST. Early enteral feeding versus "nil by mouth" after gastrointestinal surgery: systematic review an meta-analysis of controlled trials. Br Med J 2001; 323:773–776.
32. Anderson ADG, McNaught CE, MacFie J, et al. Randomised clinical trial of multimodal optimisation and standard perioperative surgical care. Br J Surg 2003; 90:1497–1504.
33. Holte K, Kehlet H. Postoperative ileus: a preventable event. Br J Surg 2000; 87:1480–1493.
34. Carli F, Mayo N, Klubien K, et al. Epidural analgesia enhances functional exercise capacity and health-related quality of life after colonic surgery: results of a randomised trial. Anesthesiology 2002; 97:540–549.
35. Makela JT, Kiviniemi H, Laitinen S. Risk factors for anastomotic leakage after left-sided colorectal resection with rectal anastomosis. Dis Colon Rectum 2003; 46:653–660.
36. Henriksen MG, Jensen MB, Hansen HV, et al. Enforced mobilisation, early oral feeding, and balanced analgesia improve convalescence after colorectal surgery. Nutrition 2002; 18:147–152.
37. Basse L, Hjorte Jakobsen D, Billesbolle P, et al. A clinical pathway to accelerate recovery after colonic resection. Ann Surg 2000; 232:51–57.
38. Basse L, Raskov HH, Hjort Jakobsen D, et al. Accelerated postoperative recovery program after colonic resection improves physical performance, pulmonary function and body composition. Br J Surg 2002; 89:446–453.
39. Hjort Jakobsen D, Sonne E, Basse L, et al. Convalescence after colonic resection with fast-track versus conventional care. Scand J Surg 2004; 93:24–28.
40. Chumbley GM, Hall GM. Recovery after major surgery: does the anaesthetic make any difference?. Br J Anaesth 1997; 78:347–349.
41. Bonnet F, Marret E. Influence of anaesthetic and analgesic techniques on outcome after surgery. Br J Anaesth 2004; 95:52–58.

23
Anesthesia for Anorectal Surgery

Irwin Foo and Damien Mantle
Department of Anesthesia, Critical Care and Pain Medicine,
Western General Hospital, Edinburgh, U.K.

INTRODUCTION

Surgical intervention for the treatment of anorectal lesions ranges from the simple incision and drainage of abscesses to more complicated procedures (e.g., resection of anorectal malignancies). A wide range of surgical techniques is available to treat anorectal conditions (Table 1). Common to all these surgical procedures is the requirement for optimal patient positioning and appropriate anesthetic technique. This can make the difference between a procedure that is difficult for the surgeon and uncomfortable for the patient and a painless one, in which visualization is excellent. Close cooperation and communication with the surgeon in order to achieve this is therefore of paramount importance.

This chapter outlines anesthetic considerations for anorectal surgical procedures with a particular emphasis on the newer surgical techniques. Relevant anatomy of the rectum and anus, various surgical approaches/techniques, and positioning commonly used are discussed. A wide range of anesthetic techniques that may be employed and common complications that may follow anorectal surgery are highlighted.

ANATOMY OF THE RECTUM AND ANAL CANAL

An understanding of the normal anatomy of the rectum and anus is helpful. It provides greater insight into what particular operations involve, thus enabling selection of the most appropriate anesthetic technique for the specific procedure. Potential complications could be anticipated and unpleasant surgical stimuli blocked effectively.

Rectum

The sigmoid colon becomes rectum in front of the third sacral segment. The distinction between sigmoid and rectum is a matter of peritoneal attachments: where there is a mesocolon, the gut is called sigmoid, where there is no mesentery, it is called rectum. The rectum itself is approximately 15 cm long and ends where its muscle

Table 1 Common Anorectal Conditions and Operative Procedures

Anorectal conditions	Operative procedures
Anal condylomata	Excision
Abscesses (perianal, intersphincteric, etc.)	Incision and drainage
Fissure	Lateral sphincterectomy
Fistula	Fistulotomy, insertion of setons (cutting or draining), endoanal mucosal advancement flap, fistulectomy with muscle repair
Pilonidal sinus	Excision
Hemorrhoids	Hemorrhoidectomy, stapled hemorrhoidopexy
Rectal prolapse	Excision including resection of bowel
Anal tags	Excision
Stricture/stenosis	Dilatation
Polyps	Excision/biopsy
Anorectal benign and malignant tumors	Transanal excision of tumor, transanal endoscopic microsurgery, endoscopic transanal resection of tumor

coats are replaced by the sphincters of the anal canal. This is the anorectal junction and it is slung in the U-loop of the puborectalis muscle, which forms a palpable landmark, the anorectal ring, on rectal examination.

The three taeniae of the large intestine, having broadened out over the sigmoid colon, come together over the rectum to invest it in a complete outer layer of longitudinal muscle. The rectum follows the posterior curve of the sacrum but also has three lateral curves as it descends. Corresponding to these three external curves are three transverse rectal folds (Fig. 1), which project into the lumen (also known as the valves of Houston). It is speculated that these folds may be involved in the separation of flatus and fecal material, allowing flatus to be passed while supporting the weight of feces. Peritoneum covers the upper third of the rectum at the front and sides, and the middle third only at the front. The lower third is below the level of the peritoneum, which is reflected forwards on to the upper part of the bladder (in males) or upper vagina to form the rectovesical or rectouterine pouch of Douglas.

Anal Canal

The anal canal makes up the last 4 cm of the alimentary tract. It consists of a tube of muscle comprising the internal and external anal sphincters, which are composed of visceral and skeletal muscles, respectively. The internal anal sphincter is a thickening of the inner, circular, muscular coat of the anal canal. The external anal sphincter is composed of three parts: deep, superficial, and subcutaneous; the deep part intermingles with the puborectalis muscle posteriorly. The longitudinal muscle layer of the rectum separates the internal and external anal sphincters and terminates in the subcutaneous tissue and skin around the anus.

Within the anal canal are 5 to 10 vertical folds of mucosa, known as the anal columns (columns of Morgagni), which are separated by anal valves. Four to eight anal glands drain into the crypts of Morgagni at the level of the dentate or pectinate line. Most rectal abscesses and fistulae originate in these glands. The dentate line divides the squamous epithelium from the mucosal or columnar epithelium. This is an important landmark because this line delineates where sensory fibers end.

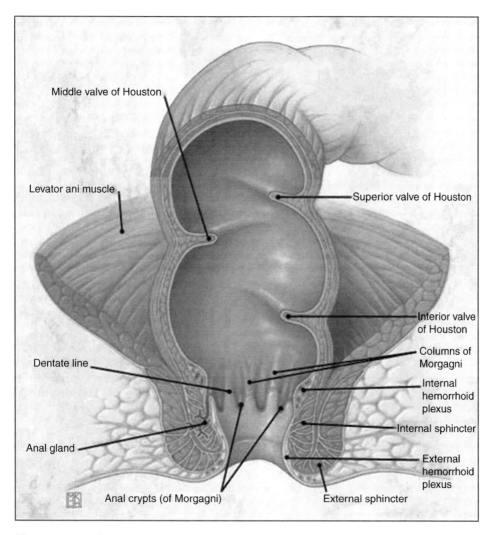

Figure 1 Anal/rectal anatomy. *Source*: From Ref. 1.

Above (proximal to) the dentate-line, the afferent innervation is visceral, thus allowing many surgical procedures to be performed without anesthesia; whereas below the dentate line, afferent innervation is somatic and there is extreme sensitivity. The perianal area is one of the most sensitive areas of the body.

Nerve Supply to the Rectum and Anus

The voluntary external anal sphincter and skin surrounding the anus are innervated by the inferior rectal nerve, a branch of the pudendal nerve (S2–S4). Direct perineal branches from S3–S4 also contribute sensory fibers to the anal canal and perianal skin. Autonomic innervation comes from the parasympathetic pelvic splanchnic nerves (S2–S4), the sympathetic hypogastric plexus (L1–L5), celiac plexus (T11–L2), and the visceral (sacral) splanchnic nerves (from the second and third sacral sympathetic ganglia). Both the sympathetic and parasympathetic fibers become intermingled in the inferior hypogastric plexus, located on the lateral wall of the rectum. The fibers are then conveyed from the plexus to the wall of the rectum and the involuntary internal anal sphincter. Functionally, parasympathetic nerves provide rectal and bladder motor function and inhibit the internal anal sphincter tone, whereas the sympathetic fibers inhibit visceral motor function and increase the tone of the internal anal sphincter (2,3).

On observing the innervation of the anorectal region, it can be deduced that for operations in the anal canal and surrounding perianal skin, a sacral block would offer adequate analgesia. However, if the operation involves traction or distension of the rectum, a block up to T10 would be desirable to avoid the effects of unblocked autonomic nerve stimulation.

SURGICAL APPROACHES AND TECHNIQUES

Many different surgical approaches and techniques are available for anorectal procedures. The commonest approach is the transanal approach and is used for a large number of intra-anal and intrarectal procedures, including biopsies, hemorrhoidectomy, fistulotomy, sphincterotomy, polyp removal, and local excision of low rectal tumors. Two other techniques [transanal endoscopic microsurgery (TEM) and endoscopic transanal resection of rectal tumors] also utilize this approach and will be discussed further below. Other approaches, such as the abdominoperineal, intersphincteric, parasacral, and trans-sacral, are required for excision of rectal tumors that are not suitable for excision via the transanal route. These other approaches require the patient to be either in the Lloyd-Davies position (abdominoperineal approach) or in the prone jackknife position (intersphincteric and parasacral approaches). These different surgical approaches will each have their own impact on patient positioning, the extent and site of postoperative pain, and specific operative complications.

Surgical techniques for anorectal surgery continue to evolve. These developments aim to minimize the invasiveness and reduce perioperative complications of open surgery. Two of these developments will be described briefly: TEM and endoscopic transanal resection of tumor (ETAR). Stapled hemorrhoidectomy will also be highlighted because this surgical procedure has gained popularity in the last ten years.

Recent Surgical Techniques

Transanal Endoscopic Microsurgery

The invasiveness of the posterior approaches to the rectum and the limited view given by the transanal approach led to the development of TEM for the excision of rectal tumors, especially the middle and upper part of the rectum (4). TEM uses an operating sigmoidoscope either 12 or 20 cm in length and 4 cm in outer diameter, which incorporates a binocular optical system with up to 6x magnification. When in place, the instrument is sealed with a gas-tight disc and operating instruments (diathermy knife and graspers) are introduced through airtight ports in the disc. Visibility is maintained by rectal distension to a pressure of 10 mmHg, using carbon dioxide as the insufflating gas with simultaneous continuous low-pressure suction. This procedure is carried out under general anesthesia and the patient is positioned such that the lesion to be excised lies at the bottom, because the instruments and optics are designed to operate downwards. Therefore, for a tumor on the posterior rectal wall, the patient is placed in the lithotomy or Lloyd-Davis position, whereas for anterior lesions, the patient is placed prone with the hips flexed and the legs apart. For lateral lesions, the patient is placed either in the left or lateral position, depending on the lesion (5).

This procedure is mainly performed in patients with localized rectal tumors for palliative symptom control or in patients who are unfit for major surgery (e.g., elderly frail patients) because the rate of complications is lower (4). However, because TEM is a technically demanding procedure, coupled with the cost of the equipment, this technique is still not universally used in the UK except by a few specialist centers.

Endoscopic Transanal Resection of Tumor

ETAR is a method of applying electrocoagulation to rectal tumors using a modified transurethral resectoscope inserted through the anal sphincter. To aid visibility, the rectum is distended with 1.5% glycine solution up to a pressure of 50 cm water, the obturator removed, and a diathermy loop inserted. The resection of the tumor is carried out under direct vision in a manner similar to a transurethral resection of the prostate (6). The technique of ETAR is particularly useful when the lesion lies below the peritoneal reflection, but not within reach of rectal examination. It has been demonstrated to be of benefit in treating benign disease and effective as a minimally invasive means of palliating patients with locally advanced malignant disease. The debulking of the rectal tumor load alleviates the symptoms of bleeding, tenesmus, mucus discharge, and diarrhea (7). This avoids the need for more invasive traditional approaches, such as trans-sacral, sphincter-splitting, or abdominal resections in an often elderly, frail group of patients.

This procedure is carried out in the lithotomy position under either regional or general anesthesia. The complication rate is lower than conventional open surgical techniques (8) (1–3% death rate vs. 21–38% when used solely for palliative purposes), and postoperative pain is minimal. The limitation of this technique includes limited histopathological information about extent of resection and tumor clearance.

Stapled Hemorrhoidopexy

Stapled hemorrhoidopexy has been developed as an alternative to the standard hemorrhoidectomy: The Milligan and Morgan technique involves ligation and excision of the hemorrhoids while leaving the wound open (favored in the United Kingdom) and the Ferguson hemorrhoidectomy involves ligation and excision of the hemorrhoids with closure of the wound (favored in the United States) to reduce pain, which is usually associated with traditional hemorrhoidectomy. This new development involves transanal, circular stapling of redundant normal fibrovascular cushions lining the anal canal with a standard circular stapling device. Redundant anorectal mucosa (fibrovascular cushion) is drawn into the stapling device and excised within the "stapled doughnut," while both the mucosal and submucosal blood flow is interrupted by the circular staple line, thus achieving a reduction in blood flow and removal of redundant tissue simultaneously. Because no incisions are made into the somatically innervated, highly sensitive anoderm, postoperative pain is less than that seen in traditional techniques (9).

This procedure is carried out in the prone/jackknifes or lithotomy position, depending on the surgical preference. General, regional, and local anesthetic techniques have all been described with this procedure. However, if local anesthesia is chosen, conscious sedation is strongly recommended, because placement of the purse-string suture into the rectal mucosa can be associated with discomfort that would not be adequately controlled by means of a local anesthetic alone (10). When compared with traditional hemorrhoid surgery, stapled hemorrhoidectomy is associated with less postoperative pain, shorter postoperative hospital stay, and quicker return to normal function (11,12).

POSITIONING OF PATIENTS DURING SURGERY

The correct positioning of the patient on the operating table for the various surgical approaches and techniques is important not only in optimizing surgical access but also in ensuring patient safety, especially while anesthetized. The main positions employed in anorectal surgery are Lloyd-Davies position, lithotomy position, lateral decubitus position, and prone position. Each of these positions exerts specific physiological changes on the patient and has its own potential risks (Table 2). These risks are magnified especially in the anesthetized patient, and a reposition check should be performed after the patient is placed in the desired position (Table 3).

Lloyd-Davies and Lithotomy Positions

The resulting physiological changes and complications of these two positions are essentially the same. The key difference between the two positions is the degree of hip and knee flexion. Lloyd-Davies position allows access to both the abdomen and the perineum and is, therefore, used in the abdominoperineal approach for low rectal tumors. Lithotomy position is used for examination under anesthesia as well as for procedures, such as incision and drainage of abscesses. Allen stirrups are used for procedures expected to take longer than a few minutes to minimize pressure injury to the peroneal nerve. Many surgeons dislike the use of the lithotomy position for anal procedures, because the anal tissues and perineum tend to become engorged with blood. This can complicate procedures such as hemorrhoidectomy and fissurectomy.

Table 2   Risk of Position-Related Injuries in Anorectal Surgery (Greatest with General Anesthesia)

Complications	Lloyd-Davies/ lithotomy	Lateral decubitus	Prone
Eye injury	Low	High	High
Brachial plexus injury	Low	High	High
Ulnar nerve injury	Low	Low	High
Soft tissue injury	Low	Low	High
Sciatic nerve injury	Medium	Low	Low
Obturator nerve injury	Medium	Low	Low
Femoral nerve injury	Medium	Low	Low
Peroneal nerve injury	High	High	Low
Saphenous nerve injury	High	High	Low
DVT	High	Low	Low
Compartment syndrome	High	Medium	Low

Abbreviation: DVT, deep venous thrombosis.

Table 3 Reposition Checklist

Airway	Endotracheal tube/LMA	Patent and in correct position
Breathing	Ventilation	Pulmonary compliance satisfactory
	Auscultation	Both axillae
	Monitoring	SaO_2
		Capnograph trace and shape
Circulation	Monitoring	Heart rate, blood pressure, electrocardiogram still functioning
	Intravascular lines	All still in situ, patent, and accessible
Disability/ neurology	Eyes	Closed and protected
	Neurovascular	Padded vulnerable areas and avoidance of excessive passive stretch
Exposure	All cables, catheters, and electrodes	Checked and removed from the patient/ operating table interface
	Access	Maintain access for review of at risk areas if possible

Abbreviation: LMA, larygeal mask airway.
Source: From Ref. 13. Reproduced with permission.

However, this position allows good access and control of the patient's airway, and is thus safer for patients with severe respiratory disease or morbid obese patients. Furthermore, this position facilitates the use of facemasks for shorter procedures.

In lithotomy and Lloyd-Davies positions, lung volumes are reduced by the cephalad movement of the abdominal contents. The resulting decrease in functional residual capacity (FRC) is detrimental to gas exchange, with an increase in ventilation–perfusion mismatching and a decrease in pulmonary compliance. Furthermore, leg elevation redistributes pooled lower limb blood centrally, which may lead to volume overload in susceptible patients. In patients whose trachea is intubated, the raising of legs invariably leads to some cephalad movement of the endotracheal tube. This may lead to unexpected bronchospasm or endobronchial intubation.

Careful limb positioning in lithotomy or Lloyd-Davies positions is important to prevent injury and neuropathies. Resting the arms by the patient's side can lead to crush injuries when the leg section of the table is replaced at the end of the operation. This can be avoided by placing one arm on an arm board for access, while placing the opposite arm over the patient's chest. Before placing a patient in lithotomy or Lloyd-Davies position, it is necessary to assess degree of hip and knee joint movements of the patients, while awake, in order to avoid excessive or damaging movements during surgery and anesthesia. Both hip and knee joints should be moved at the same time. Extreme flexion of the hip joint can cause neural damage by stretch (sciatic and obturator nerves) or by direct pressure (compression of the femoral nerve because it passes under the inguinal ligament). Distally, the common peroneal and saphenous nerves are particularly at risk of compression injury because they wind around the neck of the fibula and medial tibial condyle, respectively (13,14).

In lithotomy position, calf compression is almost inevitable and, if prolonged, may predispose the patient to thromboembolism and compartment syndrome. The risk of compartment syndrome is less in patients for anorectal surgery, because procedures are unlikely to exceed five hours. Thromboembolism is more of an issue, and appropriate measures (e.g., compression stockings and mechanical calf compressors) should be considered in susceptible patients, especially when surgery is prolonged.

Lateral Decubitus Position

This position is used commonly for drainage of pilonidal and perianal abscesses. Its effectiveness may be limited by the patient being obese or difficulty in positioning assistants at the operating table. In the anesthetized patient, the dependant lung is relatively underventilated and overperfused whereas the opposite is true for the non-dependant lung. Although this is generally well tolerated in the healthy patient, it may cause hypoxemia in the compromised patient.

The lateral position is associated with the highest number of ocular complications. These are mainly corneal abrasions and occur equally in the dependant and nondependant eye, but more serious complications, such as blindness from retinal artery thrombosis, has occurred. This can be avoided by the application of eye padding/tape and by avoiding objects, such as face masks and surgical drapes over the eyes.

Several nerve injuries are more common in the lateral position. The brachial plexus is at risk if the head and neck do not have sufficient lateral support. An axillary roll is traditionally used to support the thorax. If placement is inadequate, the neurovascular bundle can be compressed in the axilla. Even with adequate support, venous hypertension in the dependant arm is almost inevitable, due to outflow obstruction.

Padding should be placed between the legs to prevent damage to both common peroneal and saphenous nerves. Peroneal nerve injury is also possible from pressure of the dependent leg against a poorly padded operating table (13,14).

Prone Position

Nearly all anorectal procedures can be carried out using this position. Many surgeons favor this position because it offers excellent exposure, provides space for assistants, and reduces engorgement of the hemorrhoidal plexus. Many of the physiological problems that occur in this position are due to poor patient positioning. It is important to avoid pressure on the abdomen, because any increase in pressure can lead to inferior vena caval compression, causing a reduction in venous return and poor cardiac output. Furthermore, lung compliance is reduced due to an increase in transdiaphragmatic pressure, thereby increasing airway pressure in ventilated patients. However, if a patient is positioned correctly, the prone position can improve oxygenation by increasing FRC and improving ventilation–perfusion matching.

The greatest concern with this position is the access to the airway and the risk of airway dislodgement on turning the patient. Thus, prior to turning, the airway should be well secured and its position ascertained by auscultation. Often on turning prone, an endotracheal tube will migrate and endobronchial intubation may occur. A simple test to help avoid this is to carefully flex a patient's neck while still supine, watching at the same time for a rise in airway pressure or a reduction in movement of one hemithorax. This can be supplemented by auscultation. If the airway pressure rises or there is a decrease in chest wall movement with this procedure, it is wise to withdraw the endotracheal tube slightly until this no longer happens, making endobronchial intubation on turning prone less likely.

Position-related injuries are common in the prone position and can only be avoided by scrupulous attention to detail. Adequate staff members must be present for moving the patient. The head and neck need to be carefully positioned to prevent excess pressure on the nose and eyes, with the eyes having been taped shut and padded prior to turning. The position of the arms should be symmetrical, maintaining a small degree of anterior flexion with abduction and external rotation to less than 90°. Care should be taken to ensure that the chest support does not impinge on the axilla, and forearm supports/pads should be positioned to prevent direct compression of the ulnar nerve in the cubital tunnel, and indirect compression of the axillary neurovascular bundle by axial pressure from the humerus. The feet, knees, pelvic area, breasts, axilla, elbows, and face are all at risk of pressure necrosis, and care should be taken to ensure that they are properly padded and supported (13,14).

ANESTHETIC TECHNIQUES

Anorectal disease is widespread in Western countries, with conditions such as hemorrhoids, anal fissures, and fistulas being the most common. The prevalence of anorectal disease is 4% to 5% of the adult population in the United States, with approximately 10% of these cases requiring surgery (15). Fortunately, the majority of anorectal surgery is for benign disease, which is amenable to relatively simple surgery of short duration. It has been estimated that 90% of anorectal cases may be suitable for ambulatory surgery (16). A U.K. survey of 105 patients undergoing day surgery proctology revealed that 79% found day surgery convenient and 82% rated the experience good or very good. Furthermore, 75% would accept day surgery again for a similar operation in the future (17).

As with any day case procedure, preoperative screening and consistent protocols in individual units are vital. To further achieve this goal, practice parameters for ambulatory anorectal surgery have been prepared by the Standards Task Force of the American Society of Colon and Rectal Surgeons (18). These guidelines are based on best available evidence and provide information for individual units to base their practice on. Patient's day case suitability on both medical and social grounds must be assessed. They should be in good general health with any chronic disease being well controlled. Patients need to be accompanied home, have an adult carer for at least 24 hours, have access to a telephone (along with clear instructions on how to get in contact with the unit), and be able to return easily to the hospital if problems occur. An admission rate of 2% has been reported (19).

Although many anorectal procedures are relatively simple, any surgery to this area is extremely stimulating and can result in severe pain (due to its multiple nerve supply), reflex body movements, tachypnea, and laryngeal spasm (Brewer–Luckhardt reflex), if the anesthetic depth is inadequate. Any anesthetic technique chosen must, therefore, aim to effectively block these painful stimuli. This may be achieved by general, regional, or local anesthesia or a combination.

General Anesthesia

General anesthesia, either alone or combined with regional/local techniques, remains the mainstay for anorectal surgery in the United Kingdom, although the acceptance of regional or local anesthesia with sedation is gaining popularity. Due to the intense stimulation produced by these procedures, the anesthesia employed should be deep and easily controllable as well as possessing a rapid recovery profile with minimal postoperative side effects. This can be achieved through the use of either inhalational or intravenous anesthetic agents. The newer, less-soluble agents, such as desflurane and sevoflurane, appear to be superior to isoflurane, in terms of faster recovery parameters; but there is probably little difference between the two newer agents (20,21). Propofol used as a sole anesthetic agent total intravenous anesthesia (TIVA) is also appropriate and has been demonstrated to be superior to isoflurane in terms of discharge time and nausea rate (22).

Due to the intense pain associated with anorectal surgery, adequate analgesia is vital perioperatively. The use of the relatively new opioid (remifentanyl) intraoperatively is particularly suited for anorectal procedures because it is a potent analgesic that has a fast onset, is easily controllable, and is rapidly metabolized, resulting in a short and predictable context-sensitive halftime (about five minutes) when used by infusion. However, prior to stopping the remifentanyl infusion, a longer-acting opioid should be given in order to maintain postoperative analgesia.

For a large proportion of anorectal procedures, in patients who are not at increased risk of aspiration, a laryngeal mask airway (LMA) is suitable, combined with either spontaneous ventilation or mechanical ventilation if muscle relaxation is required (23). Although the LMA has been used in the prone position for selected patients, it is not without risk because the airway is not protected and dislodgement may be a problem. It is safer to use an endotracheal tube for patients who are required to be prone or those at risk of aspiration. To facilitate endotracheal intubation, for short procedures, a short-acting muscle relaxant is often used (e.g., suxamethonium or mivacurium). The use of suxamethonium is associated with a high incidence of postoperative myalgia (45–85%), especially in young, muscular adults (24). Pretreatment with small doses of a nondepolarizing muscle relaxant has been ineffective in abolishing myalgia, despite their ability to eliminate fasciculation (25).

Because a large proportion of anorectal surgery can be carried out in the day case setting, it is important to minimize postoperative side effects that may prolong hospital stay. The most common of these are residual effects of anesthetics, nausea and vomiting, and severe pain (24). The use of the faster-acting anesthetic agents (desflurane, sevoflurane, and propofol) can improve recovery characteristics and return the patient to the preoperative level of functioning as soon as possible. Anesthetic technique should also be geared toward reducing factors known to contribute toward postoperative nausea and vomiting (PONV). Thus, emetogenic agents should be avoided (e.g., nitrous oxide), hydration maintained, hypotension/hypoxemia avoided, and gastric dilatation kept to a minimum. Patients at risk for PONV would benefit from a propofol TIVA technique, although it is more effective in early PONV (26,27). It is unclear whether the technique of choice for the high-risk patient is inhalational anesthesia with combination PONV prophylaxis or TIVA with propofol.

The combined use of opioids, paracetamol, nonsteroidal anti-inflammatory drugs, and local anesthesia is widely practised (multimodal analgesia). These drug combinations, working by various mechanisms of action, generally have a synergistic effect, so that a smaller amount of a single agent can be used for pain relief, resulting in fewer side effects and increase in overall patient satisfaction (28). With the reduction in the total amount of opioid required, the troublesome side effects of opioids, notably nausea and vomiting and urinary retention (a major complication in anorectal surgery), may be reduced. Ideally, these drugs should be given as early as possible, preferably preoperatively (if possible), because this would reduce overall intraoperative need for analgesia and promote better recovery (29).

Regional Anesthesia

Regional anesthesia can be used alone or in combination with sedation or general anesthesia. If used alone, it avoids the hazards associated with general anesthesia as well as avoiding or reducing side effects, such as sore throat, airway trauma, myalgia, and PONV. Other advantages to the patient include improved postoperative pain relief, shortened recovery room stay, and the ability to communicate with staff during the operation. When performed on its own, regional anesthesia techniques can take longer in the anesthetic room, as a result of having to spend time explaining the procedure to the patient, the time involved in performing the regional technique itself and waiting for the "block" to take effect, as well as the extra time required should an incomplete "block" require supplementation or conversion to a general anesthetic. Usually, the primary obstacle in using regional anesthetic techniques is convincing the surgeon that the extra time invested is worthwhile in improving the experience for both the patient and the surgeon. Each regional technique also carries its own complications and side effects. The regional techniques used for anorectal surgery are caudal, epidural, and spinal anesthesia.

Caudal Anesthesia

Caudal anesthesia is a form of epidural blockade achieved through the sacral hiatus that is palpable between the two sacral cornua of S5. Caudal anesthesia can be performed in the lateral or prone position, both in a patient who is awake and in the anesthetized patient. It is preferable to perform this block with the patient awake, because subperiosteal injection can be reported by the patient and accidental intravenous injection can be detected before the full dose is given. Caudal anesthesia is usually performed as a single-dose technique (although continuous anesthesia can be achieved by the insertion of a catheter) with full sterile precautions.

In clinical practice, the methods used to identify the caudal space before injection of medications include the characteristic "give" or "pop" when the sacrococcygeal ligament is penetrated, the "whoosh" test (injection of 2.5 mL of air to produce the characteristic "whoosh" on auscultation with a stethoscope placed over the lumbar region) (30), or nerve stimulation (correct needle placement confirmed by the presence of anal sphincter contraction to electrical stimulation) (31). Unfortunately, even with experienced anesthetists, the failure rate can be as high as 25% (30,31). This is due to the relatively common prevalence of anatomical abnormalities of the sacrum within the population (e.g., displacement of the hiatus, pronounced narrowing of the sacral canal making needle insertion difficult, and absence of the bony posterior wall of the sacral canal due to failure of laminae to fuse). Other complications of caudal anesthesia include subperiosteal injection, intravenous injection, dural tap with subsequent spinal block, and postoperative urinary retention.

For blockade to L2–L4 (i.e., the whole of the perineal area), 30 mL of local anesthetic are required, but for uncomplicated hemorrhoids or anal fissure, 20 mL will suffice. Both bupivacaine and levobupivacaine are used (due to their long action), although lidocaine is sometimes added to speed up the onset of the block. Several adjuvants have also been used to improve the quality and duration of the block. The addition of morphine, fentanyl, epinephrine, ketamine, and clonidine have all been described. In a study on patients undergoing elective hemorrhoidectomy, the addition of clonidine (75 μg) to the caudal mixture of 0.5% bupivacaine 35 mg with 2% lidocaine 140 mg and epinephrine 5 μg/mL more than doubled the period of analgesia when compared to a control group (32).

Caudal anesthesia has several advantages when compared with spinal anesthesia. The level of the block is directly related to the volume of anesthetic injected; therefore, the height of the block is more predictable. It is possible to achieve a selective sensory and motor block in the anorectal area without a motor block of the legs, thus allowing earlier mobilization and faster discharge if performed as a day case. Furthermore, with the use of long-acting local anesthetics and adjuvants, postoperative analgesia can be prolonged up to 16 hours (32). Finally, complications, such as hypotension and postdural puncture headache, are much less common (33).

Epidural Anesthesia

Epidural anesthesia is rarely used for simple anorectal surgery, being reserved for more complicated or radical procedures, particularly those requiring an abdominal incision.

Spinal Anesthesia

Spinal anesthesia is a useful technique for anorectal surgery. Its association with rapid onset, reliable block, prompt achievement of discharge criteria, minimal side effects, and improved analgesia makes it a popular choice. The technique itself is easy to perform, with success rates of greater than 90% after only 40 to 70 supervised attempts (34). A single-dose technique tends to be used, although spinal catheters are available for multiple dosing to prolong the anesthesia and for more precise titration of central neuraxial blockade.

A "saddle block" aiming to anesthetize S2–S5 dermatomes using small volumes (0.5–1.5 mL) of 0.5% heavy bupivacaine is most commonly used for anorectal surgery. This is best performed with the patient in the sitting position to allow the patient to remain sitting for a few minutes after the injection to limit the spread of the block. This low spinal blockade has no effect on the respiratory system and produces little in the way of hypotension because cardiac sympathetic fibers (T1–T4) are not affected, although there is a small reduction in preload and afterload associated with vasodilation. However, the height of the block may increase a few segments on changing the patient's position on the operating table (e.g., on turning prone). Plain bupivacaine is also suitable for operations in the prone jackknife position in a dose of 5 mL of 0.1% bupivacaine (35).

Spinal lidocaine (hyperbaric 5% lidocaine) used to be a popular choice of local anesthetic for day case anorectal surgery, due to its rapid onset of dense anesthesia and short-to-intermediate duration of action. However, the use of spinal lidocaine has decreased, due to its association with transient radicular irritation (defined as pain or dysanesthesia or both occurring in the legs or buttocks, which appear within a few hours until 24 hours after a full recovery from spinal anesthesia) (36). There have not been any reports of transient radicular irritation involving bupivacaine.

Recent attention has focused on the use of spinal adjuncts to decrease the overall dose of local anesthetic. Opioids, such as the highly lipophilic fentanyl and sufentanil, have been used to improve the quality of spinal anesthesia through a synergistic effect. Intrathecal fentanyl with a smaller subtherapeutic dose of lidocaine has been shown to enhance analgesia and improve the duration of the sensory block without prolonging recovery of the motor block or micturition (37). The usual dose of intrathecal fentanyl ranges from 10 to 25 µg. However, there are dose-related side effects of intrathecal opioids, such as pruritus, urinary retention, and respiratory depression. The most frequent side effect is pruritus, which is easily treated; respiratory depression is rare with fentanyl doses less than 25 µg (38).

Clonidine, the alpha-2 agonist, is another useful alternative analgesic adjunct. Intrathecal clonidine (15–45 µg) increases the quality and duration of anesthesia when combined with local anesthetics (39). Low-dose clonidine is not associated with known side effects (e.g., bradycardia, hypotension, and sedation), although it may delay the time to void (40).

Finally, with the introduction and widespread use of small gauge, pencil-point needles, the incidence of postdural puncture headache has fallen to below 1%, thereby increasing its acceptance in ambulatory anorectal surgery. However, acute urinary retention remains a well-known complication of spinal anesthesia (41). With the use of smaller dosages of local anesthetics and adjuncts, faster recovery of bladder function and earlier mobilization may lead to a reduction in the incidence of acute urinary retention.

Local Anesthesia

The Standards Task Force of the American Society of Colon and Rectal Surgeons (2003) recommends that most ambulatory anorectal surgery may be safely and cost-effectively performed under local anesthesia (18). However, this requires patient and surgeon cooperation and, most importantly, patient's acceptance of the technique. Monitored anesthetic care (MAC) with intravenous sedation (conscious sedation) will enhance patient acceptability and is recommended (10). Doses of commonly used sedative and analgesic drugs used in MAC are listed (Table 4). The aim of MAC is to maintain the patient in a moderate state of sedation, during which the patient is able to respond to verbal or light tactile stimulation. In this state, no interventions are required to maintain a patent airway and spontaneous respiration is adequate (Observer's Assessment of Alertness–Sedation score of 3, with 5 = awake/alert and 1 = asleep) (43).

Various local anesthetic techniques are available for the surgeon. It is important to stress that injection in the anorectal region causes severe pain, and that the pain is caused not by the needle puncture but by the injection of the anesthetic agent itself, especially when it is distal to the dentate line. The technique described by Nivatvong (1982) causes the least pain (44). The anesthetic solution (0.25% bupivacaine with 1:200,000 epinephrine) is first injected into the submucosa proximal to the dentate line. The wheal of local anesthetic solution is then milked across the dentate line into the subdermal plane to anesthetize the sensitive anoderm. The next injection into the anoderm, thus, causes minimal or no pain to the patient. Typically, 20 to 25 mL of the local anesthetic solution is required.

Other techniques include the posterior perineal block, which involves deep blockade of the pudendal nerve and its branches. Commonly used local anesthetic agents are lidocaine 0.5% to 1% and bupivacaine 0.25% to 0.5%, which is often

Table 4 Sedative and Analgesic Drugs Used in Monitored Anesthetic Care

Drug	Bolus dose range	Infusion range ($\mu g/kg/min$)
Sedative/anxiolytic		
Midazolam	0.01–0.1 mg/kg	0.25–2.0
Propofol	0.25–1 mg/kg	10–75
Analgesics		
Alfentanil	5–10 µg/kg	0.25–1.0
Fentanyl	25–50 µg	
Remifentanil	0.10–0.35 µg/kg	0.025–0.15
Ketamine	0.15 mg/kg	

Source: Adapted from Ref. 42.

combined with epinephrine (1:200,000) to prolong the duration of action of lidocaine and to induce vasospasm of the operative field. Addition of sodium bicarbonate to the solution may help to alleviate the pain on injection (45).

The advantages of a local anesthetic technique (with MAC) is its simplicity, speed of administration, minimal recovery time, low cost, and low incidence of complications compared with regional or general anesthesia. In a study by Li et al. (2000), patient satisfaction was high with the local anesthesia sedation technique and may be related to good postoperative pain control and the absence of side effects, such as urinary retention, nausea, and vomiting, which were reported with the other two techniques (general anesthesia and spinal anesthesia) (15).

However, the local anesthetic techniques described are not suitable for procedures that involve a large operative field, procedures that invade the peritoneal cavity (e.g., perineal proctosigmoidectomy), long duration surgery, or procedures performed in the setting of severe anorectal sepsis. Furthermore, young men with large muscular buttocks, who are apprehensive of anorectal surgery, may be better with regional anesthesia to facilitate exposure and limit patient motion during sedation.

POSTOPERATIVE COMPLICATIONS

Urinary retention is a common complication following anorectal surgery, occurring with a frequency of up to 30% (41,46). Hemorrhoidectomy and the performance of multiple anorectal procedures have the highest rates of urinary retention (41,47). There are numerous reasons for this including the use of opioids, presence of postoperative pain (reflex inhibition of bladder contraction), overzealous use of intraoperative fluids, and unfamiliar hospital surroundings where privacy may be a premium. Patients who have received regional anesthesia are at increased risk, especially if adjuvant opioids were used. Good multimodal analgesia to achieve adequate pain control and limiting perioperative fluids have been shown to reduce the incidence of urinary retention (41). Other common postoperative complications include pain, PONV, bleeding, and prolonged motor blockade with spinal anesthesia, and have already been discussed.

The minimally invasive surgical techniques of TEM and ETAR possess their own unique postoperative complications. Recognized TEM postoperative complications are bleeding, transient postoperative pyrexia, perforation of the rectum, and urinary retention. In addition, the requirement for carbon dioxide insufflation of the rectum has resulted in hypercapnia, surgical emphysema, and delayed postoperative ventilatory failure in a patient (48). It is recommended that patients with arterial hypercapnia or surgical emphysema after TEM should be observed for a prolonged period in the recovery room to allow early detection of ventilatory failure. With ETAR, postoperative complications are similar and include hemorrhage, perforation, sepsis, rectovaginal fistulas, strictures, and urinary retention. The potential problem of glycine absorption leading to a "TUR syndrome" (described after transurethral resection of prostate) has not been seen after ETAR (49).

SUMMARY

The challenge in anesthesia for anorectal surgery is to provide optimal patient positioning and selection of the most appropriate anesthetic technique for the patient. Close cooperation and communication with the surgeon and patient will ensure a satisfactory patient experience and good operating conditions for the surgeon. Because the majority of anorectal procedures are suitable as day case, any anesthetic technique chosen should achieve a state of home-readiness in the shortest possible time, and measures instituted to reduce the common postoperative complications of urinary retention and pain. Furthermore, the recent minimally invasive surgical techniques present their own challenges as frailer, older patients, not suitable for radical open procedures are presented for surgery.

REFERENCES

1. Pfenninger JL, Zainea GG. Common anorectal conditions: Part I. Symptoms and complaints. Am Fam Physician 2001; 63:2391–2398.
2. McMinn RMH. Regional and applied anatomy. In: McMinn RMH, ed. Last's Anatomy 10th ed. New York: Churchill Livingstone, 1994:377–381.
3. Nicholls RJ, Dozois RR. Topographic anatomy. In: Surgery of the Colon and Rectum. New York: Churchill Livingstone, 1999:1–17.
4. Endreseth BH, Wibe A, Svinsås M, et al. Postoperative morbidity and recurrence after local excision of rectal adenomas and rectal cancer by transanal endoscopic microsurgery. Colorect Dis 2005; 7:133–137.
5. Keighley MRB, Williams NS. Surgical treatment of rectal cancer. In: Keighley MRB, Williams NS, eds. Surgery of the Anus, Rectum, and Colon. 2nd ed. WB Saunders, 1999:1119–1244.
6. Berry AR, Souter RG, Campbell WB, et al. Endoscopic transanal resection of rectal tumours: a preliminary report of its use. Br J Surg 1990; 77:134–137.
7. Sutton CD, Marshall L-J, White SA, et al. Ten year experience of endoscopic transanal resection. Ann Surg 2002; 235(3):355–362.
8. Dickinson AJ, Savage AP, Mortensen NJ, et al. Long-term survival after endoscopic transanal resection of rectal tumours. Br J Surg 1993; 80:1401–1404.
9. Longo A. Treatment of hemorrhoid disease by reduction of mucosa and hemorrhoid prolapse with a circular-suturing device: a new procedure; 777–784. Proceedings of the 6th World Congress of Endoscopic Surgery, Rome, Italy, June 3–6, 1998.
10. Corman ML, Gravié J-F, Hager T, et al. Stapled haemorrhoidopexy: a consensus position paper by an international working party—indications, contra-indications and technique. Colorect Dis 2003; 5:304–310.
11. Rowsell M, Bello M, Hemingway DM. Circumferential mucosectomy (stapled haemorrhoidectomy) versus conventional haemorrhoidectomy: randomised controlled trial. Lancet 2000; 355:779–781.
12. Nisar PJ, Acheson AG, Neal K, et al. Stapled hemorrhoidopexy compared with conventional haemorrhoidectomy: systematic review of randomised controlled trials. Dis Colon Rectum 2004; 47(11):1837–1845.
13. Knight D, Mahajan R. Patient positioning in anaesthesia. Continuing education in anaesthesia. Crit Care Pain 2005; 4(5):160–163.
14. Karulf R. Anesthesia and intraoperative positioning. In Hicks T, Beck D, Opelka F, Timmcke A, eds. Complications of Colon and Rectal Surgery. Baltimore: Williams and Wilkins, 1996:34–49.
15. Li S, Coloma M, White PF, et al. Comparison of the costs and recovery profiles of three anesthetic techniques for ambulatory anorectal surgery. Anesthesiology 2000; 93: 1225–1230.
16. Smith LE. Ambulatory surgery for anorectal disease: an update. South Med J 1986; 79:163–166.
17. Thompson-Fawcett MW, Cook TA, Baigrie RJ, et al. What patients think of day-surgery proctology. Br J Surg 1998; 85:1388.

18. Place R, Hymen N, Simmang C, et al. Practice parameters for ambulatory anorectal surgery. Dis Colon Rectum 2003; 46(5):573–576.
19. Medwell SJ, Friend WG. Outpatient anorectal surgery. Dis Colon Rectum 1979; 22: 480–482.
20. Ghouri AF, Bodner M, White PF. Recovery profile after desflurane-nitrous oxide versus isoflurane-nitrous oxide in outpatients. Anesthesiology 1991; 74:419–424.
21. Philip BK, Kallar SK, Bogetz MS, et al. A multicentre comparison of maintenance and recovery with sevoflurane or isoflurane for adult ambulatory anesthesia. The Sevoflurane Multicenter Ambulatory Group. Anesth Analg 1996; 83:314–319.
22. Visser K, Hassink EA, Bonsel GJ, et al. Randomised controlled trial of total intravenous anesthesia with propofol versus inhalation anesthesia with isoflurane-nitrous oxide: postoperative nausea with vomiting and economic analysis. Anesthesiology 2001; 95:616–626.
23. Verghese C, Brimacombe JR. Survey of laryngeal mask airway usage in 11,910 patients: safety and efficacy for conventional and non-conventional usage. Anesth Analg 1996; 82:129–133.
24. Rawal N. Analgesia for day-case surgery. Br J Anaesth 2001; 87(1):73–81.
25. Blitt CD, Carlson GL, Rolling GD, et al. A comparative evaluation of pretreatment with nondepolarizing neuromuscular blockers prior to the administration of succinylcholine. Anesthesiology 1981; 55(6):687–689.
26. Apfel CC, Kranke P, Katz MH, et al. Volatile anaesthetics may be the main cause of early but not delayed postoperative vomiting: a randomised controlled trial of factorial design. Br J Anaesth 2002; 88(5):659–668.
27. Gan TJ, Meyer T, Apfel C, et al. Consensus guidelines for managing postoperative nausea and vomiting. Anesth Analg 2003; 97:62–71.
28. Kehlet H, Dahl JB. The value of multi-modal or balanced analgesia on postoperative pain relief. Anesth Analg 1993; 77:1048–1056.
29. Michaloliakou C, Chung F, Sharma S. Preoperative multimodal analgesia facilitates recovery after laparoscopic cholecystectomy. Anesth Analg 1996; 82:44–51.
30. Lewis MPN, Thomas P, Wilson LF, et al. The "whoosh" test: a clinical test to confirm correct needle placement in caudal epidural injections. Anaesthesia 1992; 47:57–58.
31. Tsui BC, Tarkkila P, Gupta S, et al. Confirmation of caudal needle placement using nerve stimulation. Anesthesiology 1999; 91:374–378.
32. Van Elstraete AC, Pastureau F, Lebrun T, et al. Caudal clonidine for postoperative analgesia in adults. Br J Anaesth 2000; 84(3):401–402.
33. Gudaitytė J, Marchertienė I, Pavalkis D. Anesthesia for ambulatory anorectal surgery. Medicina 2004; 40(2):101–111.
34. Liu SS, McDonald SB. Current issues in spinal anaesthesia. Anesthesiology 2001; 94(5): 888–906.
35. Maroof M, Khan RM, Siddique M, et al. Hypobaric spinal anaesthesia gives selective sensory block for anorectal surgery. Can J Anaesth 1995; 42(8):691–694.
36. Schneider M, Ettlin T, Kauffman M, et al. Transient neurologic toxicity after hyperbaric subarachnoid anesthesia with 5% lidocaine. Anesth Analg 1993; 76:1154–1157.
37. Liu S, Chiu AA, Carpenter RL, et al. Fentanyl prolongs lidocaine spinal anaesthesia without prolonging recovery. Anesth Analg 1995; 80:730–734.
38. Varrassi G, Celleno D, Capogna P, et al. Ventilatory effects of subarachnoid fentanyl in the elderly. Anaesthesia 1992; 47:558–563.
39. Niemi L. Effects of intrathecal clonidine on duration of bupivacaine spinal anaesthesia, haemodynamics, and postoperative analgesia in patients undergoing knee arthroscopy. Acta Anaesthesiol Scand 1994; 38:724–728.
40. De Kock M, Gautier P, Fanard L, et al. Intrathecal ropivacaine and clonidine for ambulatory knee arthroscopy: a dose response study. Anesthesiology 2001; 94:574–578.
41. Prasad M, Abcarian H. Urinary retention following operations for benign anorectal diseases. Dis Colon Rectum 1978; 21(7):490–492.

42. Gregory J, McGoldrick K. Monitored anesthesia care for ambulatory surgery. In: Steele SM, Nielsen KC, Klein SM, eds. Ambulatory Anesthesia and Perioperative Analgesia. McGraw-Hill, 2005:223–231.
43. Chernik DA, Gillings D, Laine H, et al. Validity and reliability of the observer's assessment of alertness/sedation scale: study with intravenous midazolam. J Clin Psychopharmacol 1990; 10:244–251.
44. Nivatvong S. An improved technique of local anesthesia for anorectal surgery. Dis Colon Rectum 1982; 25:259–260.
45. McKay W, Morris R, Mushlin P. Sodium bicarbonate attenuates pain on skin infiltration with lidocaine, with or without epinephrine. Anesth Analg 1987; 66:572–574.
46. Petros JG, Bradley TM. Factors influencing postoperative urinary retention in patients undergoing surgery for benign anorectal disease. Am J Surg 1990; 159(4):374–376.
47. Zaheer S, Reilly WT, Pemberton JH, et al. Urinary retention after operations for benign anorectal diseases. Dis Colon Rectum 1998; 41:696–704.
48. Kerr K, Mills GH. Intra-operative and post-operative hypercapnia leading to delayed respiratory failure associated with transanal endoscopic microsurgery under general anaesthesia. Br J Anaesth 2001; 86(4):586–589.
49. Boyle JR, Thompson MM, Lopez B, et al. TUR syndrome and endoscopic transanal resection: no evidence for a clinically important association in 38 procedures. Br J Surg 1997; 84:831–833.

24

Anesthesia for Emergency Exploratory Laparotomy

Elizabeth C. Storey and Andrew B. Lumb
Department of Anesthetics, St. James's University Hospital, Leeds, U.K.

INTRODUCTION

Patients who require emergency exploratory laparotomy face all the same challenges as patients requiring elective surgery described in the other chapters of this book. Unfortunately, emergency patients do not have the luxury of time to have their preexisting medical conditions properly assessed and optimized, investigations completed, and any physiological derangements corrected. Because of the rapidly progressive course of the surgical presentation, patients often require surgery outside of normal operating hours, and so both the surgeons and the anesthetists responsible for the patient may be inexperienced at managing such complex cases. These are some of the factors contributing to the observation that emergency abdominal surgery exposes the patient to a high risk of morbidity and mortality.

PREOPERATIVE ASSESSMENT AND OPTIMIZATION

The principles of preoperative evaluation (Chapter 7) of the elective patient must also be applied to the emergency situation, and normally extended to include further risk assessment and preoperative management. This phase of patient management is crucial to determining whether any operation is in the patient's best interests and, if so, the optimal surgical procedure that will reverse the underlying pathological process. A team approach is required, with the anesthetist being best placed to manage the patient's acute physiological disturbance and assess their other medical conditions, while the surgeon evaluates their acute surgical condition and the options available for its management. Throughout this process, all members of the team are responsible for involving the patient and their relatives in the decision-making process.

Assessment of Risk

The recognition and evaluation of risk plays a crucial role in management planning, and anesthetists are often asked to predict the risk that an emergency laparotomy will impose on an individual patient. The risks are multifactorial and may include patient age, chronic health issues, acute physiology and preoperative condition, type of operation, time of operation, duration of operation, grade of surgeon and anesthetist, and the intensity of perioperative monitoring and care.

Comorbidity

Systemic disturbance caused by pathophysiological processes other than the condition to be treated will significantly contribute to the clinical picture and ability of the patient to respond to the acute illness. Hypertension, heart failure, valvular disease, ischemic heart disease, nonsinus ECG, acute or chronic respiratory disease, renal impairment, electrolyte disturbance and hypovolemia, diabetes, obesity, malnutrition, septicemia, and dementia or confusion are important considerations.

OUTCOME FOLLOWING EMERGENCY LAPAROTOMY

Outcome is usually measured in terms of morbidity and mortality, with estimates of mortality ranging from 10% to 55% (1). Crude measurements like these can be misleading, but scoring systems that group patients based on the severity of illness before treatment and on intraoperative timing and events can allow a meaningful analysis of morbidity and mortality. There have been some studies examining risk and outcome in emergency laparotomy using such scores (1,2). The studies highlight that increasing age and American Society of Anesthesiologists (ASA) status are strong predictors of a poor outcome. In one study (1), no patient of ASA class 4 or 5, and aged over 85 survived. Of the deaths reported to the National Confidential Enquiry into Perioperative Deaths for the period 1998–1999, 69% of patients were aged over 70, and 72% of deaths occurred in patients having emergency surgery (3). Probability of death was also shown to be increased in patients who were admitted to the intensive care unit (ICU) or had invasive hemodynamic monitoring, a likely reflection of appropriate allocation to these interventions.

PREOPERATIVE FLUID MANAGEMENT

Perioperative hypovolemia is associated with poorer clinical outcomes following elective bowel surgery (4). Hypovolemia will be even more severe in most emergency cases, so intravenous fluid resuscitation is a vital part of care for the sick laparotomy patient. Hypovolemia refers to a reduction in extracellular fluid volume, which, when severe, leads to inadequate tissue perfusion and organ dysfunction. Hypovolemia can be absolute, with actual loss of volume, or relative, with redistribution of body fluid or dilatation of the intravascular space resulting in a decrease in the effective intravascular volume.

Clinical Assessment

History-taking and clinical examination are useful tools in the diagnosis of hypovolemia, and the clinical picture of hypovolemia is shown in Table 1. However the absence of these clinical signs does not exclude hypovolemia; it may be masked by physiological compensatory mechanisms and, in such cases, significant delay in treatment may result. Several studies have shown that accurate prediction of hemodynamic status

Table 1 Clinical Features of Varying Degrees of Hypovolemia

	Severity of hypovolemia		
	Mild	Moderate	Severe
Clinical features	Thirst	Pallor	Coma
	Dry mouth	↓ Skin turgor	Breathlessness
		Confusion	
Cardiovascular response			
Clinical	Postural hypotension	↑ Heart rate	Shock
CVP	Normal	Normal/low	Low
Renal response	↑ Urine osmolality	Oliguria	Renal failure

Abbreviation: CVP, central venous pressure.

by clinical assessment alone only occurs in half the cases. More invasive procedures are therefore advisable in the diagnosis and ongoing assessment of hypovolemia, such as central venous pressure (CVP) measurement, and these are discussed later in this chapter. New techniques are being evaluated for the noninvasive assessment of fluid status (5), though these are not yet widely available.

Monitoring

CVP is the most commonly used surrogate marker of volume status, the benefit of which is its relative ease of measurement, but it is unreliable in pulmonary vascular disease, right-ventricular disease, valvular heart disease, and isolated left-ventricular failure. A tense abdomen may also lead to inaccuracies. A single CVP measurement, therefore, has little significance, but a change in CVP in response to fluid administration provides helpful information, and this is discussed in the following section. In patients with significant cardiac disease, particularly heart failure, a pulmonary artery catheter may be indicated, though recent improvements in noninvasive cardiac output measurement have reduced the popularity of pulmonary artery catheters.

Measurement of urine output is important as a method of assessing fluid status, and insertion of a urinary catheter allows precise evaluation. A volume greater than $0.5 \, \text{mL} \, \text{kg}^{-1} \, \text{hr}^{-1}$ is regarded as indicative of adequate renal perfusion.

Fluid Resuscitation

The aim of fluid resuscitation (6) is to increase intravascular volume and to improve cardiac output and organ perfusion. It is a dynamic process that requires ongoing evaluation of clinical and hemodynamic indices. The use of a fluid challenge is a method of safely restoring circulating volume according to physiological need, rather than using fixed hemodynamic end points. Because of their ability to remain in the intravascular compartment for a longer period, colloids are more appropriate than crystalloids for fluid challenge. Ideally, the response to the fluid is assessed by measuring trends in CVP or stroke volume (Chapter 8), but in the absence of these measures, clinical indices of perfusion, such as urine output, may be used.

Fluid challenges are useful for the rapid correction of intravascular volume depletion, but in patients with abdominal pathology, there is likely to be significant depletion of other fluid compartments. The choice of a replacement fluid then depends in part on the type of fluid that has been lost. Blood and blood products are indicated in patients with significant hemorrhage to maintain oxygen-carrying capacity and hemostasis. Both crystalloids and colloids can be used to replace extracellular fluid deficit. Crystalloid solutions, such as Hartmann's and normal saline solution, do not possess oncotic properties, and so only 25% of the infused volume is retained in the intravascular space, while the remainder replenishes the interstitial space. The use of large volumes of normal saline may lead to hyper-chloremia and metabolic acidosis, but it is unknown whether or not this is clinically harmful (6,7). Other advantages of crystalloid solutions include its relatively low cost and nonallergenic properties.

Colloids include plasma substitutes, such as human serum albumin, or synthetic solutions that use dextrans, gelatins, or starches as the colloid component. They contain large molecules that stay within the intravascular space and exert an oncotic force to maintain plasma volume. All the colloid solutions have particles with an average molecular weight of greater than 45 kDa, which prevents the particles from being filtered in the kidney. However, different solutions have differing ranges of particle size, with, for example, the starches having a wider range than gelatins. With a wide range in particle size, some particles will be small enough to be filtered in the glomerulus and so act as an osmotic diuretic, and some particles will be so large that even in the presence of leaky capillaries they will be retained within the circulation. Disadvantages of colloids include relatively high cost, a risk of developing coagulopathy, and rare allergic reactions.

The controversy over colloid versus crystalloid is well known (6). Both are capable of restoring circulating volume, and though colloids achieve this more rapidly, smaller volumes are required and their effects last longer. Conversely, leakage of colloid particles into the interstitial space contributes to edema formation in the presence of leaky capillaries.

WHEN TO OPERATE?

A common dilemma arises regarding the optimal time to perform surgery in very ill patients with an acute abdomen. The optimization of the patient's preexisting medical problems, the institution of invasive monitoring, and correction of fluid deficits all take some hours to achieve. In the meantime, the surgical condition may deteriorate, for example, if bowel obstruction progresses to a perforation, worsening the patient's physiological abnormalities. A compromise on the timing of surgery is therefore usually required, with the surgeon needing to accept that a period of preoperative optimization is necessary while the anesthetist must accept that the operation may need to be performed before preoperative preparation is completely optimal.

ANESTHETIC TECHNIQUE

Induction

Individual clinicians should choose between induction in the operating theater and induction in the anesthetic room, and in the United Kingdom, the vast majority choose the anesthetic room for elective cases (8). Anesthetists may still choose to induce acutely ill patients in the theater to avoid the inevitable interruption to monitoring that takes place on transferring the patient to the operating theater. Minimal standards of monitoring (see below) should be instituted before induction in all patients, with more invasive monitoring required in patients with severe cardiovascular disease or hemodynamic instability.

Induction Agents

Little evidence exists on the best technique for induction of anesthesia in emergency patients. Intravenous rapid sequence is the technique traditionally taught in emergency circumstances, although more experienced clinicians may modify or even abandon this technique in the critically ill. Rapid injection of a prejudged dose of intravenous induction agent is potentially hazardous because determination of a safe dose in the critically ill patient is difficult, and is often no more than a guess. Hypotension from relative overdose may produce myocardial ischemia and adversely influence the postoperative course. On the contrary, these patients represent a high-risk group for awareness, and failure to administer an adequate induction dose may lead to the return of consciousness in the paralyzed patient during intubation. A recent large prospective study reported an incidence of awareness of 0.18% with a slightly higher proportion of these occurrences seen after emergency rather than elective operations (9).

Intravenous induction agents are widely used in the emergency situation. Etomidate is known for its cardiovascular stability, and although peripheral vascular resistance may fall slightly, myocardial oxygen supply, contractility, and blood pressure remain largely unchanged. Etomidate has long been known to suppress adrenocortical function when used by infusion, but recent work has suggested this may also occur following its use for induction of anesthesia (10). Suppression of the adrenal gland after a bolus dose of etomidate persists for up to 48 hours, and may therefore lead to an inadequate cortisol response in the early postoperative period when patients are most at risk of developing multiorgan dysfunction syndrome. Thiopentone produces predictable and rapid loss of consciousness, but there is a dose-dependent reduction in cardiac output and systemic vascular resistance. Even so, when carefully titrated doses are used, thiopentone may compare favorably with etomidate in elective cases (11). Propofol is also associated with a dose-dependent fall in peripheral vascular resistance, blood pressure, and myocardial contractility, and bradycardia may occur. Ketamine may be used intravenously for induction, which, unlike other agents, produces sympathetic stimulation, increasing circulating levels of adrenaline and noradrenaline.

Choice of an agent is often based on user preference and experience, and some anesthetists may opt for an inhalational technique. A survey of the Royal College of Anesthetists clinical tutors in the United Kingdom revealed that 25% of tutors reported inhalational induction with sevoflurane being an acceptable technique for laparotomy for a patient in shock (12). Advantages of sevoflurane include a rapid smooth induction, less reduction in mean arterial pressure, and a minimal change in heart rate; airway assessment is possible in a spontaneously breathing patient. This must of course be balanced against the risk of aspiration of gastric contents.

Rapid Sequence Induction

A patient requiring an emergency laparotomy is at high risk of aspiration of gastric contents at the induction of, and emergence from, anesthesia. Patients with bowel obstruction or those in whom surgery is so urgent that there is insufficient time for preoperative fasting will clearly have a full stomach at induction, and are, therefore, particularly at risk of aspiration of gastric contents. Any form of acute intra-abdominal pathology may lead to reduced small bowel peristalsis and gastric stasis, which may be further impaired by the preoperative use of opioids. It is worth remembering that the stomach normally produces 2.5 L of secretions per day, with a further 8 to 10 L produced by the pancreas and small bowel; so even in a patient with adequate duration of preoperative fasting, the stomach may contain huge volumes of secretions if stomach and small bowel function is even slightly impaired. If a nasogastric tube is in place before induction of anesthesia, any gastric contents should be removed, though this does not empty the stomach sufficiently to obviate the need for airway protection. The nasogastric tube should be left in situ during induction, because it does not affect the effectiveness of cricoid pressure (13).

A rapid sequence induction (RSI) should be considered. The aim of an RSI is to minimize the time that the patient spends in the unconscious state, and, therefore, being at risk of aspiration, before being intubated with a cuffed tracheal tube. Following formal preoxygenation, predetermined doses of the induction agent and a fast-acting muscle relaxant are administered, and the trachea intubated as rapidly as possible. Potential complications of an RSI should be considered. The major risk arises from attempted intubation without assurance that it is possible to ventilate the patient, which may lead to inability of ventilating a paralyzed patient. Guidelines to deal with this life-threatening situation are available (14).

For preoxygenation to be effective, some attention to detail is required (15). The breathing system in use must be adequately flushed to remove nitrogen or other contaminants before application to the patient using a tight-fitting face mask, which must be applied with suitable force so as to prevent entrainment of room air by the patient. Three minutes of normal breathing or various vital capacity maneuvers are all described, though there is no single technique that is agreed upon to be optimal. One solution to this uncertainty is to measure expired oxygen concentration, and only when FeO_2 reaches 0.9 can preoxygenation be regarded as adequately completed. Preoxygenation provides a time cushion for dealing with any adverse responses to the induction of anesthesia or any difficulties in maintaining a patent airway or artificial ventilation. The store of oxygen to provide this reserve is mostly in the functional residual capacity (FRC) of the patient's lungs. Preoxygenation may therefore be rendered less effective either because the FRC is reduced (e.g., with lung disease, abdominal distension, or pregnancy) or if oxygen consumption is increased (e.g., in sepsis or pregnancy).

In most patients requiring a RSI, cricoid pressure should also be used to minimize the risk of regurgitation of gastric fluid. First described in 1961 (16), Sellick's maneuver involves occluding the esophagus by extension of the neck, and application of pressure over the cricoid cartilage against the body of the sixth cervical vertebra (Fig. 1). Incorrect application may lead to distortion of the larynx, difficult intubation, airway obstruction, and rarely esophageal rupture during active vomiting (17). The safe use of cricoid pressure reduces complications associated with its use, and adequate training of staff who perform cricoid pressure is vital (17,18). A force of 20 N applied to the cricoid cartilage is believed to be the minimum required to prevent regurgitation, but at 40 N, distortion of the laryngeal anatomy or airway obstruction commonly occurs. Current recommendations are that a force of 10 N should be applied while the patient is still conscious, increasing to 30 N on induction of anesthesia (17). Various methods are available to train staff in how to apply this amount of force. Descriptive methods, such as applying the same force as that required to cause discomfort while pressing on the bridge of your own nose, have been shown to be unreliable (18); however simple simulators, such as weighing scales, can be used to more formally train the staff (19).

Modified RSI is a loose term applied to a range of deviations from the standard RSI described so far, such as maintaining the cricoid pressure and using a bag and mask to ventilate the patient, while waiting for the nondepolarizing muscle relaxant

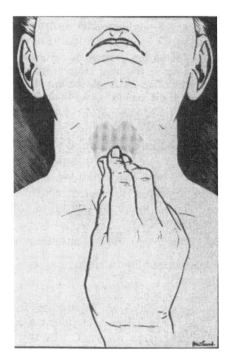

Figure 1 The correct technique for application of cricoid pressure, as illustrated in Sellick's original description in 1961. *Source*: From Ref. 16.

to produce sufficient paralysis for intubation. As a result of its rapid speed of onset, suxamethonium remains the muscle relaxant of choice for an RSI, with adequate conditions for intubation occurring in less than 60 seconds after administration. Some recently introduced nondepolarizing agents such as rocuronium can provide intubating conditions with a sufficiently rapid speed of onset to facilitate RSI (20); however, the long duration of action of these agents is of particular concern if airway maintenance or ventilation difficulties occur. Current research and development of a new reversal agent may allow safer use of rocuronium for RSI (21).

INTRAOPERATIVE CARE

Intraoperative analgesia and maintenance of anesthesia for emergency laparotomy are not significantly different from the techniques used for elective cases. Postoperative analgesia is discussed below.

Monitoring

The minimal monitoring required for a patient receiving a general anesthetic and artificial ventilation includes the continuous presence of a suitably trained anesthetist and the following monitors (22):

- Inspired oxygen concentration
- Continuous capnography, airway pressure, and expired tidal volumes to monitor the integrity of the breathing system and adequacy of ventilation

- Pulse oximetry
- Electrocardiogram
- Noninvasive blood pressure recordings

Most patients having emergency laparotomy will require more complex monitoring than these minimum standards. Measurement of core body temperature should be used routinely if active warming of the patient is to be done. Monitoring of neuromuscular blockade is advisable in laparotomy patients who require complete muscle relaxation to facilitate surgery. As described above, urine output provides a simple but effective way of monitoring the fluid status of the patient. Finally, invasive cardiovascular monitoring will be needed in a significant proportion of emergency laparotomy patients. The large shift of fluid between body compartments that occurs with major abdominal pathology and surgery will have significant repercussions in patients with cardiac disease. For example, a patient with heart failure (either currently or in the past) or a poorly functioning left ventricle is at a substantial risk of developing perioperative complications, and invasive cardiovascular monitoring is required. If abdominal sepsis progresses to septicemia, management will routinely require invasive monitoring, normally including pulmonary artery catheterization or some other assessment of cardiac output.

Fluid Administration

If fluid resuscitation, as described above, has been adequately implemented before surgery, then intraoperative requirements should be similar to those for elective patients. Three types of fluid replacement should be considered:

- Maintenance fluid, using crystalloid solutions, at approximately $2\,\mathrm{mL}$ $\mathrm{kg^{-1}\,hr^{-1}}$, remembering to include any time spent nil-by-mouth preoperatively, if fluids have not been given before theater
- Blood loss should be estimated during surgery, and the volume replaced with colloid solutions or blood products if required to maintain an adequate hemoglobin concentration and hemostatic function of the blood
- Third-space loss describes all other forms of fluid requirement, including evaporation from the wound, secretion of fluids into the bowel when abdominal pathology prevents its reabsorption, and shift of intravascular fluid into the interstitial or intracellular compartments. For elective intra-abdominal surgery, third-space losses may be estimated to be 6 to $8\,\mathrm{mL\,kg^{-1}\,hr^{-1}}$, though in emergency patients this may still be an underestimate, and monitoring of CVP and urine output is advisable

Temperature Control

Central body temperature decreases after induction of general anesthesia, due to vasodilation, causing redistribution of heat from central to peripheral body compartments, and from a reduction in metabolic heat production. During laparotomy, this heat loss is compounded by exposure of a large surface area of peritoneum. The effects of hypothermia are significant and include decreased cardiac output and oxygen delivery, an increase in oxygen consumption, an increase in bleeding tendency, and a compromised immune function. A randomized control study investigated the influence of active warming by using a forced air blanket, before and during surgery on 40 patients undergoing major abdominal surgery (23). It concluded that maintenance of normothermia reduced stay on the postanesthesia care unit, lowered the incidence of postoperative mechanical ventilation, and reduced perioperative blood loss, resulting in fewer transfusion requirements.

EMERGENCE

Extubation

Particular care is required during emergence from anesthesia in patients who have required a RSI. During their return to full consciousness, the patient passes through another period of risk of aspiration of gastric contents, when protective reflexes are impaired and the tracheal tube may have been removed. Before extubation, the patient should be fully awake and should be making purposeful movements, to ensure that they can protect their own airway after removal of the endotracheal tube. The patient may be sat up or placed in the left lateral position to further reduce risk.

POSTOPERATIVE CARE

Level of Care

Few patients who have had an emergency laparotomy will be well enough to be discharged back to a general surgical ward, and will require some degree of critical care management. Three levels of critical care beds are described (24) below:

- Level 1—an acute surgical ward, but with availability of advice and support from critical care staff
- Level 2—a high-dependency unit where more detailed and frequent monitoring may be performed, and intervention for a single organ failure is possible
- Level 3—an ICU where advanced respiratory support may be used and multiple-organ failures managed simultaneously

Patients may step progressively down these levels of care postoperatively as their condition improves, or may step up the levels of care if their condition deteriorates. Which level is required postoperatively must be decided during surgery or in the postanesthesia care unit. Hypothermia, cardiovascular instability requiring the use of inotropes, poor respiratory function, or inadequate urine output indicates that level 3 care is likely to be required (Chapter 27). In the absence of these, a patient whose immediate recovery from anesthesia has been uncomplicated may return directly to a lower level of care, though preexisting cardiorespiratory disease may require the closer monitoring afforded by level 2 or 3 care.

Analgesia

The importance of adequate postoperative analgesia has been brought to the forefront of anesthetic management in recent years. Not to treat pain adequately is firstly inhumane; secondly, may lead to adverse physiological sequelae, leading to an increased morbidity and mortality; and thirdly, it creates the possibility of the development of chronic pain. Strategies for dealing with pain associated with emergency laparotomy may involve a mixture of neuraxial blockade, systemic opioids, and other adjuncts (Chapter 25).

Epidural Analgesia

While regional anesthesia has many advantages in elective gastrointestinal surgery, in the emergency situation, the decision to perform an epidural is often complicated by the patient's clinical state. Hypovolemia is a relative contraindication to any neuraxial block, because sympathetic blockade in the presence of a low intravascular volume will lead to profound hypotension. Deranged clotting or low platelet count may occur in the critically ill patient, and introduces the risk of the rare but devastating complication of an epidural hematoma. An international normalized ratio of less than 1.5 is usually regarded as acceptable, but the potential benefit of an epidural for an individual patient should always be balanced against the risk of an epidural hematoma. Systemic sepsis should also be considered, due to the risk of bacteremia infecting any epidural hematoma that may develop, potentially causing epidural abscess and more extensive neurological damage.

The aim of a thoracic epidural is to selectively block pain fibers from the surgical site and the thoracic sympathetic chain bilaterally. Freedom from pain allows early mobilization and feeding, and reduces respiratory complications seen postoperatively; while sympathetic block has many beneficial effects described below.

Because there is a progressive increase in the width of the epidural space from 1 to 1.5 mm at C5 to 5 to 6 mm at L2, high thoracic epidurals have minimal cranial but marked caudal spread. Conversely, more cranial spread occurs after low thoracic epidurals. Thus, insertion should correspond to the middle or top of the surgical incision with low or high thoracic epidurals, respectively. Various infusion regimes are used for postoperative epidural analgesia, including local anesthetics alone, opioids alone, or a combination of the two. The last of these has been shown to provide the best analgesia on movement, with less hypotension than local anesthetic alone and half the duration of ileus compared with epidural opioid alone or patient-controlled analgesia (PCA). A stepwise optimization model investigated various combinations and found the best balance of analgesia and side effects in 190 patients receiving thoracic epidural anesthesia for major abdominal surgery (25). The optimal combinations were bupivacaine 8 mg hr^{-1} plus fentanyl 30 µg hr^{-1} at an infusion rate of 9 mL hr^{-1} or bupivacaine 13 mg hr^{-1} plus fentanyl 25 µg hr^{-1} at an infusion rate of 9 mL hr^{-1}.

Epidural analgesia also creates a sympathetic block, which may be associated with cardiac, endocrine, and gastrointestinal benefits. The cardiac effects of sympatholysis include an improvement in the myocardial oxygen supply–demand ratio, which contributes to a reduction in the incidence of postoperative ischemia and infarction in patients with existing coronary vessel disease. The neural and endocrine "stress response" to surgery is attenuated by epidural blockade and the consequent reduction in hypercoagulability and activation of inflammatory pathways, protects the patient from thromboembolic phenomena, muscle catabolism, poor glycemic control, and postoperative infection. Sympathectomy created by thoracic epidural analgesia has been shown to benefit bowel function by reducing the need for systemic opioids, reducing the duration of postoperative ileus, and improving gastric intramucosal pH. Studies of the effect of epidural anesthesia on splanchnic blood flow are contradictory (26). Several older studies demonstrated an increase in gut blood flow, but epidural block that dilates the splanchnic circulation may also have a deleterious effect on hemodynamics, because splanchnic veins contribute significantly to overall venous capacitance. Vasodilatation may therefore lead to systemic hypotension and decreased venous return, which can compromise gut mucosal integrity. Vasopressors may therefore be more effective than fluid administration in improving splanchnic blood flow (26).

Opioids

Opioids can produce very effective analgesia, particularly for visceral pain, but their use is frequently accompanied by adverse effects. The most important of these is respiratory depression—resting ventilation is reduced, with respiratory rate falling to a greater extent than tidal volume, and the sensitivity of the brainstem to carbon dioxide is reduced. Other very common adverse effects include sedation, and nausea and vomiting, which can make the recovery period unpleasant or further exacerbate the pain. Constipation is well described with opioid use and is especially undesirable following gastrointestinal surgery. Urinary retention and itching may also be troublesome.

Despite these numerous adverse effects, opioid-based analgesia is used very commonly. Morphine may be administered by a variety of routes, but following emergency laparotomy, when there will be a prolonged period of impaired gastrointestinal absorption, the intravenous route is preferred. Patient controlled analgesia (PCA) systems have become almost universal for patients not managed with an epidural, usually involving a standard regime of 1 mg boluses of morphine with a "lock out" time of five minutes, allowing a maximum of 12 mg of morphine per hour. PCA provides a safe and effective method of administering strong opioids, allowing for the wide variation in opioid requirement between patients. The technique has become very popular with both patients and staff, with patients mostly appreciative of the control over their own pain relief that PCA allows them. A substantial benefit of PCA for ward staff is the reduced workload in giving repeated injections to the patients. Some commentators have also suggested that PCA is popular with staff because it allows them to psychologically distance themselves from patients who are in pain, and pass responsibility for management of the pain onto the patient themselves (27).

Adjunctive Analgesics

As described above, opioid-based analgesia has a wide range of adverse effects, and any further analgesic techniques that can reduce the required dose of opioid drugs will attenuate these side effects. Also, whether epidural or PCA systems are used, at some point in the patients' recovery from their emergency laparotomy, usually when their paralytic ileus begins to resolve, oral analgesia needs to be introduced. A range of adjunctive analgesic drugs may be used for this purpose, and the World Health Organization's analgesic pain ladder (28) provides a logical and now widely accepted technique for deciding which drugs to use. At each level of the pain ladder, patients are provided with a combination of regular analgesic drugs and stronger "rescue" analgesics on a when-needed basis. Drugs most commonly used include the following:

- Acetaminophen, which may be administered orally, rectally, or intravenously. Although sometimes viewed as a rather weak analgesic by patients who have had major surgery, regular doses of acetaminophen have a significant effect in reducing opioid requirements, and acetaminophen's antipyretic effect is useful in postoperative patients with low-grade sepsis
- Nonsteroidal anti-inflammatory drugs (NSAIDs) have analgesic effects by inhibiting the cyclo-oxygenase (COX) pathway for prostaglandin

production. They can be effective analgesics following major surgery, but the wide range of side effects such as gastrointestinal irritation, renal impairment, and interference with hemostasis make their use hazardous in the elderly or acutely ill patient

- Coxibs have the same mode of action as NSAIDs, but they act specifically on the COX-2 isoenzyme, and so have less of the adverse effects of nonspecific NSAIDs. As fairly recently introduced drugs, the coxibs have yet to find their place in acute pain management, and recent concerns about cardiovascular complications associated with coxib use have cast further uncertainty on their safety

Choice of Analgesic Technique

A review of 141 trials comparing the effect of neuraxial block with other forms of analgesia on postoperative mortality and morbidity found a significant survival advantage to receiving an epidural or spinal technique (29). Deep vein thrombosis, pulmonary embolism, blood transfusion, and pulmonary complications all occurred less commonly in the neuraxial block patients. The Master study (30) was a prospective, randomized controlled trial of epidural analgesia versus postoperative systemic opioids in high-risk patients undergoing major abdominal surgery. This study showed no difference in overall mortality between the two groups, but again demonstrated a decreased incidence of pulmonary complications and thromboembolic events in the epidural group. Although the study did not show a difference in overall mortality, this is a fairly crude outcome measure for an analgesic technique, and the other benefits of epidural analgesia seen in the study support the continued use of the technique, particularly in subgroups that would benefit the most, such as patients at high risk of postoperative respiratory complications.

POSTOPERATIVE COMPLICATIONS

Respiratory System

Respiratory complications are common following elective abdominal surgery, with between 13% and 33% of patients having some type of respiratory problem (31). Apart from the usual risks of respiratory problems associated with general anesthesia, intraperitoneal surgery is associated with dysfunction of the respiratory muscles, particularly the diaphragm. These effects carry on for long into the postoperative period and are affected by the quality of the analgesia provided. Opioid analgesia will also affect the control of respiration, and the large doses often required after abdominal surgery require close monitoring of respiratory drive. All these deleterious effects apply to patients having either elective or emergency abdominal surgery, but those patients having emergency surgery face two further impediments to their respiratory function:

- Diaphragmatic splinting describes the impaired diaphragmatic function that occurs with abdominal distension, and was first observed by Galen in around 150 A.D. when he described breathing as "little and fast" in such conditions as pregnancy and "water or phlegm in the liver." During the use of any general anesthetic, the weight of the abdominal organs causes a cephalad shift of the dependent part of the diaphragm, which in turn compresses the lung tissue above, frequently causing localized collapse of lung tissue. Shunting of mixed venous blood through these areas of pulmonary collapse explains most of the impairment of oxygenation normally seen during routine general anesthesia. During emergency laparotomy, the abdominal organs may cause much worse diaphragmatic splinting because of either large volumes of peritoneal fluid or blood, or distension of obstructed bowel. Other physiological effects of raised intra-abdominal pressure are described below

- Acute lung injury may occur in response to abdominal sepsis, and is associated with a particularly poor prognosis. Acute lung injury may take from a few hours to a few days to develop after the initial sepsis begins. Many patients presenting for emergency laparotomy will already have been acutely ill for this length of time before surgery, so may already have some degree of acute lung injury. General anesthesia, abdominal distension, and diaphragmatic dysfunction will then seriously compound the lung injury, often precipitating the need for artificial ventilation postoperatively. It is therefore important to recognize patients with early signs of lung injury at the preoperative assessment, and dyspnea, tachypnea, and even minimal impairment of oxygenation should alert the anesthetist to potentially serious respiratory insufficiency postoperatively

Prevention of respiratory complications is more effective than attempted treatment later. Preoperative physiotherapy, if time allows, may be useful, particularly in patients with existing respiratory disease. Prompt treatment of intra-abdominal sepsis and careful fluid management may help prevent or reduce the severity of subsequent lung injury. During anesthesia, pulmonary collapse may be effectively prevented by the use of moderate amounts of positive end-expiratory pressure (5–10 cmH$_2$O). If pulmonary collapse does occur, a situation usually evidenced by the new onset of impaired oxygenation, then reexpansion maneuvers should be performed prior to emergence from anesthesia. The most effective of these involves a sustained inflation of the lungs to an inflation pressure of 40 cmH$_2$O, held for up to 10 seconds. Finally, postoperative abdominal distension should be minimized by the complete removal of intraperitoneal fluid and, if possible, by decompressing obstructed bowel before closing the abdomen.

Abdominal Compartment Syndrome

Abdominal compartment syndrome (ACS) (32,33) describes the combination of raised intra-abdominal pressure and end-organ dysfunction. Small increases in intra-abdominal pressure can have adverse effects on renal function, cardiac output, hepatic blood flow, respiratory mechanics, splanchnic perfusion, and intracranial pressure. The pressure in the abdominal cavity is normally little more than the atmospheric pressure. Organ dysfunction starts to develop with pressures of greater than 25 mmHg. Measurement of intra-abdominal pressure is usually achieved via the urinary bladder. ACS is seen in a variety of conditions, with a high incidence following repair of ruptured abdominal aortic aneurysm, abdominal trauma, pancreatitis, and bowel resection, or secondary to massive crystalloid or colloid resuscitation. It is associated with a poor prognosis—the mean survival rate of patients affected is 53%. The only available treatment is decompressive laparotomy. Optimal time for intervention is unknown and controversial. Some argue that an intra-abdominal pressure greater than 25 mmHg alone is an indication for intervention, while others would not intervene unless there were also signs of severe physiological dysfunction and clinical deterioration (e.g., oliguria, hypotension, acidosis, or decreased pulmonary compliance).

Prevention of ACS by temporary closure of the abdominal wall, leaving a tension-free and watertight coverage should be considered in high-risk patients, but benefits from this invasive intervention have not been demonstrated in clinical trials. Most surgeons adopt a wait-and-see policy, with patients at risk requiring close monitoring.

Sepsis

Systemic infection as a result of contamination of the peritoneum by bowel contents is a common and life-threatening complication of emergency laparotomy. Four grades of sepsis may be defined (34):

- Systemic inflammatory response syndrome (SIRS) describes a clinical picture that results from activation of the inflammatory cytokine cascade, and may follow any severe infection, trauma, or pancreatitis. It is defined by the presence of any two of the following:
    1. Hypothermia ($<36°$C) or hyperthermia ($>38°$C)
    2. Tachycardia (>90 beats/min)
    3. Tachypnea (>20 breaths/min)
    4. Leucopenia ($<4000/mm^3$) or leucocytosis ($<12000/mm^3$)
- Sepsis is defined as SIRS that results from an infection
- Severe sepsis is sepsis accompanied by organ dysfunction
- Septic shock describes sepsis associated with hypotension, or a requirement for inotrope in a patient who has received adequate fluid replacement

Almost all patients who have an emergency laparotomy will develop SIRS, and some will progress to the other more severe degrees of sepsis. For those who develop septic shock, mortality is still of the order of 50%. Management involves treatment for the infection, with surgical removal of the source and effective antibiotic therapy, supplemented with supportive therapy of whatever degree is required. Specific immunomodulatory treatments have shown great promise in recent years, but have so far failed to have an impact on the poor outcome from sepsis.

REFERENCES

1. Cook TM, Day CJE. Hospital mortality after urgent and emergency laparotomy in patients aged 65 yr and over. Risk and prediction of risk using multiple logistic regression analysis. Br J Anaesth 1998; 80:776–781.
2. Church JM. Laparotomy for acute colorectal conditions in moribund patients: is it worthwhile? Dis Colon Rectum 2005; 48:1147–1152.
3. National Confidential Enquiry into Perioperative Deaths. Then and Now. The 2000 Report of the National Confidential Enquiry into Perioperative Deaths. London: NCEPOD, 2000.
4. Gan TJ, Soppitt A, Maroof M, et al. Goal-directed intraoperative fluid administration reduces length of hospital stay after major surgery. Anesthesiology 2002; 97: 820–826.

5. Ackland GL, Singh-Ranger D, Fox S, et al. Assessment of preoperative fluid depletion using bioimpedance analysis. Br J Anaesth 2004; 92:134–136.
6. Grocott MPW, Mythen MG, Gan TJ. Perioperative fluid management and clinical outcomes in adults. Anesth Analg 2005; 100:1093–1106.
7. O'Connor MF, Roizen MF. Lactate versus chloride: which is better? Anesth Analg 2001; 93:809–810.
8. Bromhead HJ, Jones NA. The use of anaesthetic rooms for induction of anaesthesia: a postal survey of current practice and attitudes in Great Britain and Northern Ireland. Anaesthesia 2002; 57:850–854.
9. Sandin RH, Enlund G, Samuelsson P, et al. Awareness during anaesthesia: a prospective case study. Lancet 2000; 355:707–711.
10. Morris C, McAllister C. Etomidate for emergency anaesthesia; mad, bad and dangerous to know. Anaesthesia 2005; 60:737–740.
11. Fuchs-Buder T, Sparr HJ, Ziegenfuss T. Thiopental or etomidate for rapid sequence induction with rocuronium. Br J Anaesth 1998; 80:504–506.
12. Moore EW, Davies MW. Inhalational versus intravenous induction. A survey of emergency anaesthesia practice in the United Kingdom. Eur J Anaesthesiol 2000; 17:33–37.
13. Vanner RG, Pryle BJ. Regurgitation and oesophageal rupture with cricoid pressure: a cadaver study. Anaesthesia 1992; 47:197–199.
14. Henderson JJ, Popat MT, Latto IP, et al. Difficult airway society guidelines for management of the unanticipated difficult intubation. Anaesthesia 2004; 59:675–694.
15. Bell MDD. Routine pre-oxygenation—a new 'minimum standard' of care? Anaesthesia 2004; 59:943–947.
16. Sellick BA. Cricoid pressure to control regurgitation of stomach contents during induction of anaesthesia. Lancet 1961; 2:404–406.
17. Vanner RG, Asai T. Safe use of cricoid pressure. Anaesthesia 1999; 54:1–3.
18. Escott MEA, Owen H, Strahan AD, et al. Cricoid pressure training: how useful are descriptors of force? Anaesth Intens Care 2003; 31:388–391.
19. Clayton TJ, Vanner RG. A novel method of measuring cricoid force. Anaesthesia 2002; 57:326–329.
20. Lowry DW, Carroll MT, Mirakhur RK, et al. Comparison of sevoflurane and propofol with rocuronium for modified rapid-sequence induction of anaesthesia. Anaesthesia 1999; 54:247–252.
21. Epemolu O, Bom A, Hope F, et al. Reversal of neuromuscular blockade and simultaneous increase in plasma rocuronium concentration after the intravenous infusion of the novel reversal agent Org 25969. Anesthesiology 2003; 99:632–637.
22. Association of Anaesthetists of Great Britain and Ireland. Recommendations for Standards of Monitoring During Anaesthesia and Recovery. London: Association of Anaesthetists of Great Britain and Ireland, 2000.
23. Bock M, Müller J, Bach A, et al. Effects of preinduction and intraoperative warming during major laparotomy. Br J Anaesth 1998; 80:159–163.
24. Intensive Care Society. Levels of Critical Care for Adult Patients. London: Intensive Care Society, 2002.
25. Curatolo M, Schnider T, Petersen-Felix S, et al. A direct search procedure to optimize combinations of epidural bupivacaine, fentanyl, and clonidine for postoperative analgesia. Anesthesiology 2000; 92:325–327.
26. Gould TH, Grace K, Thorne G, et al. Effect of thoracic epidural anaesthesia on colonic blood flow. Br J Anaesth 2002; 89:446–451.
27. Salmon P, Hall GM. PCA: patient-controlled analgesia or politically correct analgesia? Br J Anaesth 2001; 87:815–818.
28. World Health Organization. Cancer Pain Relief. Geneva, Switzerland: WHO, 1986.
29. Rodgers A, Walker N, Schug S, et al. Reduction in postoperative mortality and morbidity with epidural or spinal anaesthesia: results from an overview of randomised trials. BMJ 2000; 321:1–12.

30. Rigg JRA, Jamrozik K, Myles PS, et al., and the MASTER Anaesthesia Trial Study Group. Epidural anaesthesia and analgesia and outcome of major surgery: a randomised trial. Lancet 2002; 359:1276–1282.
31. Lumb AB. Nunn's Applied Respiratory Physiology. 6th ed. London: Elsevier, 2005.
32. Moore AFK, Hargest R, Martin M, et al. Intra-abdominal hypertension and the abdominal compartment syndrome. Br J Surg 2004; 91:1102–1110.
33. Hunter JD, Damani Z. Intra-abdominal hypertension and the abdominal compartment syndrome. Anaesthesia 2004; 59:899–907.
34. Brun-Buisson C. The epidemiology of the systemic inflammatory response. Intens Care Med 2000; 26:S064–S074.

25

Postoperative Pain Management After Abdominal Surgery

Terry T. Durbin
Department of Anesthesiology, The Pennsylvania College of Medicine, and The Milton S. Hershey Medical Center, Hershey, Pennsylvania, U.S.A.

INTRODUCTION

Prior to the 1980s, pain experienced by surgical patients was normally treated by the operating surgeon, usually with routine orders for an intramuscular or intravenous injection of a weight-based dose of morphine or pethidine every four to six hours. The inadequacy of this regimen elevated the anticipation of postoperative pain to the primary fear and concern patients had for undergoing a surgical procedure (1).

Recent Advancements in Postoperative Pain Management

The past 25 years have seen a marked improvement in postoperative pain management, due to the combination of an increased understanding of the physiology of pain, the development and application of new techniques for treating pain, and the discovery of new medications. In conjunction with these new understandings and techniques, a new role for anesthesia providers was created. As a result, formalization of postoperative pain management services by anesthesia departments began in the early to mid-1980s (2). The anesthesia provider has since become the primary physician responsible for providing treatment of pain, after surgeries that result in moderate to severe pain.

Despite these developments, postsurgical pain continues to be undertreated in many medical institutions in the United States (3,4) and Britain (5,6). To help improve this situation, medical societies began publishing guidelines for the treatment and management of surgical pain (7,8). In the year 2000, the Joint Commission on Accreditation of Healthcare Organizations (JCAHO) formulated new standards for pain management, which included a mandate for the measurement of perceived pain by patients as well as its documentation as a fifth "vital sign" (9). The JCAHO is the national accreditation body for this measurement that is now routinely recorded, using a visual analogue scale (VAS) that correlates the intensity of pain to a number between 1 and 10 or, for utilization in some studies, between 1 and 100. The interpretation of the number given by patients may often prove to be difficult, due to several factors including variations in analgesic requirements, previous experience and history of opioid use, and individual subjective pain experiences. In recent years, assessment of pain has been further refined to the evaluation of pain at rest, with motion, and while coughing. Despite these limitations, the goal in many institutions is to keep the related number (VAS) below 3 in all circumstances (10).

POSTOPERATIVE PAIN AND ABDOMINAL SURGERY

Open wound abdominal surgery produces pain that is somatic, visceral, and neuropathic in nature. Flank incision, clam-shell incision, and midline laparotomy all produce moderate to severe pain, lasting several days to weeks. Judicious pain control following gastrointestinal surgery produces many benefits beyond the alleviation of patient suffering, because optimization of analgesia has the potential to decrease complications that impede the recovery of patients after surgery (11). Pain relief is especially crucial following upper abdominal surgery, in order to avoid significant respiratory dysfunction (12). Poorly controlled pain produces a neuroendocrine stress response, involving sympathoadrenal and neuroendocrine interactions, which induce a subsequent increase in catecholamine and catabolic hormone secretion (13). The resultant increase in sympathetic tone can exacerbate existing pathophysiology present in surgical patients.

Myocardial and renal functions may be adversely affected, especially in elderly patients, leading to an increase in morbidity and mortality (14). Morbidity, which may be due to poor control of postoperative pain, is summarized in Table 1.

The development and use of laparoscopic surgery for colorectal procedures have accomplished as much, if not more, in the area of reducing postoperative pain and its complications, than all of the advancements achieved by newer methods for treating pain. The laparoscopic technique for performing a cholecystectomy has become the gold standard. It is well established that there is significant reduction in postoperative pain, and thus, diminished need for intervention, when compared to an open procedure, (15) as well as decreased complication rates (16). In recent years, the use of laparoscopy has been expanded to more complicated cases for colorectal surgery, including total colectomy and abdominoperineal resection. This will undoubtedly continue to expand in the future, benefiting more patients.

Effective pain control in colorectal surgery can best be obtained by using a multimodal approach comprising opioids [both intravenously upon request and via a patient-controlled analgesia (PCA) device], nonsteroidal anti-inflammatory drugs (NSAIDs), and epidural analgesia (17).

MANAGEMENT OF POSTOPERATIVE PAIN

Opioids

For years, physicians caring for surgical patients relied solely on opioid analgesics for the treatment of postoperative pain. Although the role of opioids has been

Table 1 Increased Morbidities Encountered with Poor Post-Op Analgesia

Respiratory: hypoxia, hypercarbia, bronchospasm, pneumonia
Cardiovascular: hypertensive crisis, ischemia, infarction, heart failure
Renal: acute/chronic failure, glomerular nephritis
Hyperglycemia causing ketoacidosis and poor wound healing
Negative nitrogen balance and a catabolic state impeding recovery

diminished with the advent of the multimodal approach to care of these patients, they still have a vital role in the treatment of acute postoperative pain, but with modern ways of delivery methods.

Actions and Effects

Opioids exert their analgesic effect through microreceptors located in the limbic system, thalamus, striatum, hypothalamus, midbrain, and spinal cord. Their efficacy in the treatment of pain is limited only by each patient's individual development of untoward side effects and a tolerance to the medication.

In addition to their analgesic property, opioids exhibit numerous profound effects on the central nervous system, especially respiratory depression. This is initiated by a direct effect on the brainstem, which produces an alteration in respiratory rhythm and ventilatory control through a decrease in sensitivity to carbon dioxide tension in the blood. This action is much more rapid and profound with drugs given intravenously. Historically, fear of this particular side effect is one of the primary reasons; acute pain has not been adequately treated (18).

The patients undergoing abdominal surgery are likely to suffer more nausea and vomiting (19) (Chapter 26). Opioids can compound this problem either by directly stimulating the chemoreceptor trigger zone in the medulla oblongata or by inducing orthostatic hypotension. Opioid-induced hypotension can occur as a result of vasodilatation from histamine release or suppression of sympathetic outflow from the vasomotor medullary center.

Nausea and/or subsequent vomiting can increase incision pain, affect surgical repairs (anastomosis), and potentiate the development of wound dehiscence. Morphine can increase smooth muscle tone throughout the gastrointestinal tract (including the gastric antrum, duodenum, large bowel, and gastrointestinal and biliary sphincters), leading to increased spasmodic movements. Although pethidine has anticholinergic properties, it has much less effect on smooth muscle and sphincter tone.

Urinary flow is often impeded with the use of opioids, due to increase in bladder sphincter tone and increase in tone and contraction of the lower one-third of the ureter, leading to increased requirements of bladder catheterization. Opioids may also increase secretion of vasopressin, which may contribute to oliguria in patients with coexisting renal dysfunction and hypovolemia.

Methods of Delivery

Opioids are generally administered through intravenous, intramuscular, neuraxial, or oral routes, but transcutaneous, submucosal, and transmucosal routes have been used as well. The use of a patch to deliver transcutaneous fentanyl has been studied and is shown to require less supplementary injection of opioids (20,21). The role of this method of utilization of opioids remains unclear due to inability to control the dosage delivered and wide variations in dose and response between patients (22).

The most common routes for postoperative pain management are oral, intramuscular, intravenous, and neuraxial. Oral medication is initiated only when the patient is allowed to drink and eat. It is usually used after the immediate postoperative period, when severe pain has subsided, or used as an adjunct for breakthrough pain when utilizing neuraxial opioids. Intramuscular administration of opioid is less favored in the modern practice.

Intravenous administration via a PCA device has become the standard for delivery of opioids in the management of postoperative pain. This method has

Table 2 On-Demand Patient-Controlled Analgesia Settings for Various Medications

Drug	Bolus amount (mg)	Lockout interval (min)
Morphine	0.5–2.5	5–10
Fentanyl	10–20	5–10
Meperidine	5–25	5–15
Hydromorphone	0.05–0.2	6–10
Methadone	0.5–2.5	8–20

significantly reduced the impact of factors, such as patient variability in analgesic needs, unpredictable attainment of necessary serum levels, and administrative delays that hampere the successful treatment using traditional standing and as required orders.

The ability of the patient to self-administer opioid analgesics when needed has circumvented these issues and optimized medication delivery in a way that improves treatment, while, in many instances, decreasing the amount of drug utilized (23). The on-demand function of the PCA device allows programming a bolus amount of drug and a lockout interval (the amount of time the patient must wait to receive the next dose). However, various studies have confirmed adequate settings for both of these parameters (Table 2) (24,25).

The PCA device also has the capability of delivering a continuous infusion but is not employed. In the early days of PCA use, this was a common practice to make up for any analgesic deficits that may occur due to inadequate bolus or lockout interval. However, this practice has been shown to increase the amount of medication delivered along with unwanted side effects, without improving the quality of the analgesia (26,27).

Nonopioid Analgesics

Nonopioid analgesics are used to treat minor or moderate acute postoperative pain. NSAIDs are commonly used. Traditional NSAIDs inhibit cyclooxygenase-1 (COX-1) and COX-2 enzymes. Most of the analgesic effects of NSAIDs have been attributed to their COX-2 inhibition, whereas their undesirable side effects have been attributed to their inhibition of COX-1 enzymes. Newer agents have been introduced and they selectively inhibit COX-2 enzymes without inhibiting COX-1 enzymes. Therefore, these agents should provide analgesia equal to that of traditional NSAIDs without many of the side effects.

Nonopioid analgesics do not interrupt the transmission of painful stimulus. The effect of these agents depends on the central and inflammatory response to tissue injury. They also have little or no effect on catabolic stress hormones. They also have a narrow therapeutic range above which there is little increase in analgesia.

These drugs are commonly used in conjunction with opioids in the management of early postoperative pain, thus enhancing analgesic effects of both, and at the same time, they reduce the requirement of opioid.

Gastrointestinal upset is the most common adverse effect of the above agents. Nausea, vomiting, dyspepsia, and heartburn occur in 5% to 25% of patients who have been provided with aspirin, and in 3% to 9% of patients receiving the other NSAIDs. Ulceration and bleeding of the gastrointestinal mucosa can occur because of direct irritation by these drugs, and, thus, it is avoided in patients who suffer from ulcerative colitis.

The use of most nonopioids is avoided in patients with an indwelling epidural catheter. Prolonged bleeding may occur as a result of the action of these drugs on the COX-1 enzyme located in platelets, increasing the risk of the development of an epidural hematoma. This, however, does not appear to be a problem with the newer COX-2 enzyme inhibitor drugs.

Patients with a history of nasal polyps, asthma, and rhinitis are at a greater risk for exacerbation of bronchospasm by these drugs, and so these drugs are avoided.

Epidural Analgesia

Background

Prolonged epidural analgesia by means of a catheter was first described in 1949 by Cleland (28). At that time, the technique of providing intermittent boluses of local anesthetic agent proved to be inefficient, due to staff requirements and the cyclical pain relief achieved between injections. Continuous infusion of local anesthetic agent in concentrations and volumes high enough to alleviate pain proved to be problematic because of hypotension from intense sympathetic blockade as well as profound motor blockade, which prevented ambulation.

In 1980, a landmark article demonstrated the efficacy and safety of the administration of opioids in the epidural space for the treatment of postoperative pain (29). There are opioid microreceptors present in the spinal cord. These receptors could be blocked in the treatment of surgical pain, and this subsequently led to an increased interest. There was also marked improvement in the pumps that deliver drugs (Table 3). Continuous epidural analgesia, either alone or as part of a multimodal treatment, has become a standard technique in the management of pain in patients who have undergone major abdominal surgical procedures.

Advantages of Epidural Analgesia

A meta-analysis performed in 2003 looked at studies related to postoperative epidural analgesia, which were published from 1966 to 2002 (30). A total of 100 studies met the investigator's criteria for inclusion in the review. The conclusion drawn from their analysis was that epidural analgesia provided superior postoperative pain relief compared to parenteral opioids, irrespective of the analgesic agent used or location of the catheter insertion. Epidural analgesia has been shown to be superior to parenteral opioids in relieving postoperative pain (Table 4), specifically for abdominal surgery (31–33).

Pain is a major contributor to respiratory dysfunction following upper abdominal surgery (12). The superior pain relief provided by epidural analgesia, along with the attenuation of spinal reflex inhibition of diaphragmatic function, can result in a decreased incidence of postoperative pulmonary complications (34–36).

Table 3 Advantages of Continuous Epidural Infusion Over Intermittent Bolus

Constant level of analgesia, avoiding peaks and valleys
Less instance of motor blockade and profound sympathetic blockade by local anesthetics
Less rostral spread, minimizing side effects
Fewer breaks in sterile technique from manual injection
Decreased anesthesia personnel requirement for periodic injection

Table 4 VAS Scores After Abdominal Surgery: Epidural Versus Parenteral Opioids

Thoracic epidural: local anesthetic with or without opioid; 16 studies—2591 observations
  Mean VAS (SEM, mm) parenteral = 28.0 (0.3), epidural = 17.1 (0.2)
  Weighted mean difference = 10.9
Thoracic epidural: opioid alone; 5 studies—284 observations
  Mean VAS (SEM, mm) parenteral = 38.1 (1.1), epidural = 31.4 (0.9)
  Weighted mean difference = 6.7
Lumbar epidural: local anesthetic with or without opioid; 2 studies—342 observations
  Mean VAS (SEM, mm) parenteral = 33.9 (0.8), epidural = 16.0 (0.6)
  Weighted mean difference = 17.8
Lumbar epidural: opioid alone; 6 studies—438 observations
  Mean VAS (SEM, mm) parenteral = 34.3 (0.8), epidural = 25.8 (0.8)
  Weighted mean difference = 8.5

Abbreviations: VAS, visual analogue scale; SEM, standard error of the mean.
Source: Adapted from Ref. 30.

Postoperative analgesia via continuous thoracic epidural has been shown to decrease the incidence of postoperative myocardial infarction in patients with underlying cardiovascular disease (37,38). This may be attributed to an increase in analgesia (i.e., attenuation of the stress response to surgery) which provides a positive redistribution of coronary blood flow (39). Such myocardial sparing is not associated with lumbar epidural or epidural delivering only opioids. The utilization of thoracic epidural analgesia with a local anesthetic component has also been shown to produce an earlier return of gastrointestinal function and a decrease in ileus (40,41). This is accomplished by a decrease in sympathetic outflow, a decrease in the amount of opioids used, and attenuation of the spinal reflex inhibition of the gastrointestinal tract (42). An earlier return of normal bowel function usually translates into discharge criteria being met sooner (43).

Several dynamic metabolic disturbances detrimental to patient convalescence are observed in the immediate postoperative period (44). These disturbances include blunting of the hyperglycemic response, protein loss, and lactate production, resulting in a catabolic physiologic state. Epidural analgesia decreases the above changes, leading to improved recovery (45,46). Epidural blockade has also been shown to accentuate the stimulating effect of parenteral alimentation on whole body protein synthesis (47).

Surgery results in a hypercoagulable state that increases the risk of venous and arterial thrombosis (48). Epidural analgesia reduces peripheral vascular resistance and increases calf blood flow by raising arterial outflow and venous return. Although this has been shown to reduce venous thrombosis in patients undergoing lower extremity vascular and orthopedic surgical procedures, such an advantage has not been shown in gastrointestinal surgery (49,50).

Risks, Side Effects, and Complications of Epidural Analgesia

Although epidural analgesia can produce superior results, it is not without risks or potential serious side effects. This necessitates the need for careful patient selection, not only for the procedure itself, but also for the medications utilized and the rates at which they are delivered.

Epidural hematoma is a rare but serious potential complication associated with both the placement and removal of epidural catheter, but this usually resolves spontaneously (51). But, occasionally, immediate surgical intervention may be required in order to avoid permanent neurological damage. Most reported cases of hematoma involved patients who either had a bleeding tendency or were receiving anticoagulation therapy (52,53). The exact incidence of this serious complication remains unknown; however, there was an increase in the number of cases in the last decade in the United States with the introduction of low-molecular-weight heparins (54). New anticoagulants have been developed. These include argatroban, which is a thrombin inhibitor, and fondaparinux, which inhibits factor Xa. At present, we do not know enough about what influence these drugs have on neuraxial block.

It is, therefore, important to know the clinical history, medication list, and the results of laboratory tests prior to the initiation of epidural analgesia. American Society of Regional Anesthesia maintains up-to-date recommendations for the use of neuraxial intervention in the face of anticoagulation therapy (55).

Complications can result from inadvertent penetration of the dura, damage to neurovascular structures, or infection after epidural. In one large study, accidental dural puncture during needle insertion occurred (0.16–1.3%) in a series of 51,000 epidurals, and 16% to 86% of the patients developing a postdural puncture headache (56,57). Migration of the epidural catheter into the subarachnoid space, although rare, has been reported (58). Movement of the vertebral column and ligamentum flavum, along with respiratory-induced space pressure variations, make epidural catheters mobile. Improved catheter tip design and intact dura prevent entry into the subarachnoid space. Epidural abscess and meningitis appear to be a rare occurrence. In a review of 65,000 epidurals, only three cases of meningitis were found, and there was no incidence of epidural abscess (59).

Selection of Agents for Epidural Analgesia

Neuraxial opioids produce analgesia by binding to opioid receptors in the substantia gelatinosa, as well as by systemic redistribution. Local anesthetic agents block transmission of afferent impulses at the nerve roots and dorsal root ganglia. Coadministration of opioid and local anesthetic potentiates the analgesic effect (60), as well as reduces the necessary volume and concentration of each drug (61). This also has the added benefit of reduction and severity of unwanted side effects (62).

The optimal choice and dose of both local anesthetic agent and opioid that will provide the lowest pain score with the fewest side effects is not known. However, one study (63) supports that a combination of bupivacaine and fentanyl delivered at a rate of 8 mg/hr and 30 μg/hr, respectively, appeared to provide the most consistent level of analgesia for upper abdominal surgery.

Clonidine is an α_2 agonist that can modulate nociceptive impulses in the dorsal horn of the spinal cord as well as throughout the central nervous system. Epidural clonidine produces dose-dependent analgesia when given as a bolus (64). Respiratory depression is not seen, but its use is associated with hypotension and bradycardia, due to inhibition of preganglionic sympathetic fibers. This is more prevalent at lower doses, because increased concentrations normalize blood pressure because of systemic vasoconstriction that overrides the central hypotensive effect. Optimal ratios for combining α_2 agonists with opioid or a local anesthetic agent have not yet been determined, because these drugs exhibit a nonlinear synergism (65).

Dexmetotomidine is an α_2 agonist that is much more highly selective in comparison to clonidine. Tizanidine is an analogue of clonidine that produces analgesia with fewer cardiovascular side effects. Future trials may suggest increased use of α_2 agonists with epidural analgesia.

Side Effects and Risks from Medications Administered as Epidurals

Local Anesthetic Agent.   Local anesthetic agent, when injected through the epidural, leads to blockade of sympathetic fibers, resulting in hypotension. In a normovolemic, cardiovascularly stable individual, this is usually not critical. Hypotension can be easily treated with intravenous fluid administration or small doses of sympathomimetics (ephedrine or phenylephrine) (66). Caution must be exercised when administering the local anesthetic agent as bolus, particularly in a hypovolemic patient. Even a 3 mL test dose may cause profound hypotension. Colorectal surgical patients often come to surgery in a hypovolemic state, following bowel preparation, lack of adequate nourishment, or intravenous infusion. The elderly patients who may have decreased cardiac reserve in conjunction with a hypovolemic state may be at risk for a myocardial event should severe hypotension ensue.

The severity of hypotension induced by epidural analgesia may be reduced by lowering the concentration of local anesthetic agent, addition of an opioid to reduce the local anesthetic requirement, and appropriate placement of epidural catheter (which should limit the spread of the medication to only those dermatomes essential in providing adequate pain relief).

Lower extremity motor block is another troublesome side effect that may be encountered with local anesthetic when administered through epidural. It is well established that early postsurgical mobilization decreases the risk of thromboembolic and pulmonary complications (67). Postoperative hypoxemia is also more pronounced in the supine position, potentially contributing to pulmonary, cardiac, and cerebral dysfunction (68). In elderly patients, recovery of muscle strength is delayed after abdominal surgery. This may be less severe with forced early mobilization (69).

The incidence and severity of motor blockade may be reduced by lowering the concentration and amount of local anesthetic delivered, along with addition of an opioid to help maintain analgesic efficacy. More importantly, efforts should be made to avoid anesthetizing the lumbar plexus by proper catheter placement, which coincides with the dermatomes involved within the surgical site.

Opioids.   Respiratory depression is an uncommon but potentially serious risk of epidural administration of opioids. Early respiratory depression may be caused by systemic drug absorption when utilizing lipophilic medications, such as fentanyl and sufentanil (70). Late respiratory depression can occur up to 12 hours after administration, due to rostral spread of hydrophilic agents into the cerebrospinal fluid (71). The incidence is increased by factors, such as dose, age, posture, aqueous solubility of the drug administered, positive-pressure ventilation, and increased intra-abdominal pressure.

The incidence of respiratory depression appears to be no different, or possibly less than that seen in patients receiving parenteral opioids (72). With an appropriate monitoring in place, this therapy is considered safe enough to be utilized in a non-intensive care setting (73). In assessing patients receiving epidural opioids, the respiratory rate is not a reliable predictor of patient ventilatory status or the possibility of future respiratory depression (74).

Respiratory depression should be treated with ventilatory support as needed, and naloxone should be given in 0.1 to 0.4 mg increments. Rebound respiratory depression may occur because the duration of naloxone is short lived. A continuous infusion of naloxone (0.5–5 mg/kg/hr) may be initiated to prevent recurrence.

Nausea and vomiting are frequent side effects of epidural opioids, and are usually dose dependent (75). They occur more often with morphine than with fentanyl (76). Respiratory depression is probably caused by systemic absorption of fentanyl and rostral spread of morphine. Naloxone, droperidol, metoclopramide, and dexamethasone have all been shown to be effective in the treatment of nausea and vomiting induced by epidural opioids (77).

Urinary retention is a side effect of both neuraxial local anesthetics and opioids. Opioid receptors in the spinal cord appear to decrease strength of the detrusor muscle contraction. An indwelling urinary catheter is normally required for any patient with a continuous epidural infusion of local anesthetic or opioids.

Pruritus is another side effect of epidural opioids and occurs with greater frequency when compared to systemic opioids (78). This does not appear to be histamine release dependent because the administration of antihistamine agent rarely alleviates the condition (79). Morphine appears to cause this side effect more often than fentanyl/local anesthetic combination. The mechanism remains unclear. It is hypothesized that opioid-induced pruritus occurs secondary to direct opioid receptor binding in the spinal cord and brain or via neurotransmission stemming from opioid receptor binding. This is supported by the fact that opioid antagonists, such as naloxone, reverse this effect (80,81).

Site of Epidural Catheter Insertion

The hydrophilic nature of compounds, such as hydromorphine and hydromorphone, produces a rostral spread of these medications in such a manner that analgesia may be produced at thoracic dermatomes levels, even when administered through an epidural catheter placed at the lumbar region. This strategy, however, produces several significant shortcomings in optimizing postoperative pain management and patient recovery. First, significantly higher amounts of opioid are needed to reach thoracic dermatomes, increasing the likelihood of unwanted side effects. Second, local anesthetic agents are usually required to diminish the stress response to surgery. This also appears to be effective only with catheters located at thoracic region. Lastly, when local anesthetic agents are utilized, the lumbar plexus should be avoided whenever possible, in order to avoid motor blockade, thus allowing early ambulation of the patient.

Ideally, catheter placement should approximate the dermatome levels that correspond to the point intersecting the upper one-third and lower two-thirds of the surgical incision. Appropriate catheter placement (Fig. 1), corresponding to various surgical procedures (Fig. 2) involving the gastrointestinal tract, is of paramount importance.

The placement of a thoracic epidural is technically more difficult than the lumbar epidural. At vertebral levels above the termination of the spinal cord, the epidural needle may accidentally puncture the spinal meninges and damage the spinal cord. The epidural space at the thoracic level has a more shallow depth compared to the lumbar region. Experience must be attained in order to identify the interspinous ligaments and the ligamentum flavum by feel, and to advance the epidural needle slowly and under control. In addition, the caudally directed vertebral spinous processes often render access to the epidural space by a medial approach difficult. It is extremely helpful to gain proficiency utilizing the paramedian approach when administering thoracic epidurals (Fig. 3).

Patient-Controlled Epidural Analgesia

The delivery of epidural medications for postoperative pain through a patient-controlled device has become more popular in recent years. As in the case of

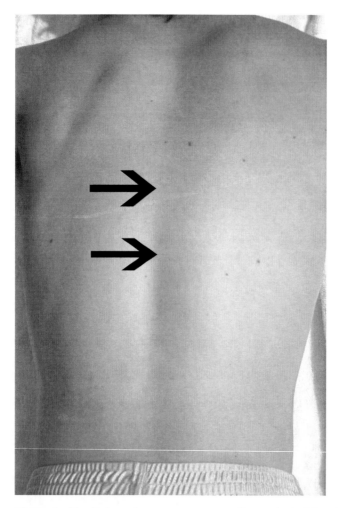

Figure 1   Needle insertion areas, corresponding to the incisional areas shown in Figure 2, for epidural placement; T-6 to 7 for upper and T-9 to 10 for lower.

PCA utilized to deliver intravenous opioids upon demand, the ability to match the amount of epidural medication delivered to the analgesic needs of the patient has been shown to have a dose-sparing effect, and, in turn, results in fewer side effects after major abdominal surgery when compared to continuous epidural, initiated alone (82).

Unlike PCA, however, a background infusion when utilizing patient-controlled epidural analgesia is shown to decrease the amount of overall medication delivered (83).

Management of Epidural Analgesia

All patients with an indwelling epidural catheter must be seen and assessed everyday. In addition, a member of the anesthesia department/acute pain service must be available at all times to intervene and make adjustments whenever problems occur. Patient mobility may be compromised by an unwanted motor block whenever a local anesthetic is utilized. This should be evaluated and infusions adjusted if this occurs. In case of excessive paresthesia, the infusion rate or local anesthetic concentration

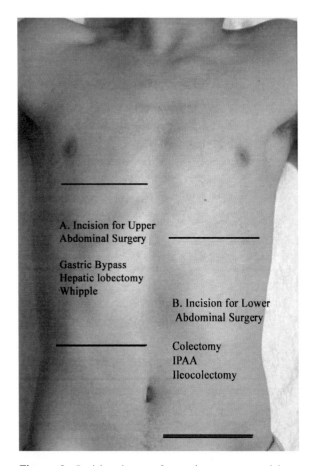

Figure 2 Incisional areas for various upper and lower abdominal surgeries. *Abbreviation*: IPAA, ideal pouch-anal anastomosis.

should be reduced. If a profound motor block is present, the infusion should be stopped. The patient should be examined to exclude epidural hematoma. Once this suspicion has been eliminated, the infusion may be restarted at a reduced rate or lower local anesthetic concentration.

Even though epidural analgesia is usually highly effective, patients may occasionally experience inadequate pain relief. A systematic approach should be initiated to either resolve problems with the indwelling epidural catheter or plan an alternate strategy (Table 5).

PAIN MANAGEMENT STRATEGIES

It is well established that epidural analgesia provides superior pain relief when compared to intravenous PCA (43; p. 757–765). In addition to superior pain relief, evidence from controlled studies indicates that epidural analgesia decreases respiratory and cardiovascular perioperative morbidity, and aids in faster recovery of bowel function, improved wound healing, and earlier hospital discharge (84). There are also strong indications that long-term quality of life benefits are gained through

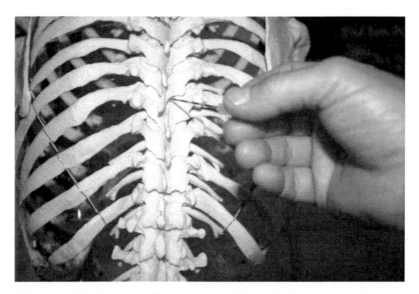

Figure 3 The large caudally directed vertebral spinous processes often make access to the epidural space via the medial approach difficult. A paramedial approach should be learned for a higher rate of success.

the proficient control of pain and decreased stress response of surgery by utilizing a continuous epidural for postoperative pain relief after colonic surgery. Due to its many advantages, except when contraindicated (Table 6), postoperative epidural analgesia should be planned for major open gastrointestinal surgical intervention. Pain scores after major colon surgery are not influenced by whether epidural analgesia is

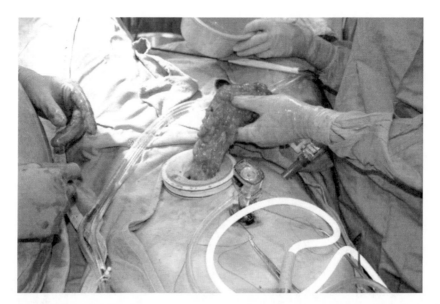

Figure 4 Laparoscopic partial colectomy. Although this approach produces much less surgical trauma and pain than an open procedure, some studies report better outcomes when postoperative epidural analgesia is utilized.

Table 5 Algorithms for Inadequate Epidural Analgesia (Pain Score 3)

Test dermatomal sensory block adequacy utilizing ice or scratch test
  No reaction
    Bolus with test dose of 5 cc 2% lidocaine with 1:200 k epi
    Repeat sensory test
      No reaction—discontinue epidural: reinsert or start IVPCA
      Positive bilateral sensory block
        Bolus 4 to 10 cc of infusion solution
        Adjust basal and demand rates
  Inadequate dermatomal coverage
    Coverage too high
      Pull back catheter if sufficient length is within space
      Sit patient up at 30°
      Bolus 4 to 10 cc of infusion solution, repeat sensory test
      If coverage is adequate, increase basal rate
        May need to decrease local anesthetic concentration
    Coverage too low
      Bolus 4 to 10 cc of infusion solution and repeat sensory test
      If coverage is adequate, increase basal rate
        May need to decrease local anesthetic concentration
        If using fentanyl, consider hydromorphone or morphine
    If dermatomal coverage still inadequate for after [b(i)] or [b(ii)] above:
      Add supplemental IV morphine either with prn orders or via a PCA
      Consider replacing epidural if addition of morphine is insufficient
  One-sided epidural coverage
    Pull back catheter if sufficient length is within space
      Bolus 4 to 10 cc of infusion solution and repeat sensory test
      If still one sided
        Add supplemental IV morphine either with prn orders or via a PCA
        Consider replacing epidural if addition of morphine is insufficient

Abbreviations: IVPCA, intravenous patient-controlled analgesia; PCA, patient-controlled analgesia; IV, intravenous.

commenced before the surgical incision is made or during wound closure (85). However, when it is initiated prior to incision, postoperative analgesic requirements have been shown to be reduced (86).

Multimodal pain therapy involves the simultaneous use of multiple analgesic techniques with different mechanisms of action. This strategy reduces the use of intravenous opioid, which has untoward side effects. This may be accomplished by the addition of nonopioid analgesic and α_2 agonists. Pain is less intense and analgesic requirements are lower after laparoscopic colon resection (Fig. 4). The duration of recovery is shortened, and the postoperative quality of life is improved

Table 6 Contraindications to Epidural Placement

Coagulation defects or concurrent anticoagulant therapy
Sepsis
Infection at the site of needle placement
Poor or a limited cardiac function (relative contraindication, consider hypotension)
Patient refusal
Lack of patient cooperation, dementia, or an unconscious patient

after laparoscopic colorectal resections. Although these findings and experiences often preclude the use of epidural analgesia for laparoscopic cases, several studies have indicated that even in laparoscopic colonic surgery, postoperative pain control (using an epidural) provides benefits, such as a significant decrease in postoperative pain, early mobilization, and reduced hospital stay when compared to that required when parenteral opioids are administered (87,88). A thorough preoperative evaluation that takes into consideration the patient's expectations, opioid history, and extent of the surgical procedure will help determine if placement of an epidural is warranted in these cases.

REFERENCES

1. Weis OF, Sriwatanakul K, Alloza JL, et al. Attitudes of patients, housestaff, and nurses toward postoperative analgesic care. Anesth Analg 1983; 62:70–74.
2. Ready LB, Oden R, Chadwick HS, et al. Development of an anesthesiology-based postoperative pain management service. Anesthesiology 1988; 68:100–106.
3. Carr DB, Jacox AK, Chapman RC, et al. Clinical Practice Guideline: Acute Pain Management: Operative or Medical Procedures and Trauma. Rockville, MD: Agency for Health Care Policy and Research, US Department of Health and Human Services, 1992.
4. Lynch EP, Lazor MA, Gellis JE, et al. Patient experience with pain after elected noncardiac surgery. Anesth Analg 1997; 61:466.
5. Dolin S, et al. Effectivness of acute postoperative pain management: I. Evidence from published data. Br J Anaesth 2002; 89:409.
6. Powell AE, Davies HTO, Bannister J, et al. Rhetoric and reality on acute pain services in the UK: a national postal questionnaire survey. Br J Anaesth 2004; 92:689.
7. American Society of Anesthesiologists. Practice guidelines for acute pain management in the perioperative setting: a report by the American Society of Anesthesiologists Task Force on pain management, acute pain section. Anesthesiology 1995; 82:1071.
8. American Pain Society Quality of Care Committee. Quality improvement guidelines for the treatment of acute pain and cancer pain. JAMA 1995; 274:1874.
9. Phillips DM. JCAHO pain management standards are unveiled. JAMA 2000; 284:428.
10. Kehlet H. Postoperative pain relief. What is the issue? Br J Anaesth 1994; 72:373.
11. Kehlet H, Holte K. Effect of postoperative analgesia on surgical outcome. Br J Anaesth 2001; 87:62.
12. Vassilakopoulos T, Mastora Z, Katsaounou P, et al. Contribution of pain to inspiratory muscle dysfunction after upper abdominal surgery: a randomized controlled trial. Am J Respir Crit Care Med 2000; 161:1372–1375.
13. Desborough JP. The stress response to trauma and surgery. Br J Anaesth 2000; 85:109.
14. Liu S, Carpenter RI, Neal JM. Epidural anesthesia and analgesia. Their role in postoperative outcome. Anesthesiology 1995; 82:1474.
15. McMahon AJ, Russell IT, Ramsay G, et al. Laparoscopic and minilaparotomy cholecystectomy: a randomized trial comparing postoperative pain and pulmonary function. Surgery 1994; 115:533–539.
16. Frazee RC, et al. Open versus laparoscopic cholecystectomy: a comparison of postoperative pulmonary function. Ann Surg 1991; 213:651–653.
17. Kehlet H, Wilmore DW. Multimodal approach to improve surgical outcomes. Am J Surg 2002; 183:630.
18. Marks RM, Sachar EJ. Undertreatment of medical inpatients with narcotic analgesics. Ann Int Med 1973; 78:173–181.
19. Benson JM, DiPiro JT, Coleman CL, et al. Nausea and vomiting after abdominal surgery. Clin Pharm 1992; 11:965–967.

20. Lehmann LJ, DeSio JM, Radvani T, et al. Transdermal fentanyl in postoperative pain. Reg Anesth 1997; 22:24–28.
21. Viscusi ER, Reynolds L, Chung F, et al. Patient controlled transdermal fentanyl hydrochloride vs. intravenous morphine pump for postoperative pain. JAMA 2004; 41.
22. Gourlay GK, Kowalski SR, Plummer JL, et al. Fentanyl blood concentration—analgesic response relationship in the treatment of postoperative pain. Anesth Analg 1998; 67:329.
23. White PF. Patient controlled analgesia—a new approach to the management of postoperative pain. Semin Anesth 1985; 4:255.
24. Macintyre PE. Safety and efficacy of patient controlled analgesia. BR J Anaesth 2001; 87:36.
25. Camu F, Van Aken H, Bovill JG. Post operative analgesic effects of three demand dose sizes of fentanyl administered by patient controlled analgesia. Anesth Analg 1998; 87:890.
26. Doyle E, Robinson D, Morton NS. Comparison of patient controlled analgesia with and without a background infusion after lower abdominal surgery in children. Br J Anaesth 1993; 71:670.
27. Parker RK, Holtmann B, White PF. Does a concurrent opioid infusion improve management after surgery? JAMA 1991; 266:1947.
28. Cleland JG. Continuous peridural caudal analgesia in surgery and early ambulation. NW Med J 1949; 48:26.
29. Bromage PR, Camporesi E, Chestnyt D. Epidural narcotics for postoperative analgesia. Anesth Analg 1980; 59:473–480.
30. Block BM, Liu SS, Rowlingson AJ, et al. Efficacy of postoperative epidural analgesia, a meta-analysis. JAMA 2003; 290(18):2455–2463.
31. Dahl JB, Rosenberg J, Hansen B, et al. Differential analgesic effects of low-dose epidural morphine and morphine-bupivicaine at rest and during mobilization after major abdominal surgery. Anesth Analg 1994; 74:362.
32. Yosunkaya A, Tavlan A, Tuncer S, et al. Comparison of the effects of intravenous and thoracic epidural patient-controlled analgesia with morphine after upper abdominal surgery. Pain Clin 2003; 15:271–279.
33. Jayr C, Beaussier U, Gustafsson Y, et al. Continuous epidural infusion of Ropivicaine for postoperative analgesia after major at abdominal surgery: comparative study with IV PCA morphine. Br J Anaesth 1998; 81:887–892.
34. Ballantyne JC, Carr DB, deFarranti S, et al. The comparative effects of post operative analgesic therapies on pulmonary outcome: cumulative meta-analysis of randomized, controlled trials. Anesth Analg 1998; 86:598.
35. Jayr C, Thomas H, Rey A, et al. Postoperative pulmonary complications: epidural analgesia using bupivicaine and opioids versus parenteral opioids. Anesthesiology 1993; 78:666.
36. Manikian B, Cantineau JP, Bertrand M, et al. Improvement of diaphragmatic function by a thoracic extradural block after upper abdominal surgery. Anesthesiology 1998; 68:379–386.
37. Beattie WS, Badner NH, Choi P. Epidural analgesia reduces postoperative myocardial infarction: a meta-analysis. Anesth Analg 2001; 93:853.
38. Kock M, Blomberg S, Emanuelsson H, et al. Thoracic epidural anesthesia improves global and regional left ventricular function during stress induced myocardial ischemia in patients with coronary artery disease. Anesth Analg 1990; 71:625.
39. Veering BT, Cousins MJ. Cardiovascular and pulmonary effects of epidural anesthesia. Anaesth Intensive Care 2000; 28:620.
40. Carli F, Trudel JL, Belliveau P. The effect of thoracic epidural anesthesia and postoperative analgesia on intestinal function after colorectal surgery. Dis Colon Rectum 2001; 44:1083–1089.
41. Ahn H, Bronge A, Johansson K, et al. Effect of continuous postoperative epidural analgesia on intestinal motility. Br J Surg 1988; 75:1176–1178.

42. Scheinin B, Asantila R, Orko R. The effect bupivicaine and morphine on pain and bowel function after colonic surgery. Acta Anaesthesiol Scand 1987; 31:161.
43. Liu SS, Carpenter RL, Mackey DC, et al. Effects of perioperative analgesic technique on rate of recovery after colon surgery. Anesthesiology 1995; 83:757.
44. Licker M, Suter PM, Krauer F, Rifat NK. Metabolic response to lower abdominal surgery: analgesia by epidural blockade compared with intravenous opiate infusion. Eur J Anaesthesiol 1994; 11:193–199.
45. Barratt McG, Smith RC, Kee AJ, et al. Epidural analgesia reduces the release of amino acids from peripheral tissues in the ebb phase of the metabolic response to major upper abdominal surgery. Anaesth Intensive Care 1999; 27:26–32.
46. Hjortso NC, Christensen NJ, Andersen T, Kehlet H. Effects of the extradural administration of local anesthetic agents and morphine on the urinary excretion of cortisol, catecholamines and nitrogen following abdominal surgery. Br J Anaesth 2002:400–406.
47. Schricker T, Wykes L, Eberhart L, et al. The anabolic effect of epidural blockade requires energy and substrate supply. Anesthesiology 2002; 97:943–951.
48. Christopherson R, Beattie C, Frank SM, et al. Perioperative ischemia randomize anesthesia trial study group: perry operative morbidity in patients randomized to epidural or general anesthesia for it lower extremity vascular surgery. Anesthesiology 1993; 79:422–434.
49. Mellbring G, Dahlgren S, Reiz S, et al. Thromboembolic complications after major abdominal surgery: effect of thoracic epidural analgesia. Acta Anaesthesiol Scand 1983; 149:263–268.
50. Modig J, Borg T, Bagge I, Saldeen T. Role of extradural and general anesthesia in fibrinolysis and coagulation after total hip replacement. Br J Anaesth 1983:629.
51. Inoue k, Yokoyama M, Nakastutka H, et al. Spontaneous resolution of epidural hematoma after continuous epidural analgesia in a patient without bleeding tendency. Anesthesiology 2002; 97:735–737.
52. Onishchuk JL, Carlsson C. Epidural hematoma associated with epidural anesthesia: complications of anticoagulant therapy. Anesthesiology 1992; 77:1221–1223.
53. Vandermeulen EP, Van Aken H, Vermylen J. Anticoagulants and spinal-epidural anesthesia. Anesth Analg 1994; 79:1165–1177.
54. Horlocker TT, Wedel DJ. Spinal and epidural blockade and perioperative low molecular weight heparin: smooth sailing on the Titanic (editorial). Anesth Analg 1998; 86:1153–1156.
55. www.asra.com.
56. Tanaka K, Watanabe R, Harada T, et al. Extensive applications of epidural anesthesia and analgesia in a university hospital: incidence of complications related to technique. Reg Anesth 1993; 18:34–38.
57. Neal JM. Management of postdural puncture headache, epidural and spinal analgesia and anesthesia: contemporary issues. In: Benumof JL, Bantra MS, eds. Anesthesiology Clinics of North America. Philadelphia: WB Saunders, 1993:163–178.
58. Kane RE. Neurologic deficits following epidural or spinal anesthesia. Anesth Analg 1981; 60:150–161.
59. Cousins MJ, Glynn CJ, Wilson PR, et al. Epidural morphine. Anaesth Intensive Care 1980; 8:217.
60. Akerman B, Arwenstrom E, Post C. Local anesthetic potentiate spinal morphine antinociception. Anesth Analg 1998; 67:943.
61. Niiyama Y, Kawamata T, Shimizu H, Omote K, Namiki A. The addition of epidural morphine to ropivacaine improves epidural analgesia after lower abdominal surgery. Can J Anesth 2005; 52:181–185.
62. Etches RC, Writer WD, Ansley D, et al. Continuous epidural ropivacaine 0.2% for analgesia after lower abdominal surgery. Anesth Analg 1997; 84:784–790.
63. Curatolo M, Schnider TW, Peterson-Felix S, et al. A direct search procedure to optimize combinations of epidural bupivacaine, fentanyl and clonidine for postoperative analgesia. Anesthesiology 2000; 92:325.

64. DeKock M, Gautier P, Pavlopaulo A, et al. Epidural clonidine or bupivacaine as the sole analgesic agent during and after abdominal surgery. Anesthesiology 1999; 90:1354.

65. Asono T, Dohi S, Ohta S, et al. Antinociception by epidural and systemic alpha-2 agonists and their binding affinity in a rat spinal cord and brain. Anesth Analg 2000; 90:400.

66. McCrae AF, Wildsmith JAW. Prevention and treatment of hypotension during central neural block. Br J Anaesth 1993; 70:672–680.

67. Harper CM, Lyles UM. Physiology and complications after bed rest. J Am Geriat Soc 1988; 36:1047–1054.

68. Mynster T, Jensen LM, Jensen FG, et al. The effect of posture on late postoperative hypoxemia. Anaethesia 1996; 51:225–227.

69. Waters JM, Clancey SM, Moulton SB, et al. Recovery of strength in older patients after a major abdominal surgery. Ann Surg 1993; 218:380–393.

70. Swenson JD, Owen J, Lamoreaux W, et al. The effect of distance from injection site to the brainstem using spinal sufentanyl. Reg Anesth Pain Med 1998; 23:252.

71. Mulroy MF. Monitoring opioids. Reg Anesth 1996; 21:89.

72. Clyburn PA, Rosen M, Vickers MD. Comparison of the respiratory effects of IV infusions of morphine and regional analgesia by extradural block. Br J Anaesth 1990; 64:446–449.

73. Rygnestad T, Borchgrevink PC, Eide E. Post operative epidural in the fusion of morphine and bupivicaine is safe on surgical wards, organization of the treatment, effects and side-effects in 2000 consecutive patients. Acta Anesthesiol Scand 1997; 41:868.

74. Bailey PL, Rhondeau S, Schafer PG, et al. Does-response pharmacology of intrathecal morphine in human volunteers. Anesthesiology 1993; 79:49.

75. Chaney MA. Side-effects of intrathecal and epidural opioids. Can J Anaesth 1995; 42:891.

76. White MJ, Berghausen EJ, Dumont SW, et al. Side effects during continuous epidural infusion of morphine and fentanyl. Can J Anaesth 1992; 39:576.

77. Tzeng JI, Hsing CH, Chu CC. Low dose dexamethasone reduces nausea and vomiting after epidural morphine: a comparison of metoclopramide with saline. J Clin Anesth 2002; 14:19.

78. Kjellberg F, Tramer MR. Pharmacological control of opioid induced pruritus: a quantitative systemic review of a randomized trials. Eur J Anaesthesiol 2001; 18:346.

79. Vrchoticky T. Nalaxone for the treatment of narcotic induced pruritus. J Pediatr Pharm Prac 2000; 5:92–96.

80. Kam P, Tan K. Pruritus-itching for a cause and relief? Anaesthesia 1996; 51:1133–1138.

81. Dello Buono F, Friedman J. Opioid antagonists in the treatment of opioid-induced constipation and pruritus. Ann Pharmacother 2001; 35:85–90.

82. Standl T, Burmeister MA, Ohnesorge H, et al. Patient controlled epidural analgesia reduces analgesic requirements compared to continuous epidural infusion after major abdominal surgery. Can J Anesth 2003; 50:258–265.

83. Komasto H, Matsumoto S, Mitsuhata H. Comparison of patient controlled epidural analgesia with and without nighttime in fusion following gastrectomy. Br J Anaesth 2001; 87:633.

84. Carli F, Mayo N, Klubien K, Schricker T, Trudel J, Belliveau P. Epidural analgesia enhances functional exercise capacity and health-related quality of life after colonic surgery. Results of a randomized trial. Anesthesiology 2002; 97:540–549.

85. Dahl JB, Hansen BL, Hjortso NC, et al. Influence of timing on the effect of continuous extradural analgesia with bupivicaine and morphine after major abdominal surgery. Br J Anaesth 1992; 69:4–8.

86. 1e-Rockemann MG, Seeling W, Bischof C, et al. Prophylactic use of epidural mepivicaine—morphine, systemic diclofenac, and metamizole reduces the morphine consumption after major abdominal surgery. Anesthesiology 1006; 84:1027–1034.

87. Danelli G, Berti M, Perotti V, et al. Temperature control and recovery of bowel function after laparoscopic or laparotomic colorectal surgery in patients receiving combined epidural/general anesthesia and postoperative epidural analgesia. Anesth Analg 2002; 95:467–471.
88. Bardram L, Funch-Jensen P, Jensen P, Crawford ME, Kehlet H. Recovery after laparoscopic colonic surgery with epidural analgesia, and early oral nutrition and mobilization. Lancet 1995; 345:763–764.

26

Postoperative Nausea and Vomiting After Abdominal Surgery

Steven Gayer and Howard Palte
Department of Anesthesiology, University of Miami Miller School of Medicine,
Miami, Florida, U.S.A.

INTRODUCTION

Postoperative nausea and vomiting (PONV) persists, both as a problem for patients and as a thorn in the anesthetist's flesh. Despite recent pharmacologic advances in antiemetic therapy, little has been achieved in altering the frequency of this complaint. The overall incidence remains at 20% to 30%, yet may be as high as 70% for high-risk patients undergoing major intra-abdominal surgery (1,2). Nausea and vomiting are rated among the most unpleasant perioperative experiences, and commonly account for poor patient satisfaction. In one survey of a schedule of undesirable postoperative outcomes, vomiting ranked supreme (incisional pain third and nausea fourth) (3). PONV causes prolonged postanesthesia care unit (PACU) stay, contributes directly to delayed hospital discharge, and augments medical expenditure. These components stress on ambulatory centers where emphasis rests on early mobilization after minor as well as major surgery.

Certain types of gastrointestinal (GI) surgery carry increased risk for PONV. In particular, laparoscopic cholecystectomy and GI surgery are associated with increased incidence of PONV. The consequences of retching may include wrap herniation and disruption of fundoplication and esophageal myotomy (4).

A functional approach to the etiology of PONV considers a factorial triad, comprising elements of anesthesia, the patient, and the surgery. Noteworthy anesthetic factors include the use of volatile agents, nitrous oxide, opioids, and high-dose neostigmine for reversing the neuromuscular blockade. Among patient factors, risk increases with female gender, nonsmoking status, and a previous history of PONV or motion sickness (1). Finally, surgical factors include length of the procedure (more than 60 minutes) and the site of surgery (particularly intra-abdominal and laparoscopic procedures).

Nausea is an unpleasant, nonpainful sensation referred to the pharynx and upper abdomen. It varies in duration, often occurring in paroxysms. Conversely, vomiting is the forceful expulsion of upper GI contents via the mouth, requiring the complex interaction of numerous muscle groups.

PHYSIOLOGY

The physiology of vomiting involves a peripheral detection system, a central integrative process, and a motor output that produces the actual emetic response (readers are advised to read a physiology textbook). The vagus is the major nerve involved in the detection of emetic stimuli. In the abdomen, it contains approximately 80% afferent fibers. Two groups of vagal afferents constitute the peripheral detection system: the mechanoreceptors and the chemoreceptors. The mechanoreceptors are located in the muscular wall of the gut and react to abdominal distension and contraction. The chemoreceptors, located in the mucosa of the upper gut, respond to alterations in the pH and temperature, and to various chemoirritants. Vagal afferent activity is relayed to the area postrema. This U-shaped structure, a few millimeters long, lies in the caudal part of the fourth ventricle. It is rich in opioid, dopamine, and 5-hydroxytryptamine (5-HT) receptors. Activation of cells of this area, termed the chemoreceptor trigger zone, transmits stimulatory impulses to the vomiting center. Further vomiting center afferents are received from the vestibular labyrinthine system. Motion stimuli activate this complex. Experimental data suggest that head position and labyrinthine activation may affect the emetic response to apomorphine (5). The clinical relevance of this vestibular influence pertains to trolley movement and head position adjustment in the postoperative period. Furthermore, inputs from other regions may also stimulate the emetic center. Unpleasant taste, dysphoric visual stimuli, tympanic stimulation, pharyngeal irritation (suctioning), and ventricular cardiac afferent activity may all induce nausea and vomiting. Although central integration of somatic afferents occurs in the brainstem, additional influences are exerted by higher cerebral stimuli.

GI motility is inhibited to a greater extent by the surgical act than by general anesthesia per se. In abdominal surgery, inhibitory GI motility influences become greater as one proceeds from skin incision to muscle division, to laparotomy, and finally, gut manipulation (6). The significance of delayed gastric emptying and impaired GI motility is twofold—intraluminal fluid accumulation may facilitate retrograde reflux of bile into the stomach (enhancing visceral afferent activation), and the actual physiologic insult of surgery may cause a protracted delay in gastric emptying and/or return of GI motility.

Laparoscopic surgery carries an independent risk for PONV development (7). The forces generated by retching can induce wrap herniation or disruption. Bradshaw et al. (4) demonstrated that laparoscopic foregut surgical patients are at higher risk of developing PONV. Notably, esophagogastric myotomy and paraesophageal herniorraphy were procedures carrying the most accelerated risk. Fundoplication did not fall into this group. These investigators speculated that vagal or hypopharyngeal nerve irritation may be the triggering factor. In this subgroup, aggressive preemptive antiemetic therapy did not impact the incidence of PONV. While the majority of PONV incidents occur in the PACU, some occur during transport back to the floor. Therefore, vestibular apparatus perturbation may play a key role in post-GI surgery nausea and vomiting.

Gastroparesis (delayed gastric emptying) further increases emesis risk in GI surgery (8). This condition often coexists secondary to underlying disease, notably, GI obstruction and chronic cholecystitis. Additionally, there is a definite association between gastroparesis and pylorospasm, antral hypomotility, and diabetic intrinsic neuropathy (9).

Table 1 Comparison of Predictors of Apfel and Koivuranta Models

Apfel et al.	Koivuranata et al.
Female gender	Female gender
History of PONV or motion sickness	History of motion sickness
Nonsmoker	History of PONV
Postoperative opioids	Procedure >60 min
	Nonsmoker

Abbreviation: PONV, postoperative nausea and vomiting.
Source: From Ref. 12.

RISK

The routine administration of antiemetics to all surgical patients is not warranted in light of side effects and expense (10). A number of scoring systems that predict PONV within 24 hours of surgery have been proposed. There are various scoring systems, but those advocated by Apfel et al. (1) and Koivuranta et al. (11) demonstrate sound predictive accuracy, and have proven invaluable in the clinical scenario (Tables 1 and 2).

It was generally accepted that PONV risk was related to the site of surgery. However, the literature contains conflicting reports on this issue; some authors claim increased risk (13) while others feel that surgical location has no relevant impact on PONV (14). Evidence suggests that certain surgical procedures may be viewed as having a higher risk, viz., craniotomy, laparotomy, laparoscopy, and ear, nose, and throat and strabismus surgery. In GI procedures, laparoscopic and foregut surgery confer greater risk, whereas abdominal wall procedures tend to a carry lower risk (15). The gut is richly invested in vagal and splanchnic afferents. It is proposed that mechanical stimulation of these afferents triggers emesis. Many others believe that gut handling stimulates the enterochromaffin cells to release 5-HT (serotonin) and other mediators (cholecystokinin, prostaglandin, and interleukin), which are all modulators of visceral afferent activity. It is not, however, universally accepted that bowel manipulation triggers 5-HT release and vagal afferent activity (16).

MANAGEMENT

Pharmacological

There are at least four very well-known major receptor systems responsible for PONV genesis, and these include serotonergic ($5\text{-}HT_3$), dopaminergic (D_2), histaminergic (H_1),

Table 2 Comparison of Positive Predictive Value (%) of Apfel vs. Koivuranta Models

No. of predictors	1	2	3	4	5
Positive predictive value (%)					
Apfel et al.	49	53	60	72	
Koivuranta et al.	48	52	61	72	89

Source: From Ref. 12.

and cholinergic (muscarinic) receptors. Many anesthetic agents interact with these receptor systems and are hence proemetogenic. Their use should be avoided in high-risk patients and procedures. These agents include opiates, neuromuscular blocking reversal agents, nitrous oxide, etomidate, and sodium pentothal. Serious consideration should be given to the use of propofol, an agent with demonstrated antiemetic properties (17). The role of neostigmine remains controversial. Joshi et al. (18) found low-dose (2.5 mg) neostigmine to have no effect on PONV incidence. Conversely, King et al. (19) attributed significant nausea/vomiting to the use of a neostigmine–atropine combination for antagonism of neuromuscular blockade. Current consensus favors higher dose neostigmine ($70 \mu g.kg^{-1}$) as PONV contributory.

There are more than a thousand publications of randomized controlled trials evaluating pharmacologic management of PONV. Serotonin ($5\text{-}HT_3$) antagonists, dexamethasone (a corticosteroid), and droperidol (a neuroleptic), are among the most recently and best-studied agents.

Droperidol, a butyrophenone, has been widely used for PONV prophylaxis in anesthesia. Structurally similar to haloperidol, it has applications in both psychiatry and anesthesia. In high doses, it has antipsychotic effects, but low doses (1.25 mg) exhibit marked antiemetic and antinausea activity. Having been available for over 35 years, the drug held a 30% market share in PONV management (20). Droperidol has a protracted duration of action (up to 24 hours), even though its half-life is short (about three hours). Dose-dependent sedation and drowsiness are important side effects. The cost of droperidol is fractional compared with newer antiemetic agents (21).

The U.K. Medicines Control Agency (MCA) expressed concern regarding reports of cardiovascular events in psychiatric patients taking chronic large oral doses (22). It is known that droperidol may prolong QT_c interval in a small proportion of the population. Torsade de Pointes and sudden death are extremely rare complications experienced with chronic high-dose usage. In response to the MCA's attentions, the manufacturer, Janssen-Cilag Ltd., decided to discontinue production of all formulations of droperidol.

In the United States, the Food and Drug Administration (FDA) received several reports of cardiac dysrhythmias associated with doses of 1 and 2.5 mg droperidol (23). This led to placement of a "Black-Box" warning on the package insert in December 2001 (24). Consequently, there has been a marked decline in both the use and availability of droperidol. This happened despite many scientific authorities in anesthesia, psychiatry, and emergency medicine favoring the use of droperidol in low dosages. They contend that acute low-dose droperidol is highly efficacious and safe (25).

White et al. (26) demonstrated droperidol (0.625 or 1.25 mg) produced a prolongation of QT_c interval when administered at the beginning of surgery. Charbit et al. (27) compared prolongation of QT_c by droperidol (0.75 mg) and ondansetron (4 mg), and found similar clinically relevant prolongations of QT_c.

Droperidol has been administered millions of times since its introduction into clinical practice in 1970, without a single case report of dysrhythmias. An analysis of FDA-reported adverse events associated with droperidol use has failed to detect a causal relationship between the arrhythmia observed and droperidol administration (28).

Metoclopramide ($1\text{--}2 \, mg.kg^{-1}$) has proven successful in controlling chemotherapy-induced vomiting. A lower dose ($0.1\text{--}0.2 \, mg.kg^{-1}$) has been preferred in an attempt to minimize dystonic and sedative side effects. This dose proved more effective than placebo in only half the studies (29). Hence, metoclopramide is not recommended as a first-line drug for the management of PONV.

Anticholinergic agents act by blocking central pontine and cortical muscarinic receptors. Scopolamine is the most potent. The transdermal preparation needs to be applied at least four hours before the conclusion of surgery. Common side effects include dry mouth, urinary retention, visual disturbances, dizziness, and agitation, particularly in the elderly. GI surgery patients undergoing major abdominal procedures are at risk of developing postoperative dehydration and hypovolemia. Caution should be exercised in the noncatheterized patient because hypovolemia may be confused with anticholinergic-induced urinary retention. Opioid premedication, by all routes, is associated with increased PONV. The addition of an anticholinergic agent may partially attenuate this effect (30).

The two major groups of antihistamines are the ethanolamines (diphenhydramine and dimenhydrinate) and the piperazines (cyclizine and hydroxyzine). Their major side effects include sedation, dry mouth, urinary retention, and visual disturbances.

The heterocyclic phenothiazines (prochlorperazine and perphenazine) display similar efficacy to the antihistamines. However, they produce greater sedation and may elicit extrapyramidal movements.

The newer 5-HT_3 receptor antagonists exert a dual effect, acting both centrally in the chemoreceptor trigger zone, and peripherally at vagal afferents in the GI tract. They are highly specific for PONV, but are generally more effective for vomiting than nausea (31). Lack of sedative effects makes them particularly suitable for ambulatory GI surgery patients. Available agents in this group include ondansetron, granisetron, tropisetron, and ramosetron.

Ondansetron was the first 5-HT_3 receptor antagonist to be marketed, and is the most widely studied. The recommended dose is 4 to 8 mg intravenous (IV) in adults and 50 to 100 $\mu g.kg^{-1}$ in children. Originally, it was postulated that antiemetic agents of this class needed early administration in order to block central and peripheral receptors. However, it has been clearly shown that duration of action is the prime concern. The greatest benefit for ondansetron is manifested when it is administered at the conclusion of surgery. Recently, pharamacogenomics have been implicated in interindividual responses to the 5-HT_3 receptor antagonists. Candiotti et al. (32) demonstrated that patients with multiple genetically encoded copies of the liver enzyme 2D6 (CYP2D6) are more likely to experience vomiting if ondansetron is administered within 30 minutes of surgical conclusion. Side effects of this medication include headache, dizziness, flushing, and elevation of liver enzyme levels.

Granisetron has been used in a dose of 1 to 3 mg for oncology patients receiving chemotherapy (33). Low-dose granisetron (0.1–0.3 mg) may be more appropriate in post-GI surgery patients (34). Because granisetron is a pure 5-HT_3 receptor antagonist, it may be particularly advantageous in patients with a history of migraine (35).

Dolasetron is structurally related to granisetron and tropisetron. It is a prodrug that must be metabolized into its final active form (36). The recommended IV dose is 12.5 mg. In contrast to ondansetron, the timing of administration has little effect on efficacy (37). Dolasetron may be associated with prolongation of the QT_c interval (38). In fact, such electrocardiograph changes may be a class effect of all 5-HT_3 receptor antagonists.

Corticosteroids are highly effective in PONV prophylaxis. Dexamethasone, administered before initiation of surgery, is effective in preventing PONV (39). This effect may, in part, be due to a reduction of surgically induced inflammation. A double-blind, placebo-controlled study of PONV post–laparoscopic cholecystectomy documented significant PONV reduction (23% vs. 63%) with the use of dexamethasone (8 mg) (40). These impressive results lead us to highly recommend the use of dexamethasone in patients scheduled for laparoscopic GI surgery. A disadvantage is the long onset latency associated with its use. Additionally, some GI surgeons may express concern over potential steroid-induced immune suppression. These surgeons should be reassured that at these antiemetic doses (4–8 mg), dexamethasone has minimal effect on immunity or postoperative infection.

Total intravenous anesthesia (TIVA) with propofol is associated with a lower incidence of PONV than balanced inhalational anesthesia (41,42). Propofol exerts its antiemetic influence in surgical procedures of short duration. However, in long duration GI surgery, the greatest conferred benefit occurs when subhypnotic doses (10–20 mg) are administered late in the case (43,44). In the PACU, patient-controlled antiemesis has been achieved using similar doses of this agent (45).

Propofol binds to a specific γ-aminobutyric acid (GABA) receptor and potentiates GABA-activated chloride flux. This impairs serotonin release in the chemoreceptor trigger zone (46). There is limited clinical data regarding the effects of propofol on GI smooth muscle. Lee et al. (47) found propofol to exhibit an inhibitory effect on spontaneous GI smooth muscle activity. Jensen et al. (48) showed no significant differences in impairment of bowel function by either TIVA (propofol) or isoflurane inhalational anesthesia. Hamman et al. found unaltered gastric emptying, but prolonged orocecal transit time after light propofol sedation (49).

Unconventional Pharmacologic Interventions

Several other unconventional pharmacologic interventions merit mention. Intramuscular ephedrine ($0.5 \, mg.kg^{-1}$) may be an effective prophylactic antiemetic (50). Premedication with IV midazolam decreases PONV in adults undergoing cholecystectomy (51). Midazolam has also been shown to be effective as a rescue medication for failed first-line PONV treatment (52). Clonidine, an α_2 adrenergic agonist, is also an antiemetic (53). The mechanism of action is due to reduced sympathetic tone or a reduction in the use of opioids (54). Intraoperative attention to fluid replacement is associated with a significant reduction in PONV (55). Colloid fluid resuscitation has been cited to produce less PONV than crystalloid-based therapy (56).

In two of three abdominal surgery studies, increasing the F_iO_2 from 0.3 to 0.8 reduced the incidence of PONV by half (57,58). This phenomenon may be explained through avoidance of intestinal ischemia and the attendant release of emetogenic factors (serotonin). The unchanged incidence of late PONV remains unexplained. In a prospective study, Larsson and Lundberg (59) found abdominal procedures to be associated with the highest levels of postoperative vomiting. Prudence dictates that the inexpensive, essentially risk-free use of supplemental oxygen should be included in any GI surgery multimodal approach.

Nonpharmacologic Methods

Nonpharmacologic techniques to manage nausea and vomiting include transcutaneous electrical nerve stimulation, acupressure, and especially acupuncture. Acupuncture produces a significant reduction in early PONV (0–6 hour) (60). In general, these alternate modalities are more efficacious at ablating nausea than vomiting. Acupuncture utilizes the sixth point on the pericardial meridian (P6)—an area lying about 5 cm proximal to the wrist between the tendons of flexor carpi radialis and palmaris longus.

The effectiveness of gastric suction in combating PONV is unclear. Although suctioning will diminish manual ventilation-induced gastric distension, it does not attenuate opioid-induced PONV. In an attempt to minimize pharyngeal stimulation, investigators recommend that a gastric tube should only be inserted after induction, and removed prior to emergence (61). A curled intragastric tube or one passed beyond the pylorus may paradoxically stimulate retching and vomiting.

Postoperative pain, per se, may be associated with nausea in more than 50% of patients (62). The presumed mechanism is brainstem activation by visceral nociceptors. Paradoxically, withholding narcotics from patients who have had major GI surgery may actually enhance the likelihood of PONV! Visceral pain stimulates gut receptors in a proemetic fashion.

MANAGEMENT STRATEGIES

Apfel et al. (41) delineated key interventions for the prevention of PONV. They suggested that the efficacy of prophylactic antiemetic therapy is dependent on each individual patient's risk of developing PONV. The use of combinations of inexpensive antiemetic medications (e.g., dexamethasone and droperidol) confers greater efficacy than the use of expensive single agents (e.g., ondansetron), and there is a diminishing yield from adding further therapies.

It is important to note that nausea and vomiting are not controlled by a single receptor population but by a defined group of different central nervous system and gut receptors. Because at least four receptor systems are involved in the physiology of emesis, a logical management approach would target multiple receptor sites. Numerous studies support the hypothesis that combination antiemetic therapy is an effective strategy (63). The most frequently studied combinations involve a 5-HT$_3$ receptor antagonist with either dexamethasone or droperidol.

Furthermore, high-risk patients may benefit from an expanded approach (Fig. 1), encompassing not only pharmacologic interventions but focusing beyond on other etiological factors. This concept is embodied in the "multimodal" approach (64). This approach has been responsible for a marked reduction in PONV following ambulatory laparoscopic surgery. An exemplary multimodal approach may include combination therapy of 5-HT$_3$ antagonist and dexamethasone, TIVA with propofol, substitution of air for nitrous oxide, high inspired oxygen, and aggressive IV hydration.

Regional anesthesia is associated with diminished PONV (65–67). Central neuraxial blockade (via postural hypotension–induced nausea and vomiting) produces greater PONV than peripheral nerve blockade. This effect is largely attenuated by administration of 100% oxygen (68). Moreover, sympathetic blockade allows unopposed vagal activity with consequent GI hyperactivity. Hence, anticholinergic agents and regional anesthesia act synergistically to enhance PONV control.

Injection of local anesthetics and/or opioids into the subarachnoid and epidural space has gained popularity in postoperative pain management. Epidural opioids provide excellent analgesia, but disadvantages include nausea, vomiting, and pruritus. The low lipid solubility of morphine, in particular, permits delayed rostral spread with central emetic activation. Intrathecal opiates, on an equipotent basis, parallel epidural opiates in emetic potential. Blocks higher than the fifth thoracic segment (T5) and the use of additives, such as epinephrine and morphine, exacerbate the likelihood of PONV. The incidence of PONV after spinal anesthesia ranges from 7% to 18% (69). This varies according to the type of additive used. Pure epidural blockade has a lower incidence (70). Contrasting considerations shift the balance in the choice of technique. An epidural's slower onset of action favors

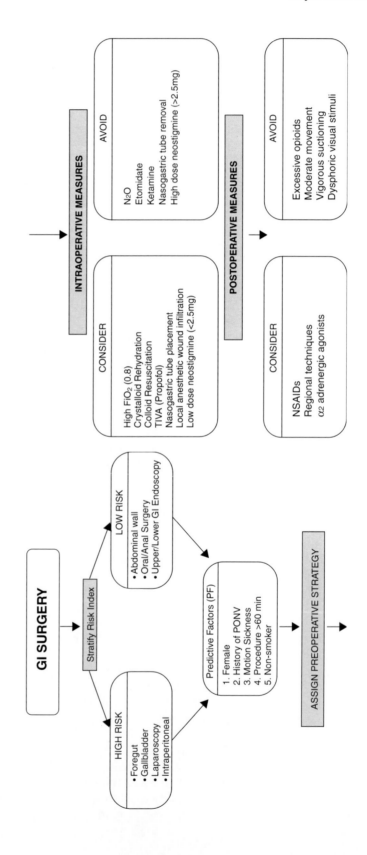

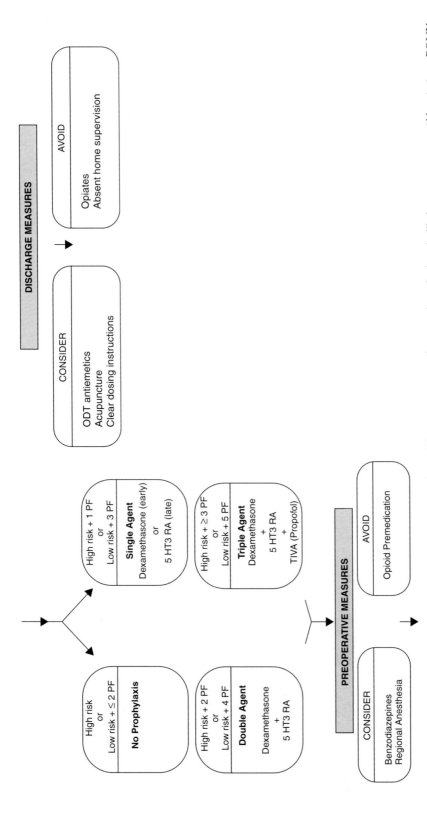

Figure 1 A multimodal approach to postoperative nausea and vomiting management in gastrointestinal and allied organ surgery. *Abbreviations:* PONV, postoperative nausea and vomiting; GI, gastrointestinal. *Source:* Courtesy of Palte H, Gayer S, and Hoa D.

hemodynamic control, while denser spinal block produces superior anesthesia and a lower demand for additional neuraxial or systemic medications (71,72).

Important considerations for neuraxial blockade include avoidance of hypotension, adequate hydration, and use of supplemental oxygen. The use of adjunctive medications produces mixed outcomes. Neostigmine, pethidine, and morphine increase PONV! Epidural fentanyl (73) and sufentanil (74) are alternatives having a lower risk. In major GI surgery, neuraxial opioids do not increase PONV risk. Finally, continuous regional anesthesia with indwelling epidural or perineural catheters should reduce systemic opiate usage and PONV.

An increasing percentage of surgery is being performed on an ambulatory basis. PONV (30–50%) often only manifest after discharge (75). One-third of PONV patients do not experience any predischarge symptomatology (76). The short half-life of most antiemetic preparations could be the underlying mechanism. The deleterious effects of this delayed phenomenon could be due to the late return to work and normal activity, and the lack of domiciliary medical supervision. Therefore, prudence censures the inclusion of an antiemetic with the discharge prescription. In this clinical setting, orally disintegrating ondansetron (ODT) has demonstrated efficacy (77). Other therapies include transdermal scopolamine (beware use in the elderly) and transcutaneous acupoint electrical stimulation.

PATIENT'S PERCEPTION AND PONV

Obviously, patients do not wish to suffer nausea, retching, and vomiting in the perioperative period. A salient question is "how dysphoric is PONV to the average patient?" Alex Macario et al. (3) asked patients to rank 10 adverse anesthesia outcomes on a scale of "least desirable" to "most innocuous." Vomiting was cited as the least desirable by almost one-quarter of the surveyed patients. Pain, gagging on the endotracheal tube, and residual weakness were all regarded as less onerous. Nausea ranked fourth. In a similar study, physicians on the other hand, ranked pain (before nausea and vomiting) as their patients' highest priority (78). This perceptual disparity is enlightening.

VALUE AND ECONOMICS OF PONV

How valuable is the avoidance of nausea and/or vomiting? Gan et al. (79) applied the "willingness to pay" model for establishing the financial benefit of medical interventions. They found that post-ambulatory surgery patients experiencing an episode of postsurgical vomiting were willing to spend $113 (mean) for "perfect" antiemetic prophylaxis. Such therapy would guarantee complete freedom from vomiting. Even those patients who did not experience nausea or vomiting were willing to contribute $61 (mean) out of their pocket toward effective prophylaxis!

The economic value of PONV prophylaxis may be expressed either as a function of quality or quantitative benefit per unit currency spent. Effective PONV prophylaxis is valuable to patients, family members, physicians, other health professionals, and hospital administrators. The real cost of antiemetic agents represents a mere 2% of global expenditure per episode of postoperative vomiting (80). In the ambulatory setting, PACU delay and potential for an inpatient admission contribute 15% to the overall expense.

THE FUTURE

Substance P, the natural ligand of the neurokinin-1 (NK-1) receptor, is found in central emetogenic zones. McLean et al. (81) found that NK-1 antagonists effectively prevent PONV. Therefore, combination of NK-1 and 5-HT receptor antagonist therapy may prove pivotal in our search to completely eliminate PONV. Additionally, selective cyclooxygenase-2 inhibitors facilitate better PONV control through reduced opioid usage.

SUMMARY

PONV is a common distressing problem for patients, anesthesia providers, and other caregivers alike. Our role as anesthetists mandates that we care for our patients in a responsible, ethical, and cost-conscious manner. We must employ evidence-based strategies in medical management. These maneuvers must balance physician and patient values with society's limited economic resources. The challenge of preventing nausea and vomiting after GI surgery confronts us daily. Morbidity defeats our clinical goal. Knowledge, rigorous attention to detail, and an appropriate application of evidence-based medicine will enable us to steer our patients on an emesis-free, "clear sailing" postoperative course.

REFERENCES

1. Apfel CC, Laara E, Koivuranta M, et al. A simplified risk score for predicting postoperative nausea and vomiting: conclusions from cross-validations between two centers. Anesthesiology 1999; 91:693–700.
2. Gan TJ, Ginsberg B, Grant AP, et al. Double-blind randomized comparison of ondansetron and intraoperative propofol to prevent postoperative nausea and vomiting. Anesthesiology 1996; 85:1036–1042.
3. Macario A, et al. Which clinical anesthesia outcomes are important to avoid? The perspective of patients. Anesth Analg 1999; 89:652–658.
4. Bradshaw WA, Gregory BC, Finley C, et al. Frequency of postoperative nausea and vomiting in patients undergoing laparoscopic foregut surgery. Surg Endosc 2002; 16: 777–780.
5. Isaacs B. The influence of head and body position on the emetic action of apomorphine in man. Clin Sci 1957; 16:215–221.
6. Livingstone EH, Passaro EP. Postoperative ileus. Digestive Diseases Sci 1990; 35:121–132.
7. Patasky AO, Kitz DS, Andrews RW, et al. Nausea and vomiting following ambulatory surgery: are all procedures created equal? Anesth Analg 1988; 67:S163.
8. Andrews PLR, Davis CJ, Binham S, et al. The abdominal visceral innervation and the emetic reflex: pathways, pharmacology and plasticity. Can J Physiol Pharmacol 1990; 68:325–345.
9. Read NW, Houghton LA. Physiology of gastric emptying and the pathophysiology of gastroparesis. Gastroenterol Clin North Am 1989; 18:359–373.
10. Watcha MF, White PF. Postoperative nausea and vomiting. Its etiology, treatment, and prevention. Anesthesiology 1992; 77:162–184.
11. Koivuranta M, Laara E, Snare L, et al. A survey of postoperative nausea and vomiting. Anaesthesia 1997; 52:443–449.
12. van den Bosch JE, Kalkman CJ, Vergouwe Y, et al. Assessing the applicability of scoring systems for predicting postoperative nausea and vomiting. Anaesthesia 2005; 60:323–331.

13. Sinclair DR, Chung F, Mezei G. Can postoperative nausea and vomiting be predicted? Anesthesiology 1999; 91:109–118.
14. Cohen MM, Duncan PG, DeBoer DP, et al. The postoperative interview: assessing risk factors for nausea and vomiting. Anesth Analg 1994; 78:7–16.
15. Lerman J. Surgical and patient factors involved in postoperative nausea and vomiting. Br J Anaesth 1992; 69:24S–42S.
16. Sirivanasandha P. Postoperative nausea vomiting (PONV): influence of bowel manipulation during intraabdominal surgery. J Med Assoc Thai 1995; 78(10):547–553.
17. McCollum JSC, Milligan KR, Dundee JW. The antiemetic effect of propofol. Anaesthesia 1988; 43:239–240.
18. Joshi GP, Garg SA, Hailey A, et al. The effects of antagonizing residual neuromuscular blockade by neostigmine and glycopyrrolate on nausea and vomiting after ambulatory surgery. Anesth Analg 1999; 89(3):628–631.
19. King MJ, Milazkiewicz R, Carli F, et al. Influence of neostigmine on postoperative vomiting. Br J Anaesth 1986; 41:635–637.
20. Fortney JT, Gan TJ, Graczyk S, et al. A comparison of the efficacy, safety, and patient satisfaction of ondansetron versus droperidol as antiemetics for elective outpatient surgical procedures. S3A-409 and S3A-410 Study Groups. Anesth Analg 1998; 86:731–738.
21. Gayer S, Lubarsky DA. Cost Effective Antiemesis. International Anesth Clin 2003; 41(4):145–164.
22. WWW.MCA.GOV.UK: Accessed March 15th, 2002.
23. Bailey P, Norton R, Karan S. The FDA droperidol warning: is it justified? Anesthesiology 2002; 97:288–289.
24. U.S. Food and Drug Administration: FDA strengthens warnings for droperidol. FDA Talk Paper 2001; T1–62.
25. Gan TJ, White PF, Scuderi PE, et al. A. FDA "Black Box" warning regarding use of droperidol for postoperative nausea and vomiting: is it justified? Anesthesiology 2002; 97:287.
26. White PF, Song D, Abrao J, et al. Effect of low-dose droperidol on the QT interval during and after general anesthesia: a placebo-controlled study. Anesthesiology 2005; 102:1101–1105.
27. Charbit B, Albaladejo P, Funck-Brentano C, et al. Prolongation of QT_c interval after postoperative nausea and vomiting treatment by droperidol or ondansetron. Anesthesiology 2005; 102:1094–1100.
28. Habib AS, Gan TJ. Food and drug administration black box warning on the perioperative use of droperidol: a review of the cases. Anesth Analg 2003; 96:1377–1379.
29. Rowbotham DJ. Current management of postoperative nausea and vomiting. Br J Anaesth 1992; 69:S46–S59.
30. Riding JE. Post-operative vomiting. Proceedings of the Royal Society of Medicine 1960; 53:671–677.
31. Tramer MR. A rational approach to the control of postoperative nausea and vomiting: evidence from systematic reviews. Acta Anaesthesiol Scand 2001; 45:4–13.
32. Candiotti KA, Birnbach DJ, Lubarsky DA, et al. The impact of pharmacogenomics on postoperative nausea and vomiting: do CYP2D6 allele copy number and polymorphisms affect the success or failure of ondansetron prophylaxis? Anesthesiology 2005; 102:543–549.
33. Taylor AM, et al. J Clin Anesth 1997; 9:658–663.
34. Frasco PE, Sharma S, Leone BJ, et al. Prevention of postoperative nausea and vomiting in outpatient surgery: a multicenter, prospective randomized, placebo-controlled clinical trial of low dose granisetron versus low dose granisetron plus dexamethasone. Anesthesiology 2004; 101:A45.
35. van Wijngaarden I, et al. Eur J Pharmacol 1990; 188:301–312.
36. Shah A, Lanman R, Bhargava V, et al. Pharmacokinetics of dolasetron following single- and multiple-dose intravenous administration to normal male subjects. Biopharm Drug Dispos 1995; 16(3):177–189.
37. Chen X, Tang J, White P, et al. The effect of timing of dolasetron administration on its efficacy as a prophylactic antiemetic in the ambulatory setting. Anesth Analg 2001; 93(4):906–911.

38. Benedict CR, Arbogast R, Martin L, et al. Single-blind study of the effects of intravenous dolasetron mesylate versus ondansetron on electrocardiographic parameters in normal volunteers. J Cardiovasc Pharmacol 1996; 28:53–59.
39. Wang JJ, Ho ST, Tzeng JI, et al. The effect of timing of dexamethasone administration on its efficacy as a prophylactic antiemetic for postoperative nausea and vomiting. Anesth Analg 2000; 91:136–139.
40. Wang JJ, Ho ST, Liu YH, et al. Dexamethasone reduces nausea and vomiting after laparoscopic cholecystectomy. Br J Anaesth 1999; 83(5):772–775.
41. Apfel C, Korttila K, Abdalla M, et al. A factorial trial of six interventions for the prevention of postoperative nausea and vomiting. N Engl J Med 2004; 350(24):2441–2451.
42. Tramer M, Moore A, McQuay H. Propofol anesthesia and postoperative nausea and vomiting: quantitative systematic review of randomized controlled studies. Br J Anaesth 1997; 78:247–255.
43. Numazaki M, Fujii Y. Antiemetic efficacy of propofol at small doses for reducing nausea and vomiting following thyroidectomy. Can J Anesth 2005; 52:333–334.
44. Kim SI, Han TH, Kil HY, et al. Prevention of postoperative nausea and vomiting by continuous infusion of subhypnotic propofol in female patients receiving intravenous patient-controlled analgesia. Br J Anaesth 2000; 85:898–900.
45. Gan TJ, El-Molem H, Ray J, et al. Patient-controlled antiemesis. Anesthesiology 1990; 90:1564–1570.
46. Cechetto DF, Diab T, Gibson CJ, et al. The effects of propofol in the area postrema of rats. Anaesth Analg 2001; 92:934–942.
47. Lee TL, Ang SB, Dambisya YM, et al. The effect of propofol on human gastric and colonic muscle contractions. Anesth Analg 1999; 89:1246–1249.
48. Jensen AG, Kalman SH, Nystrom PO, et al. Anesthesia technique does not influence postoperative bowel function: a comparison of propofol, nitrous oxide and isoflurane. Can J Anaesth 1992; 39:938–943.
49. Hamman B, Harvarfner A, Thorn E, et al. Propofol sedation and gastric emptying in volunteers. Acta Anaesthesiol Scand 1998; 42:102–105.
50. Hagemann E, Halvorsen A, Holgersen O, et al. Intramuscular ephedrine reduces emesis during the first three hours after abdominal hysterectomy. Acta Anaesthesiol Scand 2000; 44:107–111.
51. Heidari SM, Saryazdi H, Saghaei M. Effect of intravenous midazolam premedication on postoperative nausea and vomiting after cholecystectomy. Acta Anaesthesiol Taiwan 2004; 42:77–80.
52. Di Florio T, Goucke CR. The effect of midazolam on persistent postoperative nausea and vomiting. Anaesth Intensive Care 1999; 27:38–40.
53. Handa F, Fujii Y. The efficacy of oral clonidine premedication in the prevention of postoperative vomiting in children following strabismus surgery. Paediatric Anaesth 2001; 11:71–74.
54. Oddby-Muhrbec E, Eksborg S, Bergendahl H, et al. Effects of clonidine on postoperative nausea and vomiting in breast cancer surgery. Anesthesiology 2002; 96(5):1109–1114.
55. Yogendran S, Asokumar B, Cheng DC, et al. A prospective randomized double-blinded study of the effect of intravenous fluid therapy on adverse outcomes on outpatient surgery. Anesth Analg 1995; 80:682–686.
56. Moretti EW, Robertson KM, El-Moalem H, Gan TJ. Intraoperative colloid administration reduces postoperative nausea and vomiting and improves postoperative outcomes compared with crystalloid administration. Anesth Analg 2003; 96(2):611–617.
57. Greif R, Laciny S, Rapf B, et al. Supplemental oxygen reduces the incidence of postoperative nausea and vomiting. Anesthesiology 1999; 91:1246–1252.
58. Goll V, Acka O, Greif R, et al. Ondansetron is no more effective than supplemental intraoperative oxygen for prevention of postoperative nausea and vomiting. Anesth Analg 2001; 92:112–117.
59. Larsson S, Lundberg D. A prospective study of postoperative nausea and vomiting with special regard to incidence and relations to patient characteristic anesthetic routines and surgical procedures. Acta Anaesthesiol Scand 1995; 39(4):539–545.

60. Ghaly RG, Fitzpatrick KTJ, Dundee JW. Antiemetic studies with traditional Chinese acupuncture: a comparison of manual needling with electrical stimulation and commonly used antiemetics. Anaesthesia 1987; 42:1108–1110.
61. Palazzo MG, Strunnin L. Anaesthesia and emesis. Can Anaesthetists Soc J 1984; 31: 178–187.
62. White PF, Shafer A. Nausea and vomiting: causes and prophylaxis. Semin Anesth 1988; 6:300–308.
63. Eberhart LHJ, Mauch M, Morin AM, et al. Impact of a multimodal anti-emetic prophylaxis on patient satisfaction in high-risk patients for postoperative nausea and vomiting. Anaesthesia 2002; 57:1022–1027.
64. Scuderi PE, James RL, Harris L, et al. Multimodal antiemetic management prevents early postoperative vomiting after outpatient laparoscopy. Anesth Analg 2000; 91: 1408–1414.
65. Richardson MG, Dooley JW. The effects of general versus epidural anesthesia for outpatient extracorporeal shockwave lithotripsy. Anesth Analg 1998; 86:1214–1218.
66. Wulf H, Biscoping J, Beland B, et al. Ropivicaine epidural anesthesia and analgesia versus general anesthesia and intravenous patient-controlled analgesia with morphine in the perioperative management of hip replacement. Anesth Analg 1999; 89:111–116.
67. Standl T, Eckert S, Esch ISA. Postoperative complaints after spinal and thiopentone-isoflurane anesthesia in patients undergoing orthopedic surgery: spinal versus general anesthesia. Acta Anaesthesiol Scand 1996; 40:222–226.
68. Veronika G, et al. Ondansetron is no more effective than supplemental oxygen for Prevention of Postoperative Nausea & Vomiting. Anesth Analg 2001; 92:112–117.
69. Carpenter RL, Caplan RA, Brown DL, et al. Incidence and risk factors for side effects of spinal anesthesia. Anesthesiology 1992; 76:909–916.
70. Emanuelsson BMK, Zaric D, Nydahl PA, et al. Pharmacokinetics of ropivacaine and bupivacaine during 21 hours of continuous epidural infusion in healthy male volunteers. Anesth Analg 1992; 74:658–663.
71. Mulroy MF, Larkin KL, Hodgson PS, et al. A comparison of spinal, epidural, and general anesthesia for outpatient knee arthroscopy. Anesth Analg 2000; 91:860–864.
72. Seeberger MD, Lang ML, Drewe J, et al. Comparison of spinal and epidural anesthesia for patients younger than 50 years of age. Anesth Analg 1994; 78:667–673.
73. Curatolo M, Petersen-Felix S, Scaramozzino P, et al. Epidural fentanyl, adrenaline, and clonidine as adjuvants to local anaesthetics for surgical analgesia: Meta-analyses of analgesia and side-effects. Acta Anaesth Scand 1998; 42:910–920.
74. Sinatra RS, Sevarino FB, Chung JH, et al. Comparison of epidurally administered sufentanil, morphine, and sufentanil-morphine combination for postoperative analgesia. Anesth Analg 1991; 72:522–527.
75. Thagaard KS, et al. Eur J Anaesth 2003; 20(2):153–157.
76. Van den Berg AA, et al. Anaesthesia 1989; 44:110–117.
77. Gan TJ, Franak R, Reeves J. Comparison of ondansetron orally disintegrating tablet (ODT) versus placebo for the prevention of postdischarge nausea and vomiting following ambulatory surgery. Anesth Analg 2002; 94:1198–1200.
78. Macario A, Weinger M, Truong P, Lee M. Which clinical anesthesia outcomes are both common and important to avoid? the perspective of a panel of expert anesthesiologists. Anesth Analg 1999; 88:1085–1091.
79. Gan TJ, Sloan F, Dear GL, El-Moalem HE, Lubarsky DA. How much are patients willing to pay to avoid postoperative nausea and vomiting? Anesth Analg 2001; 92:393–400.
80. Hill RP, Lubarsky DA, Phillips-Bute B, et al. Cost-effectiveness of prophylactic antiemetic therapy with ondansetron, droperidol or placebo. Anesthesiology 2000; 92: 958–967.
81. McLean S, Ganong A, Seymour PA, et al. Characterization of CP-122,721; a non-peptide antagonist of the neurokinin NK1 receptor. J Pharmacol Exp Ther 1996; 277: 900–908.

27

The Role of the Critical Care Unit in Abdominal Surgery

Ian Nesbitt
Department of Perioperative and Critical Care, Freeman Hospital, Newcastle upon Tyne, U.K.

INTRODUCTION

In general, the role of critical and intensive care for abdominal surgery is similar to its role in other surgical specialties. Between 5% and 30% of intensive care admissions in the United Kingdom have undergone gastrointestinal surgery, and a similar proportion of patients having gastrointestinal surgery require postoperative ventilation (1–3).

Intensive care is a relatively new branch of medicine. The management of a poliomyelitis epidemic in Copenhagen in 1952 (4) has been widely acknowledged as the origin of the specialty. Within a few decades of its birth, intensive care has become central to hospital practice in the developed world, although it only received formal specialty recognition in the United Kingdom in June 1999.

Despite this, many operations that are carried out now only if a critical care bed is available were pioneered before the specialty existed. For example, Franz Torek carried out the first esophagectomy in 1913 (the 67-year-old patient lived for another 13 years). The first aortic graft replacement in 1951 had been preceded by aortic surgery for many decades: Albert Einstein lived for six years after aortic wrapping with reactive cellophane in 1949. Other examples of pioneering surgery carried out with minimal critical care facilities are listed in Table 1. In many parts of the world, major surgery is still carried out under basic conditions without recourse to intensive care support.

Although major surgery is possible without intensive care backup, the benefit that intensive care provides is principally one of reducing risk and improving functional outcome. For example, Ivor Lewis accepted high (but unspecified) mortality rates for two-stage esophagectomy but patients were often unable to tolerate a single-stage procedure (5), while modern in-hospital death rates for the single-stage procedure (usually in older patients) are in the order of 1% to 15% (6,7). Initial elective aortic aneurysm repair mortality rates were around 25%, compared to 5% to 10% now. Advances in critical care and surgery have also allowed survival in cases previously considered hopeless, such as liver resection for metastatic bowel cancer, liver transplantation for hepatic failure, or severe acute necrotizing pancreatitis (ANP).

Table 1 Dates of Pioneering Surgical Procedures

1881	Gastrectomy
1885	Aortic aneurysm (intraluminal wires)
1913	Esophagectomy
1938	Blalock cardiac operations
1948	Mitral valvotomy
1951	Aortic aneurysm (autologous graft)
1951	Open heart surgery (atrioseptal defect repair)
1963	Liver transplant
1966	Pancreas transplant

However, the impact of critical care alone on patient outcomes is difficult to measure against a background of other medical and surgical advances, such as stapling techniques and minimal access surgery, along with changing patterns of disease and health-care organization (8–12). Additionally, many of the reports showing benefits of critical care are written by intensive care clinicians and published in critical care literature, and may be subject to bias (publication or others).

HOW DOES CRITICAL CARE ALTER OUTCOMES?

Some of the accepted benefits of critical care are listed in Table 2. Four main aspects of critical care will be discussed in turn: staffing, organ support, monitoring and early intervention/treatment, and organizational issues.

Staffing

The initial organization of intensive care units (ICU) was planned to physically concentrate skilled staff and technology in a discrete part of the hospital where

Table 2 Factors that May Alter Critical Care Outcomes

Preoperative	Elective preoperative optimization
	Resuscitation prior to emergency surgery
Postoperative	*Monitoring*
	Early warning of physiological deterioration
	Treatment
	Mechanical ventilation
	DCS
	Tight blood sugar control
	Management of complications (sepsis, etc.) and distant organ support
	Management of the open abdomen
	Central line services (including parenteral nutrition lines)
	Selective decontamination of the digestive tract
Organization	Coordination of care
	Liaison between specialties
	Transfer for imaging and investigations
	Transfer for specialist care
Miscellaneous	Care of the organ donor
	Outreach services

Abbreviation: DCS, damage control surgery.

Table 3 Levels of Care (Department of Health Comprehensive Critical Care)

Level 0	Patients who can be managed on normal wards in acute hospitals
Level 1	Patients at risk of their condition deteriorating, or those recently relocated from higher levels of care, whose needs can be met on an acute ward with additional advice and support from the critical care team
Level 2	Patients requiring more detailed observation or intervention, including support for a single failing organ system or postoperative care, and those stepping down from higher levels of care
Level 3	Patients requiring advanced respiratory support alone or support of at least two organ systems. This level includes all complex patients requiring support for multiorgan failure

Source: From Ref. 13.

the sickest patients could be managed. The emphasis in the United Kingdom over the last few years is changing. With the publication of "Comprehensive Critical Care" in 2000 (13), the boundaries between high dependency units (HDU), ICU, and general wards have become less distinct. The terminology of ICU/HDU has been superseded by levels of care (Table 3), while critical care unit–based staff frequently lead outreach teams on general wards. However, the de facto delineation between ward care and critical care units remains. Although no nationally defined ratios exist in the United Kingdom, general wards typically have staff–patient ratios of 1 nurse for every 8 to 10 patients, compared to 1:1 or 1:2 staff–patient ratio in critical care units.

Organ Support

Respiratory support is one of the defining treatments available in critical care compared to general wards. It is useful to briefly consider the effects of surgery on the respiratory system before detailing the extent of available organ support.

Anesthesia, Surgery, and the Respiratory System

The effects of major abdominal surgery on the respiratory system have been extensively described (14–16). Abdominal surgery results in rapid shallow breathing, with a shift from predominantly abdominal breathing to increased ribcage breathing, alongside reductions in forced vital capacity, functional residual capacity, and mucociliary clearance, even in the presence of adequate analgesia. The surgical incision closer to the diaphragm has greater effects. Regional analgesia only partly reduces these detrimental effects. One study following upper abdominal surgery described normal breathing patterns in less than 30% of patients (17). Although this clinical pattern is frequently ascribed to "diaphragmatic dysfunction," the term is not universally accepted, and is too simplistic to adequately describe the complex changes in postoperative respiratory mechanics and gas exchange (18). The effects of anesthesia and surgery on the respiratory system are exaggerated in the elderly and the obese, and are more likely to cause adverse effects in those with other impaired organ systems (e.g., severe cardiac disease).

Obesity and Respiratory Functions

Obesity (body mass index, BMI, greater than 30 kg/m^2) is common and has increased from around 6% of the U.K. population in 1980 to 15% in 1990. The population with a BMI $> 35 \, \text{kg/m}^2$ (morbid obesity) is estimated to be increasing at 5% a year (19,20). Obesity and morbid obesity are associated with a myriad of complications (Chapter 13). In addition to resting cardiac and respiratory dysfunction, metabolic pathways and drug handling can be markedly impaired by anesthesia and surgery. One result is an increase in postoperative difficulties (e.g., twice the rate of respiratory complications compared to nonobese patients). Thus, aside from bariatric surgery (discussed below), obese patients will increasingly require additional postoperative resources, even if simply for monitoring of postoperative cardiorespiratory function.

Respiratory Support

Although respiratory support may be available on selected general wards (e.g., non-invasive ventilation), most forms of respiratory support require additional training and monitoring to be delivered in a safe and effective manner. Effectively, this restricts their employment to critical care units. A detailed discussion on ventilator and respiratory management is beyond the scope of this chapter. However, improvements in ventilator technologies, coupled with an increased understanding of weaning strategies and factors that influence weaning [such as modes of ventilation, tracheostomy management, sedation policies, and clinical practice guidelines (21–23)] are regarded as some of the reasons for improved critical care outcomes over the last 25 years.

Other Organ Support

The support available for other organs has undergone changes similar to those undergone by respiratory support. Early enteral feeding is now widely accepted as beneficial and selected groups of patients may benefit from enhanced feeds (24,25). Renal support has progressed from inefficient arteriovenous filtration to continuous venovenous filtration, using sophisticated technologies that provide improved homeostasis during critical illness. The roles of vasoactive drugs, appropriate hormonal support (e.g., low-dose steroids for sepsis), and more specific treatments (e.g., activated protein C as an adjunct to treat severe sepsis) have also become more widely understood and available. The net result is to allow sicker patients to recover from physiological insults that, in former years, would have proved fatal.

Monitoring

Monitoring in a controlled environment is one of the widely accepted benefits of a critical care unit. Major surgery is associated with significant intercompartmental fluid shifts, and occult hypovolemia is common. Restoring effective circulating volume is a key component in improving tissue oxygenation. Historically, cardiovascular monitoring has been pressure orientated: arterial pressure, central venous pressure, pulmonary artery pressure, etc. The relationship between measured pressures and intravascular volume is variable (26), and the evidence to show improved outcomes from pressure monitoring is scarce. For example, despite extensive study and debate, there remains significant uncertainty over the fact that the use of pulmonary artery catheters alters patient outcomes during critical illness (27,28) (although they may have a role in preoperative optimization—see below); and the limitations of central venous monitoring are well known. Rather, more evidence exists to support the use of monitoring mixed venous oxygen saturation as part of emergency treatment (29), although the correlation between the relatively easily measured central venous oxygen saturation and the true mixed venous oxygen saturation is not fully established (30).

Current interest in newer systemic monitoring techniques (e.g., esophageal Doppler and lithium dilution pulse contour analysis) is intensifying. Likewise, monitoring of regional perfusion (e.g., gastric tonometry, sublingual tissue oxygenation and capnography) is likely to become increasingly important as the technological challenges involved are overcome. There is an expanding amount of good quality evidence from clinical trials, which supports the use of such monitors in addition to traditional pressure monitoring techniques (see below). Many of these monitors can only be safely used in a well-staffed environment, such as critical care.

In addition to cardiovascular parameters, critical care is a more appropriate setting than general wards for other monitoring, often combined with treatment. For example, tight blood sugar control in the critically ill has been shown in a variety of settings to improve patient outcome, especially for those with infective complications (31,32). To accomplish these improvements, frequent monitoring and intervention, unlikely to be achievable in a general ward setting, are required. Another measurement under increasing scrutiny is that of intra-abdominal pressure (IAP). Although recognized for over 100 years, it is only recently that adequate monitoring of IAP for daily practice has been developed. Objective measurement of IAP is superior to clinical estimation, but requires attention to detail and standardization of technique, unlikely to be achieved in general wards. As understanding of IAP and the abdominal compartment syndrome increases, clinical practice will probably alter. One possible result [as with damage control surgery (DCS)—see below] is that critical care beds will be occupied by long-stay patients with a laparotomy and multiple organ dysfunction, rather than shorter stay, moribund patients with multiple organ failure.

Organization

Ideally, a critical care unit should be involved in coordinating care across ICU–HDU–Ward boundaries (e.g., by the use of outreach teams, preadmission clinics, and post–critical care follow-up). It should also coordinate specialist input and provide high-quality nursing and medical care. An indication of how this currently happens and how this affects abdominal surgical services is approached by considering the current challenges to U.K. critical care.

Challenges in Organizing Critical Care Services for Abdominal Surgery

Critical care in the United Kingdom faces increasing challenges on several fronts such as population demographics, changing patient demands, increasing medical technologies, and changing patterns of health-care delivery.

Critical care is expensive in terms of staffing, technology, and health-care finances. In the United States, approximately 6.5% of all hospital beds are classed as intensive care, although in the United Kingdom, only 2.5% of hospital beds are classified as intensive care (33,34). This is, proportionately, the lowest in Europe. The National Health Service Plan target for increasing critical care bed provision principally increased the number of level 2 (HDU) beds, rather than level 3 intensive care unit (ICU) beds. In September 2003, there were 1397 "HDU" beds, and 1731 ICU beds in U.K. hospitals (34). Critical care beds may cost £1000 to £1800 a day, with the bulk of cost going to staff salaries (each ICU bed typically requires six to seven whole time equivalent nurses to staff it); however, the long-term costs per life saved compare well with other currently accepted treatments (35,36).

There are cultural and historical differences among countries regarding the provision of critical care, which affect clinical results, and most health-care systems are under increasing strain (see below) (37–39). Currently, it seems likely that critical care in the United Kingdom will remain a scarce resource. To attempt to achieve improved outcomes and reduce some of the pressure on these beds, new approaches to patient care will be required. These will affect clinicians involved in abdominal surgery at all stages of patient stay. Possible approaches include those discussed in the following sections.

Target Critical Care at Those Who Need It.   Some of these strategies may be relatively simple (in principle at least), such as establishing efficient preassessment clinics and identifying patients who do not require critical care facilities. This may be achieved by methods such as cardiopulmonary exercise testing (40–42). Similar arguments and processes already exist for other surgical specialties traditionally reliant on critical care (e.g., carotid and aortic surgery) (43,44).

Another example is the supervision of regional analgesia postoperatively. It is still common practice in the United Kingdom for patients to be admitted to critical care units simply for management of continuous epidural analgesia postoperatively; although given sufficient, adequately trained ward staff, there is no difference in patient outcome (45). It may be more effective and attainable for a hospital to develop acute pain services than to expand existing critical care units, engage in interhospital transfers, and cancel surgery for critical care bed shortages. The actual system used in an individual hospital will depend on the capabilities and integration of pain teams, critical care, and the general wards.

Other strategies may be more difficult to implement, in part because they involve philosophical and attitudinal shifts in public and medical thinking. For example, advanced age is an independent predictor of poorer long-term outcome from critical care (46). With an increasingly aged population (20% of the U.S. population will be aged 85+ by 2030), advances in medical management which reduce the requirement for critical care for an individual patient, may be more than balanced by the increase in patients requiring critical care (47). Under such circumstances, current covert rationing of health-care resources may be made more overt. This is a difficult topic (as evidenced by the experiences in Oregon), and would involve much wider debate than amongst critical care clinicians alone. Information to inform this debate is difficult to obtain. For example, accurate prediction of short- and medium-term outcome during acute illness is extremely difficult. The Study to Understand Prognoses and Preferences for Outcomes and Risks of Treatment (SUPPORT) study showed that half of all patients assessed as likely to live another six months actually died within a week of that assessment (48). Refinements to predictive models (e.g., physiological scoring systems) may help to support clinical decision-making, but are unlikely to ever be robust enough to replace experienced judgement and adequate discussions with patients and their families. Detailed discussion about the natural history of disease states should be considered prior to critical care admission, especially for patients deemed high risk for significant complications.

Physical survival has long been the primary end point for measuring the success of critical care. More recently, the quality of life after critical illness has been recognized as a highly significant measure of the utility of critical care. It seems likely that as we understand more about the outcomes of critical illness (in terms that are meaningful to patients), decisions about referral to and continuation of critical care after major surgery will alter.

Overall, the direction in which critical care in the United Kingdom will develop is unclear—at one extreme, perhaps a more limited service for those relatively few people who society deems likely to gain benefit, and at the other, an open-ended, hugely expensive service with a high proportion of elderly (and ultimately moribund) patients. Each of these possibilities would have a significant impact on surgical services.

Optimize Patients Preoperatively. Achieving adequate oxygen delivery (goal-directed therapy) has been shown to be effective in improving outcome after high-risk surgical procedures (49–51); but this remains controversial, in part due to the heterogenicity of published trials on the subject, using disparate patient groups and different definitions, interventions, and end points on a background of rapidly changing "normal practice."

A meta-analysis of trials between 1988 and 2000 showed that for high-risk surgery, preoperative optimization before the onset of organ dysfunction was beneficial (52). After organ failure is established, the benefits are largely lost. The best timing of intervention is unknown, and although preoperative admission to critical care has been used in many of the relevant studies, it may be possible to achieve comparable results by optimization, immediately before or after surgery (53–56).

Optimize Patients Intraoperatively. As noted above, there is increasing interest in flow monitoring, in addition to traditional pressure monitoring of cardiovascular parameters. There is an expanding evidence base from well-constructed clinical trials that goal-directed therapy using such monitors can significantly improve relevant outcomes (such as time to hospital discharge) when compared to "standard" practice (53,57–59). Anesthetic techniques for specific procedures have been discussed in the relevant chapters.

Provide Enhanced Services Outside the Critical Care Unit. Expansion of services offered by theater recovery areas may be, in part, forced by lack of other critical care facilities. In some areas of the United Kingdom, this "overnight intensive recovery" (OIR) or postanesthesia care unit (PACU) is already established practice (60,61), although the ethical demarcation between establishing such "ring-fenced" elective surgical critical care beds and simply expanding an existing critical care unit is blurred. Such organizational changes may allow a relatively short period of specific preemptive treatment that may help avoid later prolonged critical care admission. For example, a European study (62) using six hours of facemask CPAP immediately following major surgery showed significantly fewer episodes of hypoxemic respiratory failure, requiring intensive care admission in the continuous positive airway pressure (CPAP) group. Adequately staffing OIR facilities will likely challenge existing theater teams' working patterns, as well as those of anesthetic and surgical medical staff.

Improve Critical Care Services. A recent report described the effect of introducing a specifically trained intensivist to an existing ICU previously managed by nonspecialist staff (63). There were numerous improvements described, such as a 4.5-fold reduction in hospital mortality, despite accepting sicker patients to fewer beds. Amongst the reasons advanced for this were improved triage of admissions, liaison with other carers, coordination of care, and different intervention strategies. The accompanying editorial noted that "the intensivist is the general practitioner for the critically ill" and estimated that intensivist-led critical care reduces mortality by 10% (64). It is increasingly accepted that successful critical care requires specialist management and a more formal structure than has historically existed (e.g., "closed" rather than "open" units) (65). Other changes in organization and delivery of critical care may be more difficult to bring about. Current admission criteria to critical care often vary widely between different centers, and depend partly on the adequacy of ward care, as well as on nonclinical issues (66–68). National standardization of critical care unit admission (and discharge) criteria is a long-term, possibly unattainable, goal.

Within the broader structure of the NHS, organizational changes impact on the delivery of critical care. NHS planning mandates the reduction of services available at peripheral hospitals and the concentration of surgical services in larger high-volume centers, where the perception is of better outcomes (69,70).

The above information is pertinent because critical care units, operating theaters, and general wards function in a dynamic interaction. Any change in one will impact on the others. Patients admitted directly to critical care following surgery have a better outcome than those who deteriorate on wards and require critical care admission. Many of these "indirect admissions" are due to respiratory failure. This may indicate insufficient critical care beds, inadequate ward care, or both (71). Deficiencies in aspects of patient management outside the critical care unit will be reflected in critical care unit use, to the extent that critical care has been termed a "backstop for a poorly performing hospital" (34). It is likely that many of the solutions to critical care bed shortages lie outside the critical care unit and will incorporate many of the aspects outlined above.

SPECIFIC SUBSPECIALTIES

The mortality rate for patients in U.K. critical care units is approximately 20%, rising to around 30% for in-hospital mortality (3). Critical care can account for around 30% of a hospital's budget; so a significant proportion of resource is expended on patients who derive little benefit from aggressive interventions before dying (72). An understanding of the natural history of disease processes and the effects of various treatments on these is useful to aid in decision-making regarding appropriate levels of intervention and support (73). This final section looks at some specific aspects of critical care related to abdominal surgery. More detailed discussions of anesthetic technique, etc. are found in the relevant chapters.

Esophagectomy and Gastric Surgery

Esophageal surgery requires an upper abdominal (transhiatal), thoracic (transthoracic), or combined thoracic and abdominal (Ivor Lewis) approach to resection (Chapters 2, 11, and 12). Previous comorbidity is a major determinant of outcome following esophagectomy, but the duration of surgery, especially the period of one-lung anesthesia and cardiovascular instability, has a profound effect on postoperative lung injury (74). Although many patients can be extubated at the end of the procedure or within a few hours of surgery, complications are common (up to 60%), including respiratory (25%), cardiac (12%), and wound breakdown (16%). In-hospital mortality is up to 15% (7,75). Longer-term survival is heavily dependent on operative resection and lymph node involvement, but typically approaches 90% five-year survival for early stage I carcinoma, falling to 15% for stage III disease (7,76).

Similar complication rates are present for patients with gastric cancer, who undergo surgery. Cardiorespiratory complications occur in around 30% of patients, and about 10% of these patients die in hospital (7).

Bariatric Surgery

For the morbidly obese (BMI > 35–40 kg/m^2), bariatric surgery is perhaps the most effective treatment option in long-term weight reduction. Typically, this involves gastric bypass or banding procedures, either by open or by laparoscopic techniques. Although elective critical care admission is rare following bariatric surgery—and the mortality rate relatively low (between 1% and 2%) principally from pulmonary embolism and cardiac causes—when complications occur, they typically result in prolonged critical care admissions (77–80).

The National Institute for Clinical Effectiveness estimates that the current 200 bariatric operations per year in the United Kingdom will increase 20-fold over the next decade (81). A key limiting step in those specialized centers providing bariatric services will be the availability of critical care beds for postoperative observation and management.

Pancreatic Surgery

The bulk of modern pancreatic surgery is carried out for malignancy. The mortality for pancreatic cancer surgery is falling [from a 30-day mortality of over 45% in one U.K. region between 1957 and 1976 to between 2% and 28% in current practice (82)]. The morbidity rate is up to 30%, with bile leakage and hemorrhage being significant reasons for critical care admission. Life expectancy following pancreatic surgery depends on the extent of resection, histopathology, and the site of tumor (worse for head of pancreas compared to ampullary carcinoma or cholangiocarcinoma). Typically, median postoperative survival is between 12 and 16 months, compared to around 50 days for nonoperated patients (83) with head of pancreas malignancy. Adjuvant chemotherapy also improves median survival following pancreatic resection (84).

The other major interaction of critical care with pancreatic diseases is the management of ANP. Patients with ANP admitted to critical care usually have severe disease. Although nationally accounting for only 20% of cases, around 95% of pancreatitis deaths in the United Kingdom are attributable to this group of patients (85). Critical care is used to sustain life in the immediate term and to prevent and manage complications, such as sepsis, pseudocyst formation, etc. The critical care management may involve laparoscopic or open necrosectomy (86), an open abdomen approach, vacuum dressings, continuous irrigation, and repeated transfers for imaging and surgery. This group of patients commonly spend significant periods in critical care units, require prolonged rehabilitation, and have a high mortality rate (around 30–40%). Long-term functional outcomes are often suboptimal, although most reports include only small numbers of patients (87–89).

Pancreatic transplantation is only carried out in specialized centers, with an annual caseload of fewer than 100 patients in the United Kingdom (compared to over 600 liver transplants). It will not be discussed further here.

Hepatobiliary Surgery

With the increase in liver resection surgery for metastatic bowel disease, there has been a concomitant increase in the requirements for critical care support. Despite advances in surgical techniques (such as ultrasound dissectors), liver resection encompasses blood loss, fluid shifts, and respiratory compromise. The clinical outcome depends partly on coexisting morbidity, but also on the extent of liver resection. Likewise, orthotopic liver transplantation (OLT) incurs additional significant metabolic derangements, often in already critically ill patients. The mortality rate for many of these procedures, without critical care backup would probably be unacceptably high.

Now, however, elective OLT in established centers is regarded as a routine procedure, frequently with a rapid step-down to level 2 care several hours postoperatively (90).

In many centers, liver resection following metastatic disease requires only level 2 care, with in-hospital mortality rates between 0% and 7%, and morbidity rates in the order of 25% to 40%, even for second or third resections (91). Five-year survival rates of over 60% have been reported, but depend heavily on the site, histology, and volume of tumor, as well as adjuvant therapies used. As with major vascular surgery, there is ongoing debate about the requirement for critical care bed use postoperatively. Selected patients (e.g., those with small-volume liver resection and good preexisting health) may be adequately managed in OIR/PACU, rather than critical care units.

Colorectal Surgery

Over 20,000 new cases of colorectal cancer are diagnosed in the United Kingdom annually, and it is the second most common cause of cancer death. In current U.K. practice, the in-hospital mortality rate following colorectal surgery is between 5.5% and 7.5% (92,93).

Although significant occult fluid losses are common in bowel surgery, these patients are often anesthetized and returned to ward care directly from recovery units, with minimal monitoring. As discussed above, pre- and intraoperative management may have a significant impact on postoperative complications and critical care use.

A risk-scoring system has been developed and validated to allow individual centers to predict outcomes and devise appropriate management pathways for their patients (94,95). The Association of Colorectal Surgeons of Great Britain and Ireland recommends critical care backup for colorectal surgery (96), but there is little information regarding what proportion of patients require level 3 care rather than level 2 care. It is likely that a significant number of these patients would be suitable for OIR/PACU management, with critical care reserved for those with significant comorbidity.

Emergency Surgery

Unlike elective surgery where an accurate diagnosis is usual, adequate discussion and patient preparation can take place, but emergency abdominal surgery is fraught with more uncertainty and physiological instability (e.g., only a minority of patients with mesenteric ischemia has an accurate preoperative diagnosis and the survival rate has remained below 50% for at least 20 years) (97). Prediction of outcome under these circumstances is difficult and many of these patients will require critical care management, sometimes preoperatively, but most often postoperatively (98). Depending on the hospital size and the population served, patients with acute abdominal problems may form the bulk of surgical admissions to critical care. Elderly patients, in particular, are more likely to undergo emergency operations than younger patients, although their physiological fitness and acute severity of illness, rather than chronological age, are often the main determinants of outcome from bowel surgery (99,100).

Damage Control Surgery

This is a staged treatment plan, where an initial limited procedure to save life is carried out, followed by definitive surgery after a period of critical care admission. The role of critical care in this case is to allow a "breathing space" to break the vicious cycle of hypothermia, blood loss, and coagulopathy, associated with prolonged emergency surgical procedures. DCS is common in trauma and military surgery, often used in conjunction with an open abdomen (laparostomy) approach, and has markedly reduced mortality rates and hospital resource use following hepatic injury and abdominal trauma (101,102). Staged abdominal closure is also an increasingly accepted means of managing other complex abdominal diseases in critically ill patients (103,104).

One result of managing patients with laparostomies is that patients who would have formerly died within hours or days of multiple organ failure may now survive with prolonged critical care length of stay (105). Again, this change in treatment may impact significantly on the availability of critical care beds.

DISTANT ORGAN SUPPORT AND CARE OF THE ORGAN DONOR

Over 2600 organs are donated in the United Kingdom annually, and a significant amount of abdominal transplant surgery depends on cadaveric donation. Care of the organ donor is a vital part of this process. The principles are broadly similar to those for organ support for other critically ill patients and will not be discussed further here.

SUMMARY

Critical care has a significant role to play in both elective and emergency abdominal surgery. With ageing populations and increasing expressed demands for medical interventions, it is likely that this role will continue to expand, and critical care services will be under increasing strain if organizational changes do not occur. These organizational and philosophical changes must occur at all levels within hospitals, not only within critical care units, but also on general wards, outpatient departments, and theater suites, and within surgical and anesthetic departments. Debate within society at large about the allocation of health-care resources will also have an effect on how critical care beds are used.

The benefits of critical care are frequently generic, rather than organ specific, namely a concentration of skilled staff, appropriate monitoring techniques, early interventions and treatments, and a focus on the coordination of care between multiple specialties and disciplines. The inclusion of critical care physicians into preoperative assessment clinics, operating theaters, and postdischarge follow-up clinics may smooth and remove traditional interspecialty boundaries and improve efficient use of scarce resources.

REFERENCES

1. Thompson JS, Baxter BT, Allison JG, et al. Temporal patterns of postoperative complications. Arch Surg 2003; 138:596–602.
2. http://www.scottishintensivecare.org.uk/AnnualReport2003_slides.ppt (accessed April 2005).
3. Harrison DA, Brady AR, Rowan K. Case mix, outcome and length of stay for admissions to adult, general critical care units in England, Wales and Northern Ireland: the Intensive Care National Audit & Research Centre Case Mix Programme Database. Crit Care 2004; 8:99–111.

4. Lassen HCA. The epidemic of poliomyelitis in Copenhagen, 1952. Proc Royal Soc Med 1954; 47:67.

5. Morris-Stiff G, Hughes LE. Ivor Lewis (1895–1982)—Welsh pioneer of the right-sided approach to the oesophagus. Dig Surg 2003; 20(6):546.

6. Visbal AL, Allen MS, Miller DL, et al. Ivor Lewis esophagogastrectomy for esophageal cancer. Ann Thorac Surg 2001; 71(6):1803–1808.

7. McCulloch P, Ward J, Tekkis PP. Mortality and morbidity in gastro-oesophageal cancer surgery: initial results of ASCOT multicentre prospective cohort study. BMJ 2003; 327:1192–1197.

8. Ghosh S, Steyn RS, Marzouk JF, et al. The effectiveness of high dependency unit in the management of high risk thoracic surgical cases. Eur J Cardio-Thoracic Surg 2004; 25(1):123–126.

9. Paw H, Vijaykumar G, Kooner T. Complications in the first 48 hours after major surgery: comparison between the general ward and high dependency unit. Clin Int Care 2000; 11(1):19–28.

10. Curran JE, Grounds RM. Ward versus intensive care management of high-risk surgical patients. BJS 1998; 85(7):956–961.

11. Lang M, Niskanen M, Miettinen P, et al. Outcome and resource utilization in gastroenterological surgery. BJS 2001; 88(7):1006–1014.

12. Simchen E, Spring C, Galai N, et al. Survival of critically ill patients hospitalised in and out of intensive care units under paucity of intensive care unit beds. Crit Care Med 2004; 32(8):1654–1661.

13. Comprehensive Critical Care: A Review of Adult Critical Care services. London: Department of Health, 2000.

14. Mills GH. Respiratory physiology & anaesthesia. CEPD Anaesth Rev 2001; 1(2):35–39.

15. Drummond GB. The abdominal muscles in anaesthesia and after surgery. BJA 2003; 91:73–80.

16. Siafakas NM, Mitrouska I, Bouros D, et al. Surgery and respiratory muscles. Thorax 1999; 54:458–465.

17. Nimmo AF, Drummond GB. Respiratory mechanics after abdominal surgery measured with continuous analysis of pressure, flow and volume signals. BJA 1996; 77:317–332.

18. Drummond GB. Diaphragmatic dysfunction: an outmoded concept. BJA 1998; 80(3):277–280.

19. Adams JP, Murphy PG. Obesity in anaesthesia and intensive care. BJA 2000; 85(1): 91–108.

20. NICE http://www.nice.org.uk/page.aspx?o=33646 (accessed April 2005).

21. Kress JP, Pohlman AS, O'Connor MF, et al. Daily interruption of sedative infusions in critically ill patients undergoing mechanical ventilation. NEJM 2000; 342:1471–1477.

22. MacIntyre NR, Cook DJ, Ely EW, et al. Evidence-based guidelines for weaning and discontinuation of ventilatory support. Chest 2001; 120(6 suppl):375S–484S.

23. The Acute Respiratory Distress Syndrome Network. Ventilation with lower tidal volumes as compared with traditional tidal volumes for acute lung injury and the acute respiratory distress syndrome. NEJM 2000; 342:1301–1308.

24. Heyland D, Dhaliwal R, Drover JW, et al. Canadian Critical Care Clinical Practice Guidelines Committee. Canadian clinical practice guidelines for nutritional support in mechanically ventilated critically ill patients. JPEN 2003; 27:355–373.

25. Heyland D, Dhaliwal R. Immunonutrition in the critically ill: from old approaches to new paradigms. Int Care Med 2005; 31(4):501–503.

26. Shippy CR, Appel PL, Shoemaker WC. Reliability of clinical monitoring to assess blood volume in critically ill patients. Crit Care Med 1984; 12(2):107–112.

27. Murdoch S, Cohen A, Bellamy M. Pulmonary artery catheterization and mortality in critically ill patients. BJA 2000; 85(4):611–614.

28. Sandham JD, Hull RD, Brant RF, et al. A randomised controlled trial of the use of pulmonary artery catheters in high risk surgical patients. NEJM 2003; 348:5–14.

29. Rivers E, Nguyen B, Havstad S, et al. Early goal-directed therapy in the treatment of severe sepsis and septic shock. NEJM 2001; 345:1368–1377.
30. Chawla LS, Zia H, Gutierrez G, et al. Lack of equivalence between central and mixed venous oxygen saturation. Chest 2004; 126(6):1891–1896.
31. Van de Berghe G, Wouters P, Weekers F, et al. Intensive insulin therapy in critically ill patients. NEJM 2001; 345:19, 1359–1367.
32. Krinsley JS. Effect of an intensive glucose management protocol on the mortality of critically ill adult patients. Mayo Clin Proc 2004; 79(8):992–1000.
33. Halpern NA, Pastores SM, Greenstein R. Critical care medicine in the United States 1985–2000: an analysis of bed numbers, use, and costs. Crit Care Med 2004; 32(6): 1254–1259.
34. Menon D, Nightingale P. On behalf of the Council of the Intensive Care Society. Critical Insight. An Intensive Care Society (ICS) Introduction to UK Adult Critical Care Services, London, 2004.
35. Stockwell M. Intensive care is not expensive compared to other treatments. BMJ 1999; 319:516.
36. Bennett D, Bion J. ABC of intensive care. Organisation of intensive care. BMJ 1999; 318:1468–1470.
37. Bennett Guerrero E, Hayam JA, Shaefi AS, et al. Comparison of P-POSSUM risk-adjusted mortality rates after surgery between patients in the USA and the UK. BJS 2003; 90(12):1593–1598.
38. Sirio CA, Tajimi K, Taenaka N, et al. A cross-cultural comparison of critical care delivery: Japan and the United States. Chest 2002; 121:539–548.
39. Values, ethics & rationing in critical care (VERICC) task force. http://www.vericc.org/02_about/index.htm (accessed April 2005).
40. ATS/ACCP statement on cardiopulmonary exercise testing. AJRCCM 2003; 167: 211–277.
41. Older P, Hall A, Hader R. Cardiopulmonary exercise testing as a screening test for perioperative management of major surgery in the elderly. Chest 1999; 116:355–362.
42. Older P, Smith R, Hall A, et al. Perioperative cardiopulmonary risk assessment by cardiopulmonary exercise testing. Crit Care Resuscitation 2000; 2:198–208.
43. Lipsett PA, Tierney S, Gordon TA, et al. Carotid endarterectomy—is intensive care unit care necessary? J Vasc Surg 1994; 20(3):403–409.
44. Bertges DJ, Rhee RY, Muluk SC, et al. Is routine use of the intensive care unit after elective infrarenal abdominal aortic aneurysm repair necessary? J Vasc Surg 2000; 32(4): 634–642.
45. Good Practice in the Management of Continuous Epidural Analgesia in the Hospital Setting. London: Royal College of Anaesthetists, 2004.
46. Keenan SP, Dodek P. Survival as an outcome for ICU patients. In: Angus DC, Carlet JC, eds. Surviving Intensive Care. Berlin: Springer-Verlag, 2004:4–20.
47. Ely EW. Understanding outcomes of critically ill older patients. In: Angus DC, Carlet JC, eds. Surviving Intensive Care. Berlin: Springer-Verlag, 2004:85–106.
48. Lynn J, Harrell FE, Cohn F, et al. Prognoses of seriously ill hospitalized patients on the days before death: implications for patient care & public policy. New Horizons 1997; 5:56–61.
49. Wilson J, Woods I, Fawcett J, et al. Reducing the risk of major elective surgery: randomised controlled trial of preoperative optimisation of oxygen delivery. BMJ 1999; 318:1099–1103.
50. Davies SJ, Wilson RJT. Preoperative optimization of the high-risk surgical patient. BJA 2004; 93:121–128.
51. Boyd O, Grounds RM, Bennett ED. A randomised clinical trial of the effect of deliberate perioperative increase of oxygen delivery on mortality in high-risk surgical patients. JAMA 1993; 270:2699–2707.
52. Kern JW, Shoemaker WC. Crit Care Med 2002; 30(8):1686–1692.

53. Pearse R, Dawson D, Fawcett J, et al. Early goal directed therapy reduces morbidity and length of hospital stay following high risk surgery. Crit Care 2005; 9(S1):45.
54. Davies SJ, Wilson RJT. Pre-operative optimisation of the high risk surgical patient. BJA 2004; 93(1):121–129.
55. Grocott MPW, Ball JAS. Consensus Meeting. Management of the high risk surgical patient. Clin Int Care 2000; 11(5):263–281.
56. Hamilton MA, Grocott MPW, Bennett ED, et al. Goal directed therapy does not have to be "pre" optimisation. Int Care Med 2002; 28(suppl 2):S41.
57. Conway DH, Mayall R, Abdul-Latif MS, et al. Randomised controlled trial investigating the influence of intravenous fluid titration using oesophageal Doppler monitoring during bowel surgery. Anaesthesia 2002; 57:845–849.
58. Laupland KB, Bands CJ. Utility of esophageal Doppler as a minimally invasive haemo-dynamic monitor: a review. CJA 2002; 49(4):393–401.
59. Grocott MPW, Mythen MG. Perioperative fluid management and clinical outcomes in adults. Anesth Analg 2005; 100:1093–1106.
60. Aps C. Surgical critical care: the Overnight Intensive Recovery (OIR) concept. BJA 2004; 92(2):164–166.
61. Jones AG, Harper SJ. "Ventilating in Recovery"—the way forward: intensive therapy or postoperative critical care? BJA 2002; 88:473–474.
62. Squadrone V, Coha M, Cerutti E, et al. CPAP for treatment of hypoxaemic respiratory ARF after abdominal surgery: a multi centre RCT. Int Care Med 2004; 30(S1):252.
63. Topeli A, Laghi F, Tobin MJ. Effect of closed unit policy and appointing an intensivist in a developing country. Crit Care Med 2005; 33(2):299–306.
64. Dorman T. Intensivists: providing primary care for critically ill patients. Crit Care Med 2005; 33(2):446–447.
65. Vincent JL. Need for intensivists in intensive care units. Lancet 2000; 356:695–696.
66. McQuillan P, Pilkington S, Allan A, et al. Confidential inquiry into quality of care before admission to intensive care. BMJ 1998; 316:1853–1858.
67. Wallis CB, Davies HTO, Shearer AJ. Why do patients die on general wards after discharge from intensive care units? Anaesthesia 1997; 52:9–14.
68. McGloin H, Adam SK, Singer M. Unexpected deaths and referrals to intensive care of patients on general wards. Are some cases potentially avoidable? J R Coll Physicians London 1999; 33(3):255–259.
69. Calman-Hine report on centralising services. Expert Advisory Group on Cancer to the Chief Medical Officers of England and Wales. A Policy framework for Commissioning Cancer Services. London: Department of Health, 1995.
70. Urbach DR, Baxter NN. Does it matter what a hospital is "high volume" for? Specificity of hospital volume-outcome associations for surgical procedures: analysis of administrative data. BMJ 2004; 328:737–740.
71. Goldhill D, Sumner A. Outcome of intensive care patients in a group of British intensive care units. Crit Care Med 1998; 26(8):1337–1345.
72. Chalfin DB, Cohen IL, Lambrinos J. The economics & cost effectiveness of critical care medicine. Int Care Med 1995; 21:952–961.
73. Murtagh FEM, Preston M, Higginson I. Patterns of dying: palliative care for non-malignant disease. Clin Med 2004; 4(1):39–44.
74. Tandon S, Batchelor A, Bullock R, et al. Peri-operative risk factors for acute lung injury after elective oesophagectomy. BJA 2001; 86(5):633–638.
75. Reasbeck PG. Treatment of oesophageal carcinoma at a small rural hospital. J Royal Coll Surg (Edin) 1998; 43:314–317.
76. Steup WH, De Leyn P, Deneffe G, et al. Tumors of the esophagogastric junction. Long-term survival in relation to the pattern of lymph node metastasis and a critical analysis of the accuracy or inaccuracy of pTNM classification. J Thorac Cardiovasc Surg 1996; 111(1):85–94.

77. Mason EE, Renquist KE, Zhang W. IBSR Data Contributors. Trends in bariatric surgery, 1986–2001. Obesity Surg 2003; 13:225.
78. Mason EE, Renquist KE, Jiang D. Perioperative risks and safety of surgery for severe obesity. Am J Clin Nutr 1992; 55:573S–576S.
79. Davidson JE, Callery C. Care of the obesity surgery patient requiring immediate-level care or intensive care. Obesity Surg 2001; 11(1):93–97.
80. Snow V, Barry P, Fitterman N, et al. Clinical Efficacy Assessment Subcommittee of the American College of Physicians. Pharmacologic and surgical management of obesity in primary care: a clinical practice guideline from the American College of Physicians. Ann Intern Med 2005; 142(7):525–531.
81. http://www.nice.org.uk/page.aspx?o=33646 (accessed April 2005).
82. Jarufe NP, Coldham C, Mayer AD, et al. Favourable prognostic factors in a large UK experience of adenocarcinoma of the head of pancreas and periampullary region. Dig Surg 2004; 21(3):202–209.
83. Wakeman CJ, Martin JG, Robertson RW, et al. Pancreatic cancer: management & survival. ANZ J Surg 2004; 74(11):941–944.
84. Alexakis N, Halloran C, Raraty M, et al. Current standards of surgery for pancreatic cancer. BJS 2004; 91(11):1410–1427.
85. Johnson CD. On behalf of the working party of the British Society of Gastroenterology. United Kingdom guidelines for the management of acute pancreatitis. Gut 2005; 54(suppl III):1–9.
86. Bosscha K, Hulstaert PF, Hennipman A, et al. Fulminant acute pancreatitis and infected necrosis: results of open management of the abdomen and "planned" reoperations. J Am Coll Surg 1998; 187(3):255–262.
87. Harrison DA, Bhanot D, D'Amico G, et al. Predicting hospital outcome for admissions to UK critical care units with severe acute pancreatitis. Int Care Med 2004; 30(suppl 1): S189.
88. Appelros S, Lindgren S, Borgstrom A. Short & long term outcome of severe acute pancreatitis. Eur J Surg 2001; 167(4):281–286.
89. Kriwanek S, Armbruster C, Dittrich K, et al. Long-term outcome after open treatment of severe intra-abdominal infection and pancreatic necrosis. Arch Surg 1998; 133(2):140–144.
90. Chen SC, Cunneen SA, Colquhoun SD, et al. Outcomes from nonemergent orthotopic liver transplantation: is postoperative care becoming routine? Am Surg 1998; 64(10):926–929.
91. Adam R, Pascal G, Azoulay D, et al. Liver resection for colorectal metastases. The third hepatectomy. Ann Surg 2003; 238(6):871–883.
92. Tekkis PP, Poloniecki J, Thompson MR, et al. Operative mortality in colorectal cancer: prospective national study. BMJ 2003; 327:1196–1201.
93. Tekkis PP, Poloniecki JD, Thompson MR, et al. ACPGBI Colorectal Cancer Study 2002. Part A. Unadjusted Outcomes. Oxfordshire: Dendrite Clinical System Ltd, 2002.
94. Fazio VW, Tekkis PP, Remzi F, et al. Assessment of operative risk in colorectal cancer surgery: the Cleveland Clinic Foundation colorectal cancer model. Dis Colon Rectum 2004; 47(12):2015–2024.
95. Tekkis PP, Kinsman R, Thompson MR, et al. The Association of Coloproctology of Great Britain and Ireland study of large bowel obstruction caused by colorectal cancer. Ann Surg 2004; 240(1):76–81.
96. Guidelines for the Management of Colorectal Cancer. London: The Association of Coloproctology of Great Britain and Ireland, 2001.
97. Mamode N, Pickford I, Leiberman P. Failure to improve outcome in acute mesenteric ischaemia: seven-year review. Eur J Surg 1999; 165(3):203–208.
98. Niskanen M, Kari A, Nikki P, et al. Prediction of outcome from intensive care after gastroenterologic emergency. Acta Anaesth Scand 1994; 38(6):587–593.

99. Kingston RD, Jeacock J, Walsh S, et al. The outcome of surgery for colorectal cancer in the elderly: a 12-year review from the Trafford Database. Eur J Surg Oncol 1995; 21(5):514–516.
100. Hessman O, Bergkvist L, Strom S. Colorectal cancer in patients over 75 years of age—determinants of outcome. Eur J Surg Oncol 1997; 23(1):13–19.
101. Pachter HL, Feliciano DV. Complex hepatic injuries. Surg Clin N Am 1996; 76(4): 763–782.
102. Asenio JA, Petrone P, Roldan G, et al. Has evolution in awareness of guidelines for institution of damage control improved outcome in the management of the posttraumatic open abdomen? Arch Surg 2004; 139(2):209–214.
103. Torrie J, Hill AA, Streat S. Staged abdominal repair in critical illness. Anaesth Int Care 1996; 24(3):368–374.
104. Scripcariu V, Carlson G, Bancewicz J, et al. Reconstructive abdominal operations after laparostomy and multiple repeat laparotomies for severe intra-abdominal infection. BJS 1994; 81(10):1475–1478.
105. Adkins AL, Robbins J, Villalba M, et al. Open abdomen management of intra-abdominal sepsis. Am Surg 2004; 7(2):137–141.

Index

411